D1071042

Postsurgical Rehabilitation Guidelines
for the Orthopedic Clinician

Section Editors

Janet B. Cahill, PT, CSCS
Section Manager
Inpatient Therapy
Department of Rehabilitation
Hospital for Special Surgery
New York, New York

John T. Cavanaugh, PT, MEd, ATC
Advanced Clinician
Sports Medicine Research and Performance Center
Department of Rehabilitation
Hospital for Special Surgery
New York, New York

Aviva Wolff, OTR/L, CHT
Section Manager
Hand Therapy
Department of Rehabilitation
Hospital for Special Surgery
New York, New York

Deborah Corradi-Scalise, PT, DPT
Section Manager
Pediatric Rehabilitation
Department of Rehabilitation
Hospital for Special Surgery
New York, New York

Holly Rudnick, PT, Cert MDT
Advanced Clinician
Sports Medicine Research and Performance Center
Department of Rehabilitation
Hospital for Special Surgery
New York, New York

Postsurgical Rehabilitation Guidelines
for the Orthopedic Clinician

Hospital for Special Surgery

Department of Rehabilitation

JeMe Cioppa-Mosca, PT, MBA
Administrative Editor
Assistant Vice President
Department of Rehabilitation
Hospital for Special Surgery
New York, New York

Janet B. Cahill, PT, CSCS
Administrative Editor
Section Manager
Inpatient Therapy
Department of Rehabilitation
Hospital for Special Surgery
New York, New York

Carmen Young Tucker, PT, BS
Administrative Editor
Director
Inpatient Division
Department of Rehabilitation
Hospital for Special Surgery
New York, New York

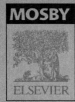
MOSBY

ELSEVIER

MOSBY
ELSEVIER

11830 Westline Industrial Drive
St. Louis, Missouri 63146

POSTSURGICAL REHABILITATION GUIDELINES FOR THE
ORTHOPEDIC CLINICIAN

ISBN-13: 978-0-323-03200-1
ISBN-10: 0-323-03200-1

Copyright © 2006 by Mosby, Inc., an affiliate of Elsevier Inc.

All rights reserved. No part of this publication may be reproduced or transmitted in any form or by any means, electronic or mechanical, including photocopying, recording, or any information storage and retrieval system, without permission in writing from the publisher. Permissions may be sought directly from Elsevier's Health Sciences Rights Department in Philadelphia, PA, USA: phone: (+1) 215 239 3804, fax: (+1) 215 239 3805, e-mail: healthpermissions@elsevier.com. You may also complete your request on-line via the Elsevier homepage (http://www.elsevier.com), by selecting "Customer Support" and then "Obtaining Permissions."

Notice

Neither the Publisher nor the Authors assume any responsibility for any loss or injury and/or damage to persons or property arising out of or related to any use of the material contained in this book. It is the responsibility of the treating practitioner, relying on independent expertise and knowledge of the patient, to determine the best treatment and method of application for the patient.

The Publisher

ISBN-13: 978-0-323-03200-1
ISBN-10: 0-323-03200-1

Acquisitions Editor: Marion Waldman
Developmental Editor: Donna Morrissey
Publishing Services Manager: Melissa Lastarria
Project Manager: Kelly E.M. Steinmann
Designer: Andrea Lutes

Printed in the United States of America.

Last digit is the print number: 9 8 7 6 5 4 3 2

Working together to grow
libraries in developing countries

www.elsevier.com | www.bookaid.org | www.sabre.org

ELSEVIER | BOOK AID International | Sabre Foundation

Dedication

This book is dedicated to all the past, present, and future therapists in the Rehabilitation Department at Hospital for Special Surgery. Their spirit and commitment to clinical excellence was, is, and will be the legacy of this book.

Preface

Postsurgical Rehabilitation Guidelines for the Orthopedic Clinician provides practitioners and students with expert, up-to-date information for developing postsurgical rehabilitation treatment plans. After reading this book, you will have a rich understanding of how you can develop individual postsurgical treatment guidelines that provide your patients with the best possible outcomes and function. Each authoritative chapter includes evidence-based research and best practices developed from years of collective clinical experience at Hospital for Special Surgery (HSS). The overlying organization of the text is based on the major orthopedic services performed at HSS. Accordingly, sections include Arthroplasty Rehabilitation, Hand Rehabilitation, Pediatric Rehabilitation, Spine Rehabilitation, and Sports Medicine Rehabilitation. Areas are further subdivided into the most common surgical procedures performed within each service area. Topics include joint replacement, tendon and ligament repair, spinal surgeries, and pediatric procedures.

Most chapters are organized uniformly with common features, such as surgical overview and rehabilitation overview, including specific phases of rehabilitation. Easy-to-follow phase-guidelines boxes encapsulate crucial information into phases/rehabilitation that incorporate goals, precautions, treatment strategies, and criteria for advancement. Clear photos and diagrams visually portray the concepts covered in the text. A one-of-a-kind DVD presents over 60 minutes and over 100 clips of video presentations demonstrating specific treatment strategies, tests, and measures. Additionally, experts from HSS are featured in the introduction and provide insight into the concept for the book as well as a history of HSS.

Founded in 1863, HSS is the world's leading specialty hospital for orthopedics and rheumatology. Ranked number one in the Northeast and with over 17,000 procedures performed per year, the hospital affords the Rehabilitation Department the remarkable opportunity to garner first-hand, in-depth experience with essentially every musculoskeletal disease known. With a commitment to the pursuit of knowledge and the advancement of rehabilitative care that it brings, the department plays an integral role in the multidisciplinary approach to patient care and research at the hospital. HSS is proud to provide a wide array of comprehensive services by a leading team of therapists.

The mission of the HSS Rehabilitation Department is to provide the highest quality of rehabilitative and restorative care to maximize patient function and promote education, clinical research, and community service. The HSS philosophy is built upon devotion to exceptional patient care, a strong belief in teamwork, and an appreciation of each employee's uniqueness. Furthermore, the department aims to excel in educating colleagues and future colleagues, and this philosophy is evident in each area of focus—patient care, education, clinical research, and community service—and, in particular, in this book.

HSS therapists have the unique opportunity to partner with world-renowned physicians, utilizing evidence-based science and research to support the HSS method of rehabilitation and restorative care. Since 1991, the Rehabilitation Department has been a regional leader in professional education symposia, providing opportunities to HSS colleagues for professional growth and development. *Postsurgical Rehabilitation Guidelines for the Orthopedic Clinician,* a collaborative effort by all of the members of the Rehabilitation Department, is the culmination of years of knowledge and treatment guidelines that have been dissected and revised by consensus of our staff and other HSS experts.

We are extremely pleased to share our collective experiences with you, our colleagues. Our book is designed to provide a guideline for therapists and health care professionals to facilitate a treatment plan, implement the program, and functionally progress the patient to the maximum level of function. It is our expectation that the therapists and health care professionals that follow these guidelines have a basic foundation of the diagnosis, special tests, and/or surgical procedures that may be warranted for these orthopedic conditions. It is imperative that each rehabilitation program is individually based on the patient's outcome to treatment, and an appropriate rationale for plan of care is necessary. This book is the result of decades of hard work, experience, and dedication on the part of HSS Rehabilitation Department therapists. We hope you derive as much insight from reading it as we did from writing it.

Acknowledgments

It is with great pride that I share with you, our fellow therapists, the rehabilitation "secrets" of Hospital for Special Surgery (HSS). I have been blessed and honored to be the Director of such an exceptional department over the past 15 years. The extraordinary talents of the team of individuals with whom I have had the privilege of working day in and day out have been the inspiration for this book.

I also have been extraordinarily lucky to be employed by such a fine institution. HSS is indeed a "special" place. It offers an incredibly supportive but challenging environment, that demands excellence and insists on the pursuit of personal growth and the development of its staff. Interwoven in this tapestry of continuous improvement is the expectation of teaching and sharing knowledge. These multiple driving forces were the genesis for this book.

Postsurgical Rehabilitation Guidelines for the Orthopedic Clinician is truly the result of a remarkable team effort, spanning 25 years of collective knowledge. Where does one begin to acknowledge the team of people whose contributions and talents have shaped postsurgical rehabilitation at HSS? First and foremost, the past and present staff (therapists and surgeons) must be recognized for the work that has been done on our guidelines over the years, beginning as early as 1979. In addition, the current HSS staff needs to be acknowledged for devoting their time and abilities so earnestly to the process of creating this book, either by writing or by covering patients for staff who were.

As in any endeavor, there are always a few people who require special mention—the names below are not listed in any particular order; it is simply a list. I would like to acknowledge the outstanding section editors who each played an immensely important role in this project. This book would never have been completed without the individual and collective strengths of Janet B. Cahill, John Cavanaugh, Holly Rudnick, Deborah Corradi-Scalise, and Aviva Wolff. Their dedication to this project, which took on a life of its own, was remarkable. They all went above and beyond to ensure the high quality and integrity of this text and accompanying DVD. Throughout the process of writing this book, these section editors have been my right hand and many times my left, too.

Secondly, I would like to thank all of the contributing authors who provided the substance for each section:

Emily Altman
Loretta Amoroso
Amy Barenholtz-Marshall
Heather M. Berns
Theresa Chiaia
Todd Cronin
Amie Diamond
Jaime Edelstein
Greg Fives
Nicole Fritz
Todd Gage
Kara Gaffney Gallagher
Sandy B. Ganz
Coleen T. Gately
Charlene Hannon
Lisa M. Kosman
Mickey Levinson
Jennifer P. Lewin
Robert Maschi
Dennis Noonan
Carol Page
Kataliya Palmieri
Adam Pratomo
Matthew Rivera
Lee Rosenzweig
Kelly Sindle
Amanda R. Sparrow
Cathi Wagner
Heather Williams
Carmen Young Tucker

Three contributing authors require special recognition: Sandy B. Ganz, Carmen Young Tucker, and Janet B. Cahill. Sandy B. Ganz has been my inspirational role model at HSS for 17 years. Her unyielding commitment to clinical excellence, education, and research is incomprehensible and continues to drive me to excel. Carmen Young Tucker was truly the behind-the-scenes coordinator. Her calm and balanced demeanor kept us all on track, especially me. Janet B. Cahill wore multiple hats during this project, and it would never have been completed without her attention to every detail.

There are also a few other people at HSS that should be recognized: Paddy Mullen and Bill Wylie in Business Development, who enabled this book to happen and who were responsible for the contract with Elsevier; Steven Portera, from the Digital Media Center, who was instrumental in coordinating the filming for our accompanying DVD; and Drs. Sculco, Root, and Levine, for their ongoing support of the Rehabilitation Department and for giving so much of their personal time for the filming of the DVD.

And finally, I'd like to thank our friends at Elsevier, especially Marion Waldman, Donna Morrissey, Dave Wisner, Christine Brown, and Kelly Steinmann.

The direction, insight, and expertise of all those mentioned here have brought this project to fruition. I am confident that *Postsurgical Rehabilitation Guidelines for the Orthopedic Clinician* will be a valued resource for our orthopedic colleagues in their treatment of postsurgical care. The knowledge in these pages was developed over years of dedication to the advancement of rehabilitative treatment, and it is a privilege to share it with you.

JeMe Cioppa-Mosca

Contents

I

ARTHROPLASTY REHABILITATION

JANET B. CAHILL, PT, CSCS

JOHN T. CAVANAUGH, PT, MED, ATC

AVIVA WOLFF, OTR/L, CHT

1

Total Hip Arthroplasty

CARMEN YOUNG TUCKER, PT

AMIE DIAMOND, PT

Total hip arthroplasty (THA) is one of the most common surgical procedures for the treatment of advanced hip arthritis. More than 254,000 THAs are performed annually. This represents 92 out of 100,000 Americans.[1,2] The Hospital for Special Surgery (HSS) performs approximately 7000 total joint arthroplasties each year, of which approximately 30% are THA. The primary goals of THA are relief of pain arising from destructive arthritis and improvement in functional mobility. Postoperative rehabilitation is an essential component in the achievement of these goals. The HSS rehabilitation guidelines following THA, which are presented in this chapter, were developed using an evidence-based approach and the clinical expertise of the rehabilitation department's physical therapist.

SURGICAL OVERVIEW

The successful outcome of a THA is based on several factors: patient selection, type of implant, method of fixation, and surgical technique. The determination of implant selection is individualized and based on specific patient characteristics (i.e., level of activity and bone quality) in addition to the experience of the surgeon.[3] There is a wide variety of implant designs and materials available. The materials most commonly used for implants are cobalt-chromium and titanium. Implant surfaces can have different finishes, such as porous-coated, plasma-sprayed surfaces, roughened titanium surfaces, and hydroxyapatite-coated surfaces. The different surfaces may enhance the strength between the implant and cement or fixation of implant to bone.[4] The type of implant component selected depends on whether the THA will be cemented, porous, or a hybrid (Figure 1-1, A–D).

The profile of the most common THA performed at HSS is a hybrid THA that combines an uncemented acetabular component and a cemented femoral component. This hybrid combination provides excellent results and is more popular in North America.[4] In addition to the standard THA procedure, HSS is currently using

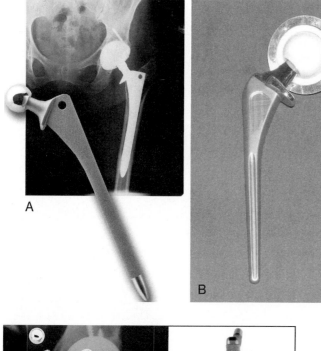

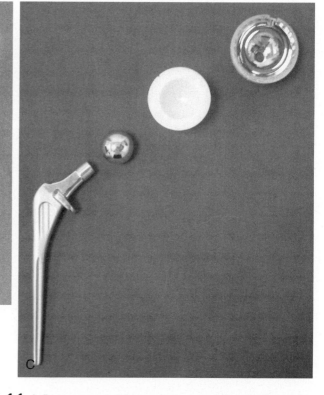

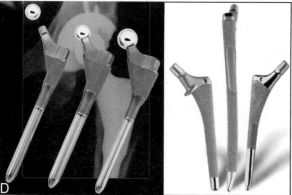

FIGURE 1-1 *A.* Pourous-coated femoral stem used for uncemented hip. (Solution System courtesy of DePuy Orthopaedics, Inc.) *B.* Cobalt-chrome femoral stem used for cemented hip with ceramic head and metal cup. (Hip components from Smith & Nephew Orthopaedicx. Photo taken by Carmen Young.) *C.* Hip components for hybrid THA. Stem used with cement, cobalt–chrome head, and porous cup. (Hip components from Smith & Nephew Orthopaedicx. Photo taken by Carmen Young.) *D.* Total hip femoral stems. (Uni-ROM Hip System courtesy of DePuy Orthopaedics, Inc. Versys Hip System courtesy of Zimmer, Inc.)

minimally invasive surgery (MIS) on a selected group of patients to perform hip arthroplasties. The minimally invasive total hip arthroplasty surgery is a modification of the standard surgical technique performed for THA. An article by Sculco et al.[5] states that "with modern techniques, implants, and instrumentation, THA could be performed safely and reproducibly through smaller incisions with increased patient satisfaction and without adversely affecting outcome." The advantages are less soft tissue damage and blood loss.

Several surgical exposures are used for THA. The posterior lateral approach is predominantly the choice at HSS. This approach spares the abductors, and a postoperative limp is uncommon.[6,7] It has been demonstrated that adequate repair of the capsule and the short external rotator hip muscles reduces the risk of hip dislocation after a posterior approach.[6,7] Longevity of the implant depends on activity level of the patient, implant type, method of fixation, and technique of insertion. At the authors' institution, patients undergoing THA are given a combination of spinal/epidural anesthesia, and a few surgeons combine the spinal/epidural anesthesia with a psoas block for enhanced postoperative pain control. A patient-controlled analgesia (PCA) pump attached via a catheter is used to control pain for the initial 24 to 48 hours.

REHABILITATION OVERVIEW

The measurement of patient progress addressing functional limitations has been documented in the acute care setting following elective THA.[8] At HSS, the patient's functional progress is documented on the HSS Rehabilitation Department Functional Milestones Form (Figure 1-2). This form was developed to measure functional progression of patients with joint replacements during their hospitalization and has been proven to be statistically valid and reliable.[8] The rehabilitation department has been using the Functional Milestones Form to collect outcome data on the total joint arthroplasty patient population for over two decades.[9] In the early 1990s the THA clinical pathway and rehabilitation guidelines for phase I were developed using data generated from the Functional Milestones Forms and with the collaboration of HSS surgeons and members of an interdisciplinary team. Phases II and III are progressive phases based on each patient's functional mobility, strength, flexibility, gait, and balance, which are objectively measured and assessed by the physical therapist.

Physical therapy management of patients who have undergone a THA is based on the theoretical framework of the disablement model addressing pathology, impairment, functional limitation, and disability. The most common impairments seen following THA are functional strength deficits in the hip musculature, decreased hip range of motion (ROM), decreased standing balance and proprioception, decreased functional activity tolerance, and increased pain during mobility activities. Functional limitations typically affect gait, transfers, stair negotiation, driving, and performing basic activities of daily living (ADLs). The disabilities that result are in the areas of self-care, social activities, sporting activities, and work.[10]

Physical therapy treatment approaches following THA are impairment based and focused on reducing pain, increasing strength and flexibility, restoring mobility, teaching adherence to precautions, addressing ADL, and educating the patient and family.

PREOPERATIVE PHASE

In 1994 HSS instituted a multidisciplinary preoperative arthroplasty education program. A major goal of this program is to prepare and educate patients and family members about the upcoming surgery and postoperative recovery. An individual assessment of the patient's functional status, psychosocial needs, and medical history can be obtained by using a custom-designed documentation tool. This information can be helpful in identifying special needs, complications, or patients who may require rehabilitation or home care after discharge.[11]

Currently, approximately 98% of THA patients attend a multidisciplinary, preoperative education class 1 week prior to surgery. The preoperative classes are instructed by an interdisciplinary team that includes a nurse, a physical therapist, and a case manager. The physical therapist explains the goals of inpatient therapy, instructing patients in a basic lower extremity exercise program consisting of ankle pumps, quadriceps and gluteal isometrics, supine hip flexion to a 45-degree angle, and hip internal rotation to neutral. Hip precautions are reviewed; transfers and gait on level surfaces and stairs with an assistive device are demonstrated. Patients are provided with a postoperative notebook containing all the information covered in the class and an ADL video to review at home before surgery. The ADL video contains information on transferring safely in and out of a chair/toilet, car, and shower and how to use assistive devices for dressing and bathing.

A preoperative evaluation to identify impairments and functional limitations would be beneficial if a patient does not have the option of a preoperative education program or cannot attend the class.

POSTOPERATIVE PHASE I: ACUTE CARE (DAYS 1 TO 4)

Phase I of the rehabilitation process focuses on restoring functional mobility, adherence to precautions while performing activities, and independence with home exercise program.

Rehabilitation following THA is initiated on postoperative day 1. Patients are instructed in a home exercise program that begins with five basic therapeutic exercises performed in supine, which include ankle pumps, quadriceps sets, gluteal sets, heel slides to 45 degrees, hip flexion with the head of the bed flat, and hip internal rotation to neutral. If the patient is already at neutral at the hip or internally rotated, the latter exercise is deferred and the patient may be instructed to work on external rotation. The therapeutic exercises are advanced from the basic five to include sitting knee extension and hip flexion maintaining THA precautions. Standing exercises include hip extension, hip abduction, and knee flexion (Figures 1-3 through 1-7). Cryotherapy is used in conjunction with oral medication for pain and swelling. Patients are also instructed

---

HSS TOTAL HIP ARTHROPLASTY—FUNCTIONAL MILESTONES FORM

REHABILITATION DEPARTMENT
PHYSICAL THERAPY
PT Initials:_____
Diagnosis:_____Age:_____
Right/Left/Bilateral
Porous/Hybrid/Cemented
Initial/Revision
WBAT   PWB   TTWB   NWB
Height_____(in) Weight_____(lbs)   **Day of Surgery:** Su M T W Th F Sa

Anesthesia: EPI   GEN
PCA: EPI   IV
Nerve Block: Psoas/Sciatic/None

Pre-op Class: YES   NO
Pre-op Amb: w/c bound   <1   1-5   6-10   >10 Blocks
Pre-op Assistive Device: Cane/Crutches/Walker/None
Need to negotiate stairs: YES   NO
Pre-op Lives Alone: YES   NO

	RR	1	2	3	4	5	6	7	8	9	10	11	12	13	14	15
BID																
Discharge																
Stairs Unassisted																
Stairs Assisted																
Cane Unassisted																
Cane Assisted																
Walker Unassisted																
Walker Assisted																
Stand Only																
Transfer Unassisted																
Transfer Assisted																
Pain Level																
Date of Surgery _____																
P.O.D.	RR	1	2	3	4	5	6	7	8	9	10	11	12	13	14	15

Discharge To: Home   Rehab   SNF
If D/c to home: Home PT   Outpatient   No PT
If D/c to home, with: Family/Friends/Other   Alone

Complications/PT Held:_____

_____
_____
_____

FIGURE **1-2** THA Functional Milestones Form.

PERTINENT PAST MEDICAL HISTORY
Please circle all that apply

Cardiovascular
1. A-fib/arrythmia
2. Angina
3. CAD
4. ↑ Cholesterol
5. HTN
6. MI
7. Tachycardia
8. Valve disease

Circulatory
9. Cellulitis
10. DVT
11. PVD
12. Phlebitis
13. PE

Endocrine
14. DM
15. Hyperthyroidism
16. Hypothyroidism
17. Renal disease

Hearing/Vision
18. Blind
19. Glaucoma
20. Cataracts
21. HOH
22. Deaf

Immunological/Infectious Disease
23. Chronic Infection
24. HIV
25. Hepatitis

Musculoskeletal
26. AVN
27. DDD
    Fractures
28. -Femur
29. -Pelvis
30. -Spine
31. -Humerus
32. -Wrist
33. -Other
34. HO
35. HNP
36. LBackP
37. OA
38. OP
39. Rotator cuff tear
40. Sciatica
41. Scoliosis
42. Spinal stenosis

Neurological
43. Alzheimers/dementia
44. CP
45. CVA/TIA
46. MS
47. Parkinsons
48. Paraparesis
49. Paraplegia
50. Polio
51. RSD
52. Seizures

Oncology
Cancer
53. -Breast
54. -Colon
55. -Leukemia
56. -Lung
57. -Lymphoma
58. -Prostate
59. -Other malignant
_____

Psychological
60. Anxiety/panic
29. Bipolar disorder
30. Depression
31. Schizophrenia

Pulmonary
64. Asthma
65. CHF
66. COPD/emphysema
67. Pneumonia
68. SOB

Rheumatological
69. Fibromyalgia
70. JRA
71. SLE
72. Psoriatic arthritis
73. RA

Other
74. Drug/substance abuse
75. Mental retardation
76. Obesity
77. Ulcer disease/gastric

Other PMH:
78. _____
_____
_____
_____
_____

PAST SURGICAL HISTORY

79. TKR
80. TKR revision
81. THR
82. THR revision
83. TSR

84. Spine
85. Arthroscopy -LE
86. Arthroscopy -UE
87. Amputee UE
88. Amputee LE
89. ORIF UE
90. ORIF LE

91. Ligament/joint reconstruction
92. CABG
93. Pacemaker
94. Valve replacement
95. Recent major abdominal surgery (within last 6 months)

Other PSH:
96. _____
_____
_____

FIGURE **1-2, cont'd**

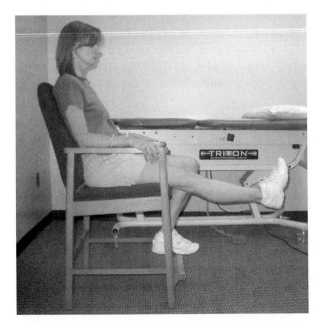

FIGURE **1-3** Knee extension sitting.

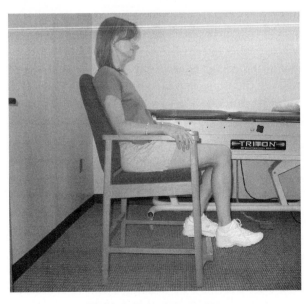

FIGURE **1-4** Hip flexion sitting.

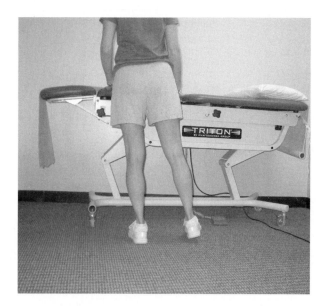

FIGURE **1-5** Hip abduction standing.

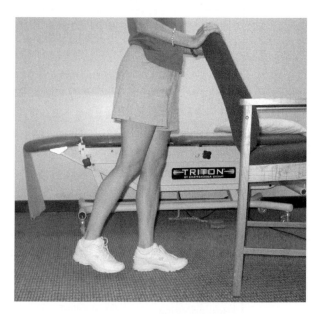

FIGURE **1-6** Hip extension standing.

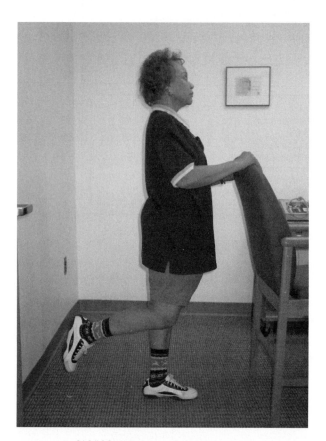

FIGURE **1-7** Knee flexion standing.

in the following total hip replacement precautions: no hip flexion greater than 90 degrees, no hip adduction past midline, and no internal rotation of the hip past neutral.

At HSS, patients who undergo a unilateral THA are instructed to transfer out of bed on the surgical side while maintaining THA precautions. This helps to keep the operated hip abducted and avoids adducting or internally rotating the operated leg. Patients who undergo bilateral hip arthroplasty can transfer out of bed on either side but are cautioned not to cross legs or internally rotate leg while pivoting to the edge of the bed. These patients may initially require more assistance getting out of bed to maintain hip precautions. The patient's ability to sit at the edge of the bed, stand, and ambulate is progressive and based on the patient's strength, motor control, and pain level. Progression from a walker to cane or crutches and stair climbing is based on the patient's pain level, ability to demonstrate symmetrical weight-bearing, and ability to ambulate with a reciprocal gait pattern. A patient who has undergone a THA will be allowed to weight-bear as tolerated (WBAT) during ambulation. Sitting in a high chair is initiated when the patient can tolerate the vertical position for prolonged periods. Ambulation to the bathroom and transfer training on and off the commode is initiated when the Foley catheter is discontinued.

Before discharge, a written home exercise program that addresses the patient's specific needs is reviewed. Patients are provided with appropriate devices, and usage of equipment is reviewed. Patients view the ADL video during the inpatient phase as well as preoperatively and postoperatively for reinforcement of precautions and use of proper technique in performing transfers and ADL. Patients are discharged to home within 4 days, when the inpatient goals are achieved. If the goals set in the acute phase are not met, patients may receive home physical therapy or be transferred to an inpatient rehabilitation facility.

Postoperative Phase I: Acute Care (Days 1 to 4)

GOALS

- Transfer unassisted and safely in and out of bed/chair/toilet
- Unassisted ambulation with cane(s) or crutches on level surfaces and stairs
- Independently perform home exercise program
- Demonstrate knowledge and adherence of total hip replacement precautions
- Independent with basic ADL

PRECAUTIONS

- Avoid hip flexion greater than 90 degrees, adduction past midline, and internal rotation of hip past neutral (for posterior-lateral approach)
- Avoid lying on operated side
- Avoid pillow(s) under knee to prevent hip flexion contracture
- Use abduction pillow when lying supine
- Reduce weight-bearing to 20–30% if concomitant osteotomy performed

TREATMENT STRATEGIES

- Instruct in strengthening exercise to include quadriceps and gluteal isometrics, ankle pumps, hip flexion to 45 degrees in supine; sitting knee extension and hip flexion with hip angle less than 90 degrees; standing hip extension and abduction and knee flexion
- Progressive ambulation with assistive device—walker to cane or crutches
- Emphasize symmetrical lower extremity weight-bearing and reciprocal gait pattern using an assistive device
- Non-reciprocal stair negotiation
- Review/instruct in hip precautions
- ADL instruction/assess equipment needs
- Cryotherapy

CRITERIA FOR ADVANCEMENT

- Progression from walker to cane or crutches when patient can demonstrate symmetrical weight-bearing and a step through non-antalgic gait pattern

Troubleshooting

Management of postoperative pain is a vital component of postoperative care and achievement of rehabilitation goals. Pain needs to be monitored closely by all of the health care providers and addressed appropriately. Educate patients about pain medication and encourage its use at regular intervals throughout the day to allow them to participate in the rehabilitation process. Instruct patients to avoid sitting for more than an hour at a time, which may cause discomfort and stiffness of hip and thereby interfere with mobility. Increase patient awareness of excessive swelling and encourage elevating or propping leg while maintaining hip precautions, using pneumatic compression pumps, or doing ankle-pump exercises. It is crucial to monitor excessive swelling in the operated leg or calf tenderness during this phase. Excessive swelling that does not subside and calf pain may be signs of a deep vein thrombosis (DVT), and the physician should be consulted. During ambulation, postoperative patients may exhibit gait deviations. Some common reasons may be pain and decreased flexibility of hip flexors. Therefore, it is important to observe ambulation and correct any gait deviation during the acute phase. With uncemented THAs, the weight-bearing status is surgeon-specific and depends on type of fixation achieved in the operating room. When a cemented/uncemented THA with a concomitant trochanteric osteotomy is performed, the weight-bearing status is usually restricted to toe-touch weight-bearing (TTWB) or 20% to 30% weight-bearing.

POSTOPERATIVE PHASE II: EARLY FLEXIBILITY AND STRENGTHENING (WEEKS 2 TO 8)

The second phase of physical therapy emphasizes monitoring wound status, monitoring pain level, restoring normal gait pattern, improving flexibility and strength, and incorporating functional activities. It is still imperative that patients continue to adhere to hip precautions. Typically, patients are discharged from the hospital and receive home physical therapy before being referred to the outpatient physical therapy setting.

The advanced exercise program given in the acute phase serves as a foundation for advancement during this time. Flexibility is addressed by assessing the hamstrings, quadriceps, hip internal rotators, and plantar flexors. The patient is then instructed in the appropriate exercises to target any deficits. Flexibility exercises, such as the supine butterfly stretch and the modified Thomas

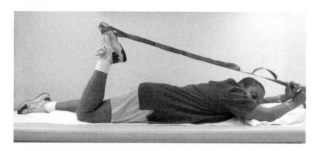

FIGURE **1-8** Prone knee extension with strap.

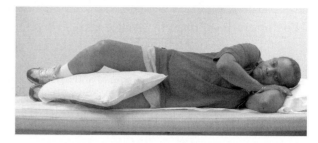

FIGURE **1-9** Side-lying clam shell with abduction pillow.

test stretch, will assist in lengthening internal rotators and hip flexors. The prone position, with knee flexion, enhances hip flexor and quadriceps length (Figure 1-8). Shortened calf muscles are stretched by standing on a wedge or lowering the heel off a step.

The short crank bike is integrated into the treatment plan once patients can negotiate transfers onto and off of the bike. The smaller-sized crank (90 mm) allows for improvements in ROM within hip precaution parameters.[12] It also provides a cardiovascular challenge in conjunction with lower extremity strengthening while avoiding the impact of gravity. Strengthening is accomplished by increasing pedal resistance.

An important treatment strategy during this phase is gait training, which aims to eliminate compensatory patterns and improve stride length, velocity, and distance. When evaluating gait, it is important to consider that abnormalities develop as compensatory patterns preoperatively. Training initially focuses on achieving a heel-toe gait pattern, with emphasis on hip extension. Tactile cues by the therapist and visual feedback from a mirror give important information to the patient when trying to achieve a symmetrical gait pattern.

The retro treadmill training at slow speeds is used to facilitate hip extension and strengthen the quadriceps and hamstrings, as well as normalizing step length and challenging coordination.[13] In this phase it is important to keep in mind that the joint contact forces in the hip can reach up to seven times the body weight as speed and stride length increase.[14] These variables should be progressed slowly during this phase. When normalized gait is achieved, the assistive device is no longer necessary.

Therapeutic exercises to target strength deficits are introduced. Side-lying clam shell with abduction pillow (Figure 1-9) and bridging strengthen gluteus medius and hip extensors. As soon as a normalized gait is demonstrated, standing exercises, such as hip abduction and hip extension, are transitioned to the nonoperative leg for strength and balance development. Heel raises will assist with calf strengthening and carry over to gait training and facilitate toe-off.

Hip flexor strengthening is initiated when a supine heel slide is tolerated without pain. This is advanced to seated hip flexion. A straight leg raising (SLR) in the supine position is not emphasized at this time because a force of three times the body weight is generated at the hip joint when performed.[14]

Closed kinetic chain (CKC) exercises are used for strengthening and return to function due to the low impact on knee and hip joints.[15] The leg press is initiated at an arc of 0 to 80 degrees or less, and equal weight-bearing through both extremities is stressed. Emphasis should be placed on both eccentric and concentric control, progressing from bilateral to unilateral activities, adjusting the resistance accordingly.

The forward step-up program is introduced once ambulation without a device is achieved. This progression (4-inch to 6-inch to 8-inch steps) is advanced once the patient is able to demonstrate pain-free negotiation with proper alignment and control.

Osteoarthritis in weight-bearing joints has been shown to have a strong correlation with diminished joint position sense or proprioception.[16,17] Wolfson[17] found that proprioception and balance decline as age progresses. These factors can place THA patients at risk for falling and can alter gait patterns.

As patients progress from phase I to phase II, weight-shifting activities should be performed until ambulation without a device is accomplished. Bilateral activities need to be mastered prior to initiating unilateral activities. An unstable surface, such as a unidirectional rocker board (Figure 1-10), is initially introduced in the sagittal plane and then progressed to the coronal plane. Dynamic stabilization is progressed when appropriate to a commercial balance system. The Biodex Balance System (BBS) (Biodex Inc., Shirley, NY) further challenges balance by training in multiple planes and simultaneously providing visual feedback (Figure 1-11). The machine's software is used to test and document the patient's progress.

Assessment of functional reach (Figure 1-12) and the timed "get-up and go" (TUG) test is done at the conclusion of this phase to establish a baseline and serve as objective balance measures for goal setting and documenting progress through phase III.[18,19] These two tests have a high reliability and validity for the prediction of falls in older adults and are useful in assessing deficits present in this patient population.[18,19] Normative values for both tests have been well documented throughout

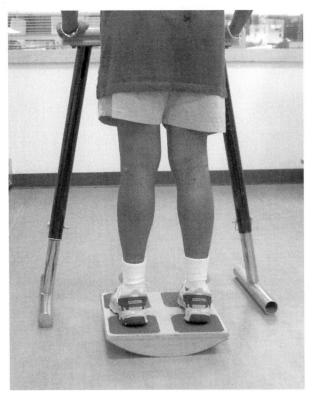

FIGURE **1-10** Unidirectional rocker board in sagittal plane.

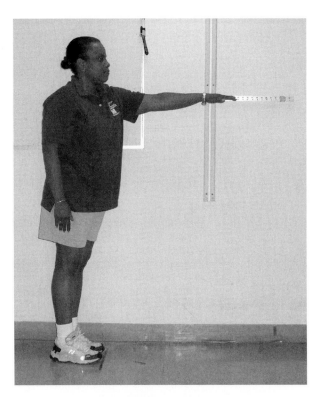

FIGURE **1-12** Functional reach test.

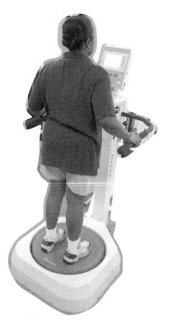

FIGURE **1-11** Balance/proprioception on Biodex. Patient is maintaining target within bull's-eye on screen.

| TABLE **1-1** | Functional Test Normative Values |

FUNCTIONAL REACH			
MALES		FEMALES	
AGE RANGE	DISTANCE (cm)	AGE RANGE	DISTANCE (cm)
41–69	38	40–49	40
70–87	33	50–59	38
		60–69	37
		70–79	34

TIMED UP AND GO				
Age Range	40–49	50–59	60–69	70–79
Time (sec)	6.2	6.4	7.2	8.5

Adapted from Podsiadlo, D., Richardson, S. *The Timed "Up & Go": A Test of Basic Functional Mobility for Frail Elderly Persons.* J Am Geriatr Soc 1991;39(2):142–148; Isles, R.C., Choy, N.L., Steer, M., Nitz, J.C. *Normal Values of Balance Tests in Women Aged 20–80.* J Am Geriatr Soc 2004;52:1367–1372.

the literature and are used to identify the level of impairment (Table 1-1).[19,20] Single limb stance time is also assessed once patients demonstrate the criteria to begin unilateral activities. Normal stance time for healthy individuals is considered 30 seconds. Continuing edu-cation in the principles of edema control is emphasized. Edema and pain levels should be steadily declining as healing progresses and mobility improves. Cryotherapy is valuable for pain management and edema control, especially posttreatment.

Pool therapy can be initiated when the incision is well healed. Patients should be cautioned about the added buoyancy of the water in relation to maintaining THA precautions.

Postoperative Phase II: Early Flexibility and Strengthening (Weeks 2 to 8)

Note—This phase continues until precautions are cleared by the surgeon and is based on a general THA population that is WBAT and ambulatory prior to surgery

GOALS
- Minimize pain
- Normalize gait without assistive device
- Hip extension 0–15 degrees
- Control edema
- Independence with ADLs

PRECAUTIONS
- Avoid hip flexion greater than 90 degrees, adduction past neutral, and internal rotation past neutral (for posterior-lateral approach)
- Avoid heat
- Avoid sitting for prolonged intervals (greater than 1 hour)
- Avoid pain with therapeutic exercise and functional activities
- Avoid reciprocal stair climbing until both ascending and descending step progression has been accomplished

TREATMENT STRATEGIES
- Continuation and progression of advanced home exercise program (HEP)
- Ice
- Prone exercises
- Short crank ergometry (90 mm)
- Gait training
- Retro treadmill
- Proximal hip stengthening progression
- CKC: leg press/eccentric leg press
- Forward step-up progression (4″ to 6″ to 8″)
- Proprioception/balance training: bilateral dynamic activities and unilateral static stance
- ADL training
- Pool therapy
- Determine baseline measurements for functional reach, TUG, unilateral stance time

CRITERIA FOR ADVANCEMENT
- MD script clearing hip precautions after 6–8 weeks postop visit
- Edema and pain controlled
- Hip extension 0–15 degrees
- Normalized gait pattern without assistive device
- Ascend a 4″ step
- Independence with ADLs

Troubleshooting

Lower extremity edema can result from increased mobility. It is important to examine both the peri-incisional area and the distal extremity for increased swelling and pitting edema. Compression stockings are useful in minimizing swelling of the lower extremities and in the prevention of DVT.[21] These stockings are worn during the day to assist the venous system as mobility is increased.

Younger or advanced patients may be ready for additional challenges during this time period. All exercises and functional activities should be advanced according to patient tolerance and ability, provided that the precautions of this phase are observed. For example, advanced balance activities may be performed during phase II if the criteria for each of these activities are met prior to initiation. Exercises throughout the rehabilitation program should be pain free. Reports of discomfort during a particular exercise require modification or elimination of that activity.

A perceived leg length discrepancy is very common. Preoperative muscle shortening and joint height destruction, combined with normal postoperative edema, influence how the operative limb is experienced by the patient. These factors can take up to 12

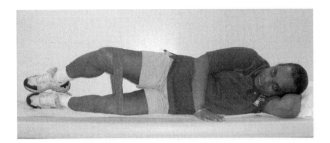

FIGURE **1-13** Clam-shell exercise with elastic band.

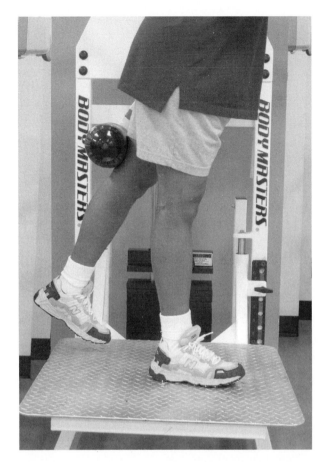

FIGURE **1-14** Hip extension exercise on the multihip machine.

weeks to resolve and are therefore not addressed at this time.

Patients should wait at least 8 weeks postoperatively before returning to physically demanding occupations, such as construction and farming, and physician consultation is necessary.

POSTOPERATIVE PHASE III: ADVANCED STRENGTHENING AND RETURN TO FUNCTION (WEEKS 8 TO 14)

At 8 weeks, THA precautions are lifted after follow-up with the surgeon. Patients often advance their activity level without sufficient lower extremity strength and control. Therefore, it is imperative for the physical therapist to educate the patient in the correct progression and its timeline. ROM/flexibility gains are typically met before strength return. Decreased flexibility is a result of adaptive tissue shortening that has taken place due to precautions that have been adhered to for 2 months.

Gentle hip flexion ROM in both sitting and supine are initiated beyond 90 degrees. Supine single knee to chest with a towel is introduced, and an unmodified Thomas test stretch is performed bilaterally. All mat exercises introduced in phase II are continued and progressed when appropriate. During this phase, a supine SLR can be initiated when it is performed in a pain-free range. Prone hip extension and knee flexion can be performed with ankle weights for additional strengthening. Once the clam shell is demonstrated with proper alignment and control an elastic band can be added to further strengthen hip abductors and external rotators (Figure 1-13). Side-lying straight leg raise will provide an additional challenge to isolate the gluteus medius. The stationary bike (170 mm) is now appropriate for increasing hip flexibility, lower extremity strength, and cardiovascular endurance. Progressive resistance exercise (PRE) machines, such as the multihip, are useful for targeting extensors, abductors, and flexors (Figure 1-14).

Functional exercises are the primary tool during this phase for restoring strength and normal function. CKC

exercises, such as the leg press, are now advanced by increasing the arc to 90 degrees or less and transitioned to squatting. Initially, squats in standing are performed against a wall with a physioball behind the back and can then be progressed to free standing once proper form and control have been achieved. Light hand weights may be added, provided that proper alignment can be maintained.

The forward step-up exercise continues to progress toward an 8-inch step (Figure 1-15). A 4-inch step down is introduced when lower extremity strength is adequate to allow a controlled, aligned negotiation. Knee and hip alignment need to be consistently evaluated by the physical therapist to protect against injury. Light hand weights can be used to advance quadriceps, hamstring, and hip extensor strength and prepare the patient for performing reciprocal stairs and carrying loads (Figures 1-15 and 1-16).

Proprioception and balance training continue to be emphasized in this phase. Goals and treatment strategies are tailored according to the deficits ascertained during testing at the end of phase II. Contralateral standing exercises using elastic bands for extension and

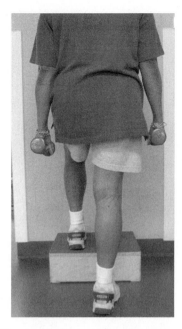

FIGURE **1-15** Forward step-up progression initiated with 4-inch step and progressed to 8-inch step.

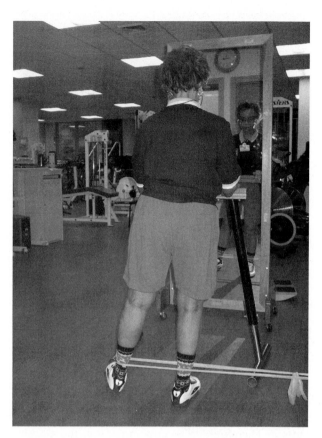

FIGURE **1-17** Contralateral hip abduction with elastic band.

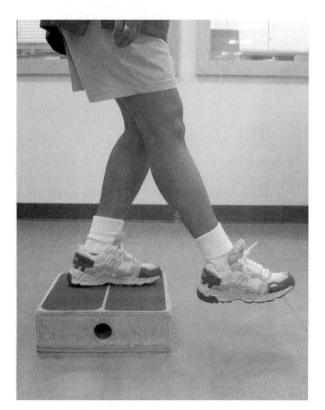

FIGURE **1-16** Forward step-down progression initiated with 4-inch step.

abduction are performed to challenge static strength and balance (Figure 1-17). Balance and proprioception exercises are advanced by performing standing exercises without upper extremity support. The patient is then progressed to unstable surfaces, such as a foam roll or rocker board. Single leg stance is performed with eyes closed and/or balancing on a multidirectionally unstable surface. Taking away visual input isolates the vestibular and central nervous systems, creating a greater challenge. All of these exercises are performed on the BBS, which provides a graded, unstable surface and visual feedback.

Encouraging normal functional tasks, such as donning/doffing shoes and socks during the day, assists the return of flexibility. These are usually the last functional goals to be achieved because they require adequate hip external rotation in tandem with flexion. Pool exercises can be advanced during this phase to include swimming for strengthening and aerobic challenge. Patients are advised to perform freestyle and backstroke, and they may use the kickboard as tolerated. Walking in the water will improve strength and endurance due to the inherent resistance provided for both upper and lower extremities.

Postoperative Phase III: Advanced Strengthening and Return to Function (Weeks 8–14)

GOALS

- Ascending/descending stairs reciprocally
- Ability to independently perform lower extremity dressing, including donning/doffing shoes and socks
- Functional reach, TUG, single leg stance times, all within age-appropriate norms
- Ability to return to patient-specific functional activities

PRECAUTIONS

- Avoid pain with ADL and therapeutic exercise
- Monitor volume with activity

TREATMENT STRATEGIES

- Stationary bike (170 mm)
- Treadmill
- Lower extremity stretching
- CKC exercises
- Continue forward step-up
- Initiate forward step-down progression
- Progressive resistive exercises of the lower extremity
- Contralateral hip exercises
- Advanced proprioception and balance activities
- Proximal PRE machines
- Pool therapy
- Reassessment of functional reach, TUG, single limb stance times
- Activity-specific training

CRITERIA FOR DISCHARGE

- Reciprocal stair climbing
- Independent donning/doffing of shoes and socks without aid
- Functional reach, TUG, single leg stance times, within age-appropriate limits
- Patient return to sport or advanced functional activities

The most significant risk for hip replacement patients after return to sport is wear of the components.[22] Patients who golfed preoperatively are permitted to return to play, as long as adequate strength and ROM goals are achieved. Patients are instructed in proper shoe wear (no cleats, initially) and to have at least 1 day of rest between rounds.

Functional reach, TUG, and single limb stance times are reassessed and compared to age-appropriate norms (see Table 1-1).[19,20] These test results should fall within age-appropriate limits. Often many therapy goals are not achieved before discharge from therapy. Patients should be independent with specific home exercises to target any deficits at the time of discharge.

Troubleshooting

Driving an automatic car for left THAs can be resumed once narcotics are no longer indicated. Driving reaction time has been evaluated and determined to be impaired until at least 6 weeks postoperative.[23] HSS surgeons generally suggest that patients refrain from driving until precautions are lifted.

Return to other recreational activities, such as doubles tennis, croquet, and ballroom dancing, can be accomplished upon meeting the criteria of discharge from this phase and with physician consultation. Patients should be reminded to initiate all new activities gradually and to discontinue or modify schedule based on symptoms. HSS surgeons typically discourage return to high impact sports, such as singles tennis, running, racquetball/squash and hockey.

At times, there will still be a measurable leg length discrepancy at the conclusion of this phase (12 to 14 weeks). A discrepancy greater than 10 mm should be addressed with a heel lift.[24] This will help restore normal hip alignment and protect the spine and other joints from excess stress due to misalignment.

REFERENCES

1. NIH Concensus Statement. Paper presented at NIH Consensus Development Conference on Total Hip Arthroplasty, September 12–14, 1994, Washington, DC.
2. U.S. Department of Health and Human Services, Center for Disease Control and Prevention, National Center for

Health Statistics. *Health Care in America: Trends in Utilization.* Available online at http://www.edc.gov/nehs/data/misc/healthcare.pdf. Accessed April 9, 2004.

3. Harkess, J.W. Arthroplasty of Hip. In Canale, T.P. (Ed). *Campbell's Operative Orthopaedics.* Mosby, St. Louis, 1998, p. 311.

4. Berry, D.J. Primary Total Hip Arthroplasty. In Chapman, M.W. (Ed). *Chapman's Orthopaedic Surgery.* Lippincott Williams & Wilkins, Philadelphia, 2001, pp. 5–10.

5. Sculco, T.P., Jordan, L.C., William, W.L. *Minimally Invasive Total Hip Arthroplasty: The Hospital for Special Surgery Experience.* Orthop Clin North Am 2004;35:137–142.

6. Berry, D.J. Primary Total Hip Arthroplasty. In Chapman, M.W. (Ed). *Chapman's Orthopaedic Surgery.* Lippincott Williams & Wilkins, Philadelphia, 2001, pp. 13, 17.

7. Masonis, J.L., Bourne, R.B. *Surgical Approach, Abductor Function, and Total Hip Arthroplasty Dislocation.* Clin Orthop Relat Res 2002;405:46–53.

8. Kroll, M., Ganz, S., Backus, S., Benick, R., MacKenzie, C., Harris, L. *A Tool for Measuring Functional Outcomes after Total Hip Arthroplasty.* Arthritis Care Res 1994;7(2):78–84.

9. Ganz, S. *A Historic Look at Functional Outcome Following Total Hip and Knee Arthroplasty.* Top Geriatr Rehabil 2004;20(4):236–252.

10. American Physical Therapy Association. *Guide to Physical Therapist Practice.* Phys Ther 2001;77:1163–1650.

11. Dunbar, C. *Making Cents—What Patient Education Can Do.* Nurs Spectr 2002;14A(15):5.

12. Schwartz, R., Asnis, P.D., Cavanaugh, J.T., Asnis, S.E., Simmons, J.E., Lasinski, P.J. *Short Crank Cycle Ergometry.* J Orthop Sports Phys Ther 1991;13(2):95–100.

13. Cipriani, D., Armstrong, C.W., Gaul, S. *Backward Walking at Three Levels of Treadmill Inclinations: An Electromyographic and Kinematic Analysis.* J Orthop Sports Phys Ther 1995;22(3):95–102.

14. Davy, D.T., Kotzar, G.M., Brown, R.H., Heiple, K.G., Goldberg, V.M., Heiple, K.G., Berilla, J., Burnstein, A.H. *Telemetric Force Measurements Across the Hip after Total Arthroplasty.* J Bone Joint Surg 1981;70(1):45–50.

15. Snyder-Mackler, L. *Scientific Rationale and Physiological Basis for the Use of Closed Kinetic Chain Exercise in the Lower Extremity.* J Sports Med 1995;5(1):24–34.

16. Barrack, R.L., Skinner, H.B., Cook, S.D., Haddad, R.J. *Effect of Articular Disease and Total Knee Arthroplasty on Knee Joint-Position Sense.* J Neurophysiol 1983;50:684–687.

17. Wolfson, L. *Gait and Balance Dysfunction: A Model of the Interaction of Age and Disease.* Neuroscientist 2001;7(2):178–183.

18. Duncan, P.W., Weiner, D.K., Chandler, J., Studenski, S. *Functional Reach: A New Clinical Measure of Balance.* J Gerontol 1990;45:M192–M197.

19. Podsiadlo, D., Richardson, S. *The Timed "Up & Go": A Test of Basic Functional Mobility for Frail Elderly Persons.* J Am Geriatr Soc 1991;39(2):142–148.

20. Isles, R.C., Choy, N.L., Steer, M., Nitz, J.C. *Normal Values of Balance Tests in Women Aged 20–80.* J Am Geriatr Soc 2004;52:1367–1372.

21. Pierson, S., Pierson, D., Swallow, R., Johnson, G. *Efficacy of Graded Elastic Compression in the Lower Leg.* J Am Med Assoc 1983;249(2):242–243.

22. Healy, W.L., Iorino, R., Lemos, M.J. *Athletic Activity after Joint Replacement.* Am J Sports Med 2001;29(3):377–388.

23. Ganz, S.B., Levin, A.Z., Peterson, M.G., Ranawat, C.S. *Improvement in Driving Reaction Time after Total Hip Arthroplasty.* Clin Orthop Relat Res 2002;413:192–200.

24. Maloney, W.J., Keeney, J.A. *Leg Length Discrepancy after Total Hip Arthroplasty.* J Arthroplasty 2004;107(6):475–482.

2

Total Knee Arthroplasty

JANET B. CAHILL, PT, CSCS

LISA M. KOSMAN, MSPT

Total knee arthroplasty (TKA) is a common surgical procedure to treat osteoarthritis (OA)/degenerative joint disease (DJD) of the knee joint. Over 300,000 TKAs are performed annually in the United States.[1] The Hospital for Special Surgery (HSS) performs over 1700 TKAs per year. Patients with OA of the knee typically present with the following impairments: decreased knee range of motion (ROM), decreased knee strength, gait deviations, decreased balance, and decreased proprioception. These impairments result in functional limitations, including difficulty ambulating due to abnormal biomechanics at the knee joint, difficulty transferring in and out of bed, difficulty ascending and descending stairs, and difficulty with activities of daily living (ADL). The goal of TKA is to restore soft tissue balance, optimize biomechanics of the knee, maximize function, and relieve pain. Rehabilitation following TKA is a crucial component to the success of the surgery to address all preoperative and postoperative impairments and maximize function. It is imperative that the patient has an understanding of the expectations throughout the continuum of care. The patient's participation in his or her own rehabilitation program is essential. This chapter presents the HSS postoperative rehabilitation guidelines following TKA.

SURGICAL OVERVIEW

Surgical techniques in TKA have made significant advances in the past 3 decades to treat advanced degenerative arthritis of the knee. Technology has allowed surgeons to replace the entire anatomical knee joint or replace either the medial or lateral portions of the knee, known as a unicondylar knee replacement. Minimally invasive surgery and high-flex knee prostheses are a few of the most recent technological advancements in joint replacement surgery. Standard TKA designs allow for bicondylar surface replacement, with either a posterior cruciate retaining (PCR) design or posterior cruciate substituting (PCS) design[2] (Figure 2-1). Other prosthetic designs are either constrained or semi-constrained, which provide different levels of stability and varying degrees of freedom.[3] The tibial and femoral components are commonly made of titanium alloy, and the tibial tray and the patella button are made of polyethylene.

A midline or parapatellar incision is commonly used for joint exposure. Osteotomies of the proximal tibia, distal femur, anterior and posterior aspect of the femoral condyles, and retropatellar surface are performed.[4] The anterior cruciate ligament (ACL) is resected to provide greater joint exposure during the procedure. The posterior cruciate ligament (PCL) may be resected if severe damage from degenerative osteophytes is found or if the surgeon prefers a PCS design. The medial and lateral collateral ligaments are retained; however, their anatomical positions may be surgically altered to

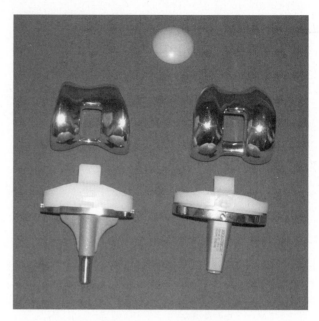

FIGURE 2-1 TKA posterior cruciate substituting components: titanium alloy femoral/tibial components and polyethylene tibial tray and patella button.

achieve optimal varus or valgus alignment. If a knee flexion contracture is found, posterior condylar osteophytes may be removed, or the posterior capsule may be released.[5]

Once soft tissue balance is achieved, a trial reduction is performed, and stability and alignment of tibiofemoral and patellofemoral joints are checked in both flexion and extension.[4,6] When optimal joint kinematics are achieved, the components are fixated with methylmethacrylate cement (Figure 2-2, A, B). The majority of patients who undergo TKA at HSS receive a combination spinal/epidural anesthesia, with a local femoral nerve block (FNB). General anesthesia is no longer used routinely at HSS. Williams-Russo et al.[7] have shown that patients progress at a faster rate, using epidural anesthesia than general. Postoperative pain is managed primarily by a patient-controlled analgesia (PCA) pump through the epidural catheter.

REHABILITATION OVERVIEW

The postoperative TKA rehabilitation program at our institution is designed and individually based on functional ability, clinical research, objective measurements, and the clinical expertise of the physical therapist. The HSS TKA rehabilitation guideline incorporates three progressive phases of postoperative rehabilitation to maximize patient outcomes. These guidelines include a general timeline of expected goals, which patients may achieve at a faster or slower rate, depending on age, comorbidities, pain, or surgical complications.

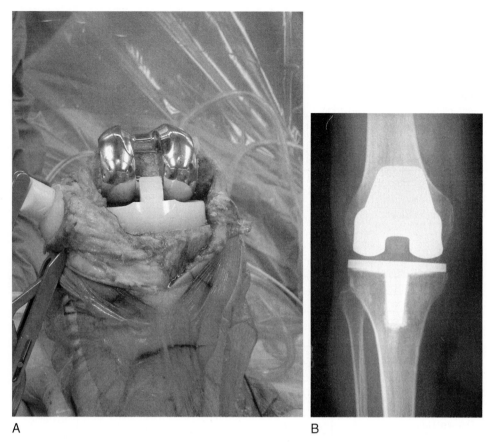

A   B

FIGURE **2-2** *A.* TKA components: intraoperative view *B.* Postoperative TKA radiograph demonstrating proper alignment.

Postoperative phase I of the inpatient TKA guideline was developed in part from functional outcome data that have been collected on over 10,000 patients who have undergone TKA over the past 15 years at the HSS, using a valid and reliable Functional Milestones Form[8] (Figure 2-3). This valuable information enabled us to benchmark functional status and design treatment interventions and goals in the early postoperative or inpatient phase. The subsequent postoperative phases II and III of the TKA guideline are based on progression and changes in function, ROM, gait, strength, flexibility, and balance that are measured objectively.

PREOPERATIVE PHASE

Preoperative education enhances patient outcomes, satisfaction, and success.[9] A preoperative physical therapy (PT) evaluation is beneficial to implement a home exercise program, including ROM and flexibility exercise, strength training, and gait training with an assistive device, if appropriate. Emphasis is placed on flexion and extension ROM prior to surgery because preoperative ROM is the ultimate postoperative predictor of ROM following TKA.[10,11] Because a preoperative PT evaluation may not always be feasible, patients are encouraged to attend a multidisciplinary education class prior to surgery. The TKA Pathway to Recovery Preoperative Education class has a 98% attendance rate. Topics discussed in the program include surgical procedure, anesthesia/pain control, nursing, rehabilitation, and discharge planning. The class is instructed by an interdisciplinary team that includes a nurse, physical therapist, and a case manager. The physical therapist explains the overall goals of inpatient physical therapy, the use of continuous passive motion (CPM) machine, initial therapeutic exercise program, functional progression, and use of assistive devices. Comprehensive written instructions regarding all topics covered in this class are provided in the preoperative notebook. Patients are encouraged to implement the functional techniques and therapeutic exercises into their daily regime in the weeks prior to surgery.

HSS TOTAL KNEE ARTHROPLASTY–FUNCTIONAL MILESTONES FORM

REHABILITATION DEPARTMENT

PT Initials:_____

Diagnosis:_____ **Age:**_____

Right/Left/Bilateral   Initial/Revision

Unicondylar ☐

WBAT   PWB   TTWB   NWB

Height_____(in) **Weight**_____(lbs) | **Day of Surgery:** Su M T W Th F Sa

Anesthesia: EPI   GEN   **Pre-op Class:**   YES   NO

PCA: EPI   IV   **Pre-op Amb:** w/c bound   <1   1-5   6-10   >10 Blocks

Femoral Nerve Block: YES   NO   **Pre-op Assistive Device:** Cane/Crutches/Walker/None

Need to negotiate stairs: YES   NO

Pre-op Lives Alone: YES   NO

	RR	1	2	3	4	5	6	7	8	9	10	11	12	13	14	15
BID																
Discharge																
Stairs Unassisted																
Stairs Assisted																
Cane Unassisted																
Cane Assisted																
Walker Unassisted																
Walker Assisted																
Stand Only																
Transfer Unassisted																
Transfer Assisted																
Dangle Unsupported																
Dangle Supported																
CPM																
Active Ext R																
Active Flex R																
Active Ext L																
Active Flex L																
Pain Level																
Date of Surgery _____																
P.O.D.	RR	1	2	3	4	5	6	7	8	9	10	11	12	13	14	15

Discharge To: Home   Rehab   SNF

If D/c to home: Home PT   Outpatient   No PT

If D/c to home, with: Family/Friends/Other   Alone

Complications/PT Held:_____

_____

_____

_____

FIGURE **2-3** TKA Functional Milestones Form.

POSTOPERATIVE PHASE I: ACUTE CARE (DAYS 1 TO 5)

Rehabilitation in the first phase focuses on minimizing edema, optimizing knee flexion and extension, restoring functional independence, and achieving independence in a comprehensive home exercise program (HEP).

Initial patient assessment at our facility begins on the day of surgery in the Post-Anesthesia Care Unit (PACU). An evaluation is completed that includes tests and measures of the following: mental status, barriers to learning, wound status, pain, upper extremity (UE) ROM/strength/sensation, and lower extremity (LE) ROM/strength/sensation. These measures are re-assessed daily. Effects that the epidural analgesia and the FNB have on motor control and sensation in the first 24 to 48 hours after surgery are monitored closely because they will impact objective measurements and functional performance. Patients are educated in a bedside exercise program that includes ankle dorsiflex-ion and plantar flexion and quadriceps and gluteal isometrics. Although research findings regarding the effectiveness of the CPM to increase ROM after TKA are inconclusive,[12] it is used at our institution in this earli-est phase. The CPM is applied in the PACU with ROM set at −5 to 60 degrees, or as directed by the orthopedic surgeon (Figure 2-4). The patient is instructed to use the CPM for 4 to 6 hours daily. The CPM flexion angle is increased as tolerated by the patient daily. Use of the CPM is discontinued if the patient can actively achieve 90 degrees of flexion for 2 consecutive days. Positioning to promote knee extension is an important component of phase I. Patients are instructed to maintain a position of passive extension for 10 to 15 minutes four to six times daily (Figures 2-5, A, B). Cryotherapy is a vital component of the postoperative rehabilitation program from the day of surgery through the continuum of care to reduce edema and pain.

The therapeutic exercise program is progressed within the first 5 postoperative days, from the initial bedside exercises to an advanced program, including straight leg raising (SLR), active-assisted range of motion (AAROM) knee flexion, active range of motion (AROM) knee extension, hamstring isometrics, sitting hip flexion, stair stretch, and passive extension with a

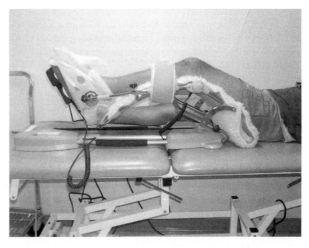

FIGURE **2-4** Continuous passive motion machine. Lateral view demonstrating proper alignment with joint axis.

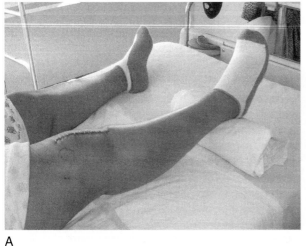

A

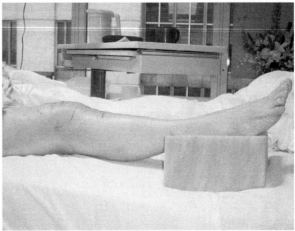

B

FIGURE **2-5** *A.* Passive knee extension with towel roll on soft surface In the acute care setting, a towel roll is placed under the ankle, while the patient is in bed, to add an extension stretch. Towel roll size may be adjusted to accommodate tolerance to the stretch. *B.* Passive knee extension with foam support maintains knee extension while controlling hip rotation.

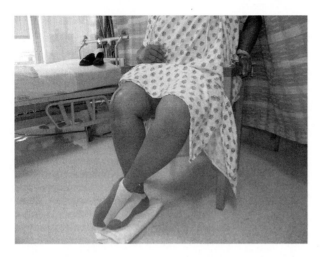

FIGURE **2-6** Patient performing active-assistive knee flexion exercise in a sitting position. Patient sits with foot supported on floor, with towel under foot. Patient actively bends involved knee as tolerated. Patient provides static stretch with contralateral LE.

towel roll (Figure 2-6). Progression of passive, active-assisted and active knee ROM is determined primarily by pain level, soft-tissue swelling, and strength of the operated limb. Bed mobility, transfer training, gait training on level surfaces and stairs, and ADL training are an integral part of phase I rehabilitation. Progression from use of walker to a cane is based on assessment of pain level, ability to demonstrate symmetrical weight-bearing, and ability to perform nonanalgic, step-through gait pattern.

All patients at discharge are provided with a comprehensive, independent exercise program. This exercise program is tailored to the specific needs and status of the patient. Patients are discharged to home when functional independence is achieved, the patient is able to ambulate household distances, and adequate social support exists in the home environment. Patients are discharged to an acute/subacute rehabilitation facility if additional rehabilitation is required to achieve independence with functional activities.

Postoperative Phase I: Acute Care (Days 1 to 5)

GOALS

- Unassisted transfers
- Unassisted ambulation with appropriate device on level surfaces and stairs
- Ability to perform independent home exercise program
- A/AAROM range of motion: active flexion > = 80 degrees (sitting)
                                          extension = < 10 degrees (supine)

PRECAUTIONS

- Avoid prolonged sitting, standing, and walking
- Severe pain with walking and ROM exercises

TREATMENT STRATEGIES

- CPM—Initiate at 60 degrees knee flexion and advance as tolerated
- Transfer training
- Gait training weight bearing as tolerated (WBAT) with appropriate assistive device
- ADL training
- Cryotherapy
- Elevation to prevent edema
- HEP to include—Strengthening exercises: quadriceps, gluteal, and hamstring isometrics, SLR, AROM knee extension, sitting hip flexion; ROM exercises: A/AAROM knee flexion in sitting, passive knee extension with towel roll under ankle, stair stretch

CLINICAL CRITERIA FOR ADVANCEMENT

- Patients are discharged home within 5 days when all the Inpatient Phase I goals are achieved.
- Gait progression from rolling walker to cane when patient demonstrates symmetrical step through gait, symmetrical weight-bearing.
- CPM is discontinued when AROM is greater than 90 degrees for 2 consecutive days.

*Note: Patients are discharged to an inpatient rehabilitation facility within 3–4 days if the patient requires progressive and additional rehabilitation to achieve independence with all functional activities.

Troubleshooting

Progression of ROM should be monitored closely. ROM deficits may be due to various factors, including poor pain management, preoperative ROM impairments or contracture, postoperative edema, and/or muscle guarding. Excessive edema and pain may result from rapid increases in ambulatory distances and frequency. Pain control needs to be addressed immediately, and pain medication should be taken as needed for the patient to be able to tolerate the rehabilitation program. Prolonged positioning of the operative extremity in a dependent position can also contribute to excessive edema and impede patient's functional progress. In addition, quadriceps inhibition may persist if edema is not effectively managed.

POSTOPERATIVE PHASE II (WEEKS 2 TO 8)

The second phase of physical therapy following TKA continues to focus on reducing edema, maximizing knee ROM, improving lower extremity strength, minimizing gait and balance impairments, optimizing independence in all functional activities, and continuing independence in the home exercise program. As the soft tissue structures of the knee continue to heal during this phase, pain level and edema need to be closely monitored as the physical therapy program is progressed. As healing progresses during weeks 2 to 8, a corresponding reduction in edema should be appreciated. Reduced levels of edema will allow active, active-assistive, and passive ROM of the knee to be optimized.

During phase II, maximizing available knee flexion and extension ranges of motion is critical to prevent arthrofibrosis. Joint mobilization techniques of the patella-femoral joint are incorporated in the rehabilitation program to restore patellar mobility. Superior and inferior gliding of the patella is essential to restore normal knee extension and flexion, respectively.[13] In addition, a short crank ergometer (90 mm) may be initiated as an effective and dynamic modality to address ROM and strength impairments[14] (Figure 2-7, A, B). Gastrocnemius stretching should also be incorporated in this phase to promote optimal knee extension.

Therapeutic exercises to address impaired strength include open chain leg raises in multiple planes and proximal hip strengthening, using a multihip machine. Closed kinetic chain (CKC) exercises, using a leg press or arc ball squats, are incorporated into the program

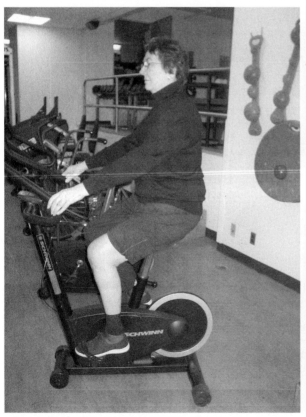
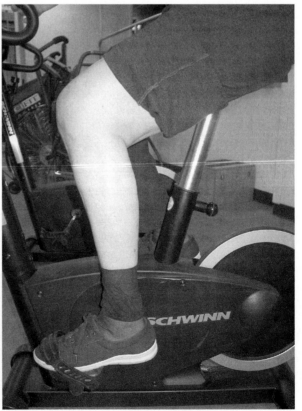

A   B

FIGURE **2-7** *A, B.* Short crank ergometer (90 mm) to promote early knee ROM.

when objective measures of strength and pain tolerance allow for symmetrical weight-bearing. A step-up program (2-inch or 4-inch step) can be initiated when a patient demonstrates improved quadriceps strength and greater than 83 degrees of knee flexion ROM.[15] When a patient can achieve full passive knee extension and lacks full active knee extension, closed chain terminal knee extension exercises are incorporated (Figure 2-8). Electrical stimulation and biofeedback may be used early in this phase for quadriceps muscular reeducation.[16,17]

Focus also continues on restoring a normalized gait pattern with or without an assistive device, restoring independence in all ADLs, and educating patients on activity modification. Cipriani et al.[18] demonstrated that retro treadmill training assists with quadriceps reeducation, as well as emphasizes extension during gait. Although balance and proprioception has been shown to improve slightly after TKA, impairments still exist.[19–21] To reestablish neuromuscular and proprioceptive control, bilateral static balance activities are initiated and progressed to unilateral static activities and bilateral dynamic activities using the NeuroCom system, the Biodex balance system, or traditional uniplanar balance boards (Figure 2-9). Functional testing, including the "timed get-up and go" (TUG)[22] and functional reach,[23] will provide objective performance-based measures regarding balance, postural control, and locomotor ability.[24] An updated HEP program is provided for the patient on a continual basis to address individual needs.

Postoperative Phase II (Weeks 2 to 8)

GOALS

- Range of Motion: active assistive knee flexion ≥ 105 degrees
- Active-assistive knee extension = 0 degrees
- Minimize postoperative edema
- Ascend 4" step
- Independence in home exercise program
- Normalize gait pattern with/or without assistive device
- Independent with ADLs

PRECAUTIONS

- Avoid ambulation without assistive device if gait deviation present
- Avoid prolonged sitting and walking
- Avoid pain with therapeutic exercise and functional activities
- Avoid reciprocal stair climbing until adequate strength/control of operated limb is achieved

TREATMENT STRATEGIES

- Passive extension with towel extensions, prone hangs
- Active knee flexion/extension exercise
- AAROM knee flexion: manual, heel slides, wall slides
- Short crank ergometry (90 mm) for ROM > 90 degrees
- Cycle ergometry (170 mm) for ROM > 110 degrees
- Cryotherapy/elevation/modalities for edema control
- Patellar mobilization (once staples/sutures removed, incision stable)
- Electrical stimulation or biofeedback for quadriceps reeducation
- SLR (all planes) PREs
- CKC: leg press
- Forward step-up progression (2" → 4")
- Proximal resistive exercises: multihip machine
- CKC terminal knee extension exercise
- Balance/proprioceptive training: unilateral static stance, bilateral dynamic activities
- Determine baseline measurements for functional tests: TUG and functional reach as appropriate
- Gait training with assistive device: emphasize active knee flexion, extension, heel-strike, reciprocal pattern, symmetrical weight-bearing
- ADL training in/out of tub/shower, car transfers

CRITERIA FOR ADVANCEMENT

- Flexion >105 degrees
- Absence of quadriceps lag
- Normal gait pattern on level surfaces with/without assistive device
- Ascend 4" step

FIGURE **2-8** *A, B.* Closed chain exercises: terminal knee extension with elastic tubing. Patient stands with operative knee slightly flexed and actively extends the knee against the resistance of the elastic band.

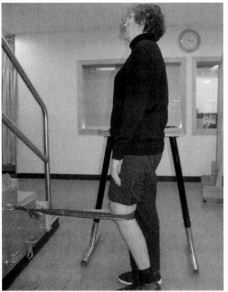
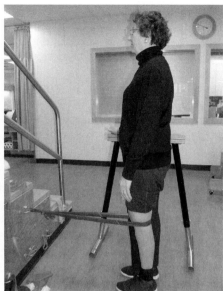

A

B

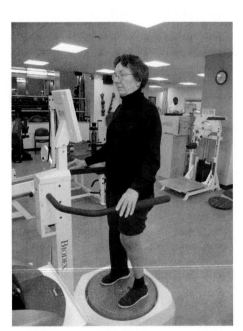

FIGURE **2-9** Biodex balance master: patient performing bilateral proprioceptive exercise with visual feedback.

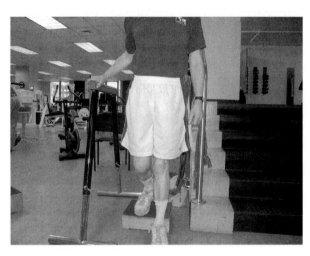

FIGURE **2-10** Patient performing 4-inch forward step-down. Patient slowly steps down on uninvolved LE, making initial contact on heel and controlling the motion with the involved LE.

Troubleshooting

Impaired knee ROM may continue to be a significant problem, at this time, as a result of edema, soft tissue adhesions, pain, and decreased strength. The physical therapist may emphasize techniques, such as contract relax, patella mobilization, soft tissue mobilization, CPM machine, and cycle ergometry to promote ROM. "Aggressive" or forceful ROM by the physical therapist may lead to soft tissue swelling and delayed achievement of optimal ROM for normal gait and functional activities. A tight rectus femoris will limit knee flexion in a prone position and may cause soft tissue irritation and swelling; therefore, to optimize flexion ROM, exercises should be performed in a sitting or supine position. Treatment strategies to address passive knee extension impairments include splinting, prone hangs with moist heat posteriorly, and/or superior patella mobilizations. A manipulation under anesthesia (MUA) may be performed by the orthopedic surgeon, if ROM is a limiting factor in the rehabilitation program.

POSTOPERATIVE PHASE III (WEEKS 9 TO 16)

During phase III, focus continues on maximizing ROM to allow the patient to perform advanced functional tasks, including ascending and descending steps, and ADL with normal movement patterns. Laubenthal et al.[15] determined that at least 117 degrees of knee flexion is required to squat and lift an object; this value is used as a benchmark for goal-setting in this phase (Table 2-1).[15,25] As ROM improves during this phase, a quadriceps stretching program may be implemented. Maximal ROM and quadriceps strength should enable a patient to ascend a 6- to 8-inch step using a reciprocal gait pattern and transfer from sit to stand from a standard height surface without deviation by the end of phase III. Advanced quadriceps strengthening exercises to achieve this goal include step-up (6 inches to greater than 8 inches) and step-down (4 inches to greater than 6 inches) (Figure 2-10) progression, ball squats, and eccentric to unilateral leg press exercise (Figure 2-11). Static and dynamic bilateral balance and proprioception exercises are progressed to dynamic unilateral activities based on the patient's ability. Functional tests are reassessed and compared to phase II initial performance. Newton[26] determined that a TUG score of 15 seconds or less represented an independent level of function in older adults. Duncan et al.[27] reported functional reach scores of 10 inches or greater to be associated with community-dwelling elderly male veterans who were non-fallers. These scores are used at HSS as phase III goals and to determine the efficacy of balance interventions. Upon the surgeon's discretion, a patient may return to work and/or athletic activities, including golf, cross-country skiing, hiking, doubles tennis, horseback riding, and cycling. Recreational activity training should be initiated, incorporating components of the specific dynamic movements that are required. High-level sport activities, including jogging, singles tennis, squash, and rock climbing, are not recommended following TKA.[28]

| TABLE 2-1 | Range of Motion Required For Functional Activities |

ACTIVITY	KNEE FLEXION ROM
Walking	*67°
Ascending/Descending Stairs	^83°
Sitting	^93°
Tying Shoe	^106°
Lifting an Object	^117°

*Data from Kettlekamp et al.
^Data from Laubenthal et al.
Adapted from Kettlekamp, D., Johnson, R.J., Smidt, G.L., Chao, E.Y., Walker, M. *An Electrogoniometric Study of the Knee Motion Normal Gait.* J Bone Joint Surg 1970;52A:775.
Adapted from Laubenthal, K.N., Schmidt, G.L., Kettlekamp D.B. *A Quantitative Analysis of Knee Motion During Activities of Daily Living.* Phys Ther 1972;52:34–42.

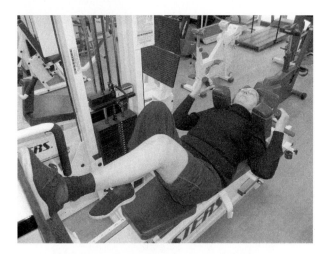

FIGURE **2-11** Eccentric leg press exercise: patient performs concentric contraction bilaterally and eccentric contraction unilaterally.

Postoperative Phase III (Weeks 9 to 16)

GOALS

- Range of motion: active assistive knee flexion >115 degrees
- Transfer sit to stand with equal limb symmetry and equal weight-bearing
- Independence with ADLs including tying shoelaces and putting on socks
- Reciprocal stair negotiation: Ascending 6"–8"
  Descending steps 4"–6"
- Maximize quadriceps/hamstring strength, control and flexibility to meet the demands of high level ADL activities
- Functional test scores: Timed get-up and go: <15 seconds
  Functional reach: 10"

PRECAUTIONS

- Avoid reciprocal stair negotiation if pain or deviations are present
- No running, jumping, plyometric activity unless allowed by the MD

TREATMENT STRATEGIES

- Patella mobilizations/glides
- Cycle ergometry 170 mm
- Quadricep stretching
- Hamstring stretching
- Leg press/eccentric leg press/unilateral leg press
- Forward step-up 6" → 8"
- Forward step-down 4" → 6"
- Ball/wall squats
- Retro treadmill on incline
- Functional ball squats
- Balance/proprioceptive training: bilateral and unilateral dynamic activities

CRITERIA FOR DISCHARGE

- Patient has achieved all goals and functional outcomes.
- Functional test measures within age-appropriate parameters.
- Ascend 6"–8" forward step up/descend 4"–6" forward step down

Troubleshooting

In this final phase the physical therapist should prepare the patient to meet the demands of his or her daily activities. Improvements in strength may continue after discharged from therapy. Physical therapy may continue beyond this timeline, if functional limitations, objective measures, and patient complaints indicate ongoing intervention. Patients are encouraged to continue a maintenance program that will address residual impairments, including decreased end range flexion or extension range of motion, decreased quadriceps strength, and decreased balance.

REFERENCES

1. Statistics, N.C.F.H. *Nation Wide Inpatient Survey 1997,* UDOHAH Services, Editor. 1997.
2. Insall, J. Historical Development, Classification and Characteristics of Knee Prostheses. In Insall, J.N., Kelly, M.A., Scott, W.N., Anglietti, P. (Eds). *Surgery of the Knee.* Churchill Livingstone, New York, 1993, pp. 677–717.
3. Burke, D., O'Flynn, H. Primary Total Knee Arthroplasty. In Chapman, M. (Ed). *Chapman's Orthopaedic Surgery.* Lippincott Williams & Wilkins, Philadelphia, 2001.
4. Lotke, P. Primary Total Knees: Standard Principles and Techniques. In Lotke, P. (Ed) *Knee Arthroplasty.* Raven Press, New York, 1995, pp. 65–92.
5. Guyton, J. Arthroplasty of Ankle and Knee. In Canale, T. (Ed). *Campbell's Operative Orthopaedics.* Mosby, St. Louis, 1998, pp. 232–295.
6. Insall, J. Surgical Techniques and Instrumentation in Total Knee Arthroplasty. In Insall, J.N., Kelly, M.A., Scott, W.N., Anglietti, P. (Eds) *Surgery of the Knee.* Churchill Livingstone, New York, 1993, pp. 739–804.
7. Williams-Russo, P., Sharrock, N.E., Haas, S.B., Insall, J., Windsor, R.E., Laskin, R.S., Ranawat, C.S., Go, G., Ganz, S.B. *Randomized Trial of Epidural Versus General Anesthesia.* Clin Orthop Relat Res 1996;331:199–208.
8. Kroll, M., Ganz, S., Backus, S., Benick, R., MacKenzie, C., Harris, L. *A Tool for Measuring Functional Outcomes After Total Hip Arthroplasty.* Arthritis Care Res 1994;7(2): 78–84.
9. Dunbar, C. *Making Cents—What Patient Education Can Do.* Nurs Spectr 2002;14A(15):5.

10. Ritter, M., Stringer, E.A. *Predictive Range of Motion After Total Knee Arthroplasty.* Clin Orthop 1979;143:115–119.

11. Ritter, M., Harty, L.D., Davis, K.E., Meding, J.B., Berend, M.E. *Predicting Range of Motion After Total Knee Arthroplasty: Clustering Log-Linear Regression, and Regression Tree Analysis.* J Bone Joint Surg 2003;85A(7):1278–1285.

12. Lachiewicz, P. *The Role of Continuous Passive Motion After Total Knee Arthroplasty.* Clin Orthop Relat Res 2000;1(380):144–150.

13. Edmond, S. *Manipulation and Mobilization: Extremity and Spinal Techniques.* Mosby, St. Louis, 1993.

14. Schwartz, R., Asnis, P.D., Cavanaugh, J.T., Asnis, S.E., Simmons, J.E., Lasinski, P.J. *Short Crank Cycle Ergometry.* J Orthop Sports Phys Ther 1991;13(2):95–100.

15. Laubenthal, K.N., Schmidt, G.L., Kettlekamp, D.B. *A quantitative analysis of knee motion during activities of daily living.* Phys Ther 1972;52:34–42.

16. Gotlin, R., Hershkowitz, S., Juris, P.M., Gonzalez, E.G., Scott, W.N., Insall, J.N. *Electrical Stimulation Effect on Extensor Lag and Length of Hospital Stay After Total Knee Arthroplasty.* Arch Phys Med Rehabil 1994;75:957–959.

17. Haug, J., Wood, L.T. *Efficacy of Neuromuscular Stimulation of the Quadriceps Femoris During Continuous Passive Motion Following Total Knee Arthroplasty.* Arch Phys Med Rehabil 1988;69:423–424.

18. Cipriani, D., Armstrong, C.W., Gaul, S. *Backward Walking at Three Levels of Treadmill Inclination: An Electromyographic and Kinematic Analysis.* J Orthop Sports Phys Ther 1995;22(3):95–102.

19. Barrett, D., Cobb, A.G., Bentley, G. *Joint Proprioception in Normal, Osteoarthritic and Replaced Knees.* J Bone Joint Surg Br 1991;73(1):53–56.

20. Fuchs, S., Thorwestern, L., Niewerth, S. *Proprioceptive Function in Knees With and Without Total Knee Arthroplasty.* Am J Phys Med Rehabil 1999;78(1):39–45.

21. Swanik, C., Lephart, S.M., Rubash, H.E. *Proprioception, Kinesthesia, and Balance after Total Knee Arthroplasty with Cruciate-Retaining and Posterior-Stabilized Prostheses.* J Bone Joint Surg Am 2004;86A(2):328–334.

22. Podsiadlo, D., Richardson, S. *The Timed "Up & Go": A Test of Basic Functional Mobility for Frail Elderly Persons.* J Am Geriatr Soc 1991;39(2):142–148.

23. Duncan, P., Weiner, D.K., Chandler, J., Studenski, S. *Functional Reach: A New Clinical Measure of Balance.* J Gerontol 1990;45(6):M192–M197.

24. Lusardi, M., Pellecchia, G.L., Schulman, M. *Functional Performance in Community Living Older Adults.* J Geriatr Phys Ther 2003;26(3):14–22.

25. Kettlekamp, D., Johnson, R.J., Smidt, G.L., Chao, E.Y., Walker, M. *An Electrogoniometric Study of the Knee Motion Normal Gait.* J Bone Joint Surg 1970;52A:775.

26. Newton, R. *Balance Screening of an Inner City Older Adult Population.* Arch Phys Med Rehabil 1997;78(6):587–591.

27. Duncan, P., Studenski, S., Chandler, J., Prescott, B. *Functional Reach: Predictive Validity in a Sample of Elderly Male Veterans.* J Gerontol 1992;47(3):M93–M98.

28. Healy, W., Iorio, R., Lemos, M.J. *Athletic Activity After Joint Replacement.* Am J Sports Med 2001;29(3):377–388.

3

Total Shoulder Arthroplasty

JOHN T. CAVANAUGH, PT, MED, ATC

JANET B. CAHILL, PT, CSCS

Total shoulder arthroplasty (TSA) has become the management of choice for many patients with debilitating glenohumeral injury or disease. A current estimate of over 10,000 shoulder arthroplasties are performed annually in the United States.[1] The primary indication for a total shoulder replacement is pain from an arthritic or incongruous glenohumeral joint that is unresponsive to conservative treatment. Other less common indications may include severe fractures or osteonecrosis. Contraindications for a TSA include paralysis of the deltoid and rotator cuff musculature, active infection, or a patient who is unwilling or unable to participate in the extensive rehabilitation necessary for success. TSA requires meticulous surgical skill and is a technically challenging operation. The variations in shoulder components (constrained, semiconstrained, unconstrained, and modular designs) (Figure 3-1, A, B) provide the surgeon with the flexibility to anatomically restore the shoulder joint. Many factors contribute to the outcome of shoulder arthroplasty, including quality of bone, integrity of soft tissues, underlying etiology of disease, and the rehabilitation program. The Hospital for Special Surgery (HSS) rehabilitation guidelines following TSA are presented.

SURGICAL OVERVIEW

Many variations exist to the surgical procedure of a TSA. A surgeon's surgical experience and preference, as well as a patient's soft tissue and bone quality, are integral factors to the technique of choice. Described is a surgical overview for patients undergoing primary TSA.

TSA is performed using either an interscalene regional block or general anesthesia, depending on the surgeon's preference. The patient is typically in a beach chair position and passive range of motion (PROM) is assessed under anesthesia, which will enable the surgeon to determine the expected postoperative ROM outcomes.

A deltopectoral incision is commonly used to attain exposure of the shoulder joint. Superficial soft tissue structures are identified and retracted at the level of the deltopectoral interval. The cephalic vein can be preserved and retracted, with the pectoralis major, or ligated and removed.[2] The clavipectoral fascia is incised superiorly to the level of the coracoacromial ligament. This allows medial retraction of the "strap muscles" (the short head of the biceps, coracobrachialis, and pectoralis minor). The coracoacromial ligament may be released (assuming there is an intact rotator cuff with good quality tissue) to more effectively expose the rotator interval.[2] The superior third of the pectoralis major tendon may be released and tagged for later repair, if necessary, for exposure as well. Adhesions between the rotator cuff and deltoid should be released if present.[3]

The subscapularis is identified, and the surgeon assesses external rotation ROM. To obtain greater exposure of the glenohumeral joint, the subscapularis tendon can be divided just medial to its insertion on the lesser tubercle, or a release of the tendon from its insertion into the lesser tuberosity may be performed (Figure 3-2, A). If an internal rotation (IR) (40 degrees) contracture is present, a lengthening of the tendon may be performed.[4]

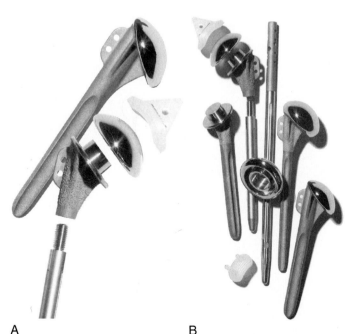

A   B

FIGURE **3-1** *A.* Integrated shoulder system. *B.* TSA modular humeral head and stem.

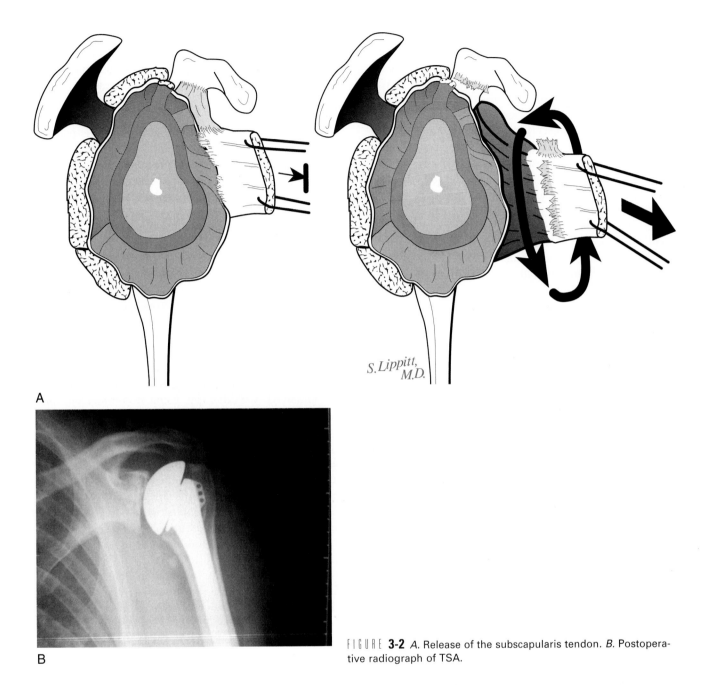

A

B

S. Lippitt, M.D.

FIGURE **3-2** *A.* Release of the subscapularis tendon. *B.* Postoperative radiograph of TSA.

Once soft tissue dissection is complete, the shoulder joint is dislocated; an osteotomy of the humeral head is performed, and degenerative bone and osteophytes are excised from the humerus and glenoid. When trial components are fitted and joint mechanics are restored, final components of titanium alloy humeral stem and head and polyethylene glenoid are cemented with methyl methacrylate. The humeral and glenoid versions are restored to provide stability and ROM. Appropriate sizing is critical to avoid mechanical impingement or "overstuffing" of the joint and ensure that the stability of the joint is not sacrificed. Final components are fitted, the subscapularis tendon is repaired, or reattached, to

the humerus and secured with heavy nonabsorbable sutures, and the wound is closed and the patient is placed in a shoulder immobilizer (postoperative X ray; Figure 3-2, *B*).

REHABILITATION OVERVIEW

Rehabilitation following TSA is a long and arduous course. Secondary to the amount of bone dissection during the procedure, pain management becomes an important treatment intervention in the early days and weeks following the procedure. Early mobilization is encouraged to prevent shoulder contractures and adhesions from developing. Therapeutic interventions are progressed following the guidelines that follow. Each patient, however, is treated individually because preoperative ROM, bone quality, and soft tissue integrity will have an influence on the progression of the program. Communication with the referring orthopedic surgeon to ascertain this information is imperative to ensure a safe and effective response to the rehabilitation program. A surgeon's prognosis, determined by the success of the procedure, should be considered when establishing rehabilitation goals. ROM, flexibility, and strengthening exercises are progressed via a criteria based approach, based on basic science principles, healing response of surgically repaired tissues, and rehabilitative experience. Patient education is essential throughout the rehabilitative course. Compliance to home therapeutic exercises as well as functional restrictions should be continually reinforced. Goals following TSA include maximizing ROM, flexibility, and muscle strength necessary for the pain-free performance of activities of daily living (ADL).

PREOPERATIVE PHASE

Before undergoing TSA, the patient is encouraged to attend a preoperative physical therapy evaluation and education session. The goals of the session are to alleviate patient apprehension toward the upcoming surgery and patient education. The postoperative rehabilitation course is described to the patient and/or family, as is the length of the rehabilitative process, with expected outcomes. The patient is educated on postoperative activity modifications, including ROM, positioning, and function restrictions. The patient is measured for a postoperative sling and is instructed in its proper use (donning and doffing). Instruction in postoperative exercises and the administration of cryotherapy are performed, and a booklet describing the information covered during the visit is provided to the patient for

review. The "Pathway to Recovery" booklet follows a multidisciplinary approach to rehabilitation. Contributors include orthopedic surgeons, physical and occupational therapists, nurses, and anesthesiologists.

POSTOPERATIVE PHASE I (WEEKS 0 TO 4)

Following TSA, a 1- to 2-night hospital stay is usually required. Before discharge, the patient is instructed in a home therapeutic exercise program to include the following:

1. Codman/pendulum exercises (Figure 3-3)
2. Dowel exercise for external rotation (Figure 3-4)
3. Active-assistive (AA) forward flexion (Figure 3-5)
4. Active ROM exercises for the elbow, wrist, and hand.

Exercises 2 through 4 are performed in a supine position in the scapular plane (Figure 3- 6) during this phase because this position is reported to yield decreased capsular stress and provides the greatest degree of conformity between the humeral head and the glenoid.[5]

Proper donning and doffing of the sling immobilizer are reviewed. Cryotherapy, using a commercial cold device (Figure 3-7) and pain medication, is encouraged for pain control. Speer et al.[6] demonstrated that postoperative shoulder patients who received cryotherapy slept better and used less pain medication in comparison with those patients in a noncryotherapy group.

The patient begins his or her formal outpatient rehabilitation within the first 2 postoperative weeks. Sling immobilization is enforced during this phase. However, the patient is encouraged to remove the sling for home therapeutic exercises and light ADL. The clinician performs a comprehensive evaluation that includes a thorough history of present condition. Limitations in preoperative ROM have been associated with compromised motion following TSA.[7] Rotator cuff degeneration will also negatively influence outcome.[8]

Preoperative Phase

GOALS
- Patient education
- Independence with donning and doffing sling
- Independence with home exercise program and precautions

TREATMENT STRATEGIES
- Measure for postoperative sling
- Instruct patient in donning/doffing the sling
- Instruct patient in necessary ADL (dressing, cooking, self-care)
- Instruct patient in and provide with written precautions
- Instruct patient in cryotherapy application
- Instruct patient in appropriate exercises (MD specific) to address ROM and strength deficits

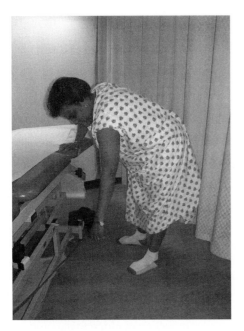

FIGURE **3-3** Codman exercises.

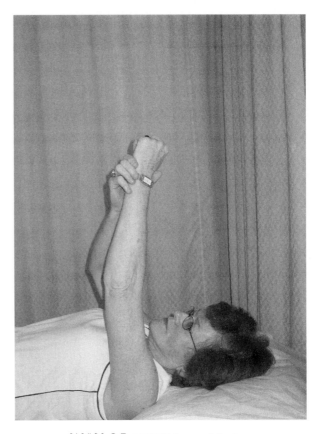

FIGURE **3-5** AAROM forward flexion.

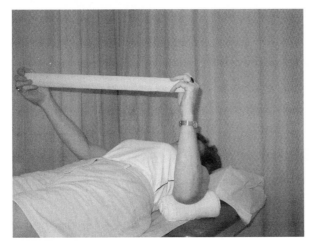

FIGURE **3-4** AAROM external rotation (ER) with dowel. Arm supported with towel roll under the elbow.

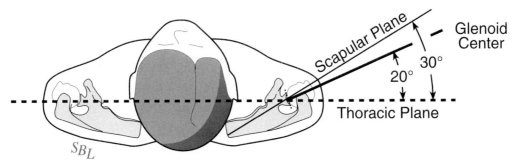

FIGURE **3-6** Plane of the scapula. The scapula plane is defined as 30 degrees from the coronal plane.

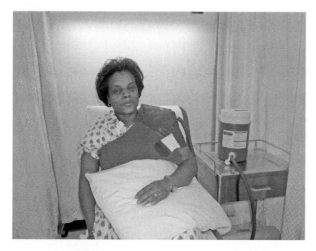

FIGURE **3-7** Cold therapy with commercial cold device.

This maximal protection phase of rehabilitation is dedicated to maximizing glenohumeral ROM within the range of motion restrictions identified at the time of surgery. Surgical detachment and subsequent repair of the subscapularis muscle necessitates limiting active and passive external rotation to 30 degrees during this phase. Elevation is limited to 120 degrees. Surgeon pref-

erence and/or concomitant rotator cuff repair may further necessitate ROM restrictions.

Scapulothoracic mobility is assessed in a side-lying position. Scapula mobilizations can be performed in this position, when restrictions are evident (Figure 3-8). A cornerstone of all shoulder rehabilitation programs at the authors' institution is scapular strengthening. By creating a stable base, the proper inclination angle of the glenoid is maintained and thus allows for an optimal length-tension relationship of the shoulder girdle musculature and decreases undo stress on the glenohumeral structures.[9] Scapula strengthening is initiated with the patient in the side-lying position, with the involved extremity supported by pillows in a neutral rotation position. Active ROM in the directions of protraction/retraction and elevation/depression is preceded by manual resistance supplied by the clinician. When tolerated, seated scapular retraction is added to the daily therapeutic exercise program. In other words, seated scapular retraction is added to the program when it can be performed without pain.

Pain management during this phase is monitored closely. Modalities used to assist in pain control include cryotherapy and transcutaneous electrical nerve stimulation (TENS).

Postoperative Phase I (Weeks 0 to 4)

GOALS
- Pain and edema control
- ROM to 120 degrees of elevation, ER to 30 degrees
- Independent home exercise program (HEP)
- Independent light activities of daily living

PRECAUTIONS
- Avoid unnecessary lifting beyond normal ADL
- Avoid ranges of motion beyond MD direction

TREATMENT STRATEGIES
- Sling immobilization except for light ADL and therapeutic exercises
- Codman/pendulum exercise
- Passive ROM exercises
- Active-assisted ROM exercises
  - External rotation (supine with wand, in the plane of the scapula, MD directed ROM limit)
  - Forward flexion (supine with contralateral limb)
- Scapulothoracic mobilization
- Scapula strengthening
  - Side-lying active range of motion → active manual resistive strengthening
  - Scapula retraction (sitting)
- Distal active range of motion exercises (elbow, wrist, hand)
- Cryotherapy/TENS as needed

CRITERIA FOR ADVANCEMENT
- Pain controlled
- Range of motion, elevation to 120 degrees, external rotation to 30 degrees
- Independent light ADL
- Independent home exercise program

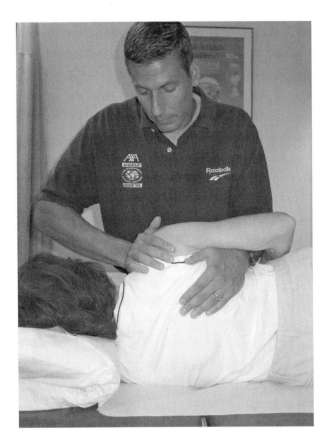

FIGURE **3-8** Scapula mobilization. Patient positioned side-lying. Clinician manually assisting scapula elevation and depression and gradually providing resistance.

Troubleshooting

External rotation (ER) ROM should follow the limits prescribed by the surgeon. Lack of progress in achieving the desired glenohumeral ROM is a common problem during the first postoperative phase. Muscle guarding and poor pain control may inhibit motion. Pain medication and relaxation techniques may reduce apprehension and muscle guarding. Furthermore, the shoulder continuous passive motion (CPM) machine may be used in conjunction with an AAROM program to facilitate controlled ROM. This may be a factor when TSA is performed with a rotator cuff repair and ROM must be restricted and monitored. The therapist should also be aware of excessive gains in external ROM during this phase because this finding may indicate a failure of the subscapularis repair. Elbow or hand swelling may occur distal to the shoulder, if patient does not use the sling as recommended by the clinician. Encourage sling usage, and maintain hand elevation to minimize swelling.

POSTOPERATIVE PHASE II (WEEKS 4 TO 10)

During phase II of the rehabilitation program following TSA, postoperative restrictions are gradually lifted.

Sling immobilization is required for only crowded or dangerous situations (e.g., subways, malls). The patient is encouraged to use his or her involved extremity in routine ADL. ROM restrictions are lifted, and the patient's ROM is progressed as tolerated. ROM goals of this phase are 150 degrees of forward elevation and 45 degrees of ER. Upon demonstrating improved control of the patient's involved arm during the supine AA elevation exercise with hands clasped, the overhead elevation exercise is progressed to using a wand/dowel. As continued humeral head control is demonstrated with the wand exercise, and range of motion exceeds 120 degrees of elevation, pulley exercises are added to the program. The shoulder should be in neutral rotation when performing pulley exercises to avoid impingement. The clinician should monitor the presence of scapular substitution in the form of "hiking" during the pulley exercise (Figure 3-9, *A*). Verbal cues to maintain the shoulder in a more neutral/depressed position will aid in truer gains in elevation. Active IR is avoided until 6 weeks postoperative, secondary to allow sufficient subscapularis muscle healing. Active IR is initiated at 6 weeks postoperative by having the patient pass a rolled towel or light object around his or her back from one hand to the other hand. Hydrotherapy, using a therapeutic pool, is used to further assist in ROM gains, normalizing scapulohumeral rhythm and strength development.[10] Buoyancy-assisted elevation, in the plane of the scapula (Figure 3-9, *B*), and horizontal abduction and adduction movements are performed *while at the same time* assessing scapulohumeral rhythm.

Strengthening programs assume a more active role during this phase. Deltoid isometrics are initiated at 4 weeks postoperative, upon demonstration of the criteria listed for advancement to this phase. Posterior, anterior, and middle deltoid submaximal isometrics are performed with the elbow position at 90-degree flexion (short lever arm) in neutral humeral rotation (Figure 3-10). The clinician should manually assess the patient performing isometric exercises to ensure that appropriate submaximal contraction is initiated. In this way, the patient should clearly understand the term "submaximal." The rotator cuff musculature is initially stimulated by the introduction of humeral head control exercises.[11] These exercises are performed in supine with the humerus positioned in the scapular plane in neutral rotation. Gentle, manual force is supplied by the clinician as the patient attempts to maintain neutral rotation. Neuromuscular training is further challenged by advancing this activity to a position of 100-degree elevation in the scapular plane (Figure 3-11). Submaximal rotator cuff strengthening is progressed to ER/IR isometrics in a modified neutral position at 6 weeks postoperative. This position approximates the scapular

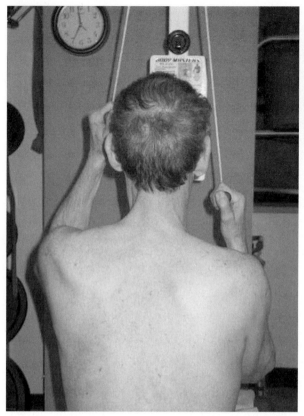

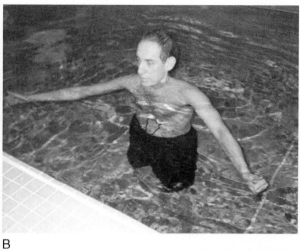

B

A

FIGURE **3-9** *A.* Pulley exercise. "Shoulder hiking" should not occur during this exercise. *B.* Forward flexion in the scapular plane in the pool.

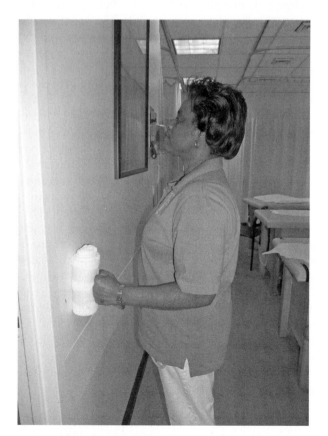

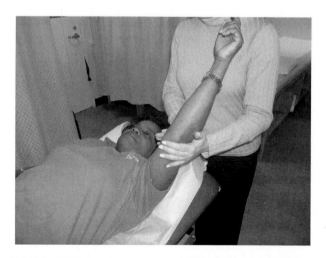

FIGURE **3-11** Humeral head stabilization exercises. Patient positioned supine and asked to maintain arm in 100-degree elevation. The clinician provides resistance as the patient maintains constant position.

FIGURE **3-10** Forward flexion deltoid isometrics (short lever arm).

plane and has been shown to improve vascular supply to the rotator cuff tendons.[5,12,13] Scapular stabilization exercises, using a closed kinetic chain, are added to promote stability and stimulate proprioception of the glenohumeral joint.[14,15] Examples of this closed chain concept include having the patient perform weight-shifting against a table and later progress to stabilizing a physioball on an inclined trampoline (Figure 3-12). Scapula strengthening is further advanced by adding elastic band resistance to the scapular retraction exercise

introduced in phase I. The posterior deltoid and latissimus dorsi are strengthened by having the patient perform elastic band extension. An airdyne bicycle or upper body ergometer is used to address muscular endurance.

Cryotherapy in the form of ice application is recommended after each exercise session, or as needed based on symptoms. Home therapeutic exercises are continually updated. Compliance to home exercise program and activity modifications is emphasized.

Postoperative Phase II (Weeks 4 to 10)

GOALS

- Pain control 0/10 with ADL
- Passive range of motion
  Elevation to 150 degrees
  External rotation to 45 degrees
- Independent HEP

PRECAUTIONS

- Avoid painful activities in activities of daily living
- Avoid ranges of motion beyond MD direction

TREATMENT STRATEGIES

- Passive range of motion exercises
- Active–assisted range of motion exercises
  - ER wand
  - Advance forward flexion to using wand in neutral rotation
  - Pulleys (ROM > 120 degrees/good humeral head control)
- Active range of motion
  - Forward flexion (supine)
  - Internal rotation at 6 weeks (towel pass)
- Humeral head control exercises
  - ER/IR (supine/scapular plane)
  - Elevation at 100 degrees
- Hydrotherapy
  - Pool exercises: forward flexion (scapular plane), horizontal abduction/adduction
- Isometrics
  - Deltoid in neutral
  - ER (modified neutral) ROM > 30 degrees
  - Internal rotation (IR) (modified neutral) at 6 weeks
- Closed kinetic chain exercises
  - Ball stabilization, weight shifting
- Scapular retraction with elastic bands
- Extension with elastic bands
- Airdyne or upper body ergometry
- Modalities as needed
- Modify home exercise program as appropriate

CRITERIA FOR ADVANCEMENT

- 0/10 pain with activities of daily living
- ROM (150 degrees elevation, 45 degrees external rotation)
- Good humeral head control
- Independent home exercise program

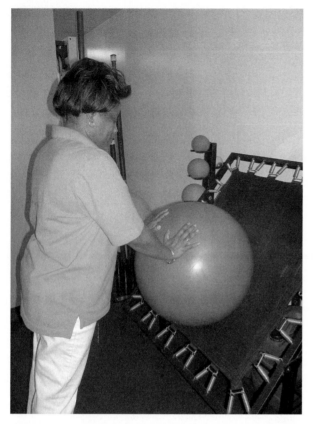

FIGURE **3-12** Closed chain scapula stabilization exercises with ball inclined trampoline.

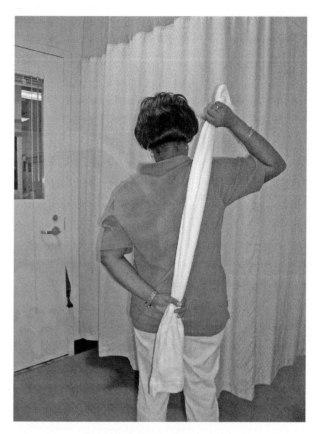

FIGURE **3-13** IR towel stretch.

Troubleshooting

Pain control should continuously be monitored and addressed to maximize daily function. If severe pain persists and limits shoulder progression, the surgeon should be consulted. ROM deficits may continue to be a limiting factor in this phase. Scapula mobility needs to be continually addressed to maximize and maintain shoulder girdle motion. Also, scapula humeral disassociation may lead to compensatory patterns. Pulley exercises, when initiated too early in the rehabilitation program, can cause compensatory muscle firing during shoulder elevation. Compito et al.[16] have shown that initiating pulley exercises early in the rehabilitation program for TSA as a result of proximal humeral fractures has caused the greater tubercle to be displaced off the humerus. IR isometric strengthening exercises may not be initiated before the sixth week to avoid potential rupture of the subscapularis.

POSTOPERATIVE PHASE III (WEEKS 10 TO 16)

Upon meeting the criteria for advancement, the patient enters the third phase of rehabilitation. The goals in this

phase are to gradually improve ROM, restore normal scapulohumeral rhythm below 90-degree elevation, and restore muscle strength so as to improve overall function in ADL.

ROM activities continue as previously described. Flexibility exercises to address tightness of the internal rotators and posterior capsule are added to the program. Specific activities include towel stretching (Figure 3-13) and a posterior capsule stretch, where the patient horizontally adducts his or her involved shoulder with light overpressure from the noninvolved arm lying supine (scapula stabilized). Gentle joint mobilizations are performed during this phase to address capsular restrictions.

As gains in ROM are demonstrated, strengthening exercises are advanced. Deltoid isometrics are progressed to use a longer lever arm (elbow extended). Forward flexion in the scapular plane below horizontal is prescribed when normal scapulohumeral rhythm is demonstrated. This is evaluated by having the patient perform forward elevation in the scapula plane in the "thumbs up" position and observe scapula movement below 90-degree elevation. This preferred hands position allows the greater tubercle to clear the acromion and minimize the chance of impinging the subacromial space. Increased electromyography (EMG) activity of the supraspinatus, infraspinatus, and deltoid has been demonstrated with this exercise.[17,18] Progression to this exercise requires significant strength and functional gains because the calculated force through the shoulder joint at 90 degrees of arm elevation is approximately 10 times the weight of the extremity, or about half the body weight.[19,20]

Light weights are added as tolerated. Progressive resistive equipment is used to further increase upper extremity strengthening. Machines include seated rows, chest press, and cable column pulldown. Isolated serratus anterior strengthening is performed supine by having the patient protract his or her scapula, with the involved arm flexed and maintained at 90 degrees. Light weights are added as tolerated. Neuromuscular training continues with rhythmic stabilization exercises being performed in multiple angles.

Modalities are continued to be administered as needed. Compliance to home therapeutic exercises and activity modification in daily life is continued to be reinforced.

Postoperative Phase III (Weeks 10 to 16)

GOALS

- Pain control 0/10 with advanced ADL
- Passive range of motion
  - Elevation to 160 degrees
  - External rotation to 60 degrees
- Internal rotation to T12
- Restore normal scapulohumeral rhythm <90-degree elevation
- Improve muscle strength 4/5
- Independent in current HEP

PRECAUTIONS

- Avoid painful activities in activities of daily living
- Avoid ranges of motion that encourage scapular hiking, poor biomechanics

TREATMENT STRATEGIES

- Progress range of motion as tolerated
- Flexibility exercises: towel stretch, posterior capsule stretch
- Hydrotherapy exercises
- Isometrics
  - Deltoid away from neutral
- Scapular stabilization
- Rhythmic stabilization
- PREs for scapula, elbow (biceps/triceps)
- Forward flexion (scapular plane)
- Airdyne/upper body ergometry
- Progressive resistive equipment: row, chest press (light weight)
- Modalities as needed
- Modify HEP

CRITERIA FOR ADVANCEMENT

- Pain control 0/10 with advanced ADL
- Passive range of motion
  - Elevation to 160 degrees
  - External rotation to 60 degrees
- Internal rotation to T12
- Restore normal scapulohumeral rhythm <90-degree elevation
- Muscle strength 4/5
- Independent in current HEP

Troubleshooting

Patients who demonstrate poor scapula humeral control should avoid overhead movements above 90 degrees to prevent increased shoulder pain. If pain continues to persist, the clinician needs to carefully reassess the patient's rehabilitation program and modify accordingly. Criteria should be demonstrated to advance to higher level activities.

POSTOPERATIVE PHASE IV (WEEKS 16 TO 22)

The final phase of rehabilitation following TSA is dedicated toward optimizing function. Goals include maximizing ROM, establishing functional muscle strength throughout the involved upper extremity, restoring normal scapulohumeral rhythm (>100-degree elevation), and developing the flexibility needed for normal ADL and selected sports activities.

Full ROM is not expected following TSA.[21-23] ROM exercises, however, are continued in this phase to maximize outcome. If a patient attains 160 degrees or more of shoulder flexion, a wall stretch is performed, with the humerus in ER to enhance range of motion and flexibility (Figure 3-14).

Strengthening with dumbbells and exercise machines continues to progress, as tolerated, emphasizing proper technique and form. Rotator cuff strengthening is advanced to IR and ER exercises, with elastic bands, when normal scapulohumeral rhythm and scapula strength *are* demonstrated. A modified neutral position is again used (Figure 3-15).

As upper extremity strength and ROM are progressed, proprioceptive neuromuscular facilitation (PNF) patterns are initiated.[24] These diagonal patterns are first performed actively by the patient in a supine position. Progression of these exercises include manual resistance from the clinician preceding resistance from elastic bands or light dumbbells. Neuromuscular control is further challenged during this phase by rhythmic stabilization exercises at multiple angles above 120-degree elevation.

For active, athletic individuals who undergo TSA, contact sports and activities that load the glenohumeral joint are not recommended. The consensus of an American Shoulder and Elbow Surgeons survey recommended or allowed participation in jogging, swimming, doubles tennis, bowling, and low-impact aerobics. The physicians also allowed their patients to participate in golf, ice skating, shooting, and downhill skiing, if they had prior experience with those sports.[25] If the patient should aspire to return to one of these activities, the *cli-*

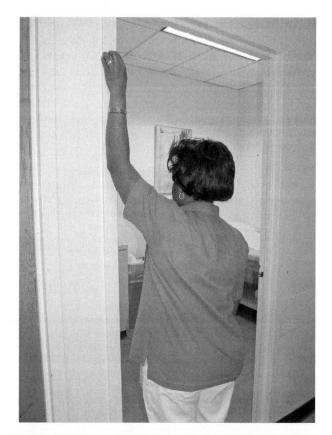

FIGURE **3-14** Wall stretch for end-range elevation. Patient positions involve arm at maximum forward flexion and leans forward, allowing body weight to provide a low-load prolonged stretch.

nician must prepare the patient to meet the strength and flexibility needs of that sport. Lower extremity and core strengthening should be addressed during rehabilitation for individuals who desire a return to sports. Sport-specific movements can also be addressed, for instance, mechanics of swimming stroke, tennis stroke, and golf swing. Golfers are encouraged to start swinging a club with low irons and gradually progress to higher irons as symptoms allow. Grounding of the club face is not recommended.

Discharge from outpatient rehabilitation is considered when ROM gains plateau and when the patient demonstrates independence in home and gym therapeutic exercise programs. Upon discharge, the patient is strongly encouraged to continue with his or her therapeutic exercise routine, performing ROM and flexibility exercises 5 days per week and strengthening exercises three times per week (not on consecutive days).

Postoperative Phase IV (Weeks 16 to 22)

GOALS

- Maximize ROM
- Achieve adequate strength and flexibility to meet demands of activities of daily living
- Functional muscle strength throughout the involved upper extremity
- Normal scapulohumeral rhythm >100-degree elevation
- Independent in home and gym therapeutic exercise programs

PRECAUTIONS

- Avoid painful activities in activities of daily living
- Avoid lifting heavy objects

TREATMENT STRATEGIES

- Assess and address any remaining deficits in ROM, flexibility, strength
- Active, active-assisted, and passive ROM exercises
- Flexibility program
  - Posterior capsule stretching
  - Towel stretch (IR)
- Progressive resistive exercises program
  - Dumbbells
  - Progressive resistive equipment
  - Elastic band IR/ER (modified neutral)
- Rhythmic stabilization
- Proprioceptive neuromuscular facilitation patterns
- Modalities as needed
- Modify home exercise program
- Individualize program to meet the specific needs of the patient
  - Sports-specific training
- Discharge planning for maintenance and advancement of gains achieved during rehabilitation

CRITERIA FOR DISCHARGE

- Maximize range of motion
- Full independence in ADLs
- Normal scapulohumeral rhythm >100-degree elevation
- Functional muscle strength throughout the involved upper extremity

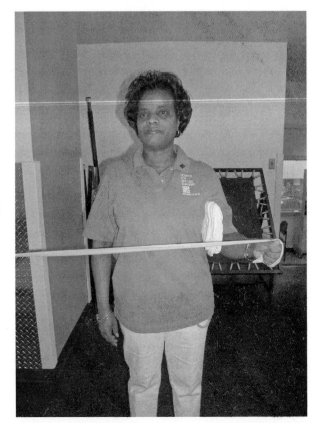

FIGURE **3-15** Modified neutral ER strengthening with elastic tubing.

Troubleshooting

The clinician should ensure that adequate strength and flexibility are met to ensure a safe return to sport progression. Sport-specific activities and mechanics should be reviewed and monitored to avoid overuse and aggressive force on the anterior capsule. To maintain and improve upon the goals achieved in rehabilitation, the patient is encouraged to comply with the therapeutic exercise program provided at discharge.

REFERENCES

1. Matsen, F.A., Rockwood, C.A., Wirth, M.A., Lippitt, S.B. Glenohumeral Arthritis and its Management. In Rockwood, C.A., Matsen, F.A. (Eds). *The Shoulder*, 2nd ed. WB Saunders, Philadelphia, 1998, pp. 840–964.

2. Marx, R.G., Craig, E.V. Primary Arthroplasty of the Shoulder. In Chapman, M.W. (Ed). *Chapman's Orthopedics.* Lippincott Williams & Wilkins, Philadelphia, 2001, pp. 2630–2664.

3. Personal communication, F. Cordasco, December 2004.

4. Fenlin, J.M., Frieman, B.G. *Indications, Technique and Results of TSA in Osteoarthritis.* Orthop Clin North Am 1998;29(3): 423–434.

5. Johnston, T.B. *The Movements of the Shoulder Joint. A Plea for the Use of the "Plane of the Scapula" as the Plane of Reference for Movements Occurring at the Humeri-scapular Joint.* Br J Surg 1937;25:252–260.

6. Speer, K.P., Warren, R.F., Horowitz, L. *The Efficacy of Cryotherapy in the Postoperative Shoulder.* J Shoulder Elbow Surg 1996;5(1):62–68.

7. Iannotti, J.P., Norris, T.R. *Influence of Preoperative Factors on Outcome of Shoulder Arthroplasty for Glenohumeral Osteoarthritis.* J Bone Joint Surg Am 2003;85A(2):251–258.

8. Kempf, J.F., Walch, G., Edwards, B., Lafosse, L., Boulaya, A. *Influence of the Rotator Cuff on Results after TSA for Centered Degeneration.* J Bone Joint Surg Br 2004;86B(Suppl 1):30.

9. Kibler, W.B. *The Role of the Scapula in Athletic Shoulder Function.* Am J Sports Med 1998;26:325–336.

10. Speer, K.P., Cavanaugh, J.T., Warren, R.F., Day, L., Wickiewicz, T.L. *A Role for Hydrotherapy in Shoulder Rehabilitation.* Am J Sports Med 1993;21(6):850–853.

11. Wilk, K.E., Arrigo, C., Andrews, J.R. *Closed and Open Chain Kinetic Exercise for the Upper Extremity.* J Sports Rehab 1996;5: 88–102.

12. Rathburn, J., MacNab, I. *The Microvasculature Pattern of the Rotator Cuff.* J Bone Joint Surg 1970;52B:540–553.

13. Saha, K. *Mechanism of Shoulder Movements and Plea for Recognition of the "Zero Position" of the Glenohumeral Joint.* Clin Orthop 1983;173:3–10.

14. Tippett, S. *Closed Chain Exercise.* Orthop Phys Ther Clin North Am 1992;1:253–268.

15. Wilk, K.E., Arrigo, C. *Current Concepts in the Rehabilitation of the Athletic Shoulder.* J Orthop Sports Phys Ther 1993;18(1): 365–378.

16. Compito, C.A., Self, E.B., Bigliani, L.U. *Arthroplasty and Acute Shoulder Trauma.* Clin Orthop 1994;307:27–36.

17. Burke, W.S., Vangsness, C.T., Powers, C.M. *Strengthening the Supraspinatus. A Clinical and Biomechanical Review.* Clin Orthop 2002;402:292–298.

18. Takeda, Y., Kashiwaguchi, S., Endo, K., Matsuura, T., Sasa, T. *The Most Effective Exercise for Strengthening the Supraspinatus Muscle: Evaluation by Magnetic Resonance Imaging.* Am J Sports Med 2002;30(3):374–381.

19. Poppen, N.K., Walker, P.S. *Normal and Abnormal Motion of the Shoulder.* J Bone Joint Surg Am 1976;58:195–201.

20. Popper, N.K., Walker, P.S. *Forces at the Glenohumeral Joint in Abduction.* Clin Orthop 1978;135:165–170.

21. Mansat, P., Mansat, M., Bellmore, Y., Rangers, M., Bonneville, P. *Mid-term Results of Shoulder Arthroplasty for Primary Osteoarthritis.* Rev Chir Orthop Reparatrice Appar Mot 2002; 88(6):544–552.

22. Norris, T.R., Iannotti, J.P. *Functional Outcome after Shoulder Arthroplasty for Primary Osteoarthritis: A Multimember Study.* Shoulder Elbow Surg 2002;11(2):130–135.

23. Sperling, J.W., Cofield, R.H., Rowland, C.M. *Minimum Fifteen-year Follow-up of Near Hemiarthroplasty and TSA in Patients Aged Fifty Years or Younger.* Shoulder Elbow Surg 2004;13(6): 604–613.

24. Knott, M., Voss, D. *Proprioceptive Neuromuscular Facilitation.* Harper and Row, New York, 1968.

25. Healy, W.L., Iorio, R., Lemos, M.J. *Athletic Activity after Joint Replacement.* Am J Sports Med 2001;29(3):377–388.

CHAPTER 4

Total Elbow Arthroplasty

AVIVA WOLFF, OTR/L, CHT

The primary goal of total elbow arthroplasty (TEA) is pain relief with restoration of stability and functional motion (arc of 30 to 130 degrees). An elbow replacement is considered when the joint is painful, is restricted in motion, and has destroyed articular cartilage. Patients who are elderly or have low demands that present with rheumatoid arthritis, advanced posttraumatic arthritis, advanced degenerative arthritis or nonunion, and comminuted, distal humeral fractures are good candidates for this surgery. A total elbow replacement is contraindicated in situations where there is active sepsis in the joint, prior infection or open wounds at the elbow, poor soft tissue envelope, skeletal immaturity, and paralysis of biceps or triceps. Complications of this surgery include delayed wound healing, infection, ulnar neuritis, triceps insufficiency, instability, and mechanical failure.[1]

ANATOMICAL AND SURGICAL OVERVIEW

TEA includes three types of implants: constrained, nonconstrained, and semiconstrained. The first prosthesis developed was rigid and fully constrained. It had a metal-to-metal interface and provided immediate stability but had a high failure rate with loosening occurring after several years. This was followed by a nonconstrained implant, which is composed of two separate units and is a resurfacing of the distal humerus and proximal ulna. This design requires strong ligaments, good bone quality, and adequate soft tissue support and is therefore only indicated in a select group of patients.[2] Examples include capitellocondylar,[3] Kudo,[4] and Souter[5] implants. The latest semiconstrained design, referred to as a "sloppy hinge," is the most popular. Although it provides stability similar to the constrained implant, its "toggle" characteristic allows for varus-valgus play and axial rotation. This type of design reduces some of the problems related to the constrained device.[2,6,7] Examples include the Coonrad-Morrey[7] and GSB 3 (Gschwend[8]) implants. The choice for a specific implant is based on the extent and cause of the disease, the specific needs of the patient, and the surgeon's preference.[2,7] At the Hospital for Special Surgery (HSS), the Coonrad-Morrey semiconstrained total elbow prosthesis (Zimmer, Warsaw, IN) is most frequently used (Figure 4-1). When a nonconstrained implant is indicated, the capitellocondylar implant is most often used.

REHABILITATION OVERVIEW

Progression of therapy is based on the stages of wound healing and is affected by implant type, skin integrity, rate of healing, and the preoperative and postoperative condition of the triceps. Time frames may be delayed to

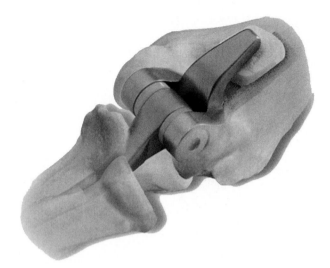

FIGURE 4-1 Coonrad-Morrey semiconstrained elbow implant (Zimmer, Warsaw, IN).

allow for wound closure and adequate healing of the triceps in patients with poor soft tissue quality, as is common in rheumatoid arthritis. Each surgeon has different preferences in the type of implant, surgical technique, and postoperative treatment. The referring surgeon is consulted for specific range of motion (ROM) restrictions and time frames. The guidelines below are for semiconstrained total elbow replacements performed with the triceps sparing approach.[9,10] This technique was developed to avoid complications such as triceps avulsion, triceps weakness, and wound healing problems. Notes in italic refer to guideline modifications for nonconstrained TEA. Time frames may be delayed in these implants to allow for adequate stability.

POSTOPERATIVE PHASE I: INFLAMMATION/ PROTECTION (WEEKS 0 TO 2)

Postoperatively, the elbow is wrapped in a bulky dressing and a plaster cast, and the wound is surgically closed with staples or sutures, which are removed 2 weeks after surgery and replaced with Steri-Strips. Drainage lines are left in for 24 to 48 hours. On postoperative day 2 or 3 the patient is referred for therapy. The bulky dressing is removed; a sterile, nonadherent dressing is applied; and bulk is kept at a minimum to ensure a close and precise fit in the splint.[7]

Immobilization Splinting

An immobilization splint or brace is provided on the first postoperative visit. Several options are available based on the preference of the surgeon and the experience of the therapist. Some surgeons prefer a brace such as the Bledsoe brace (Bledsoe Brace Systems,

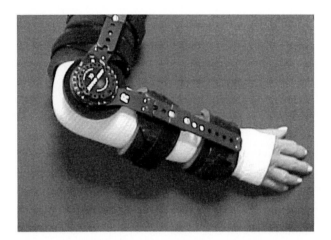

FIGURE **4-2** Bledsoe Brace (Bledsoe Brace Systems, Grand Prairie, TX).

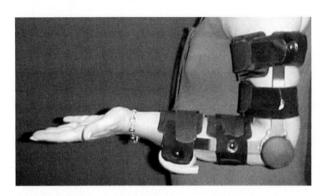

FIGURE **4-3** Universal Mayo Clinic Elbow Brace (Aircast, Summit, NJ).

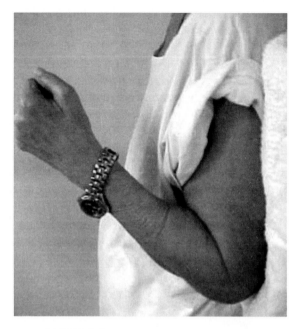

FIGURE **4-4** Active isolated elbow flexion.

Grand Prairie, TX) (Figure 4-2) or the Universal Mayo Clinic Elbow Brace (Aircast, Summit, NJ (Figure 4-3). The brace provides medial and lateral stability while allowing flexion and extension of the elbow. The parameters of the brace are preset to limit end ROM in both flexion and extension: Extension is set to tolerance, and flexion is determined by the condition of the triceps muscle and surgical repair. Protected ROM exercises are initiated with the brace on for 2 to 3 weeks.

Another common option is a posterior elbow immobilization splint (see Figure 7-2), a custom-molded thermoplastic splint positioned in 80- to 90-degree flexion. The advantages of this splint are that it fits well by conforming to the patient's elbow and that it can be remolded to accommodate changes in edema. Disadvantages of the splint include posterior pressure at the incision site and development of an elbow flexion contracture, if the splint is not removed regularly for exercise. The splint is removed three to four times daily for the performance of protected ROM exercises. In the presence of infection or instability, the splint is worn continuously and for a longer period.

Many surgeons prefer not to use a splint. The arm is instead wrapped lightly in an Ace bandage and positioned in a sling. This approach encourages early functional use and is comfortable and well tolerated. The rationale is that pain and postsurgical swelling will limit the end ROM.[11]

Motion

The patient is instructed in gentle-active and active-assisted elbow ROM exercises, with and without a dowel. Positioning a towel behind the arm against the wall is helpful in isolating elbow ROM (Figure 4-4). To avoid triceps attenuation, elbow motion is often limited to 90 degrees. Limits to elbow flexion and extension are established by the surgeon based on the surgical approach and the condition of the triceps muscle. Gentle, passive elbow extension to tolerance is permitted to maintain joint extension while avoiding active use of the repaired triceps. Gentle, active pronation and supination may commence; however, this should be delayed if stability is in question. Proximal and distal joint ROM must be maintained throughout this phase because this population is prone to develop stiffness. An elbow continuous passive motion (CPM) device may be appropriate for patients who cannot perform exercises independently and for patients with a history of prior elbow contracture. The therapist sets the parameters at 90 degrees of flexion and extension to tolerance and then instructs patients to use the CPM for 2 consecutive

Postoperative Phase I: Inflammation/Protection (Weeks 0 to 2)

GOALS
- Protective immobilization
- Wound healing and closure
- Control of edema and inflammation
- Full ROM of proximal and distal joints
- Full elbow ROM within protected arc

PRECAUTIONS
- Monitor wound carefully (increased potential for delayed wound healing and infection in RA)
- Triceps precautions: active elbow flexion to 90 degrees, passive elbow extension (gravity assist)
- Nonconstrained implants: no combined shoulder abduction and elbow extension (may lead to implant dislocation); extension limited to 30 degrees

TREATMENT STRATEGIES
Immobilization Options
- Bledsoe brace
- Static posterior elbow splint: custom molded at 90 degrees
- Static anterior elbow splint
- Sling

Wound Care
- Monitor wound, dressing changes (no bulky dressings that restrict motion)

Edema Control
- Cold packs/ice, elevation, retrograde massage, light Ace wrapping, Isotoner glove; avoid tight elastic sleeves

Proximal and Distal ROM
- A/AAROM of digits, wrist, and shoulder
- No shoulder abduction with elbow extension in nonconstrained implants

Protected Elbow ROM (Begin POD 2 with MD Approval)
- Active/gentle active-assisted elbow flexion to 90 degrees
- Elbow extension passively via gravity
- Gentle active pronation and supination
  - *Elbow flexed at 90 degrees with arm at side to maintain stability in nonconstrained implants*
- CPM if patient is unable to perform exercises: 30 to 90 degrees, 2 consecutive hours, three times daily

CRITERIA FOR ADVANCEMENT
- Wound closure
- Sufficient healing of triceps and stability of implant to withstand greater stresses

hours, three times daily. Between CPM sessions the elbow rests in the splint.[11]

Troubleshooting

The wound should be assessed for color, temperature, drainage, and tissue integrity. Excess drainage, delayed healing, and infection require prolonged immobilization. If any of these factors are present, an anterior splint is indicated to avoid pressure over the wound (Figure 4-5). Immobilization is usually prolonged and ROM delayed. It is important to note that these patients often present with poor skin quality, prolonged healing, and increased risk of infection from prolonged steroid use.[2]

POSTOPERATIVE PHASE II: FIBROPLASIA (WEEKS 2 TO 6)

The treatment focus during this phase is to increase active and passive elbow ROM, minimize development of adhesions, control scar formation, isolate triceps muscle contraction, and encourage functional use of the extremity. Proximal strengthening of scapular and shoulder muscles and postural reeducation are also addressed.

ROM limitations are addressed according to the needs of each patient. Some patients have full functional ROM in the early phases of treatment, whereas others require frequent and prolonged therapy to regain motion. Moist heat is applied before exercise. Co-contraction of the

Postoperative Phase II: Fibroplasia (Weeks 2 to 6)

GOALS

- Maximum active elbow ROM
- Minimal adhesion formation and decreased scar development
- Isolated active triceps muscle contraction
- Functional use of the extremity

PRECAUTIONS

- Obtain MD approval prior to D/C of triceps precautions
- No forceful active elbow extension, including during ADL (i.e., pushing up from a chair)
- No lifting over 1 pound or other ADL stressful to elbow
- No resistive exercises
- *Avoid varus/valgus stress in unconstrained implants*

TREATMENT STRATEGIES

ROM/Isometrics

- A/AAROM
  - Progress elbow flexion to tolerance
  - Active extension with gravity assist, gradually progressing to other planes
  - Place and hold exercises at comfortable end range
- Submaximal isometrics to isolate triceps throughout range
- Education to avoid compensatory motions (shoulder shrug, protraction)

Modalities

- Massage, moist heat to biceps and triceps to inhibit co-contraction
- Biofeedback to inhibit co-contraction and isolate triceps
- Cold packs and other edema reduction measures

Scar Management

- Scar massage when sutures/staples have been removed and incision is dry and closed
- Soft tissue mobilization and cross-friction massage to triceps tendon insertion
- Silicone/otoform insert with light compression for night use

Functional Use

- Gradually wean splint and promote performance of light ADL/self-care

CRITERIA FOR ADVANCEMENT

- Sufficient stability and soft tissue healing to withstand light resistive exercise and static progressive/serial static splinting

---

biceps muscle may limit elbow extension. Massage to the biceps muscle belly following application of heat is helpful in inhibiting co-contraction. Exercises are continued from the previous phase and are upgraded to gradually increase active elbow flexion beyond 90 degrees. Three weeks after surgery, the triceps is strong enough to tolerate gentle, passive flexion and active-assisted extension. Passive elbow flexion is increased by increments of 10 degrees per therapy session. Active and active-assisted elbow extension exercises are performed first in a gravity-assisted plane and upgraded as tolerated. Toward the end of this phase, overhead pulleys can be used to increase ROM. Early use of pulleys is avoided because the joint may not be stable enough to withstand the traction force.[11]

Troubleshooting

Triceps tendon adhesions and weakness may prevent isolated elbow extension. Graded active extension is first initiated in a gravity-eliminated plane, as in a table-top towel stretch. Exercises should be performed in a position that avoids compensatory use of the latissimus dorsi and teres major muscles or eccentric use of the biceps. Biofeedback is used to inhibit co-contraction by providing feedback to the patient who cannot actively fire the triceps muscle[11,12] (Figure 4-6). Occasionally, patients may be unable to activate the triceps to adequately extend the elbow, despite the best therapy attempts. In these situations it is important to determine, with the surgeon, the integrity of the tendon and explore surgical options, if appropriate.

POSTOPERATIVE PHASE III: SCAR MATURATION (WEEK 6 TO MONTH 6)

As the collagen decreases during this phase, the wound becomes stronger and can tolerate increased stress.[12,13] Treatment during this phase concentrates on obtaining and maintaining maximum ROM and functional

Postoperative Phase III: Scar Maturation (Week 6 to Month 6)

GOALS

- Maximum stable passive elbow ROM
- Adequate strength required for elbow AROM to equal PROM
- Functional strength required for independent use of UE for ADL, work, and leisure
- Awareness of lifetime precautions and potential complications

PRECAUTIONS

- No aggressive stretching; no joint mobilizations
- Avoid dynamic splints (these apply to excessive, uncontrolled force to elbow)
- Do not sacrifice stability to gain ROM
- Lifetime precautions:
  - Five-pound maximum for lifting or carrying
  - No weight-bearing on extended elbow
  - No impact sports such as golf and tennis

TREATMENT STRATEGIES
Splinting/PROM for maximum stable ROM

- Static progressive elbow flexion: worn intermittently during the day
- Serial static extension splint: worn at night and/or intermittently during the day
- Alternative to splints previously mentioned: Universal Mayo Clinic Elbow Brace (Aircast)
- PROM/gentle stretching at end range

Gentle Strengthening

- Elbow extension exercises against gravity (overhead)
- Isometrics
- Light resistive exercises for triceps, biceps, and scapular muscles: light Thera Band (mid-range), 1 pound free weights or cable column
- NMES to triceps if weakness and adhesions persist

Restoration of Function

- Encourage resumption of functional activities while observing lifetime precautions

CRITERIA FOR DISCHARGE

- Achievement of functional ROM and strength for all light ADL
- Independence in home exercise program, joint protection, and awareness of precautions

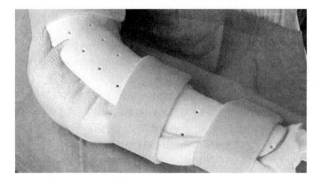

FIGURE **4-5** Anterior elbow splint.

strength to enable functional independence. Patients are educated and made aware of lifetime precautions, limitations, contraindications, and possible complications. It is important to remember that full ROM is not the goal and is often not achievable. Stability of the joint can never be compromised to achieve greater mobility. Joint mobilization and aggressive passive ROM are never appropriate and are strictly forbidden on an elbow implant.

Troubleshooting

If stiffness persists at end ROM, static progressive elbow flexion or extension splinting is used to gain end ROM by providing a low load prolonged stretch (see Chapter 9, Treatment Guidelines for Contractive Release of the Elow).

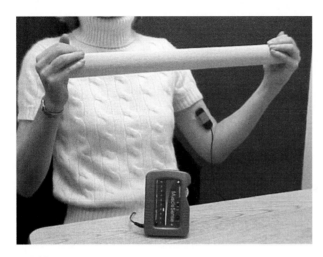

FIGURE **4-6** Biofeedback to decrease co-contraction of the biceps muscle.

REFERENCES

1. Morrey, B. Complications of Elbow Replacement Surgery. In Morrey, B. (Ed). *The Elbow and Its Disorders,* 2nd ed. WB Saunders, Philadelphia, 2000.
2. Cooney, W. Elbow Arthroplasty: Historical Perspective and Current Concepts. In Morrey, B.F. (Ed). *The Elbow and Its Disorders,* 3rd ed. WB Saunders, Philadelphia, 2000.
3. Ewald, F. *Total Elbow Replacement.* Orthop Clin North Am 1975;6:685.
4. Kudo, H., Iwano, K., Watanabe, S. *Total Replacement of the Rheumatoid Elbow with a Hingeless Prosthesis.* J Bone Joint Surg 1980;62A:277.
5. Souter, W.A. *Arthroplasty of the Elbow: With Particular Reference to Metallic Hinge Arthroplasty in Rheumatoid Patients.* Orthop Clin North Am 1973;4:395.
6. Ferlic, D. *Total Elbow Arthroplasty for Treatment of Elbow Arthritis.* J Elbow Shoulder Surg 1999;75:367–378.
7. Morrey, B.F., Adams, R.A., Bryan, R.S. *Total Replacement for Post-traumatic Arthritis of the Elbow.* J Bone Joint Surg 1991;73:607–612.
8. Gschwend, N., Lowhr, J., Ivosevic-Radovanovic, D., Scheler, H. *Semi-constrained Elbow Prosthesis with Special Reference of the GBS III Prosthesis.* Clin Orthop 1988;232:104.
9. Bryan, R.S., Morrey, B.F. *Extensive Posterior Approach of the Elbow: A Triceps Sparing Approach.* Clin Orthop 1982;166: 188–192.
10. Pierce, T.D., Herndon, J.H. *The Triceps Preserving Approach to Total Elbow Arthroplasty.* Clin Orthop 1998;354:144–152.
11. Wolff, A. *Postoperative Management after Total Elbow Replacement.* Tech Hand Up Extrem Surg 2000;4(3):213–220.
12. Smith, K. Wound Healing. In Tribuzi, S., Stanley, B.J. (Eds). *Concepts in Hand Rehabilitation.* Davis Publishing, Philadelphia, 1992.
13. Madden, J.W., Peacock, E.E. Jr. *Studies on the Biology of Collagen During Wound Healing: Dynamic Metabolism of Scar Collagen and Remodeling of Dermal Wounds.* Ann Surg 1971;174:511.

5

Metacarpophalangeal Joint Arthroplasty

CAROL PAGE, PT, DPT, CHT

Rheumatoid arthritis (RA) is a chronic, progressive, autoimmune disease that causes joint destruction. It affects women more than men and increases in prevalence with aging. An estimated 0.5% to 1% of adults are affected.[1]

Unlike osteoarthritis and traumatic arthritis, which rarely affect the metacarpophalangeal (MP) joints of the fingers, RA commonly affects these joints. Soft tissue and bony destruction lead to deformities that are often severe. Ulnar drift of the fingers at the MP joint level (Figure 5-1) results from attenuation of the radial collateral ligament and joint capsule, with ulnar dislocation of the extensor tendon. The ulnar collateral ligament, capsule, and intrinsic muscles become contracted. The metacarpal heads are usually subluxed palmarly.[2]

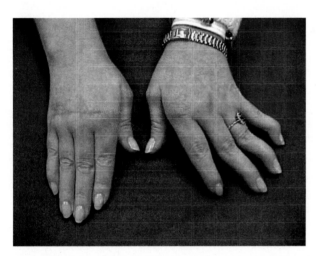

FIGURE **5-1** Left hand with ulnar drift of the MP joints; right hand after MP arthroplasty.

ANATOMICAL AND SURGICAL OVERVIEW

Although arthrodesis may be indicated for deformities of the proximal and distal interphalangeal (IP) joints, arthrodesis is rarely indicated for MP joint deformities because it is so functionally limiting. Arthroplasty is the treatment of choice. Surgery consists of a replacement of the MP joint, with an implant (typically made of silicone), and soft tissue rebalancing.[2]

MP joint arthroplasty necessitates excision of the head of the metacarpal, the hypertrophied synovium, and the base of the proximal phalanx. The medullary canals of the metacarpal and proximal phalanx are reamed and trial implants inserted to determine the best fit. Soft tissue releases are performed to correct ulnar deviation, palmar subluxation, and ulnar intrinsic tightness. Residual laxity of the radial structures is corrected and the extensor tendon centralized over the MP joint.[2,3]

Many approaches to MP arthroplasty have been taken, including joint resurfacing and hinged, semiconstrained, and constrained implants. Awareness of the particular implant used is helpful to the therapist in setting goals for motion. Silicone arthroplasty is currently the most commonly performed procedure.[4] The Swanson (Dow Corning, Midland, MI), NeuFlex (Depuy Inc., Warsaw, IN), and Avanta (Avanta Orthopedics, San Diego) MP implants are all one-piece, flexible prostheses of this type. However, differences between them may result in different, potential motion ranges. Because the NeuFlex MP joint prosthesis rests in 30-degree flexion, greater flexion may result than with use of the Swanson MP implant, which rests in 0-degree extension.[2] The Avanta MP implant, unlike the Swanson and NeuFlex implants, has a volar axis designed to increase potential for MP flexion.[5]

REHABILITATION OVERVIEW

The primary purpose of rehabilitation is to promote functional motion of the implanted MP joints, while preserving correct alignment as healing occurs. Stability of the implanted MP joints depends on the formation of a fibrous pseudo-capsule around the implants, a process known as encapsulation.[6] Protection is provided both through splinting and through patient education, in avoidance of deforming forces during exercises and functional activities. Lifelong adherence to joint protection principles is critical to preserve the implants and maximize joint stability. Metacarpophalangeal joint arthroplasty is widely considered to be effective in improving motion, cosmesis, function, and pain.[7] However, implant fracture and deformation have been shown to be common with long-term follow-up, performed at an average of 14 years postoperatively.[4]

POSTOPERATIVE PHASE I: INFLAMMATION/ PROTECTION (WEEKS 0 TO 3)

Referral to therapy occurs 5 to 7 days postoperatively, after the bulky postoperative splint has been removed. The hand is inspected to assess wound healing, edema, and digital alignment. Instruction is given in daily dressing changes with the hand and wrist supported. The surgical incision is covered with a sterile nonadherent dressing, over which sterile gauze is applied. If the patient is unable to perform dressing changes at home without assistance, they are completed in therapy several times weekly.

Several options are available for splinting in phase I, depending on the preference of the surgeon and the condition of the patient's soft tissues. The three splints most commonly used during this phase are the dynamic MP extension outrigger splint, the static MP extension

Postoperative Phase I: Inflammation/Protection (Weeks 0 to 3)

GOALS
- Provide correct protective splinting
- Protect repaired structures
- Reduce edema and pain
- Achieve full wound closure
- Protective mobilization of involved joints
- Maintain AROM of uninvolved joints, including wrist and thumb

PRECAUTIONS
- No use of involved digits for functional activities
- Protect MP joints from ulnar deviation forces
- No forceful PROM, stretching or resistance
- Never attempt to perform joint mobilizations on implants
- Modify treatment for additional surgeries performed, such as fusions of the thumb MP and IP joints, and finger IP joints

TREATMENT STRATEGIES
- Splinting options
  - Dynamic MP extension outrigger splint: MP joints extended to neutral with 10 degrees radial deviation, wrist extended 15 degrees
  - Static MP extension splint: MP joints extended to neutral with 10 degrees radial deviation, IP joints extended, wrist extended 15 degrees
  - Static MP flexion splint: MP joints flexed to a maximum of 70 degrees with 10° radial deviation, IP joints extended, wrist extended 15 degrees
- Edema and pain reduction: instruct patient in elevation, cold modalities, retrograde massage (avoiding surgical incision until fully closed)
- Wound care: Change dressings, monitor surgical incision
- A/AAROM of involved digits: Tendon gliding, thumb opposition to index and middle fingers, radial digit walking
- Gentle PROM by therapist: MP flexion, avoiding ulnar deviation; gentle intrinsic stretching
- ROM exercises for uninvolved joints: Thumb, wrist, elbow, forearm, shoulder

CRITERIA FOR ADVANCEMENT
- Edema and pain well controlled
- Surgical incision fully closed
- MP joint stability

splint, and the static MP flexion splint. The dynamic MP extension outrigger splint (Figure 5-2) allows active MP joint flexion and provides assisted MP joint extension, while maintaining slight radial alignment of the MP joints. Slings supporting the proximal phalanges are connected through a dorsal outrigger via elastic threads or rubber bands to the proximal dorsal portion of the splint. The splint is fabricated to position the MP joints in full extension (avoiding hyperextension), with 10 degrees of radial deviation at rest, and allow MP flexion. Because the elasticity of the elastic threads or rubber bands decreases over time, the position of the MP joints requires frequent checking and adjusting. The splint is dorsally based, supporting the wrist in 15 degrees of extension. Radial deviation of the wrist is avoided in the outrigger and static splints because this is the most common position of wrist deformity in RA. The outrig-

ger splint is worn during the day, and a static MP extension splint is worn at night.

Alternatively, if preferred by the surgeon, a static MP extension splint (Figure 5-3) can be used full-time for individuals with adequate soft tissue quality. The splint is removed for daily dressing changes and for exercises several times daily. The extension splint can be alternated with a static MP flexion splint (Figure 5-4), if MP flexion is particularly limited. The splint is serially remolded to gradually increase MP flexion to a maximum of 70 degrees. Care must be taken not to overstretch the extensor system, creating an extensor lag. The MP extension and flexion splints are volar-based and position the MP joints in 10-degree radial deviation, blocking ulnar deviation. The IP joints are positioned in extension in both splints. The wrist is in 15 degrees of extension, avoiding radial deviation. Because the exer-

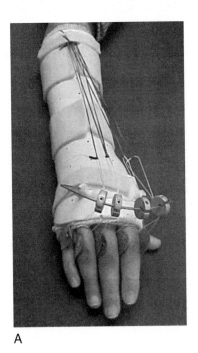

A

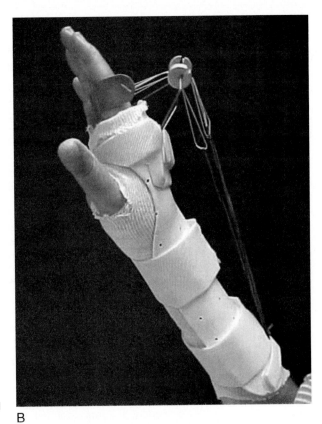

B

FIGURE **5-2** Dynamic MP extension outrigger splint. *A.* Dorsal view. *B.* Lateral view.

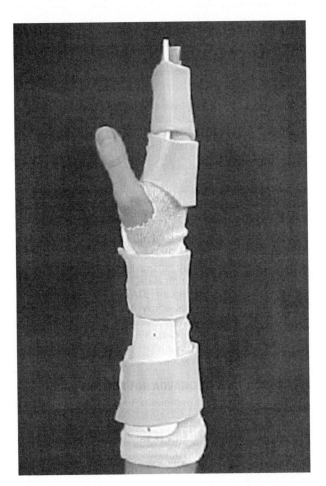

FIGURE **5-3** Static MP extension splint.

FIGURE **5-4** Static MP flexion splint.

cises, in this case, are performed without the support of the splint, extra care must be taken that ulnar deviating forces are strictly avoided. Recent research suggests that use of static splints for this patient population is an effective alternative to the dynamic extension outrigger splint.[8]

Additional protective splinting may be indicated if other surgeries, such as fusion of the thumb MP or IP joint or finger IP joints, are performed concomitantly with MP arthroplasty. A thumb component is added to both the static splints and the stationary dorsal portion of dynamic outrigger splints for protection of thumb MP or IP fusion. Proximal interphalangeal (PIP) and distal interphalangeal (DIP) joint fusions of the fingers are protected by inclusion in the static splints described. If a dynamic outrigger splint is used, individual finger gutters are fabricated for protection of finger IP fusions. Similarly, a dorsal gutter splint is fabricated to block the PIP joint in slight flexion to protect a corrected swan neck deformity.

Edema and pain are controlled in phase I by consistent elevation of the involved upper extremity above the level of the heart. Propping on pillows is encouraged. Overdependence on a sling can lead to elbow and shoulder stiffness. In addition, cold packs are used intermittently during the day, including after exercises. Light compression wraps are used, only if edema is excessive.

Active and active-assisted motion exercises are initiated during the first postoperative week, once the acute postoperative inflammation has diminished. Digit exercises are either performed while wearing the outrigger splint, or if static splints are being used exclusively, after removal of the splint. Motion exercises are modified to protect any concomitant fusions, with individual finger gutter splints left in place. "Hook" fisting (IP joint flexion and extension with the MP joints maintained in extension) is important to avoid recurrence of intrinsic contractures. "Duck" fisting (MP joint flexion and extension with IP joints maintained in extension) isolates motion of the implants. Composite finger flexion and extension prevents extrinsic extensor tightness and adhesion formation, and facilitates gross grasp. Opposition of the thumb to the tips of the index and middle fingers serves as a foundation for correct functional pinch activities in phases II and III. Radial finger walking, with the fingers supported in extension on a tabletop, is added as phase I progresses, to promote correct alignment and strengthen the radial intrinsic muscles (Figure 5-5). Additional range of motion (ROM) exercises include flexion and extension of the wrist (with splint removed and fingers supported), thumb IP and MP flexion, and forearm, elbow, and shoulder joint motion. Exercises are typically performed 10 repetitions each, four times daily. At 2 weeks postoperatively,

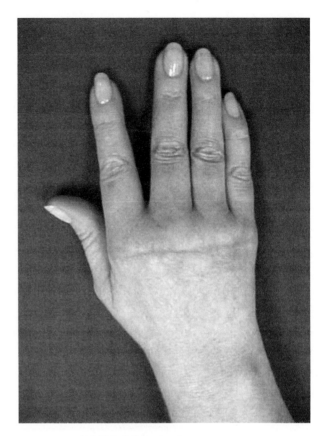

FIGURE **5-5** Radial finger walking.

gentle, passive motion performed by the therapist, strictly avoiding ulnar deviating forces to the MP joints, is added to promote MP flexion. The goal is a functional range of MP flexion, up to 70 degrees, obtained while preserving stability. For most individuals, the ring and small fingers require more MP flexion for function than the index and middle fingers. During phase I, the involved hand is not used for functional activities. Patient education in joint protection principles is initiated for future use.

Troubleshooting

Signs of infection or delayed wound healing are reported to the referring physician. Wound healing is often compromised in patients with RA. If soft tissue is of poor quality or if infection and wound healing are problematic, motion is delayed for as long as 3 weeks postoperatively, with the hand resting in a static MP extension splint. Another option, in cases of poor soft tissue quality, is to initially limit MP flexion through the application of stops to the lines of the dynamic outrigger splint.

Intrinsic tightness is common, despite surgical release. If poor IP flexion, with the MP joints extended, persists postoperatively, the therapist may passively flex

Postoperative Phase II: Fibroplasia (Weeks 3 to 6)

GOALS

- Protect MP arthroplasties through continued splinting and activity modification
- Reduce residual edema and pain
- Minimize scar adhesions
- Achieve functional AROM of MP joints
- Perform light functional activities while adhering to joint protection principles

PRECAUTIONS

- No resistive activities or exercises
- Protect MP joints from ulnar deviation forces

TREATMENT STRATEGIES

- Splinting
  - Continue protective splinting
  - Serial static or static progressive MP flexion splinting as necessary to regain functional flexion
- Continue phase 1 edema treatments, adding light compression wrapping if necessary (avoiding overly tight application)
- Precondition soft tissues with superficial heat modalities prior to ROM and scar techniques
- Scar management when incision has healed: scar massage, silicone pad
- A/AA/PROM: digits (avoiding ulnar deviation of MP joints), wrist
- Light functional activities while adhering to joint protection principles

CRITERIA FOR ADVANCEMENT

- Minimal pain with light activities and motion exercises
- Patient cleared by MD for strengthening exercises

the IP joints with the MP joints supported in extension and radial deviation.

Some individuals use IP joint flexion to compensate for difficulty flexing the MP implants. The fifth MP joint is commonly stiffer than the other MP joints.[3] To promote MP flexion, emphasis should initially be placed on isolated MP flexion, with the IP joints extended (duck fist). Individual gutter splints, which hold the IP joints in extension, may be used during this exercise. The resting position of the MP joints in the dynamic outrigger splint is checked frequently to ensure proper positioning, and hyperextension, if present, is corrected to neutral extension.

POSTOPERATIVE PHASE II: FIBROPLASIA (WEEKS 3 TO 6)

Protective splinting continues during phase II. If, at 3 weeks after surgery, MP flexion is not adequate for function, serial static or static progressive MP flexion splinting is added. Specifically, the volar-based MP flexion splint described in phase I can be serially remolded to increase MP joint flexion. Alternatively, a splint with finger cuffs over the dorsum of the proximal phalanges can be used to progressively increase MP flexion. For all splints, the MP joints are positioned in slight radial deviation.

Scar management begins when the surgical incision has fully closed. Scar massage is performed with oil or thick lotion, taking care not to reopen the incision. A silicone pad worn over the scar at night facilitates scar-remodeling.[9]

Edema control measures are continued as needed. Light compression is added if the phase I treatments do not adequately control edema. Care is taken to avoid overly constrictive compression.

The patient continues with the motion exercises of phase I, both at home and in therapy. The therapist increases passive range of motion (PROM) techniques, as needed, to increase motion, while avoiding MP joint ulnar deviation and aggressive stretching. As the joint encapsulation progresses, stability must not be sacrificed in an attempt to gain more motion. Superficial heat modalities are used before motion and scar management techniques to precondition soft tissues.

Light, functional activities are initiated in phase II, with an emphasis on education in joint protection techniques. For example, during performance of pinch activities, the three-point pinch (opposition of the thumb to the index and middle fingertips) is encouraged, whereas the lateral pinch is avoided. The lateral pinch (opposition of the thumb against the side of the index finger) applies a strong ulnar deviating force to

Postoperative Phase III: Scar Maturation (Weeks 6 to 12)

GOALS

- Maximize stable digital AROM and PROM
- Achieve functional hand strength
- Preserve correct digital alignment
- Promote safe hand function with awareness of joint protection principles
- Restore independent activities of daily living while maintaining joint protection

PRECAUTIONS

- MP joint stability should not be sacrificed to maximize ROM
- Resistive exercises must be used with caution
- Lateral pinch and other activities which promote MP radial deviation are avoided
- Patient must adhere to lifetime joint protection principles, with avoidance of all excessive forces to the implants, especially into ulnar deviation

TREATMENT STRATEGIES

- Gradually wean from splint during day at 6–8 weeks postoperatively with concurrence of MD
- Continue static MP extension splint at night for ongoing joint protection
- Consider neoprene anti-ulnar deviation splint for use during functional activities
- Continue edema control and modalities as needed
- Continue scar management until scar is mature
- Maximize stable AROM and PROM through therapeutic exercise, gentle stretching, and addition of flexion splinting if needed (serial static or static progressive), protecting MP joints from ulnar deviation
- Light resistance for grip and three point-pinch strengthening; avoid lateral pinch
- Reinforce patient education in joint protection principles
- Promote independence in safe performance of functional activities

CRITERIA FOR DISCHARGE

- Independence in home program of splinting, scar management, joint protection, and therapeutic exercise
- Understanding and application of joint protection principles
- Functional hand ROM and strength
- Independence in light activities of daily living with adherence to joint protection principles

---

the index MP and through the index to the other MP joints.

Troubleshooting

Common problems during phase II are inadequate MP joint flexion and MP joint extensor lag. Flexion splinting, as described previously, is the most effective treatment to improve MP flexion. To avoid development of an extensor lag, MP flexion exercises should be balanced with MP extension exercises. If a lag develops, increased time in a static MP extension splint is indicated. In addition, specific extensor digitorum exercises, such as composite fist to hook fist (EDC glides), isolated digit extension, and gentle resistive extension exercises, such as putty rolling, are emphasized.

POSTOPERATIVE PHASE III: SCAR MATURATION (WEEKS 6 TO 12)

Gradual weaning from protective splinting during the day begins at 6 to 8 weeks postoperatively, with con-

currence of the referring surgeon. Individuals who are moderately active benefit from prefabricated neoprene anti-ulnar deviation splints or other functional splints that promote correct alignment. Use of the static extension splint is continued at night during sleep. Many individuals continue using night splints throughout their lives to provide protection to the implants, other joints of the digits, and wrists. Serial static or static progressive MP flexion splinting is continued until MP flexion is adequate for function. Edema control measures are continued if needed. The scar management techniques described in phase II are continued until scar maturity is achieved, usually 6 months to a year after surgery. The motion exercises and techniques from phases I and II are continued. Light, resistive exercises may be added cautiously to avoid uncontrolled forces to the implants. Sponge-squeezing and light isometric grip strengthening, such as putty stamping with a dowel, improve grip strength and promote MP joint flexion. Light, resistive three-point pinch exercises and activities are performed to build strength and reinforce avoidance of lateral pinch during function. Light, resistive dowel-rolling strengthens the extensors. Education on joint protection is continually reinforced. Therapy and home exercises continue for 12 or more weeks postoperatively. After 12 weeks, with increased functional use of the hand, the frequency of home exercises can be reduced. When functional motion and strength have been achieved, and the individual's daily functional activities can be performed while observing joint protection principles, discharge from therapy is indicated.

Troubleshooting

MP joint stiffness is most easily treated when noted and addressed early. Stiffness persisting into phase III is treated with continued serial static or static progressive splinting. Aggressive stretching techniques are contraindicated because they may create instability or damage implants. If MP joint extensor lag continues into phase III, progression of treatment is slowed, extension exercise emphasized, and extension splinting continued. Recurrence of MP ulnar drift is more easily avoided than treated. Once it occurs, it should be addressed with prolonged protective splinting in radial deviation and carefully monitored exercises.

References

1. Kvien, T.K. *Epidemiology and Burden of Illness of Rheumatoid Arthritis.* Pharmacoeconomics 2004;22(Suppl 1):1–12.
2. Berger, R.A., Beckenbaugh, R.D., Linscheid, R.L. Arthroplasty in the Hand and Wrist. In Green, D.P., Hotchkiss, R.N., Pederson, W.C. (Eds). *Green's Operative Hand Surgery,* 4th ed. Churchill Livingstone, New York, 1999, pp. 156–161.
3. Stirrat, C.R. *Metacarpophalangeal Joints in Rheumatoid Arthritis of the Hand.* Hand Clin 1996;12(3):515–529.
4. Goldfarb, C.A., Stern, P.J. *Metacarpophalangeal Joint Arthroplasty in Rheumatoid Arthritis. A Long-term Assessment.* J Bone Joint Surg 2003;85A:1869–1878.
5. The Avanta Soft Skeletal Hand Implant System. Available online at http://www.avanta.org/arthroplasty/hand.htm. Accessed 20 Jan, 2006.
6. Swanson, A.B. Flexible Implant Arthroplasty for Arthritic Finger Joints. J Bone Joint Surg 1972;54A(3):435–455.
7. Chung, K.C., Kowalski, C.P., Kim, H.M., Kazmers, I.S. *Patient Outcomes Following Swanson Silastic Metacarpophalangeal Joint Arthroplasty in the Rheumatoid Hand: A Systemic Overview.* J Rheumatol 2000;27:1395–1402.
8. Burr, N., Pratt, A.L., Smith, P.J. *An Alternative Splinting and Rehabilitation Protocol for Metacarpophalangeal Joint Arthroplasty in Patients with Rheumatoid Arthritis.* J Hand Ther 2002;15:41–47.
9. Ahn, S.T., Monafo, W.W., Mustoe, T.A. *Topical Silicone Gel for the Prevention and Treatment of Hypertrophic Scars.* Arch Surg 1991;126(4):499–504.

6

Hip Fractures

SANDY B. GANZ, PT, DSc, GCS

Hip fractures are associated with significant morbidity and mortality in the United States, resulting in 350,000 hospitalizations annually.[1] This number is an increase of 23% from 1988.[2,3] Census trends indicate that the fastest rate of growth occurs in those populations over age 85 and those most susceptible to sustain a hip fracture. It is estimated that by 2040, the annual number of hip fractures will surpass 500,000 and that one in four women and one in eight men will sustain a hip fracture by age 90.[4]

Since the inception of the prospective payment system (PPS), the care of elderly patients who have sustained a hip fracture has changed dramatically. Hospital length of stay for Medicare recipients decreased from 21.9 days in 1981 to 12.4 days in 1986,[5] and patients enrolled in managed care programs had a hospital length of stay of 7.3 days.[5] Discharge to skilled nursing facilities for short-term rehabilitation rose from 38% to 60%.[5]

For those individuals who have sustained a hip fracture, returning to their prefracture functional status is a primary goal. Rehabilitation following hip fracture occurs along a continuum.[6] Patients improve along a line of increasing functional status and may transition from the acute care setting to a free-standing rehabilitation hospital or a subacute facility, such as a nursing home for short-term rehabilitation where physical therapy services are provided daily.[7] Patients may be discharged directly home following surgery and receive physical therapy services at home, or they are discharged home and receive physical therapy services in an outpatient facility.[8,9]

The rehabilitation program following hip fracture is begun immediately following surgery. The clinician must take into consideration the type of surgical repair—whether it is an open or closed reduction and internal fixation or type of total hip arthroplasty (THA) or hemiarthroplasty—and surgical approach used (i.e., anterior/posterior approach) to set realistic short- and long-term goals and deliver appropriate postoperative care. The choice of settings in which rehabilitation is provided following hip fracture is most often determined by the physician, insurance coverage, patient factors, and the health care delivery system.[10,11] Patients improve along a continuum. It is not uncommon for patients to receive therapy up to 6 months following fracture, and it is crucial for physical therapists to know the expected rate of recovery throughout this continuum of care.[1,12] The purpose of this chapter is to describe the postoperative rehabilitation following internal fixation after hip fracture along a trajectory.

SURGICAL OVERVIEW

The rehabilitation following femoral neck, intertrochanteric, and subtrochanteric hip fractures that were

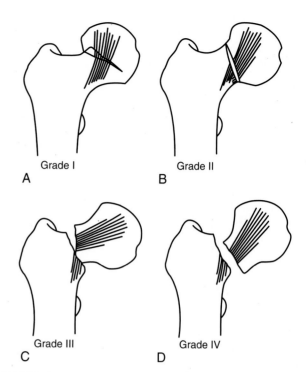

FIGURE **6-1** The Garden classification of femoral neck fractures with various misalignment. *A.* Incomplete fracture. *B.* Non-displaced fracture. *C.* Incompletely displaced fracture. *D.* Completely displaced fracture.

surgically repaired using an open/closed reduction and internal fixation, will be discussed in this chapter.[13]

The femoral neck fracture is a fracture that occurs proximal to the intertrochanteric line in the intracapsular region of the hip and is classified as nondisplaced or minimally displaced. Figure 6-1 represents the Garden classification of femoral neck fractures.[13]

Nondisplaced or minimally displaced femoral neck fractures are commonly repaired using cannulated screws. Cannulated (hollow) screws are typically inserted through fluoroscopy aided placement for nondisplaced or minimally displaced fractures through a limited or percutaneous lateral approach. The hollow screws are placed over thin wires, which are removed from the screws after bone alignment has been made. Using this approach, the subcutaneous fat, vastus lateralis, and deep fascia of the fascia lata are affected (Figure 6-2).

An intertrochanteric fracture is a fracture that occurs between the greater and lesser trochanter along the intertrochanteric line outside the capsule and is classified as stable or unstable[13] (Figure 6-3). The intertrochanteric region connects the femoral shaft and femoral neck at an angle of about 130 degrees. This angular moment created by weight-bearing is greatest at this angle. The most common instrumentation used for a stable intertrochanteric fracture is a sliding compres-

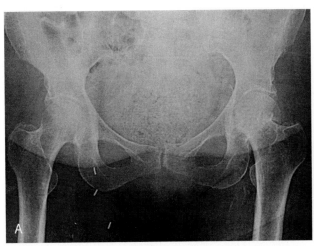 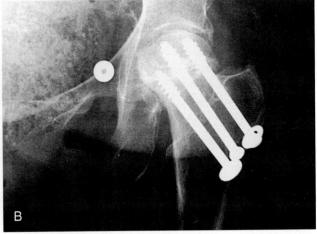

FIGURE **6-2** Repair of femoral neck fractures utilizing cannulated screws. *A.* Femoral neck fracture. *B.* Cannulated screws.

FIGURE **6-3** Intertrochanteric fracture. *A.* Stable. *B.* Unstable.

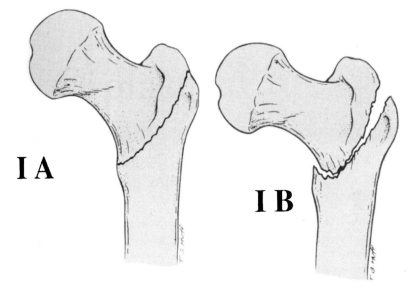

sion screw and side plate (Figure 6-4). The instrumentation holds the bone fragments in their proper position while fracture healing occurs. A lateral approach is used, violating skin, subcutaneous tissue, fascia lata, vastus lateralis fascia, and muscle belly. Using this type of instrumentation, the distance is shortened between the insertion of the hip abductors in the greater trochanter and the center of rotation of the hip, which creates a mechanical disadvantage for the abductors. This may lead to a Trendelenburg gait pattern.

A subtrochanteric fracture is a fracture that occurs between the lesser trochanter and the adjacent proximal third of the femoral shaft and may extend proximally to the intertrochanteric region[13] (Figure 6-5). Subtrochanteric fractures have been extremely difficult to fix because of the extreme angular force in the subtrochanteric region. The bone type in the subtro-

chanteric region is cortical. Cortical bone has poor blood supply and decreased osteogenic activity; therefore, the two preferred methods of fixation are an extended compression screw device and intermedullary nail. Fixation using a Richards compression screw-plate device is to repair a subtrochanteric fracture, as illustrated in Figure 6-6.

The type of surgical intervention is determined by the severity, type, and location of the hip fracture. Four types of instrumentation are commonly used in surgical intervention following hip fracture. Internal fixation may be either open (ORIF) or closed (CRIF), bipolar hemiarthroplasty, hemiarthroplasty, or THA.[13] Rehabilitation following THA was discussed previously in Chapter 1. This chapter will focus on the rehabilitation management of a hip fracture following open reduction and internal fixation.

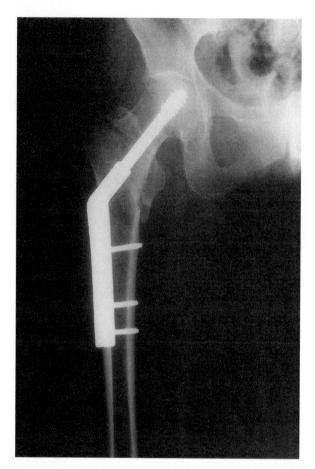

FIGURE **6-4** Repair of intertrochanteric fracture, using sliding hip screw.

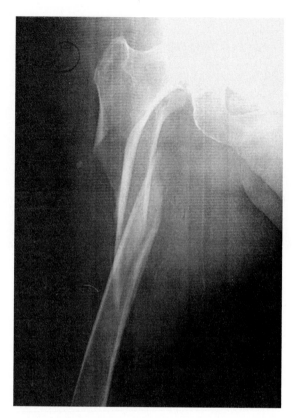

FIGURE **6-5** Subtrochanteric fracture.

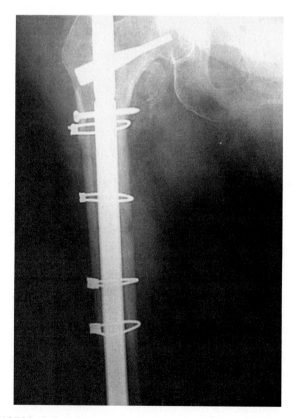

FIGURE **6-6** Subtrochanteric fracture, using intramedullary rod with locking screw.

It is important for physical therapists to have an understanding of the phases of bone healing, as well as an understanding of the types of instrumentation and the principles of the fixation devices used in the surgical management of patients who have sustained a hip fracture. These concepts are pivotal because rehabilitation is guided by the phases of bone healing, type of fracture, and surgical procedure performed. Fixation devices used in fracture repair are either stress-sharing or stress-shielding devices.[14] Stress sharing implies that the fixation device permits partial transmission of a load across the fracture site, and micromotion occurs at the fracture site, which induces secondary bone healing with callus formation. Examples of stress-sharing devices are rods, pins, and screws. A dynamic hip screw was used in the repair of an intertrochanteric fracture, as illustrated in Figure 6-4. The dynamic hip screw slides, causing micromotion at the fracture site and inducing secondary fracture healing. Cannulated screws were used in the repair of a femoral neck fracture, as illustrated in Figure 6-2.[14]

Stress-shielding devices, such as the Gamma nail or Richards intermedullary hip screw, as illustrated in Figure 6-6, shield the fracture site from stress and trans-

TABLE 6-1 | Hip Fracture Disablement Model

PATHOLOGY	IMPAIRMENT	FUNCTIONAL LIMITATIONS	DISABILITY	SOCIAL
Hip fracture	↓ hip strength ↓ hip ROM ↓ endurance ↓ balance ↑ pain	↓ gait speed ↓ ambulation ↓ transferring ↓ stair climbing	Basic ADL Instrumented ADL	Community Work

fer the stress to the rod, and primary bone healing occurs without callus.[14]

Regardless of the type of hip fracture or internal fixation performed, the principles of both fracture healing and rehabilitation are the same.[13]

REHABILITATION OVERVIEW

The rehabilitation goals following hip fracture are to have a successful outcome. A successful outcome is often defined as the return to prefracture level of function. This is a daunting task because less than 50% of patients who have sustained a hip fracture do not return to their prefracture level of function.[1] Following hip fracture, the following impairments are commonly seen: functional strength deficits, functional activity intolerance, impaired balance and coordination, decreased walking speed, and decreased ability to perform activities of daily living (ADL). The goals of rehabilitation following hip fracture are to increase muscle strength, endurance, and balance coordination, in an effort to improve the ability to transfer, walk, stair climb, and perform ADL. According to the guide to physical therapist practice, for the practice pattern 4G: Impaired joint mobility, muscle performance, and range of motion associated with fracture; and 4H: Impaired joint mobility, motor function, muscle performance, and range of motion associated with joint arthroplasty relating to the International classification of disease (ICD)9 code 820 (fracture of the neck or femur), the expected numbers of therapy visits throughout the continuum of care range from 6 to 70 visits.[15]

POSTOPERATIVE PHASE I: HOSPITALIZATION (DAYS 1 TO 7)

A physical therapy initial evaluation is performed the day after surgery. Following an assessment of pain level, cognitive status, wound status, gross upper and lower extremity strength, range of motion (ROM), sensation, and physical performance, physical therapy treatment is initiated. Emphasis of treatment is based upon the disablement model (Table 6-1).

Treatment is impairment-based and focuses on bed mobility, transfer training, gait training, and muscle reeducation. Before initiating physical therapy, the pa-

tient's pain must be well controlled. Timing of pain medication is pivotal to ensure that pain medications reach their peak effectiveness during therapy sessions. The therapist must have an understanding of medications that may affect mobility and rehabilitation. Table 6-2 illustrates medications that may have adverse drug reactions that affect rehabilitation.

In the first phase of the postoperative rehabilitation program, emphasis is on regaining muscle control of the limb. It is not uncommon for patients who have sustained a hip fracture to have difficulty moving their leg and repositioning themselves in bed, which can lead to a heel pressure ulcer. Once a patient has a pressure ulcer on his or her heel, rehabilitation is prolonged.[1] Once a pressure ulcer has developed, it is imperative that a pressure-relieving device be used during ambulation to avoid any pressure on the heel during gait training and ADL that

TABLE 6-2 | Medications That May Affect Rehabilitation

DRUG CATEGORY	DRUG	ADVERSE DRUG REACTIONS
Antihypertensives	Atenolol Lisinopril Lopressor	Orthostatic Hypotension Dizziness Fatigue Musculoskeletal pain
Antiarrhythmics	Inderal Accupril Digoxin	Hypotension Dizziness Fatigue Bradycardia Weakness
Diuretics	Lasix	Orthostatic Hypotension Weakness Fatigue Confusion Muscle cramps
Antidepressants	Prozac Remeron Wellbutrin	Sedation Weakness Poor muscle performance Tachycardia

Epocrates.com

involve weight-bearing. Typically, pressure-relieving footwear devices, such as a Multi-Podus boot, are used.

Beginning ROM exercises and muscle strengthening early in the postoperative period enables the patient to gain the mobility necessary to perform bed mobility activities, transfers in and out of bed, and transfers on and off a commode. The specific muscle groups that affect following hip fracture vary according to the location of fracture and surgical repair.

Functional testing using performance-based measures are initiated as soon as the patient is able to stand to obtain baseline measurements of physical function. The following performance-based measures have been shown to be valid and reliable instruments to measure functional performance in elderly patients[16-19]: Tinetti gait and balance test[19] (Figures 6-7 and 6-8), timed "get-up and go" test,[20] functional reach test,[16] and six-minute walk test.[21]

Gait Tests

Initiation of Gait (immediate initiation)
a. Any hesitancy or multiple attempts to start = 0
b. No hesitancy = 1 _____

Step Length and Height
a. Right Swing Foot _____
- Does not pass left stance foot with step = 0
- Passes left stance foot = 1

- Right foot does not clear floor = 0 _____
- Right foot completely clears floor = 1

b. Left Swing Foot _____
- Does not pass right stance foot with step = 0
- Passes right stance foot = 1

- Left foot does not clear floor = 0 _____
- Left foot completely clears floor = 1

Step Symmetry _____
a. Right and left step length not equal (estimate) = 0
b. Right and left step length appear equal = 1

Step Continuity _____
a. Stopping or discontinuity between steps = 0
b. Steps appear continuous = 1

Path (estimate 12-inch floor tiles over 10 feet) _____
a. Marked deviation = 0
b. Mild/moderate deviation or uses walking aid = 1
c. Straight without walking aid = 2

Trunk _____
a. Marked sway or uses walking aid = 0
b. No sway but flexion of knees or back or spreads arms = 1
c. No sway, no flexion, no use of arms or aid = 2

Walking Time _____
a. Heels apart = 0
b. Heels almost touching while walking = 1

Gait   /12

FIGURE 6-7 Tinetti gait scale.

Balance Tests

Sitting Balance
    a. Leans or slides in chair = 0
    b. Steady, safe = 1
                                           ____

Arises
    a. Unable without help = 0
    b. Able, uses arms to help = 1
    c. Able, without using arms = 2
  ____

Attempts to Arise
    a. Unable without help = 0
    b. Able, requires > 1 attempt = 1
    c. Able to rise, 1 attempt = 2
  ____

Immediate Standing Balance (first 5 seconds)
    a. Unsteady (swaggers, moves feet, trunk sways) = 0
    b. Steady but uses cane or other support = 1
    c. Steady without walker or other support = 2
  ____

Standing Balance
    a. Unsteady = 0
    b. Steady but wide stance (medial heels > 4" apart)
       and uses cane or other support = 1
    c. Narrow stance without support = 2
  ____

Nudged (subject at max position with feet as close as possible,
examiner pushes three with palm on subject's sternum)
    a. Begins to fall = 0
    b. Staggers, grabs, catches self = 1
    c. Steady = 2
  ____

Eyes Closed (same as position 6)
    a. Unsteady = 0
    b. Steady = 1
  ____

Turning 360 Degrees
    a. Discontinuous Steps = 0
    b. Continuous = 1
  ____

    c. Unsteady (grabs, staggers) = 0
    d. Steady = 1
  ____

Sitting Down
    a. Unsafe (misjudged distance, falls into chair) = 0
    b. Uses arms or not a smooth motion = 1
  ____
    c. Safe, smooth motion = 2

Balance	/16
Gait	/12
Total	/28

FIGURE **6-8** Tinetti balance scale.

The Tinetti gait and balance test is a 28-point scale: 12 points address gait, and 16 points address balance. A score of less than 19 indicates a high fall risk.[19] The timed "get-up and go" test, created by Podsiadlo and Richardson,[20] measures dynamic balance and gait. The patient rises from an 18-inch arm chair, walks 3 meters, turns and walks back to the chair, and sits down. A score of less than 10 seconds is normal, but a score greater than 32 seconds indicates dependence in ADL. The functional reach test, developed by Duncan et al,[16] measures how far one can reach out of his or her base of support without taking a step. Less than 6 inches indicates a high fall risk. A yardstick is placed on the wall at the level of the acromion. The patient stands parallel to a wall and extends his or her arm to the level of the yardstick, reaching as far forward as possible, without taking a step or touching the wall.[16] The six-minute walk test addresses functional activity tolerance.[21] The patient walks for 6 minutes and rests for as many minutes as necessary. The time does not stop until 6 minutes. The total distance walked is recorded.[21]

Refer to Chapter 1 for the postoperative guidelines for hip fracture management following THA.

Impairments commonly seen following hip fracture are functional strength deficits, functional activity intolerance, decreased ROM, and increased pain. These impairments result in the following functional limitations: difficulty moving about in the bed (bed mobility), difficulty in transferring in and out of bed (and variable surface transfers), difficulty in ambulation on level surfaces, and stair climbing. Treatment is impairment-based, and emphasis during phase I is on pain control, muscle reeducation, muscle strengthening, and therapeutic exercises aimed to optimize lower extremity motor control for transfers, ambulation, and ADL retraining.[22,23]

Postoperative Phase I: Hospitalization (Days 1 to 7)

GOALS

- Assisted transfers in and out of bed
- Assisted ambulation with walker
- Assisted lower body dressing
- Unassisted upper body dressing
- Ability to cover a distance of 100 feet with walker in 6 minutes
- Ability to score 5/28 on Tinetti gait and balance
- Gait speed of 0.60 feet per second
- A score of 75 seconds on the timed "get-up and go" test
- Independent with bedside exercise program

PRECAUTIONS

- Femoral neck
  Protected weight-bearing, if fracture is unstable
  Avoid passive ROM on fractures that have been reduced
- Intertrochanteric fracture
  Protected weight-bearing, if fracture is unstable
  Avoid passive ROM on fractures that have been reduced
  Avoid strengthening the adductors because of increased stress at the fracture site
- Subtrochanteric
  Protected weight-bearing, if fracture is unstable
  Avoid passive ROM on fractures that have been reduced
  Avoid active adduction/abduction because of increased stress (torque on fracture site)
  No isometric exercises to quadriceps or hamstrings (1 week)

TREATMENT STRATEGIES

- Bed mobility training
- Transfer training in and out of bed, on and off toilet
- Gait training with walker
- Regaining muscle control of the operated limb through hip, knee, and active ankle ROM; isometric exercises such as quadriceps and gluteal sets
- Prevention of pressure ulcers, specifically on the heel, through positioning or pressure-relieving device
- Upper extremity strengthening
- ADL retraining

CLINICAL CRITERIA FOR ADVANCEMENT

- Patients are typically discharged to a subacute facility when independence in bed mobility, transfers, and ambulation have not been achieved.
- Gait progression from assisted ambulation with rollator walker to unassisted ambulation with rollator walker
- Weight-bearing is advanced, depending on stability of fracture.

Troubleshooting

It is not uncommon for patients who have sustained a hip fracture to avoid moving their operated limb. This can result in acquiring a pressure ulcer on the heel. Elevating the heel off the bed prevents heel pressure ulcers. If a patient develops a pressure ulcer on the heel, a pressure-relieving device to eliminate pressure on the heel should be used during ambulation[24,25] (Figure 6-9).

POSTOPERATIVE PHASE II (WEEKS 2 TO 6)

Following acute care hospitalization for a hip fracture, more patients are admitted to rehabilitation centers or nursing homes for subacute rehabilitation.[1,22,26] Some patients are discharged home and receive home care services inclusive of physical therapy, whereas others are discharged home and receive physical therapy on an outpatient basis. The determinant of discharge disposition following hip fracture from the acute care setting is multifactorial: The first priority for all health profes-sionals treating patients who have sustained a hip fracture is a safe discharge to the most appropriate setting while adhering to fiscal and insurance constraints. Typically, patients who are not able to ambulate independently, transfer independently on and off the toilet and in and out of bed, and independently perform upper and lower body dressing and could actively participate in over 3 hours of therapy daily may be discharged to an acute rehabilitation facility. Those patients who are not independent upon discharge from the hospital and are unable to tolerate at least 3 hours of therapy a day may be transferred to a subacute facility, such as a nursing home that provides short-term rehabilitation. Focus of treatment during this phase of rehabilitation is on normalizing gait, restoring functional independence in basic and instrumented ADL. The ratio of Medicare recipients to managed care recipients varies from institution to institution. Transfer from acute hospitalization to an acute rehabilitation center, or skilled nursing facility, is dependent upon insurance coverage. Medicare guidelines for facility placement are described in Table 6-3.

Regardless of the location where the patient will be receiving therapy, the primary goal is the same—to return the patient to a safe environment at the highest possible functional level.[26]

Physical therapy management is impairment-based. As patients gain motor control of the lower extremity, and ROM of the hip continues to improve, lower extremity strengthening exercises are performed using both open and closed kinetic chain. Figure 6-10 represents an example of open kinetic chain on the right lower extremity and closed kinetic chain on the left lower extremity.

Crucial to a comprehensive rehabilitation program is the integration of balance and coordination exercises into the postoperative rehabilitation program. Patients are progressed from a lower level activity of muscle strengthening, such as sitting hip flexion without weights (Figure 6-11), to a more advanced functional activity combining standing hip flexion with bilateral upper extremity support (Figure 6-12) to a unilateral upper extremity support firm surface (Figure 6-13). When patients achieve adequate balance that is unsupported, they may advance to more complex activities,

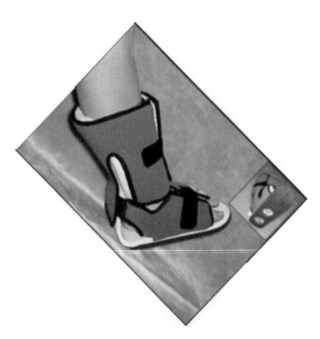

FIGURE 6-9 Walkassist AFO™—heel pressure–relieving device.

TABLE 6-3	Medicare Guidelines for Therapy Services		
	ACUTE REHABILITATION CENTER	**SUBACUTE**	**HOME**
Medicare guidelines for discharge disposition	Patient must be able to tolerate at least 3 hours of therapy daily.	Patient must be able to tolerate at least 30 minutes of therapy daily.	Home care is authorized by Medicare for homebound patients or if leaving the home would be an undue hardship.

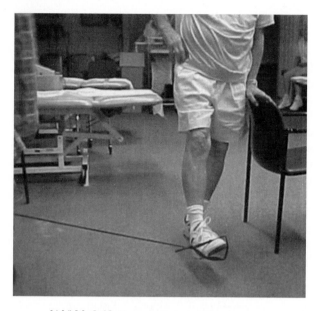

FIGURE **6-10** Open and closed kinetic chain.

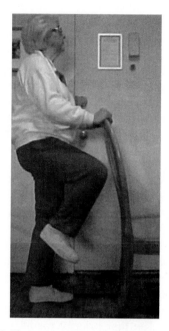

FIGURE **6-12** Standing hip flexion without weights.

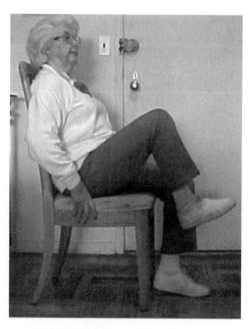

FIGURE **6-11** Seated hip flexion.

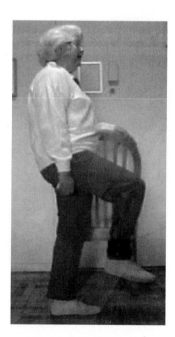

FIGURE **6-13** Standing hip flexion with weights and one upper extremity support.

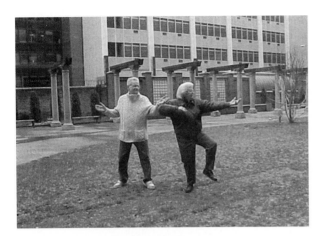

FIGURE **6-14** Tai chi.

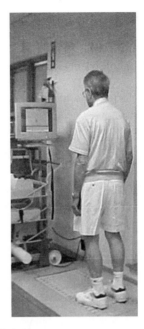

FIGURE **6-16** NeuroCom Balance Master®.

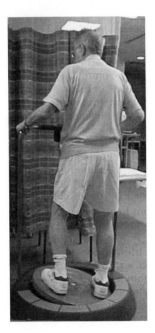

FIGURE **6-15** Kinesthetic awareness trainer (KAT).

such as tai chi (Figure 6-14). Patients then progress to more dynamic activities, such as unilateral lower extremity weight-bearing during a kickball activity. It is important for patients to incorporate functional activities into their exercise program. For example, slow dancing with a partner encourages multidirectional movement in many planes.

Once patients demonstrate their ability to function without a device, advanced levels of balance retraining and proprioception are incorporated into their rehabilitation program. Examples are the kinesthetic awareness trainer (KAT) and the balance master (Figures 6-15 and 6-16).

Studies have shown that 40% to 70% of patients who sustain a hip fracture do not return to their prefracture functional status.[1,11] Studies have also shown that a substantial number of patients who sustain a hip fracture used assistive devices before their hip fracture.[7,27] Regardless of whether patients ambulated with or without a device before their hip fracture, the goal is for patients to return to their optimal level of function. Patients are initially progressed from a walker to a cane to no device, if they are able to maintain a symmetrical gait pattern and a limp is not present.[28] According to Blount,[28] patients should not discontinue the use of a cane if there is a muscle imbalance that results in an asymmetrical gait pattern. The functional recovery during postoperative phase II (weeks 2 to 6) has been categorized into two levels: those who remain on a walker and those who advance to a cane.[22]

Troubleshooting

Patients with cognitive impairment who have difficulty comprehending limitations or precautions in weight-bearing (if the fracture is unstable) may benefit from the Multi-Podus boot used for patients with pressure ulcers. The Multi-Podus boot does not allow for pressure at the heel, essentially limiting a patient's weight-bearing status, because only the forefoot and the toes strike the floor during stance phase of gait. We have used this technique for cognitively impaired patients for almost a decade, with good results and no loss of fixation.

Increased activity may cause an increase in swelling of the affected extremity. Patients should be advised to elevate their legs, increase rest periods, wear compression hose, and apply a cold or ice pack to the swollen area.

Postoperative Phase II: Patients Who Remain on a Walker and Do Not Advance to a Cane (Weeks 2 to 6)

GOALS

- Independent transfers in and out of bed
- Independent transfers on and off toilet
- Independent ambulation with wheeled walker
- Independent lower body dressing
- Increase AROM of hip to 90 degrees (for sitting)
- Independent with bedside exercise program

(Week 2)
Ability to ambulate 150 feet with wheeled walker during six-minute walk test
Ability to score 7/28 on Tinetti gait and balance
Gait speed of 0.46 feet per second
Timed "get-up and go" test of 60 seconds

(Week 3)
Ability to ambulate 225 feet with wheeled walker during six-minute walk test
Ability to score 9/28 on Tinetti gait and balance
Gait speed of 0.63 feet per second
Timed "get-up and go" test of 55 seconds

(Week 4)
Ability to ambulate 270 feet with wheeled walker during six-minute walk test
Ability to score 12/28 on Tinetti gait and balance
Gait speed of 0.75 feet per second
Timed "get-up and go" test of 49 seconds

(Week 5)
Ability to ambulate 340 feet with wheeled walker during six-minute walk test
Ability to score 14/28 on Tinetti gait and balance
Gait speed of 0.94 feet per second
Timed "get-up and go" test score of 43 seconds

(Week 6)
Ability to ambulate 500 feet with wheeled walker during six-minute walk test
Ability to score 16/28 Tinetti gait and balance
Gait speed of 1.40 feet per second
Timed "get-up and go" test score of 32 seconds

PRECAUTIONS

Femoral neck fracture
- Passive hip ROM for 6 to 8 weeks

Intertrochanteric fracture
- Muscle strengthening of the adductors causes stress to the fracture site\implant: Avoid strengthening until fracture is stable
- Torsion or twisting at the fracture site (6 weeks)
- Passive hip ROM (6 to 8 weeks)
- *Caution should be used when prescribing strengthening exercises to patients who are not full weight-bearing.*

Subtrochanteric fracture
- No adduction/abduction to hip (2 weeks)

TREATMENT STRATEGIES

- Stair training using bilateral upper extremity support nonreciprocally
- Outdoor ambulation on variable surfaces using wheeled walker
- Gait speed >1.18 feet per second to cross 33 feet of city street
- AROM of hip in supine, standing, side-lying, and prone if tolerated
- Strengthening exercises using cuff weights (1 repetition max.—60%)
- Strengthening exercises using elastic tubing exercises in supine, sitting
- Balance retraining/perturbation activities on unleveled surfaces (foam/carpet) with bilateral upper extremity support
- Isotonic exercise machines
- Kinetron, Nu-Step
- KAT, balance board with bilateral upper extremity support
- Progressive resistive exercises and functional activities

Postoperative Phase II: Patients Who Advance to a Cane (Weeks 2 to 6)

GOALS

- Independent transfers in and out of bed
- Independent transfers on and off toilet
- Independent ambulation with cane on level surfaces
- Independent ambulation with cane on variable surfaces
- Independent lower body dressing
- Increase AROM of hip to 90 degrees (for sitting)
- Independent with bedside exercise program

(Week 2) Ability to ambulate 260 feet with cane during six-minute walk test
Gait speed of 0.72 feet per second
Timed "get-up and go" test score of 36 seconds
Tinetti gait and balance score of 10/28

(Week 3) Ability to ambulate 400 feet with cane during six-minute walk test
Gait speed of 1.11 feet per second
Timed "get-up and go" test score of 34 seconds
Tinetti gait and balance score of 12/28

(Week 4) Ability to ambulate 410 feet with cane during six-minute walk test
Gait speed of 1.14 feet per second
Timed "get-up and go" test score of 30 seconds
Tinetti gait and balance score of 15/28

(Week 5) Ability to ambulate 460 feet with cane during six-minute walk test
Gait speed of 1.28 feet per second
Timed "get-up and go" test score of 27 seconds
Tinetti gait and balance score of 17/28

(Week 6) Ability to ambulate 550 feet with wheeled walker during six-minute walk test
Gait speed of 1.53 feet per second
Timed "get-up and go" test score of 24 seconds
Tinetti gait and balance score of 19/28

PRECAUTIONS

Femoral neck fracture
- Passive hip ROM for 6 to 8 weeks

Intertrochanteric fracture
- Muscle strengthening of the adductors causes stress to the fracture site and implant: Avoid strengthening until fracture is stable
- Torsion or twisting at the fracture site (6 weeks)
- Passive hip ROM (6 to 8 weeks)
- *Caution should be used when prescribing strengthening exercises to patients who are not full weight-bearing.*

Subtrochanteric fracture
- No adduction/abduction to hip (2 weeks)

TREATMENT STRATEGIES

- Stair training using unilateral upper extremity support and cane reciprocally
- Outdoor ambulation on variable surfaces using cane
- Gait speed >1.18 feet per second to cross 33 feet of city street
- AROM of hip in supine, standing, side-lying, and prone if tolerated
- Strengthening exercises using cuff weights (1 repetition max.—60%)
- Strengthening exercises using elastic tubing exercises in standing
- Balance retraining/perturbation activities on unleveled surfaces (foam/carpet) with unilateral upper extremity support
- Isotonic exercise machines
- Kinetron
- Nu-Step
- Kinesthetic awareness trainer with unilateral upper extremity support
- Heel rises
- Progressive resistive exercises and functional activities

CLINICAL CRITERIA FOR ADVANCEMENT

- Independent ambulation without a device on leveled and variable surfaces
- Able to perform balance activities without external support

POSTOPERATIVE PHASE III (WEEKS 12 TO 26)

During phase III, patients should transition to advanced functional activities, if they demonstrate adequate hip and knee strength that enables them to perform these activities without marked gait deviations. The following data for the goals described in postoperative phase III were the results of a randomized, controlled trial performed at the Hospital for Special Surgery (HSS), addressing functional outcome following hip fracture.[23]

Troubleshooting

Many physicians do not like to prescribe shoe lifts immediately following surgery when patients complain of leg length discrepancies. It is important to allow the weak muscles to be strengthened and alleviate specific gait impairments before a shoe insert or lift is recom-mended. It is expected that an increase in activity along the rehabilitation continuum may produce increased discomfort, muscle soreness, and pain. If there is persistent hip or thigh pain without relief, the surgeon should be contacted because there may be loss of fixation. If the persistent pain is accompanied by swelling, redness, and/or fever, it may indicate an infection, and it would be imperative that the patient seek medical attention immediately.

HIP FRACTURE PREVENTION

It is important to discuss the factors that contribute to hip fractures and provide patients with written instructions on fall prevention. Table 6-4 represents a fall prevention handout that illustrates home hazards that are common causes of hip fractures and rationale for corrections to prevent falls.

Postoperative Phase III (Weeks 12 to 26)

GOALS

(Week 12)
Ability to ambulate 862 feet during six-minute walk test
Timed "up and go" score of 16 seconds
Gait speed of 2.4 feet per second
Functional reach test score of 9 inches

(Week 26)
Ability to ambulate 980 feet during six-minute walk test
Gait speed of 2.7 feet per second
Timed "up and go" test score < 13 seconds
Functional reach test score of 10 inches

PRECAUTIONS

If femoral neck, intertrochanteric, subtrochanteric fractures are generally healed and precautions are lifted.

TREATMENT STRATEGIES

- Stair training without upper extremity support nonreciprocally
- Outdoor ambulation on variable surfaces without device
- Gait speed > 1.74 feet per second
- Stationary bicycle
- Isotonic hip and knee machines
- Isokinetic machines
- Kinetron
- Nu-Step
- Balance Master
- Progressive resistive exercises and functional activities in preparation for return to sport

TABLE 6-4 Home Hazards—Fall Prevention

CORRECTION	RATIONALE
GENERAL HOUSEHOLD	
Lighting	
Too dim — Provide ample lighting in all areas	Increased illumination improves visual acuity
Too direct creating glare — Reduce glare with evenly distributed light, indirect lighting, or translucent shades	
Inaccessible light switches — Easily accessible upon entering room	Reduces risk of falling when walking across darkened room
Carpets, Rugs	
Slippery — Rugs should be tacked down to prevent curling; nonskid backing should be used	Prevents trips and slips in persons with decreased step height
Chairs	
No arm rests — Arm rests should extend forward enough to provide leverage when rising or sitting down	Assists persons with lower extremity weakness
Unstable, wheels — Legs must be stable to support weight of person rising	Chairs should have stable legs when transferring to and from standing to avoid a fall
BATHROOM	
Bathtub	
Slippery tub floor — Install skid-resistant strips or rubber mat, tub or shower chair. Use shower shoes.	Prevents sliding on wet tub floor. Sitting while showering prevents falls
Side of bathtub used for support or transfer — Use portable grab bar on side of tub or on wall (DO NOT USE TOWEL RACK)	Grab bars aide in safe transfer. Portable grab bar can be taken along when traveling
Standing in shower — Use a shower chair	The heat of the shower in combination with various medications may result in a fall
Sinks	
Towel rack, sink tops used for transfers — Install secure grab bar into wall studs next to toilet. Obtain 3 in 1 commode and place over standard toilet	Prevents falls using safe transfer technique. 3 in 1 commode provides elevation of toilet and armrests on both sides of the commode
Toilet	
Low toilet seat — Use elevated toilet seat or commode placed over toilet	Requires less lower extremity strength to rise from a higher surface. Ease in transferring to standing
KITCHEN	
Cabinets, shelves too high — Keep frequently used items at waist level, on low shelves in cabinets.	Reduces risk of falling due to reaching or standing on unstable ladders or chairs
Floor wet or waxed — Place rubber mat in sink area. Use nonslip or buff paste wax.	Prevents slipping and falling
STAIRWAYS	
Configuration	
Stair rise too high — Stair rise height <6 inches requires less strength in lower extremities to perform.	Reduces risk of tripping for persons with decreased steppage height and decreased leg strength
Staircase is too long — Stairways with intermediate landings are best.	Rest stop is convenient for cardiac or patients with pulmonary impairments
Handrails	
Missing — Install and anchor well on both sides of stairs. Ends should turn inward.	Handrails give increased support.
Improper shape — Rail should be cylindrical and should be placed 1–2″ from the wall.	Cylindrical rail is easier to grasp with hand.
Improper length — Rails should extend beyond top and bottom step.	Inward turn of rail signals that the top or bottom step has been reached if visually impaired.
Condition	
Slippery — Place non-skid tread strips securely on all steps	Prevents slipping
Lighting Inadequate — Install adequate lighting at the top and bottom of stairway. Night lights or bright colored adhesive strips may be used to clearly mark each step	Location of steps should be outlined especially for those who are visually impaired

REFERENCES

1. Eastwood, E.A., Magaziner, J., Wang, J., Silberzweig, S.B., Hannan, E.L., Strauss, E., Siu, A.L. *Patients with Hip Fracture: Subgroups and Their Outcomes.* J Am Geriatr Soc 2002;50(7):1240–1249.

2. Ray, W., Griffin, M., Baugh, D. *Mortality Following Hip Fracture Before and After Implementation of the Prospective Payment System.* Arch Intern Med 1990;150:2109–2114.

3. *National Center for Health Statistics. Health, United States, with Health and Aging Chartbook.* Hyattsville, MD, National Center for Health Statistics, 1999.

4. Morris, A., Zuckerman, J. *National Consensus Conference on Improving the Continuum of Care for Patients with Hip Fracture.* Washington, DC, 2001.

5. Fitzgerald, J., Moore, P., Dittus, R. *The Care of Elderly Patients with Hip Fracture: Changes Since Implementation of the Prospective Payment System.* N Engl J Med 1988;319(21):1392–1397.

6. Studenski, S., Duncan, P.W. *Measuring Rehabilitation Outcomes.* Clin Geriatr Med 1993;9(4):823–830.

7. Guccione, A.A., Fagerson, T.L., Anderson, J.J. *Regaining Functional Independence in the Acute Care Setting Following Hip Fracture.* Phys Ther 1996;76(8):818–826.

8. Jette, A.M., Harris, B.A., Cleary, P.D., Campion, E.W. *Functional Recovery After Hip Fracture.* Arch Phys Med Rehabil 1987;68(10):735–740.

9. Harada, N.D., Chun, A., Chiu, V., Pakalniskis, A. *Patterns of Rehabilitation Utilization After Hip Fracture in Acute Hospitals and Skilled Nursing Facilities.* Med Care 2000;38(11):1119–1130.

10. Clancy, T., Kitchen, S., Churchill, P., Covingto, D., Hundley, J., Maxwell, J.G. *DRG Reimbursement: Geriatric Hip Fractures in the Community Hospital Trauma Center.* South Med J 1998;91(5):457–461.

11. Coleman, E.A., Kramer, A.M., Kowalsky, J.C., Eckhoff, D., Lin, M., Hester, E.J., Morgenstern, N., Steiner, J.F. *A Comparison of Functional Outcomes After Hip Fracture in Group/Staff HMOs and Fee-for-Service Systems.* Eff Clin Pract 2000;3(5):229–239.

12. Alarcon, T., Gonzalez-Montalvo, J.I., Barcena, A., Saez, P. *Further Experience of Nonagenarians with Hip Fractures.* Injury 2001;32(7):555–558.

13. *Wheeless' Textbook of Orthopaedics.* Available online at http://www.medmedia.com/oo1/238.htm. Accessed 23 Jan, 2006.

14. McRae, R. *Practical Fracture Treatment,* 3rd ed. Churchill Livingstone, New York, 1994.

15. *Guide to Physical Therapist Practice.* Phys Ther 2001;77:1163–1650.

16. Duncan, P.W., Weiner, D.K., Chandler, J., Studenski, S. *Functional Reach: A New Clinical Measure of Balance.* J Gerontol 1990;45(6):M192–M197.

17. VanSwearingen, J., Brach, J. *Making Geriatric Assessment Work: Selecting Useful Measures.* Phys Ther 2001;81(6):1233–1252.

18. Harada, N., Chiu, V., Stewart, A. *Mobility-related Function in Older Adults: Assessment with a 6 Minute Walk Test.* Arch Phys Med Rehabil 1999;80(7):837–841.

19. Tinetti, M.E. *Performance-oriented Assessment of Mobility Problems in Elderly Patients.* J Am Geriatr Soc 1986;34(2):119–126.

20. Podsiadlo, D., Richardson, S. *The Timed "Up & Go": A Test of Basic Functional Mobility for Frail Elderly Persons.* J Am Geriatr Soc 1991;39(2):142–148.

21. Guyatt, G., Sullivan, M.J., Thompson, P.J., Fallen, E.L., Pugsley, S.O., Taylor, D.W., Berman, L.B. *The 6-minute Walk: A New Measure of Exercise Capacity in Patients with Chronic Heart Failure.* Can Med Assoc J 1985;132:919–923.

22. Ganz, S., Peterson, M. *Measuring Functional Outcomes Following Hip Fracture in the Subacute Setting* (abstract). J Am Geriatr Soc 2004;52(4 Suppl S1–S246):146.

23. Peterson, M. *High Intensity Exercise Training Following Hip Fracture.* Top Geriatr Rehabil 2004;20(4):273–284.

24. Sae-Sia, W., Wipke-Tevis, D. *Pressure Ulcer Prevention and Treatment Practices in Inpatient Rehabilitation Facilities.* Rehab Nurs 2002;27:192–198.

25. *Pressure Ulcers in America. Prevalence, Incidence, and Implications for the Future. An Executive Summary of the National Pressure Ulcer Advisory Panel Monograph.* Adv Skin Wound Care 2001;14(4):208–215.

26. Parker, M. *Mobilization Strategies After Hip Fracture Surgery in Adults.* Cochrane Database Syst Rev 2004;CDOO1704.

27. Cree, M., Carriere, K., Soskolne, C., Suarez-Almazor, M. *Functional Dependence After Hip Fracture.* Am J Phys Med Rehabil 2001;80(10):736–743.

28. Blount, W. *Don't Throw Away the Cane.* J Bone Joint Surg Am 1956;38(3):695–708.

II

HAND
REHABILITATION

AVIVA WOLFF, OTR/L, CHT

7

Elbow Fractures and Dislocations

AVIVA WOLFF, OTR/L, CHT

The elbow joint consists of three bones: distal humerus, olecranon, and radial head. Elbow trauma can result in a simple one-bone fracture or a complex fracture/dislocation involving a combination of bones. These injuries vary by the bones and structures involved and the extent of the injury. Elbow dislocations occur in isolation or along with a fracture. Both fractures and dislocations often include concomitant soft tissue injury, such as ligament, muscle, or nerve. Seven percent of all fractures are elbow fractures,[1] and one third of those involve the distal humerus. The mechanism of injury is a posterior force directed at the flexed elbow, often a fall to an outstretched hand, or axial loading of an extended elbow. Thirty-three percent of all elbow fractures occur in the radial head and neck by axial loading on a pronated forearm, with the elbow in more than 20 degrees of flexion.[2] Radial head fractures are often associated with ligament injuries. Radial head fractures that are associated with interosseous membrane disruption and distal radial ulnar joint dislocation are termed *Essex-Lopresti lesions*. Twenty percent of elbow fractures occur in the olecranon as a result of direct impact or a hyperextension force.[3] When the radial head dislocates anteriorly along with an ulnar fracture, the result is a *Monteggia* fracture. Another common fracture location along the proximal ulna is the *coronoid process*.[4]

ANATOMICAL OVERVIEW

The elbow joint is composed of three complex articulations: ulna-humeral, radio-capitellar, and proximal radio-ulnar (Figure 7-1). The joint capsule is thin, translucent, and has an exaggerated response to injury.[5] The radial head, along with the medial and lateral ligaments, plays a major role in the stability of the elbow joint by preventing dislocation. The joint is highly congruent and has limited joint play. The elbow is particularly prone to contracture and stiffness because of the high congruity, multiple articulations, and the close relationship of ligaments and muscle to the joint capsule.[6] Types of fixation range from rigid to tenuous. *Rigid* fixation allows early active and passive motion with minimal pain. *Stable* fixation allows early protected motion, and *tenuous* fixation requires delayed protected mobilization.[7,8]

REHABILITATION OVERVIEW

General rehabilitation goals are to restore motion and strength for optimal function while protecting injured and repaired structures and preventing joint stiffness. The trend in rehabilitation has been toward early mobility with less immobilization. The greatest challenge facing therapists is determining the balance between mobility and stability. Often, attention is given to mobil-

ity and strength at the expense of stability and comfort, but clinicians must consider mobility and stability of equal importance and not strive for progress in one while sacrificing gains in the other. Range of motion (ROM) is initiated as early as possible within safe parameters to prevent the development of stiffness. In cases where fractures and dislocations are considered unstable, ROM should not be ignored, but rather delayed or performed in a protective position.[7] The following guideline outlines appropriate treatment to restore joint motion and function after elbow fractures, while avoiding damage to repaired and injured structures. The phases of wound healing are correlated to treatment so that techniques are used appropriately to augment healing and avoid inflammation.

POSTOPERATIVE PHASE I: INFLAMMATION/PROTECTION (WEEKS 0 TO 2)

Splinting

In phase I, therapy focuses on protection of repaired or injured structures. Healing structures are protected in a brace, cast, or custom-molded thermoplastic splint to maintain alignment and prevent deformity. Splint designs vary and are based on the surgeon's preference, therapist's experience, and the patient's needs. The protective splint is worn for as long as 2 to 8 weeks postoperatively, depending on the stability of the fracture/joint and the severity of the injury. The position and angle of immobilization is based on the type of fracture. Distal humeral fractures are immobilized in 90 degrees of elbow flexion, with the forearm in neutral rotation (Figure 7-2). Olecranon and proximal ulna fractures may be immobilized, with the elbow in 60 to 75 degrees of flexion, the forearm in neutral, and the wrist in slight extension (Figure 7-3). Complex radial head fractures/dislocations and radial head replacements may be immobilized in up to 120 degrees of flexion to stabilize the radial head (see Figure 8-2).

Motion

Active and active-assistive ROM is initiated as soon as stability of the fracture is achieved via fixation or bone healing. The elbow splint is removed for the performance of exercises three to four times daily. The patient is instructed in elbow ROM as tolerated, within the safe prescribed arc, that is, 12 days postoperatively, if *rigid* fixation is achieved. If the fixation or joint is considered *stable*, a program of early-protected motion is begun (see Chapter 8). In cases of *tenuous* fixation and joint instability, protected motion is delayed. Elbow flexion and extension is performed with the shoulder resting on a towel roll against a wall (see Figure 4-4). Forearm ROM, if permitted, is performed with the arm at the side and

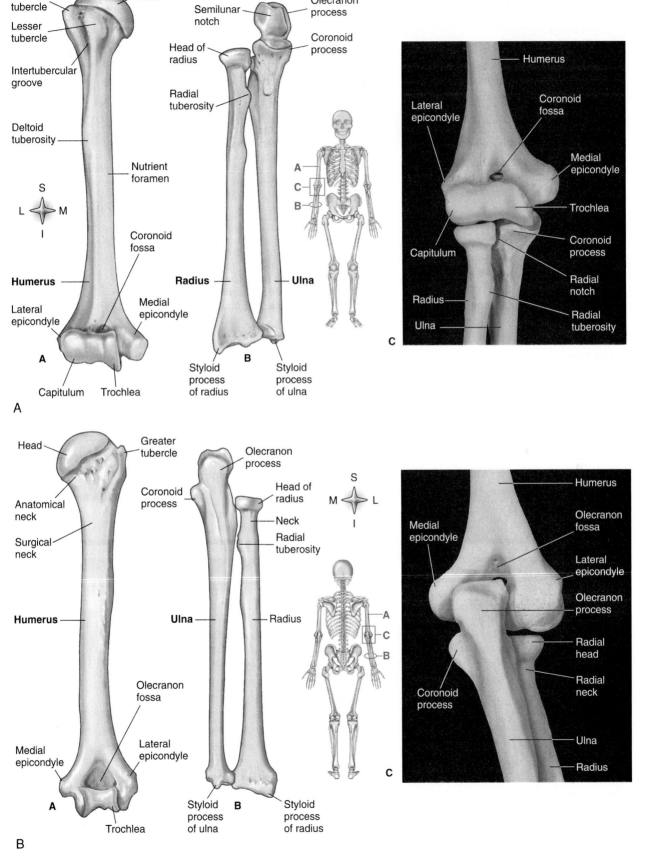

FIGURE 7-1 Elbow joint. *A.* Anterior view. *B.* Posterior view. *(From Thibodeau and Patton [Eds].* Anatomy and Physiology, *5th ed.)*

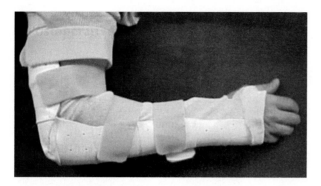

FIGURE **7-2** Posterior elbow shell at 90 degrees.

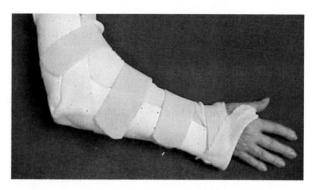

FIGURE **7-3** Posterior elbow immobilization splint in 60 to 75 degrees.

the elbow flexed to 90 degrees. Shoulder, wrist, and forearm ROM, and active and passive stretches are performed to the forearm flexor and extensor muscle groups to avoid muscle tightness. Tendon gliding exercises are performed to avoid tendon tightness and joint stiffness.

Precautions

Specific precautions apply to particular fractures. Radial head fracture dislocations are least stable in combined elbow extension and forearm supination. Extension is limited to 75 degrees and progressed slowly, as the joint becomes more stable. Olecranon fractures that are un-

stable should not be flexed beyond 90 degrees, until fracture union is achieved. Fractures that involve triceps rupture/reattachment follow tendon-healing precautions. Active elbow extension and active and passive elbow flexion beyond 90 degrees is contraindicated for the first 3 weeks to avoid tension at the repair site.

Troubleshooting

Complications of these surgeries include risk of redislocation and failure of fixation. Any unusual symptoms are reported to the surgeon for further investigation. Joint stiffness in the uninvolved joints is common and should be monitored closely and treated accordingly.

Postoperative Phase I: Inflammation/Protection (Weeks 0 to 2)

GOALS
- Protective immobilization
- Edema and pain control
- Full ROM in uninvolved joints
- A/AAROM of elbow within safe parameters
- Awareness and understanding of repair process and precautions
- Independence in HEP

PRECAUTIONS
- Exercise only within safe prescribed arc
- Monitor pressure areas over posterior aspect of elbow from prolonged splinting
- No passive manipulation or stretching
- No aggressive motion, which can cause inflammation and pain
- Avoid neurovascular compromise

TREATMENT STRATEGIES
Protection Options
- Custom thermoplastic splint
  - Adequate padding over the olecranon, medial/lateral epicondyles, and ulnar styloid

Pin and Wound Care for ORIF/CREF
- Solution of 50% hydrogen peroxide and sterile water daily to pin sites
- Standard sterile wound care procedures to ORIF
- Use of nonadherent dressing with minimal bulk to allow for early motion

Postoperative Phase I: Inflammation/Protection (Weeks 0 to 2)—cont'd

Edema/Pain Management

- Elevation, correct positioning, cryotherapy, light compression wrap (Ace bandage), safe early active ROM

Uninvolved Joint ROM

- Hand: tendon gliding (full composite flexion to DPC), thumb all planes
- Wrist: MD approval required, gravity eliminated flexion, extension, deviation
- Shoulder: in supine, wearing splint, AAROM exercises—all planes
- Avoid use of sling or posturing in the sling position

Elbow ROM

Only appropriate for **stable** *fractures/dislocations and within limits of repaired structures*
- Removal of splint to allow early active-assisted ROM exercises
- Exercise only in safe prescribed arc, in gravity-eliminated or gravity-assisted positions
- Forearm pronation/supination if permitted

CRITERIA FOR ADVANCEMENT

- Clinical union at fracture site or stability via surgical fixation
- Joint stability throughout full arc of motion at ulna/humeral and radio-ulnar joints

POSTOPERATIVE PHASE II: FIBROBLASTIC/ FRACTURE STABILITY (WEEKS 2 TO 8)

Phase II may commence as early as day 1, if fracture and joint stability is achieved.

Splinting

In the early part of this phase, the protective splint is removed frequently for exercises and light, functional activities. The splint is gradually weaned during the day so that by the end of this phase, the splint is worn for sleep and protection. The splint is usually discharged by the sixth postoperative week.

Motion

Controlled stress to the healing tissue is most effective during the fibroplastic phase. The goal is to achieve maximum active and passive elbow ROM. Communication with the surgeon is imperative to define precautions and establish realistic goals. When significant stiffness presents at an early stage, static progressive splinting is considered with the approval of the physician. Early joint stiffness is treated with serial static or static progressive elbow mobilization splints. These splints are described in detail in Chapter 9. When splints are provided in this phase, the joint is held at the *active* end range for a prolonged stretch. Passive end range stretch is delayed until phase III to avoid an inflammatory response. Treatment sessions begin with moist heat followed by an elbow flexor, extensor, and forearm compartment stretch (Figure 7-4). Applied force is steady and prolonged to gain tissue length. Passive stretching is applied to the point of discomfort. Total

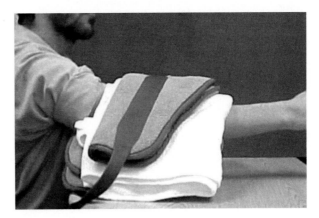

FIGURE **7-4** Moist heat applied at end range elbow extension.

end range time (TERT) is emphasized over several repetitions.[9] At no point should motion be forced. Forced motion can damage tissue or trigger an inflammatory response.

Precautions

Specific precautions apply to each fracture type. Combined elbow extension and supination are contraindicated for radial head fracture/dislocations. Elbow extension is increased gradually as the joint becomes more stable. Elbow ROM exercises are performed with the shoulder in slight external rotation in cases with lateral ligament involvement to avoid stress to the healing ligament. For olecranon fractures with concomitant triceps repair, aggressive elbow flexion is avoided.

Troubleshooting

Significant pain at end range with a hard end feel may indicate heterotopic bone formation and warrant reevaluation by the surgeon. Elbow stiffness is a common complication of trauma to the elbow. To avoid stiffness, strict adherence to the home program is imperative. Compliance and commitment to the home program are crucial for a good outcome. It should be noted that sometimes, even with the best therapy and compliance, stiffness is inevitable because of the nature of the injury and the length of immobilization required to achieve stability. In these situations, it is important to give the patient hope. The patient needs to be aware that further procedures (see Chapter 9) are available to increase elbow motion and function farther down the road.

Postoperative Phase II: Fibroblastic/Fracture Stability (Weeks 2 to 8)

GOALS
- Maximize active/passive ROM of the elbow and forearm in a pain-free range
- Control of edema and inflammation
- Decrease scar adherence
- Increase distal strength and proximal stabilization strength
- Improved muscle-tendon unit length
- Return to light, functional tasks with use of involved extremity

PRECAUTIONS
- Full arc active/passive ROM with MD approval
- Monitor response to ROM: avoid inflammatory episodes and/or exacerbation of pain
- No dynamic elbow splinting
- Monitor for early forearm and/or elbow joint contractures
- No grade III or IV joint mobilization
- No resistive exercises or activities

TREATMENT STRATEGIES
Protection
- Use thermoplastic splint for travel, sleep, or at-risk activities
- D/C sling, avoid posturing in "sling" position

ROM Program
- Active, active-assisted, and gentle passive ROM exercises, against gravity
- Emphasize total end range time (TERT) over several repetitions
- Gentle distraction, grades I & II joint mobilizations only
- Use of moist heat before exercising, heat on stretch
- Contract/relax exercises
- Biofeedback and/or NMES

Edema Control
- Cold pack, retrograde massage, moist heat before retrograde massage, light compression wrapping or sleeve, overhead ROM exercises

Scar Management
- Scar massage and silicone gel sheeting following removal of sutures/staples and complete closure of the wound
- Decrease scar adherence with cross-friction massage at scar interface
- Deep muscle massage to flexor/extensor muscle groups
- Compression sleeves (Tubigrip) to minimize hypertrophic scarring

Light, Functional Activities
- Restoration of normal movement patterns and encouraged use of extremity for light ADL
- Encourage functional splinting (holding phone to increase flexion, swinging arm while walking, and/or using keyboard)
- PNF patterns encouraged

CRITERIA FOR ADVANCEMENT
- Evidence of radiographic union or confirmation by MD of fracture, joint, and repaired structures to withstand resistance/stress

POSTOPERATIVE PHASE III: SCAR MATURATION AND FRACTURE CONSOLIDATION (WEEK 8 TO MONTH 6)

The primary goal in this phase is to achieve maximum ROM, increase strength and endurance, and resume normal activity. There are no longer precautions that limit motion. If stiffness persists, capsular stretching, soft tissue mobilization, joint mobilization, and low load prolonged stretch via static progressive splints are used (see Chapter 9).

Graded strengthening begins when the fracture union is stable and soft tissue is healed. Isometric exer-cises are progressed to progressive resistive exercises (i.e., elastic bands, pulleys, and free weights). Functional retraining and work conditioning is performed in this phase.

Troubleshooting

Complications of elbow fractures include reflex sympathetic dystrophy, heterotopic bone formation, malunion, nonunion, nerve compression, flexion or extension contractures, and joint stiffness.[6] If any of these are suspected, the patient should be referred back to the surgeon for further evaluation.

Postoperative Treatment Phase III: Scar Maturation and Fracture Consolidation (Week 8 to Month 6)

GOALS
- Full functional ROM
- Full functional strength and endurance
- Full participation in all functional activities, work, and leisure

PRECAUTIONS
- Hard end feel indicating a bony or hardware block; notify MD
- Failure of hardware, joint incongruity
- Nonunion or malunion
- PRE is contraindicated if patient is unable to isolate specific muscle group

TREATMENT STRATEGIES

ROM Program
- Focus on end range parameters and quality of motion
- Continue previous exercises; goal: passive ROM = active ROM

Strength and Endurance
- PRE to all muscle groups
- Free weights, wall pulleys, Thera-Band, weight well, MULE, BTE, PNF patterns with resistance

Splinting Program
- Continue splinting program overnight and intermittently during the day
- Upgrade splint parameters to passive end range position
- Continue functional splinting throughout the day

Return to Function
- Encourage return to ADL, work, and leisure activities
- Activity analysis
- BTE

CRITERIA FOR DISCHARGE
- Achieved full or functional ROM and strength
- Returned to previous level of function
- Independence in home exercise program and splinting program
- Progress has plateaued, and status has not changed over 6 weeks

REFERENCES

1. Jupiter, J., Morrey, B. Fractures of the Distal Humerus in Adults. In Morrey, B. (Ed). *The Elbow and Its Disorders,* 3rd ed. WB Saunders, Philadelphia, 2000, p. 293.
2. Morrey, B. Radial Head Fractures. In Morrey, B. (Ed). *The Elbow and Its Disorders,* 3rd ed. WB Saunders, Philadelphia, 2000, p. 341.
3. Cabanela, M.F., Morrey, B. Fractures of the Olecranon. In Morrey, B. (Ed). *The Elbow and Its Disorders,* 3rd ed. WB Saunders, Philadelphia, 2000, p. 365.
4. Regan, W. Coronoid Process and Monteggia Fractures. In Morrey, B. (Ed). *The Elbow and Its Disorders,* 3rd ed. WB Saunders, Philadelphia, 2000, p. 396.
5. Morrey, B. Anatomy of the Elbow Joint. In Morrey, B. (Ed). *The Elbow and Its Disorders,* 3rd ed. WB Saunders, Philadelphia, 2000, p. 13.
6. Hotchkiss, R. Fractures and Dislocations of the Elbow. In Rockwood, C., Green, D.P. (Eds). *Rockwood and Green's Fractures in Adults,* 4th ed. Lippincott-Raven, Philadelphia, 1996, p. 929.
7. Barenholtz, A., Wolff, A. *Elbow Fractures and Rehabilitation.* Orthop Phys Ther Clin North Am 2001;10(4):525–539.
8. Hotchkiss, R., Davila, S. Rehabilitation of the Elbow. In Morrey, B., Nickel, V.N. (Eds). *Orthopedic Rehabilitation.* Churchill Livingstone, New York, 1992, p. 157.
9. Flowers, K.R., LaStayo, P. *Effect of Total End Range Time on Improving Passive Range of Motion.* J Hand Ther 1994;7(3): 150–157.

8

Radial Head Replacement

AVIVA WOLFF, OTR/L, CHT

ELBOW STABILITY

In the normal elbow, stability is provided by the bony anatomy, ligaments, and muscle forces surrounding the joint. The joint surfaces are highly congruent, thus contributing to the overall stability.[1] The biceps and brachialis create a posterior force vector at the elbow, which is counteracted by the coronoid and radial head creating a joint reaction force at the elbow[2] (Figure 8-1). Stability is further provided by the medial and lateral ligament complexes and the anterior capsule (Figure 8-2). Historically, much attention has been devoted to the role of the medial collateral ligament, but in recent years descriptions of the anatomy of the lateral ligament complex have been discussed, expanded, and studied.[1,3–6] Sojberg et al.[7] have further studied the role of the lateral ligament complex in elbow stability. Findings of these investigators indicate that the lateral liga-

ment complex, specifically the lateral ulnar collateral ligament, is a major stabilizer of the elbow joint. Elbow instability results when these structures are injured or disrupted (Figure 8-3).

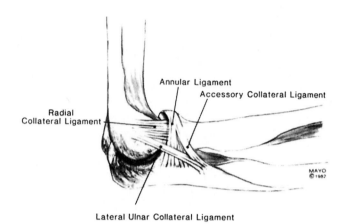

FIGURE **8-2** Lateral ligament complex of the elbow. *(Reprinted from the Mayo Foundation, Morrey, B.F. The Elbow and Its Disorders, 2nd ed. WB Saunders, Philadelphia, 1993, with permission.)*

ELBOW INSTABILITY

Elbow instability results from a dislocation of the ulnohumeral joint and injury to the varus and valgus stabilizers of the elbow and the radial head.[5] This injury often results from a forceful fall on an outstretched hand. The impact drives the head of the radius into the capitellum of the humerus,[5,8] which may result in radial head and coronoid process fracture, medial collateral, posterolateral, and/or lateral collateral ligament disruption. When all of the previous structures are injured, the condition is described as the "terrible triad."[8]

SURGICAL/MEDICAL MANAGEMENT

The surgical treatment of complex unstable elbow injuries may include titanium radial head replacement, open reduction internal fixation to the radial head, primary repair of the posterolateral ligament, and open reduction internal fixation to the ulnohumeral joint.[5] Nonsurgical treatment in the form of immobilization may be appropriate in less complex injuries. Radial head excision vs radial head replacement has long been debated among surgeons.[7] Radial head replacements have evolved over the years to include a metallic head, silicone head, allograft head, and most recently the titanium head replacement,[9–11] and the titanium head replacement has been used effectively in the treatment of complex radial head fractures and fracture disloca-

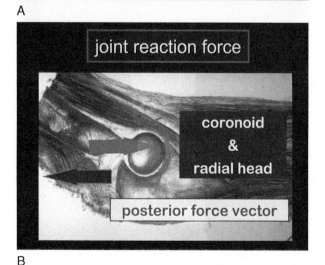

FIGURE **8-1** Joint reaction force. *(Adapted from diagram of Robert N. Hotchkiss, with permission.)*

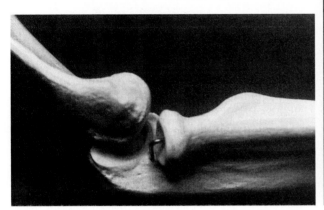

A   B

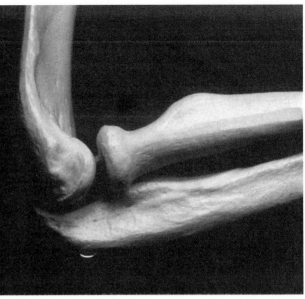

FIGURE **8-3** Lateral photograph of the elbow skeleton. In cases of posterolateral rotatory instability, the radial head lies posterior to the capitellum, and the lateral aspect of the ulnohumeral articulation is widened. Supination, valgus, and compressive force applied to the elbow in extension will cause this pattern of subluxation following injury to the lateral ulnar collateral ligament *A*. Gradual flexion of the joint will result in reduction of the radius and ulna onto the humerus *(B)*. *(From Mackin, E.J., Callahan, A.D., Shirven, T.M., Schneider, L.H., Osterman, A.L. Rehabilitation of the Hand, 5th ed., St. Louis, Mosby, 2002.)*

tions. The annular ligament is repaired surgically to reinforce lateral stability of the elbow.

POSTOPERATIVE PHASE I: INFLAMMATION/ PROTECTION (WEEKS 0 TO 3)

The challenge facing surgeons and therapists in the rehabilitation process is how do they successfully initiate early range of motion (ROM) to avoid joint stiffness without jeopardizing the stability of the elbow joint? Traditionally, the unstable elbow was immobilized until adequate stability had been achieved, and ROM exercises commenced at that point. This resulted in significant limitations in both forearm supination and elbow extension. The authors have developed a protocol that allows for early motion while protecting the stability of the joint. Postoperative management begins as early as 2 days postoperatively and involves splint fabrication and protected ROM exercises. The treatment goals during this phase are to maintain stability of the elbow and begin early protected motion in a safe overhead position to avoid joint stiffness.

Splint Fabrication and Management

The treatment plan begins with fabrication of a custom thermoplastic posterior elbow shell, with the elbow positioned in 120 degrees or more of flexion and the forearm in full pronation (Figure 8-4). The wrist is

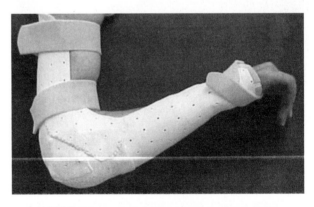

FIGURE **8-4** Posterior splint—position of stability.

included and splinted in neutral. A figure-eight strap may be added to further stabilize the elbow in 120 degrees for a larger framed individual (Figure 8-5). The splint is worn at all times and removed three to five times daily for protected exercises. The elbow must be in 120 degrees or more of flexion to ensure approximation of the radial head. If this is not achieved, an instability may occur (Figure 8-6). An alternative to the thermoplastic splint, and a preference of some surgeons, is a Bledsoe brace (Bledsoe Brace Systems, Grand Prairie, TX) or the Mayo Clinic elbow universal brace

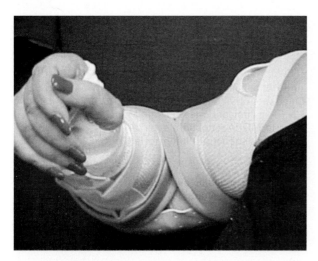

FIGURE 8-5 Figure-eight strap to secure elbow in splint.

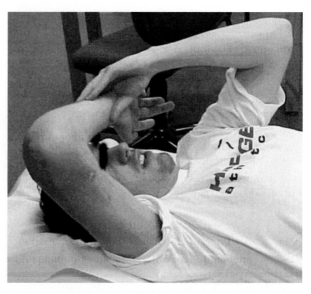

FIGURE 8-7 Overhead stable position for radial head.

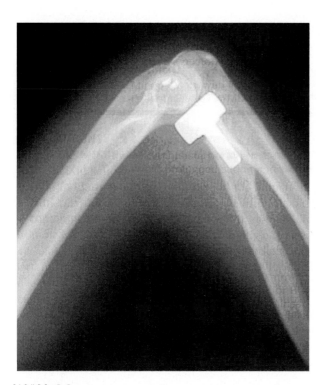

FIGURE 8-6 Radial head subluxes posteriorly if joint is not approximated.

(Aircast, Summit, NJ). The brace is locked in 120 degrees of elbow flexion and neutral forearm rotation. The brace is worn at all times, and exercises are performed within protected range. Some surgeons immobilize the elbow in 90 degrees of flexion, if adequate stability was achieved intraoperatively.

Therapeutic Exercises

The patient is instructed in two basic exercises, usually by the second postoperative day. Early protected ROM exercises are performed in a supine overhead position to decrease the effects of gravity by minimizing posterior vector forces at the elbow. This places the elbow in a stable position while allowing early motion to avoid joint stiffness (Figure 8-7).

In the supine position with the shoulder in 90 degrees of forward flexion and forearm maintained in pronation (forearm resting on forehead), gentle, active-assisted supination and pronation is performed (Figure 8-8). The second exercise is performed in the same position. The shoulder is placed in 90 degrees of forward flexion and the elbow in 90 degrees or more of flexion. Gentle, active, and active-assisted elbow flexion to full range and elbow extension is performed as tolerated, not to exceed 30 degrees (Figure 8-9).

Troubleshooting

Elbow stiffness is a common complication of elbow trauma. Maintaining the balance between mobility and stability is a constant challenge during this phase. Successful treatment of this injury requires diligence, expertise, skill, and ongoing communication with the referring surgeon, and compliance and accuracy with the home program are paramount to achieving good results. In rare instances, the joint may be unstable even in the overhead position. In such situations, motion is delayed until some degree of stability is achieved. Dynamic hinged fixation may be indicated in cases of extreme instability.

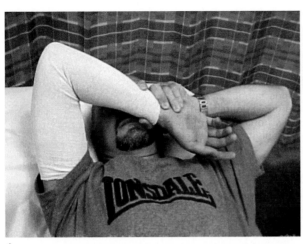

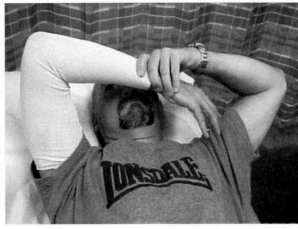

A   B

FIGURE **8-8** *A, B.* Supine overhead protected forearm pronation/supination.

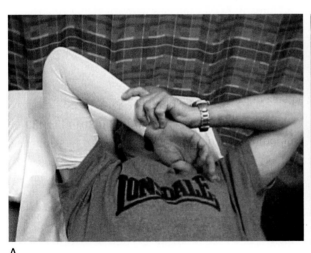

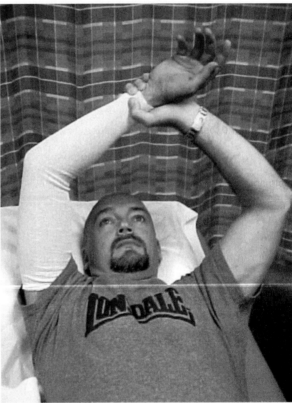

A

FIGURE **8-9** *A, B.* Supine overhead protected elbow flexion/extension.

B

Postoperative Phase I: Inflammation/Protection (Weeks 0 to 3)

GOALS

- Maintain stability of the elbow in a *safe position* elbow splint.
- Begin early, protective ROM exercises to the elbow and forearm in a *safe overhead position* to avoid joint stiffness.
- Minimize edema of the hand.
- Maintain AROM of the uninvolved joints.

PRECAUTIONS

Maintain the shoulder position in neutral to external rotation and the forearm in pronation to avoid stress to the lateral elbow when the patient is not in the splint or performing the specific exercises described below.

TREATMENT STRATEGIES

Protective Immobilization

- Choice is based on surgeon's preference, therapists, experience, and specific injury
- Posterior elbow shell or Bledsoe brace

Early Protected Motion

- Protected active and active-assisted elbow and forearm ROM exercises performed in a supine overhead position
- Protected forearm supination
- Protected elbow extension:
  Maintain full pronation throughout ROM at the elbow.

Range of Motion Exercises

- AROM exercises to the uninvolved joints
- Active and active-assisted ROM shoulder forward flexion and abduction are performed in supine with the splint on.
- Active and active-assisted wrist ROM exercises and hand tendon gliding exercises

Edema Control and Wound Care

- Standard wound care procedures and edema management is followed.

CRITERIA FOR ADVANCEMENT

- Joint stability determined by the surgeon

POSTOPERATIVE PHASE II: FIBROPLASTIC/EARLY REMODELING (WEEKS 3 TO 6)

Phase II of therapy commences as soon as joint stability is achieved. The splint is remolded to a position of 90 degrees of flexion and neutral forearm rotation. The protected (supine-overhead) ROM exercises are replaced by active and active-assisted elbow and forearm ROM in sitting or standing within the safe prescribed arc. Elbow flexion and extension is performed with the shoulder resting on a towel roll against a wall and the forearm positioned in neutral rotation (see Figure 4-4). The shoulder is positioned in slight external rotation to avoid stress on the lateral ligament. Forearm ROM is performed with the arm at the side and the elbow flexed to 90 degrees (see Figure 7-4). Combined elbow extension and supination is the most unstable position and is therefore avoided until clearance is received from the physician. Likewise, passive elbow extension and passive forearm supination is avoided.

Scar management in the form of scar massage and silicone gel sheets is added once the incision is fully closed and sutures or staples have been removed. Manual edema mobilization and soft tissue mobilization techniques are effective in reducing elbow edema. Gentle wrist and grip strengthening begins at 4 weeks. Specific strengthening activities include weight well, putty, and hand-helper exercises.

Troubleshooting

Elbow stiffness continues to be a challenge during this phase. Specific treatment strategies are discussed in detail in Chapters 7 and 9. Occasionally, instability persists postsurgery for longer than the usual 2 to 3 weeks. In those situations, the progression of treatment is delayed until further instructions from the physician.

Postoperative Phase II: Fibroplastic/Early Remodeling (Weeks 3 to 6)

GOALS

- Wean from splint over a 2- to 6-week time period
- Initiate scar management
- Achieve full AROM of the elbow and forearm
- Begin gentle grip and wrist strengthening
- Initiate light ADL

PRECAUTIONS

- The shoulder is positioned in slight external rotation during exercises to avoid stress to the lateral ligaments of the elbow.
- Passive ROM for elbow extension and for forearm supination is avoided.

TREATMENT STRATEGIES

Splint Adjustment and Management

- The posterior elbow shell splint is adjusted to 90 degrees of flexion and the forearm in neutral rotation.
- The splint is weaned from the patient during the day for self-care and light ADL.
- Splinting is continued for sleeping and for protection.

Scar Management

- Scar massage is initiated when the wound is fully healed.
- Silicone gel sheet or otoform is provided for use at night.

Active/Active-Assisted and Passive ROM Exercises

- Phase II ROM exercises are performed in sitting or standing.
- Active and active-assisted ROM for elbow extension and forearm pronation is progressed as tolerated.

Gentle Grip and Wrist-Strengthening Exercises

- Wrist PREs using 1-pound and 2-pound weights for forearm pronation and elbow flexion at 4 weeks.
- Grip strengthening: Isometrics, putty, and hand-helper exercises may be initiated gradually.

CRITERIA FOR ADVANCEMENT

- Joint stability determined by surgeon

POSTOPERATIVE PHASE III: SCAR MATURATION (WEEKS 6 TO 12)

The goals in this phase are to achieve maximum ROM, increase strength and endurance, and resume normal activity. There are no longer precautions that limit motion. If stiffness persists, capsular stretching, soft tissue mobilization, joint mobilization, and low load prolonged stretch via static progressive splints are used (see Chapter 9). Graded strengthening begins when the elbow joint is stable and the soft tissue is healed. Isometric exercises are progressed to progressive, resistive exercises: elastic bands, pulleys, and free weights. Func- tional retraining and work conditioning is performed in this phase.

Troubleshooting

Persistent pain that does not respond to conservative treatment may be indicative of a more serious complication, particularly when accompanied by loss of motion. Any unusual symptoms are reported to the physician. Complications associated with radial head dislocations have been reported in the literature and include infection, redislocation, and prosthetic failure.[3,12]

Postoperative Phase III: Scar Maturation (Weeks 6 to 12)

GOALS

- To achieve full active and passive elbow and forearm ROM
- To achieve functional upper extremity strength
- Independence in ADL and other activities

TREATMENT STRATEGIES

Range of Motion Exercises

- Prolonged end range stretching for elbow flexion and extension, forearm supination, and pronation.
- Combined elbow extension and forearm supination active and passive ROM exercises.
- Static progressive elbow and forearm splints to achieve end ROM.

Progressive Resistive Exercises

- Elbow flexion/extension: Thera-Band exercises, dumbbell PREs.
- Wrist and forearm: Thera-Band and dumbbell PREs.
- Grip strengthening: hand-helper and putty exercises.

Functional and Sports-Specific Activities Training

REFERENCES

1. An, K., Morrey, B.F. *Biomechanics of the Elbow.* In Morrey, B.F. (Ed). *The Elbow and Its Disorders.* WB Saunders, Philadelphia, 2000.
2. Hotchkiss, R.N. Fractures and Dislocations of the Elbow. In Rockwood, C.A., Green, D.P., Bucholz, R.W., Heckman, J.D. (Eds). *Rockwood and Green's Fractures in Adults.* Lippincott, Philadelphia, 1996.
3. Birkedal, J.P., Deal, D.N., Ruch, D.S. *Loss of Flexion After Radial Head Replacement.* J Shoulder Elbow Surg 2004;13: 208–213.
4. Hotchkiss, R.N., Kai-Nan, A., Sowa, D.T., Basta, S., Weiland, A.J. *An Anatomic and Mechanical Study of the Interosseous Membrane of the Forearm: Pathomechanics of Proximal Migration of the Radius.* J Hand Surg 1989;14A:256–261.
5. Morrey, B.F., An, K.N. *Functional Anatomy of the Ligaments of the Elbow.* Clin Orthop 1985;201:84.
6. O'Driscoll, S.W. Elbow Dislocations. In Morrey, B.F. (Ed). *The Elbow and Its Disorders.* WB Saunders, Philadelphia, 2000.
7. Sojberg, J.O., Ovesen, J., Nielsen, S. *Experimental Elbow Stability After Transection of the Annular Ligament.* Arch Orthop Trauma Surg 1987;106:248.
8. Gupta, G.G., Lucas, G., Hahn, D.L. *Biomechanical and Computer Analysis of Radial Head Prostheses.* J Shoulder Elbow Surg 1997;6:37–48.
9. Beredjiklian, P.K., Nalbantoglu, U., Potter, H.G., Hotchkiss, R.N. *Prosthetic Radial Head Components and Proximal Radial Morphology: A Mismatch.* J Shoulder Elbow Surg 1999;8: 471–475.
10. Frankle, M.A., Koval, K.J., Sanders, R.W., Zuckerman, J.D. *Radial Head Fractures Associated with Elbow Dislocations Treated by Immediate Stabilization and Early Motion.* J Shoulder Elbow Surg 1999;8:355–360.
11. Furry, K.L., Clinkscales, C.M. *Comminuted Fractures of the Radial Head: Arthroplasty versus Internal Fixation.* Clin Orthop Relat Res 1998;353:40–42.
12. Harrington, J., Seky-out, A., Barrington, T.W., Evans, D.C., Tuli, V. *The Functional Outcome of Metallic Radial Head Implants in the Treatment of Unstable Elbow Fractures: A Long-Term Review.* J Trauma 2001;50(1):46–52.

9

Contracture Release of
the Elbow

AVIVA WOLFF, OTR/L, CHT

EMILY ALTMAN, PT, CHT

Elbow contractures have many causes. The choice of intervention for the stiff elbow is dictated by the cause of stiffness and the specific pathophysiology.[1] Posttraumatic stiffness following elbow fractures and dislocations is the most common cause of elbow contracture. Other causes include osteoarthritis or inflammatory arthritis, congenital or developmental deformities, burns, and head injury. The elbow joint is prone to stiffness for several reasons. Anatomically, the joint is highly congruent. In most joints of the body, the *tendinous portions* of the muscles that act on the joint lie over the joint capsule. In the elbow, however, the brachialis muscle *belly* lies directly over the anterior joint capsule, making adhesion formation between the two structures inevitable following injury. The elbow is often held in 70 to 90 degrees of flexion postinjury because that is the position of greatest intracapsular volume for accommodation of edema. The thin joint capsule responds to trauma by thickening and becoming fibrotic, and quickly accommodating to this flexed position of the elbow. This results in a tethering of joint motion, particularly in the direction of extension. Biomechanically, the strong (and often co-contracting) elbow flexors overpower the weaker elbow extensors, which challenges the ability to regain extension.[2] Last, the elbow joint is prone to heterotopic ossification following trauma and surgery.

Elbow contractures are classified as intrinsic or extrinsic. Extrinsic contractures result from extra-articular pathology, involving the skin, neurovascular structures, joint capsule, ligaments, muscle tendon units, and heterotopic bone. Intrinsic contractures result from intra-articular pathology, such as joint incongruity, fracture, deformity, and intra-articular heterotopic bone.[2]

Posttraumatic elbow contractures that are of short duration may respond well to conservative treatment. Typically, extrinsic contractures that are 6 to 12 months postinjury have minimal articular incongruity and a soft or firm end feel that will improve with therapy. When conservative intervention fails, surgical release is indicated. Surgical options for releasing the joint range from simple arthroscopy to the placement of hinged, external fixation (see Chapter 10).

Arthroscopic release is generally reserved for patients with minimal joint stiffness, small osteophytes at the coronoid or olecranon, or loose bodies. The anterior joint capsule is well visualized arthroscopically.[3] An open release is indicated for more involved cases that may require any one or combination of the following: anterior and posterior capsulectomy, ulnar nerve transposition, removal of large osteophytes, and removal of hardware. The open release is performed via a medial, lateral, or posterior incision, or any combination of the three. The approach selected is determined by the type of contracture and location of pathology. The lateral approach is selected for simple flexion contractures, such as those that result from radial head fractures. The lateral approach is the most simple to perform, yet it provides the least exposure. Situations that present with ulnar nerve involvement require medial exposure. A medial "over-the-top" approach has been advocated by Hotchkiss.[3] This technique allows exposure of the joint, while protecting the ulnar nerve, anterior collateral ligament, and posterolateral ulnohumeral ligament complex. It also allows both anterior and posterior access to the joint. If heterotopic bone is present on the lateral side, a combined medial and lateral approach is used. Heterotopic bone that is present on the olecranon warrants a posterior approach.

REHABILITATION OVERVIEW

Rehabilitation following any type of elbow contracture release focuses on regaining functional, pain-free, active range of motion (ROM) of the elbow joint. Therapy must be initiated immediately after surgery, and the three members of the patient care team (surgeon, therapist, and patient) must work closely together for an optimal outcome. The treatment guidelines for arthroscopic and open contracture releases are similar conceptually, but arthroscopic releases generally require less intervention through all of the phases and progress more quickly. Patient compliance is crucial for a successful outcome. Patient selection by the surgeon and patient education by the surgeon and therapist is very essential. The patient must be an active participant in every aspect of his or her rehabilitation program.

POSTOPERATIVE REHABILITATION

POSTOPERATIVE PHASE I: INFLAMMATORY PHASE (DAYS 1 TO 7)

Arthroscopic

Arthroscopic releases are usually done as an ambulatory surgery so that patients are not seen as inpatients, and postoperative and home continuous passive motion (CPM) use is not required. Immediately after surgery, patients are instructed in a home exercise program of active, active-assisted, and passive ROM for the elbow and in the edema reduction techniques of ice and elevation. Outpatient therapy is initiated as soon as possible. Therapeutic intervention in this phase includes edema reduction (gentle retrograde massage, elevation, and cryotherapy) and active, active-assisted, and passive ROM for elbow flexion/extension and forearm pronation/supination. Active range of motion (AROM) exercises are performed in standing and/or supine. A dowel or cardboard tube is held between the two hands

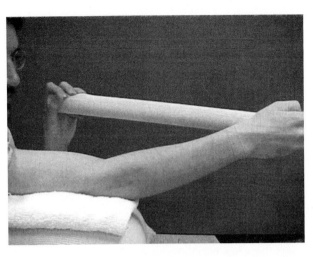

FIGURE **9-1** Passive elbow extension stretch with dowel.

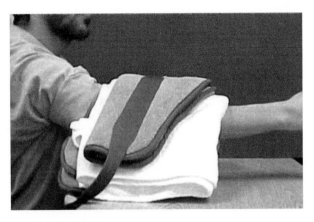

FIGURE **9-3** Moist heat applied at end range.

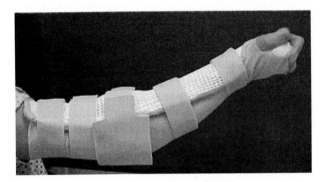

FIGURE **9-2** Night extension splint.

for active-assisted elbow flexion and extension. The same tube is used for an elbow extension stretch in sitting (Figure 9-1). The contralateral hand assists in an elbow flexion stretch. Pulleys and the Nu-Step recombent crosstrainer or upper body exercise (UBE) are used to improve the arc of elbow motion. Creative reaching tasks, using pegs/pegboard, cones, clothespins, rolling pins, and so on, are initiated in this phase as well. Any type of active pronation and supination exercises are permitted.

Splinting. If needed, a thermoplastic serial static elbow extension splint (Figure 9-2) is fabricated for use at night. This provides low load, prolonged positioning at the end range of elbow extension. It is remolded into greater extension as tolerated.

Open

After an open release, patients generally stay 2 nights in the hospital. On postoperative day 1, the postoperative plaster splint and dressing are removed, a thermoplastic serial static night extension splint is fabricated, and CPM use is initiated. The CPM protocol calls for a goal

of three 2-hour sessions (total 6 hours) of CPM use. During each session the patient alternates between 20 minutes of static positioning in maximum tolerable flexion and 20 minutes of static positioning in maximum tolerable extension. Between each 20-minute period, the patient can let the CPM run through several cycles of flexion and extension. Only the slowest speed should be used. The static extension splint is worn in between the 2-hour CPM sessions. On postoperative day 2, the patient is instructed in a series of active and active-assisted flexion/extension and pronation/supination exercises. For the first 24 to 48 hours, a continuous axillary block or coracoid indwelling catheter is used for pain control. Arrangements for home CPM may or may not be necessary.

Outpatient therapy is initiated immediately. Therapeutic intervention in this phase includes standard wound care and edema reduction, and active, active-assisted, and gentle passive ROM of the elbow and forearm. The therapeutic exercise program consists of the dowel active/active-assisted ROM program outline mentioned previously in the arthroscopic release section. Therapeutic exercises are preceded with moist heat application in the end range position of greater limitation (Figure 9-3). Activities, such as the Nu-Step recombent crosstrainer and UBE, are usually too difficult in this early phase. The patient should also be instructed in an AROM program for the shoulder to prevent the development of a stiff shoulder.

Splinting. The static elbow extension splint that was immediately fabricated postoperatively should be used at night. The use of a static progressive elbow flexion and/or extension splint is sometimes initiated as early as postoperative day 2 or 3, but more commonly not until a week to 10 days postoperative. It can be difficult to tolerate during the immediate postoperative inflammatory period.

Postoperative Phase I: Inflammatory Phase (Days 1 to 7)

GOALS

- Effective edema reduction
- Thorough patient education
- Independence in ROM home program
- Light functional use of the involved elbow and entire UE

PRECAUTIONS

- Wound

TREATMENT STRATEGIES

- Comprehensive HEP for elbow and forearm A/AAROM
- Shoulder AROM
- Elbow CPM (generally for open releases only)
- Edema reduction: light compression, retrograde massage, elevation, ice
- Creative functional tasks that involve reaching and placing. Tasks should use the entire UE and can include the contralateral UE as well. Pegs, cones, clothespins, and rolling pins are useful tools. Some of these tasks may be too difficult for involved open releases.
- UBE and Nu-Step for endurance (for arthroscopic release)
- Pulleys for increased ROM
- Static progressive splinting for flexion, extension, pronation, and supination, as indicated.

CRITERIA FOR ADVANCEMENT

- Wound closure
- Edema reduction
- Pain reduction
- Independence and compliance in comprehensive exercise and splinting program

Troubleshooting

After open contracture release, pain control can be difficult, limiting progress in therapy. Patients are encouraged to take their pain medication before therapy. Decreasing the number of repetitions per exercise session and promoting more rest, ice, and elevation is often helpful. It is important not to push through excessive pain. The skin over the posterior aspect of the elbow heal tends to heal poorly secondary to limited vascularity and repetitive tensioning of the skin with elbow flexion. It may be necessary to temporarily limit the amount of flexion to allow definitive healing.

POSTOPERATIVE PHASE II: FIBROPLASTIC PHASE (WEEKS 2 TO 6)

Therapy in postoperative phase II focuses on increasing the active ranges of elbow and forearm motion. The immediate postoperative issues of edema and pain should be under control, allowing increased use of the elbow for activities of daily living (ADL).

Arthroscopic

Scar massage to the portal site is initiated as soon as the wound is fully closed. The basic A/AAROM exercises of phase I are continued. Passive ROM becomes a greater focus of the exercise program. Beginning each therapy session with moist heat is very effective. The functional reaching tasks and endurance activities introduced in phase I are continued and progressed. Functional tasks involving the entire upper extremity are also emphasized. Throughout this phase, the patient is encouraged to use the involved upper extremity in all possible self-care activities.

Splinting. Static night extension splint use is continued. Fabrication of static progressive flexion or extension splints is indicated if AROM is not progressing. Off the shelf, prefabricated *static progressive* (not dynamic) flexion/extension splints, such as the Universal Mayo Clinic Elbow Brace (Aircast, Summit, NJ), are currently available and effective in many cases (see Figure 4-3).

Open

Scar massage and management techniques, including silicone gel sheeting, are initiated when the surgical wound is fully closed. Edema control techniques are continued, including light compression, retrograde massage, and elevation. Therapeutic exercise interventions are essentially the same as those outlined previously for arthroscopic releases. However, patients tend to progress more slowly and initially have less tolerance for exercise after open releases than after arthroscopic releases. Home use of a CPM machine is continued until pain and swelling are reduced enough to replace CPM use with AROM exercises, which is usually about 2 to 3 weeks postoperative.

Splinting. Static night extension splint use is continued. It is often necessary to fabricate static progressive flexion and/or extension splints and forearm rotation splints, depending on the ROM deficits of the patient. Patients are instructed to wear the splint for 2-hour intervals for a total of 6 hours daily. Initially, only short intervals are tolerated. The goal is to develop a tolerance for longer intervals. Patients are instructed to adjust the tension as tolerated. When more than one splint is required, the patient may alternate the splints during the day or wear one during the day and the other at night for sleeping. The splint regimen is highly individualized and tailored to meet the specific needs and limitations of each patient. Dynamic splinting is often not well tolerated and therefore not recommended. Off the shelf, prefabricated static progressive flexion/extension splints are currently available and are effective in many cases. The shape of the patient's arm, the degree of joint stiffness, and the firmness of joint end feel all impact the fit (and therefore effectiveness) of commercial splints.

Troubleshooting

Challenges encountered in phase II include the onset of symptoms of ulnar nerve compression or entrapment. Scar tissue formation can tether and/or compress the ulnar nerve. If this happens, the patient's progress will be severely impacted. Patient complaints will include tingling in the ulnar nerve distribution distal to the wrist and/or sharp "electric" pain in the forearm with end range elbow flexion. This same pain with end range extension is occasionally reported. If left untreated, ulnar nerve motor deficits will manifest as intrinsic wasting with IV and V digit clawing. The surgeon should be made aware of any changes in neurological status.

Co-contraction of the biceps muscle with attempted, voluntary elbow extension will significantly limit progress in regaining elbow extension.[6] The use of a biofeedback machine is useful in helping the patient effectively isolate the triceps as an agonist (Figure 9-4). Moist heat, gentle soft tissue techniques, and contract/relax techniques are also effective in quieting the biceps muscle.

Postoperative Phase II: Fibroplastic Phase (Weeks 2 to 6)

GOALS
- Full surgical wound closure
- Functional active elbow flexion/extension and forearm pronation/supination
- Pain <1/10
- Full use of involved UE for light functional ADL

PRECAUTIONS
- Exacerbation of pain with overactivity
- Monitor for potential ulnar nerve irritation/compression/entrapment

TREATMENT STRATEGIES
- A/AA/PROM elbow flexion/extension and forearm A/AA/PROM
- Shoulder AROM
- Home CPM (open releases only)
- Continued edema reduction: light compression, retrograde massage, elevation, ice
- Creative functional tasks that involve reaching and placing. Tasks should use the entire UE and include the contralateral UE as well. Pegs, cones, clothespins, and rolling pins are useful tools.
- UBE and Nu-Step recombent crosstrainer for endurance
- Pulleys for increased ROM
- Static progressive splinting for flexion, extension, pronation, and supination, as indicated
- Surface biofeedback for decreasing biceps co-contraction (see Troubleshooting)

CRITERIA FOR ADVANCEMENT
- No pain control issues
- Functional AROM
- MD clearance

Postoperative Phase III: Scar Maturation Phase (Week 6 and Beyond)

GOALS

- Return to vocational and avocational tasks
- Obtain and maintain intraoperative elbow and forearm ROM
- Independence in comprehensive scapular, shoulder, elbow home exercise program or gym program

PRECAUTIONS

- Heterotopic ossification
- Ulnar nerve irritation/compression/entrapment

TREATMENT STRATEGIES

- Continue A/AA/PROM exercises
- Continue/progress endurance activities: Nu-Step, UBE
- Continue static and static progressive splinting
- Initiate elbow/forearm/shoulder/scapular strengthening with dumbbells and Thera-Band
- Progression to gym program if appropriate for individual

CRITERIA FOR DISCHARGE

- Independence in ROM and strengthening program appropriate for individual's activity level and the functional demands of his or her life
- Achievement and maintenance of intraoperative ROM
- No pain impairments

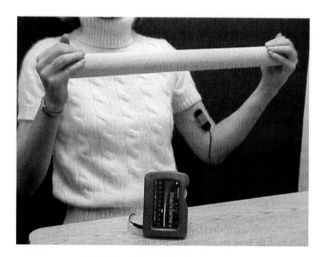

FIGURE **9-4** Use of biofeedback.

Pain control is sometimes a problem in this phase. Generally, it is an indication of excessive performance of the exercises or use of the elbow. Modification of the exercise program should resolve these issues.

Pain and loss of motion together may be indicative of heterotopic bone formation (heterotopic ossification, H-O). The surgeon is made aware of these findings to determine the presence of H-O, using X rays if necessary.

POSTOPERATIVE PHASE III: SCAR MATURATION PHASE (WEEK 6 AND BEYOND)

Postoperative phase III focuses on the return to all vocational and avocational tasks, the initiation of a strengthening program, and the maintenance of the ROM that was obtained intraoperatively. Scar management is continued. Moist heat continues to be a very effective way to start therapy sessions. The therapeutic exercise program continues to include active and passive ROM of the elbow and forearm and endurance exercises for the upper extremities. Strengthening is added to the program. This includes elbow flexion/extension, forearm pronation/supination, and shoulder and scapular strengthening. Standard Thera-Band and dumbbell exercises are initially appropriate. Progression to a gym program is optimal if the patient is an active, high demand individual.

Splinting. The night extension and static progressive splinting initiated in phases I and II is continued until maximum elbow and forearm ROM is obtained *and* maintained.

Troubleshooting

The ulnar nerve issues outlined in the Troubleshooting Phase II section continue to be a concern in the initial part of phase III. The surgeon must be made aware of any ulnar nerve symptoms, motor, or sensory. Permanent ulnar nerve damage can be a result of untreated symptoms.

Loss of ROM coupled with pain must also be addressed. It may be an indication of heterotopic ossification in the joint. The patient's therapist should communicate with the surgeon and inform him or her of any findings.

REFERENCES

1. Mansat, P., Morrey, B., Hotchkiss, R.N. *Extrinsic Contracture: "The Column Procedure," Lateral and Medial Capsular Release.* In Morrey, B. (Ed). *The Elbow and Its Disorders,* 3rd ed. WB Saunders, Philadelphia, 2000.

2. Griffith, A. *Therapist's Management of the Stiff Elbow.* In Griffith, A., Mackin, E.J., Skirven, T.M., Schneider, L.H. (Eds). *Rehabilitation of the Hand and Upper Extremity,* 5th ed. Mosby, St. Louis, 2002, pp. 1245–1262.

3. Hotchkiss, R. *Elbow Contracture.* In Hotchkiss, R., Green, D.P., Pederson, W.C. (Eds). *Green's Operative Hand Surgery,* 4th ed. Churchill Livingstone, New York, 1999, p. 667.

4. Blackmore, S.M. *Splinting for Elbow Injuries and Contractures.* Atlas Hand Clin 2001;6(1):21–50.

5. Schultz-Johnson, K. *Static Progressive Splinting.* J Hand Ther 2002;15:163–178.

6. Page, C., Backus, S.I., Lenhoff, M.W. *Electromyographic Activity in Stiff and Normal Elbows During Elbow Flexion and Extension.* J Hand Ther 2003;16:5–11.

10

Hinged Dynamic External Fixation of the Elbow

AVIVA WOLFF, OTR/L, CHT

EMILY ALTMAN, PT, CHT

Flexion and extension contractures of the elbow are common complications following injury and trauma to the joint. Open contracture release, closed manipulation, and distraction arthroplasty are three options used to regain functional elbow range of motion (ROM) in the stiff elbow population. Pain, swelling, and adaptive shortening of the soft tissue and muscle tendon unit can prevent a patient from maintaining the ROM obtained during these procedures. Unfortunately, the skilled use of comprehensive therapy, early active motion, static progressive splinting, and continuous passive motion (CPM) machines does not always guarantee success.

Dynamic hinged external fixation offers a solution for cases that responded poorly to other methods of contracture release.[1] *Dynamic hinged external fixation* is defined as a hinged device that separates and distracts the ulna from the humerus while providing varus and valgus stability to the elbow.[2] The hinged fixator allows active and passive motion of the elbow joint and stretches the soft tissue capsule at the end range of both flexion and extension. Currently, two dynamic hinged fixators are widely used: the Mayo dynamic joint distractor[3] and the Hotchkiss compass hinge[4] (Figures 10-1 to 10-3). Use of a dynamic fixator may be indicated in several situations, including acute trauma with complex instability, recurrent instability after collateral ligament release, contracted stiff elbow that is mature and has failed conservative therapy, extreme tightness in the muscle tendon unit following a capsular release, and posttraumatic arthritis of the elbow.[1,5] Following a contracture release, the hinged device is applied to maintain the ROM gains achieved intraoperatively and provide elbow stability if it was compromised during the contracture release surgery. Application of the hinge allows scar tissue to remodel in an environment that permits joint distraction, joint stability, joint motion, and promotes the healing of the articular surface. Through smooth, progressive adjustments of the device while in its locked position, the soft tissue is maintained at its available end range. Motion is performed to condition the muscles with the hinge unlocked.[6]

Once the underlying pathology has been addressed via contracture release or resurfacing of the joint, the hinge is applied. In most trauma cases, a posterior incision is made and the joint is exposed medially and laterally, depending on the pathology. For a stiff elbow both a posterior and an anterior incision may be required for a complete capsular release. A temporary axis pin is placed through the distal humerus to align the hinge with the axis of rotation. The frame is preassembled so it can freely slide medial to lateral on the axis pin. Two humeral pins (medial and lateral) are placed to secure the humerus in two planes. Two pins are placed in the ulna anterior and posterior to the axis of rotation. Once all of the pins have been placed and the joint adequately reduced, distraction is applied.

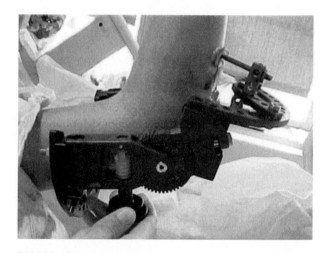

FIGURE **10-2** Medial view of the Hotchkiss compass hinge.

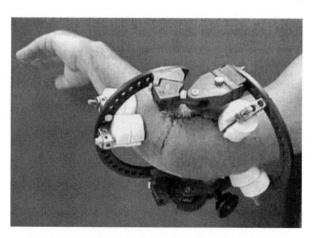

FIGURE **10-1** Lateral view of the Hotchkiss compass hinge.

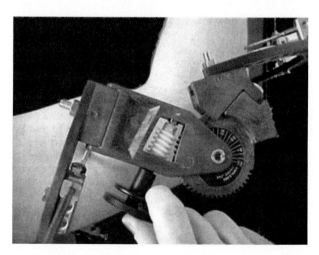

FIGURE **10-3** Hotchkiss compass hinge illustrates how worm gear is disengaged (pinching two discs together).

Both sides of the hinge should be distracted equally.[1,2] Complications of dynamic hinged fixation include compression neuropathy of the ulnar nerve, pin tract infections, heterotopic ossification, pin fractures, and delayed healing.[7]

REHABILITATION OVERVIEW

Dynamic hinged fixators are used following complex elbow dislocation, traumatic elbow fracture, and complex contracture release. Despite the various indications for placing a dynamic hinge, the role of the hinge is always the same, that is, to stabilize the joint and permit immediate postoperative movement. The therapist *must* communicate with the surgeon and obtain the details of the original injury and the operative procedure, and confirm an appropriate plan of care. Thorough knowledge of exactly what structures were involved and/or repaired is crucial to managing the rehabilitation of these patients. Examples of common key pieces of information include ligament repair/reconstruction, vascular repair, nerve repair, ulnar nerve transposition, triceps/biceps tendon repair or protection issues, and joint and fracture stability. The therapist must also be aware of associated injuries of the shoulder and wrist.

EVALUATION

During the initial therapy visit, the following are evaluated: ROM of the entire upper extremity (shoulder, wrist, forearm, and digits), edema, wound status (surgical incisions and pin sites), pain level, and sensation.

POSTOPERATIVE REHABILITATION

POSTOPERATIVE PHASE I: INFLAMMATORY/PROTECTIVE (WEEKS 0 TO 2)

The initial phase of postoperative rehabilitation focuses on patient education, splinting (if needed), wound and pin care, edema control, passive range of motion (PROM) program for the elbow joint using the hinge's gear system, and active range of motion (AROM)/PROM of the uninvolved joints of the upper extremity. The patient is seen at bedside on postoperative day 1 and is provided with detailed written instructions on the hinge protocol. The patient is directed to turn the worm gear in the direction of elbow extension in small increments through the day and sleep in maximum tolerated extension. AROM exercises of the uninvolved joints of the upper extremity are also taught. Edema reduction techniques of elevation, digit AROM, and cryotherapy (bags of ice) are emphasized. The patient is provided with a commercial wrist splint for support. Over the course of postoperative day 2, the patient gradually turns the worm gear in the direction of flexion and sleeps with the elbow in maximum tolerated flexion. On postoperative day 3 the patient begins to alternate between maximum extension and maximum flexion several times during the day and sleeps with the elbow in the position that was most limited preoperatively. The PROM program continues for 10 days to 2 weeks. Also on postoperative day 3, the patient is instructed in submaximal elbow flexion and extension isometrics with the hinge positioned at 90 degrees of flexion. Five to 10 repetitions of the isometric contractions are performed four to six times per day. Gentle, active forearm pronation and supination exercises are performed as tolerated. Before discharge from the hospital, the patient is instructed in the surgeon's preferred pin care protocol. In cases of extreme instability, a sugar tong splint may be ordered to position the forearm in pronation (Figures 10-4, *A* and *B*). This is fabricated before discharge from the hospital. Extrinsic flexor stretcher splints (resting hand splints) for night use can be fabricated as needed during phase I.[1,6]

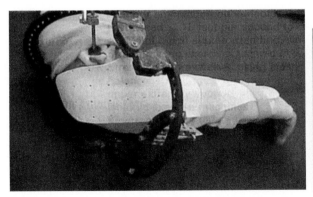
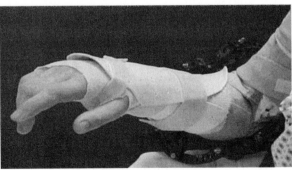

A   B

FIGURE **10-4** Compass hinge with pronation splint. *A.* Lateral view. *B.* Medial view.

Postoperative Phase I: Inflammatory/Protective (Weeks 0 to 2)

GOALS

- Edema and pain control
- Full ROM of uninvolved joints
- Maximum passive elbow flexion and extension

PRECAUTIONS

- Ulnar nerve compression at elbow
- Pin tract infection

TREATMENT STRATEGIES

- Edema control: ice, elevation, compression
- Wound care, pin care (monitor for infection) draining is common (especially at the medial pin)
- Uninvolved joint ROM: emphasize forearm pronation/supination

SPLINTING

- Wrist support
- Extrinsic flexor/extensor stretcher (resting hand splints) as needed for night
- Sugar tong splint to position forearm in pronation in cases of extreme instability

ELBOW RANGE OF MOTION PROTOCOL

Continuous axillary block for 24 to 48 hours
Worm gear is turned in small increments for PROM
- Postoperative day 1: patient instructed to turn worm gear in direction of extension gradually throughout the day and sleep in maximum tolerated extension
- Postoperative day 2: patient instructed to turn worm gear in direction of flexion gradually throughout the day and sleep in maximum tolerated flexion
- Postoperative day 3: flexion and extension are alternated several times during the day, and nighttime position is alternated between maximum flexion and extension for sleep, or patient is instructed to sleep in the position that is more limiting
- Postoperative day 4: submaximal elbow flexion and extension isometrics with the hinge locked

This program continues for 2 weeks.

Troubleshooting

Pain, persistent edema, pin tract infections, drainage at the pin sites, and poor tolerance of the PROM protocol are not uncommon in this phase. Patients should be closely monitored during this phase, with frequent visits to outpatient therapy.

POSTOPERATIVE PHASE II: FIBROPLASTIC (WEEKS 2 TO 8)

Phase II begins with the initiation of elbow AROM (unlocking the hinge fixator) and ends with the removal of the hinge. Initially, the worm gear is disengaged four times per day, and 10 repetitions of flexion and extension are performed (Figure 10-5, *A* and *B*). Active forearm pronation and supination exercises are continued, with an emphasis on end ROM. By postoperative week 3 or 4, the hinge is unlocked for longer periods of time and functional use of the extremity is encouraged. Overhead pulleys and reaching tasks that require elbow flexion and extension and object grasp are initiated (Figure 10-6). Once the wounds are closed, treatment sessions can be started with the application of a moist hot pack to the anterior elbow area. The passive program that was initiated immediately postoperatively continues through this phase. Night splinting to address extrinsic forearm muscle shortening can be initiated as needed.

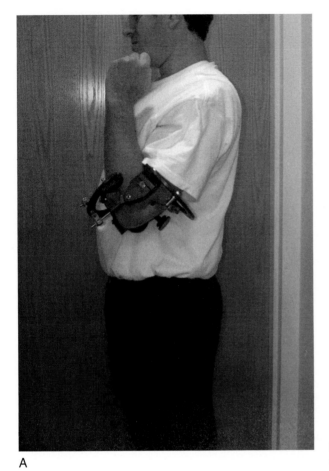

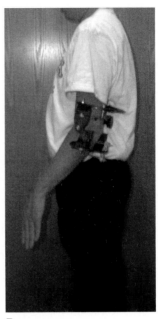

B

A

FIGURE **10-5** *A* and *B.* AROM elbow flexion and extension with worm gear disengaged.

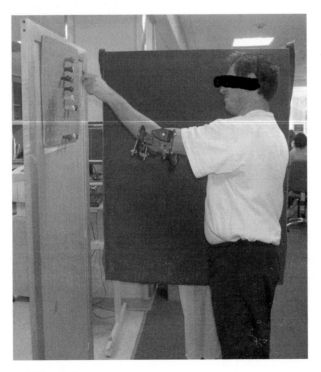

FIGURE **10-6** Pegboard AROM activity-functional forward reach.

Postoperative Phase II: Fibroplastic (Weeks 2 to 8)

GOALS

- Edema reduction
- Wound closure
- Full AROM of uninvolved joint
- Maximum active and passive elbow flexion and extension

PRECAUTIONS

- Ulnar nerve compression at the elbow
- Pin tract infection

TREATMENT STRATEGIES

- Wound care
- AROM elbow flexion and extension, forearm pronation and supination
- Uninvolved joint AROM
- Functional use of upper extremity for light ADL

SPLINTING

- As needed for
  - Wrist support
  - Maintenance of extrinsic forearm muscle length
  - Maintenance of elbow stability (forearm pronation)

ELBOW ROM PROTOCOL

- Continue PROM protocol initiated in phase I
- Initiate AROM elbow flexion and extension (unlock hinge gear), beginning with 10 repetitions, four times a day and progressing to 50% to 70% of the day spent with the hinge unlocked
- Encourage functional use of the upper extremity

Troubleshooting

Difficulty achieving acceptable increases in elbow flexion and extension ROM and the development of shoulder adhesive capsulitis can be seen in this phase. It is important to encourage the patient to perform reaching/overhead activities and limit time spent in static, protective postures of the upper extremity. Patients benefit from frequent therapy visits to address elbow ROM. Compliance with the home exercise program is critical.

POSTOPERATIVE PHASE III: SCAR MATURATION (WEEKS 6 TO 8, POST-HINGE REMOVAL)

Phase III begins with the hinge removal. Residual edema continues to be addressed. Scar mobilization and management techniques are initiated at the incisions. Pin sites are monitored and dressed as needed until closure. Therapy intervention now includes moist heat with prolonged end range stretch to improve soft tissue extensibility and prepare the muscles for exercise, AROM, active-assistive range of motion (AAROM), PROM, soft tissue mobilization and massage, contract/relax techniques, prolonged end range stretches, techniques to inhibit biceps co-contraction at the elbow, and functional activities, including the Baltimore therapeutic equipment (BTE) work simulator (Baltimore, MD). Progressive resistive exercises are initiated, using Thera-Band, dumbbells, and cable column exercise equipment. An overall, upper extremity conditioning and endurance program is also appropriate at this time, using equipment such as the Nu-Step recombent crosstrainer, Schwinn Airdyne Exerciser, and upper-body exercise bicycle. Splinting will include serial static night extension splints and static progressive elbow flexion/extension and forearm pronation/supination splints. These splints are designed to maintain motion gains and mimic the PROM role of the dynamic fixator (see Chapter 9).

Postoperative Phase III: Scar Maturation (Weeks 6 to 8, Post-Hinge Removal)

GOALS

- Regain full functional use of the elbow
- Achieve full wound closure and promote mobile scars
- Achieve independence in comprehensive strengthening and conditioning home exercise program
- Obtain maximum elbow flexion and extension ROM

PRECAUTIONS

- Ulnar nerve compression neuropathy
- Heterotopic ossification
- Persistent joint contracture

TREATMENT STRATEGIES

- AROM, AAROM, PROM stretching
- Thermal modalities
- Soft tissue massage/mobilization
- Contract/relax techniques
- Functional use of upper extremity for all ADL
- Progressive resistive exercise
- Comprehensive serial static/static progressive splinting program
- General conditioning

SPLINTING

- Serial static night extension splint
- Static progressive elbow flexion/extension and forearm rotation splints

Troubleshooting

The challenges of phase II continue in phase III. Obtaining acceptable elbow AROM can present a significant challenge for the patient, therapist, and surgeon. Patients often continue the comprehensive splinting regimen introduced in phase III for many months.

REFERENCES

1. Hotchkiss, R. *Compass Universal Hinge: Surgical Technique.* Smith and Nephew, Memphis, 1998.
2. Morrey, B.F., Hotchkiss, R. External Fixators of the Elbow. In Morrey, B.F. (Ed). *The Elbow and Its Disorders*, 3rd ed. WB Saunders, Philadelphia, 2000.
3. Morrey, B. *Post-traumatic Operative Procedures of the Elbow.* J Bone Joint Surg 1990;72(8):601.
4. Kasparyan, N.G., Hotchkiss, R. *Dynamic Skeletal Fixation of the Upper Extremity.* Hand Clin 1997;13:643.
5. Hotchkiss, R. Elbow Contracture. In Hotchkiss, R., Green, D.P., Pederson, W.C. (Eds). *Green's Operative Hand Surgery*, 4th ed. Churchill Livingstone, New York, 1999, p. 667.
6. Griffith, A. *Therapist's Management of the Stiff Elbow.* In Callahan, A.D., Osterman, A.L., Mackin, E.J., Skirven, T.M., Schneider, L.H. (Eds). *Rehabilitation of the Hand and Upper Extremity*, 5th ed. Mosby, St. Louis, 2002, pp. 1245–1262.
7. McKee, M., Bowden, M.D., King, G.J., Patterson, S.D., Jupiter, J.B., Bamberger, H.B., Paksima, N. *Management of Recurrent Complex Instability of the Elbow with Hinged External Fixation.* J Bone Joint Surg 1998;80B:1031.

11

Distal Radius Fractures

COLEEN T. GATELY, PT, DPT, MS

Epidemiological studies indicate that distal radius fractures are the most common fractures of the forearm.[1,2] The mechanism of injury usually involves a fall on an outstretched hand (FOOSH). Distal radius fractures resulting from this type of low energy injury are more common than those sustained secondary to high energy trauma, such as a motor vehicle accident.[3] The incidence of distal radius fractures in the 35- to 64-year-old population is greater in women than men.[4]

SURGICAL OVERVIEW

The distal radius articulates with the ulna and proximal row of carpal bones. The radius, ulna, and carpal bones make up the wrist complex. The medical management of distal radius fractures varies depending on the extent of the injury. Common procedures include closed reduction with casting, closed reduction with external fixation (CREF), percutaneous pinning, open reduction with internal fixation (ORIF), or any combination of these techniques.[5] Reduction may be combined with a graft, depending on the level of comminution or defect. The goal of reduction is to maintain the bone in alignment so that the fracture may heal properly.

REHABILITATION OVERVIEW

As the fracture progresses through the phases of healing, the focus of rehabilitation is to help the patient regain functional use of the hand and upper extremity. The stability of the fracture, strength of fixation, and extent of soft tissue trauma will determine the progression of therapy in each phase of healing. Direct communication with the doctor is essential to define precautions and set realistic goals. Treatment is tailored to the specific needs of the patient and the type of fixation used.

POSTOPERATIVE PHASE I: PROTECTIVE (WEEKS 0 TO 6)

The goals of phase I include maintaining correct protective immobilization, minimizing edema and pain, and maintaining full range of motion (ROM) of the uninvolved joints. Edema is addressed during the first therapy visit. Excess edema can damage the uninjured cells of surrounding tissues and delay healing time.[6,7] The principle of "rest, ice, compression, and elevation" (RICE) is reviewed. In addition, patients may be instructed in retrograde massage and use of compression wraps, such a Coban, Tubigrip stockinette, and Isotoner gloves. Active overhead fisting has been found to assist in the reduction of edema.[8,9]

Active range of motion (AROM) of the uninvolved joints—fingers, elbow, forearm, and shoulder—begins

immediately post-surgery. Distal radial ulnar joint (DRUJ) stability must be confirmed before the initiation of forearm AROM. Patients are encouraged to use their uninvolved joints for light, functional activities to decrease the risk of arthrofibrosis, which may result from immobility.[6,7]

Patients with external fixators or protruding Kirschner's wires are instructed in pin care to reduce the risk of infection. The use of a solution of hydrogen peroxide and sterile water (1 : 1 ratio) to clean the pin sites, two times per day, has been advocated.[10]

The postoperative dressing is removed within 1 to 2 weeks and replaced with a thermoplastic volar or bivalve wrist splint. The wrist is positioned in 0 to 20 degrees of wrist extension. The thenar crease and distal palmar crease are cleared to allow full thumb and digit ROM (Figure 11-1). Patients with stable fixation (ORIF) may begin AROM during the second postoperative week. The thermoplastic splint is removed for wrist and forearm AROM exercises.

Troubleshooting

A stiff shoulder and hand is a common complication of distal radius fractures. Joint stiffness is often a result of immobilization, trauma, and guarding of the injured extremity.[11-14] Participation in light, functional activities is encouraged to avoid stiffness. Special attention must

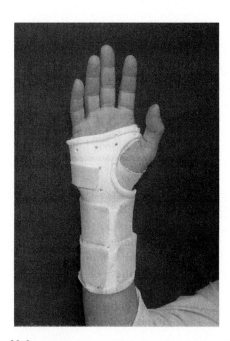

FIGURE 11-1 Custom thermoplastic volar: 0- to 20-degree wrist extension; thenar crease and distal palmar crease are cleared to prevent thumb web space and metacarpophalangeal joint stiffness.

be given to the digits and thumbs of distal radius fractures that are treated by external fixation. Flexor and extensor tendon adhesions may develop. Tendon gliding exercises (see Figures 14-18 through 14-20) are provided to encourage differential gliding of the flexor digitorum superficialis (FDS) and flexor digitorum profundus (FDP) tendons. Extensor digitorum communis (EDC) glides are also performed to encourage isolated digit extension and address intrinsic tendon shortening. Flexion gloves can be used to increase passive metacar-pophalangeal and interphalangeal joint flexion. If extrinsic flexor tightness is present, a static resting extension splint is provided for night use. The splint can be gradually remolded to increase extension over time. Pain that is extreme in nature and accompanied with unresolved joint stiffness, swelling, hypersensitivity, and shiny skin may indicate early signs of complex regional pain syndrome (CRPS).[15] Any unusual symptoms noted should be reported immediately to the referring surgeon.

Postoperative Phase I: Protective (Weeks 0 to 6)

GOALS

- Maintain correct protective immobilization
- Minimize edema and pain
- Maintain full ROM of uninvolved joints

PRECAUTIONS

- Obtain MD approval before beginning gentle forearm AROM
- Early motion of the shoulder is critical to prevent adhesive capsulitis
- Report early symptoms of CRPS to MD for early intervention

TREATMENT STRATEGIES
Protection Options

- Custom thermoplastic volar or bivalve wrist splint: 0- to 20-degree wrist extension; thenar crease and distal palmar crease are cleared to prevent thumb web space and metacarpophalangeal joint stiffness (Figure 11-1)

Pin and Wound Care (for CREF, ORIF)

- Pin care regimens may vary: Follow MD's specific protocol, for some may not request pin care at all (50% H_2O_2 and sterile water two times per day)
- Standard wound care procedures are followed for ORIF

Edema/Pain Management

- Elevation, rest, ice/cold, compression
- Light, compressive garment or wrap, that is, Isotoner gloves, Coban, Tubigrip stockinette
- Active overhead fisting

Uninvolved Joints ROM

- Tendon gliding exercises
- Hand intrinsic muscle exercises: lumbrical, interossei, thenar, and hypothenar muscles
- Differential tendon gliding exercises to prevent tendon adherence to the fracture site, hardware, or pins, that is, FDS, FDP, EPL, FPL
- Elbow, shoulder ROM is initiated on postoperative day 1
- Gentle forearm rotation in a pain-free range with MD approval (Figure 11-2)

Involved Joint ROM (for Stable/Rigid Fixation)

- Gentle wrist ROM: wrist flexion/extension, radial/ulnar deviation

CRITERIA FOR ADVANCEMENT

- Clinical union at fracture site or stability via surgical fixation

POSTOPERATIVE PHASE II: STABILITY (WEEKS 6 TO 8)

Progression to phase II occurs when either clinical union at the fracture site or stability through surgical fixation is achieved. The time frame can vary from 1 to 8 weeks, depending on the extent of the fracture and type of fixation used. Goals from the previous phase continue to be addressed. In cases in which the wrist has been completely immobilized, when the cast or fixator is removed, the custom thermoplastic splint described previously is fabricated and gentle, active wrist ROM may commence.

ROM exercises are progressed as follows. Gentle, active wrist and forearm exercises are allowed when clinical union or stability through fixation is achieved. This is followed by active-assisted range of motion (AAROM). As the bone callus forms and strengthens the fracture site, passive motion and stretching is allowed. Clearance should be obtained from the surgeon before assuming passive motion.

Scar management is initiated when the incisions are closed and healed. This will include manual massage to the scar. Silicone gel sheeting (Figure 11-3), such as Cica-Care and Mepiform, has been found to prevent and improve hypertrophic and keloid scars.[16-22] It is believed that through compression and hydration the scar becomes soft and flexible.[23] This theory has not been confirmed by prospective, randomized clinical trials.[24]

Troubleshooting

Restoration of wrist and forearm ROM is crucial during phase II. Although aggressive passive range of motion (PROM) and splinting techniques may be used during phase III to achieve further gains in motion, the greatest gains in motion can occur in phase II. Therapeutic interventions focus on restoring ROM with an emphasis on function. Several studies define functional forearm ROM as 50-degree pronation and 50-degree supination, wrist extension 30 to 45 degrees, wrist flexion 5 to 40 degrees, and radial and ulnar deviation as an arc of 20 to 40 degrees.[25-27] Hume et al[28] reported functional ROM of the fingers to be metacarpophalangeal joints, 61 degrees; proximal interphalangeal joints, 60 degrees; distal interphalangeal joints, 39 degrees; thumb metacarpophalangeal joints, 21 degrees; and the interphalangeal joints, 18 degrees.

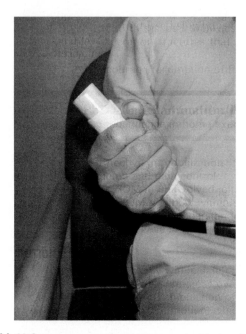

FIGURE **11-2** Forearm rotation is performed with the elbow in 90 degrees and the humerus close to the body to prevent substitution with shoulder rotation.

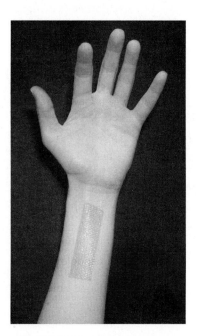

FIGURE **11-3** Silicone gel sheet.

Postoperative Phase II: Stability (Weeks 6 to 8)

Note: Phase II may begin as early as postoperative week 2, if fracture stability is achieved through ORIF

GOALS

- Maximize ROM of the wrist and forearm in a pain-free range
- Restore light, functional use of the involved extremity
- Continue phase I goals as needed

PRECAUTIONS

- Fracture stability must be obtained through bony healing or surgical fixation before initiating wrist ROM or gentle joint mobilization techniques.

TREATMENT STRATEGIES
Protection Options

- Custom thermoplastic volar or bivalve wrist splint: remove for wound and skin care
- Splint is weaned based on fracture stability and bony healing, and following MD's orders.
- External fixator is removed; splinting may be necessary to allow further protection with gradual weaning.

SCAR MANAGEMENT

- Scar massage and silicone gel sheeting may be initiated once the wound is fully healed (to avoid infection).

EDEMA/PAIN MANAGEMENT

- Cold pack
- Retrograde massage
- Gentle heat or contrast baths may be used as edema becomes brawny.
- Light, compressive garment or wrap, that is, Isotoner gloves, Coban, and Tubigrip stockinette

AROM WRIST AND FOREARM

- Initiation of wrist and forearm AROM and gentle AAROM
- Isolated wrist extension exercises are begun early to prevent assistance of the long finger extensors in wrist extension and promote a more functional grip.
- Forearm rotation is performed with the elbow in 90 degrees and the humerus close to the body to prevent substitution with shoulder rotation (Figure 11-3).
- Gentle distraction and grades I and II joint mobilizations may be initiated in this phase if fracture stability allows.

LIGHT FUNCTIONAL ACTIVITIES

- Fine motor coordination activities, that is, small object manipulation, writing, and typing
- Restoration of normal movement patterns and ADL, such as eating, dressing, hygiene

CRITERIA FOR ADVANCEMENT

- Evidence of radiographic union or determination by MD of ability of fracture to withstand resistance/stress

POSTOPERATIVE PHASE III: FRACTURE CONSOLIDATION (WEEKS 8 TO 12)

Treatment is progressed to phase III when the fracture is able to withstand stress and resistance. This happens usually by 8 to 12 weeks. The physician determines this based on radiographic union. Passive stretching techniques and joint mobilization are added to achieve maximum ROM. In addition, progressive strengthening to achieve return to function, work, and sport can begin.

Troubleshooting

Distal radial ulnar joint stiffness and limited wrist ROM are common complications of distal radius fractures. When motion does not improve, low-load, prolonged stretching accomplished by serial splinting can be used to improve PROM.[27-31] Some examples include serial static dorsal wrist extension splint (Figure 11-4), static progressive wrist splint, and static progressive pronation/supination splint.

Postoperative Phase III: Fracture Consolidation (Weeks 8 to 12)

GOALS

- Restore strength for return to functional activities and work
- Continue phase II goals as needed

PRECAUTIONS

- Progress strengthening exercises gradually, avoiding pain and compensations

TREATMENT STRATEGIES

PROM and Splinting

- PROM
  - Examples: prayer stretch
- Stretching
- Joint mobilization to achieve end range potential
- Serial static and static progressive splints to achieve end range potential
- Examples: serial static dorsal wrist extension splint, static progressive wrist splint, and static progressive pronation/supination splint

Strengthening

- Isometric and dynamic grip and pinch strengthening
  - Examples: putty, hand-helper, BTE PRIMUS, Biometrics Ltd. ULE
- Wrist and forearm PREs
  - Examples: gradual progression from weight well to Thera-Band to free weights
- Work conditioning: activity-specific functional activities, BTE
- Return to sport

CRITERIA FOR DISCHARGE

- Restoration of functional AROM and strength, and return to prior ADL, including work
- Independence in home exercise program

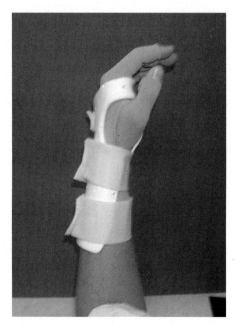

FIGURE **11-4** Static progressive dorsal wrist extension splint.

REFERENCES

1. Alffram, P.A., Bauer, G.C. *Epidemiology of Fracture of the Forearm: A Biomechanical Investigation of Bone Strength.* J Bone Joint Surg 1962;44A:105.
2. Benger, U., Johnell, O. *Increasing Incidence of Forearm Fractures: A Comparison of Epidemiologic Patterns 25 Years Apart.* Acta Orthop Scand 1985;56:158.
3. Melton, L.J. III, Amadio, P.C., Crowson, C.S., O'Fallon, W.M. *Long-term Trends in the Incidence of Distal Forearm Fractures.* Osteoporos Int 1998;4(8):341–348.
4. Owen, R.A., Melton, L.J. III, Johnson, K.A., Ilstrup, D.M., Riggs, B.L. *Incidence of Colles' Fracture in North American Community.* Am J Public Health 1982;72:605–607.
5. Seitz, W.H. Jr., Froimson, A.I. *Reduction of Treatment Related Complications in the External Fixation of Complex Distal Radius Fractures.* Orthop Rev 1991;2:169–177.
6. Flowers, K.R. Edema: Differential Management Based on Stages of Wound Healing. In Hunter, J.M., Mackin, E.J., Callahan, A.D. (Eds). *Rehabilitation of the Hand*, 4th ed. Mosby, St. Louis, 1995, pp. 87–91.
7. Hunter, J., Mackin, E.J., Callahan, A.D. Edema: Techniques of Evaluation and Management. In Hunter, J., (Eds). *Rehabilitation of the Hand*, 4th ed. Mosby, St. Louis, 1995, pp. 77–85.
8. Buncke, H.J., Jackson, R.L., Buncke, G.M. Surgical and Rehabilitative Aspects of Replantation and Revascularization of

the Hand. In Hunter, J.M., Schneider, L.H., Mackin, E.J., Callahan, A.D. (Eds). *Rehabilitation of the Hand: Surgery and Therapy*, 4th ed. Mosby, St. Louis, 1995, p. 1075.

9. Sorenson, M.K. *The Edematous Hand.* Phys Ther 1989;69:1059.

10. Leibovic, S.J. *Bone and Joint Injury in the Hand: Surgeon's Perspective.* J Hand Ther 1999;2(12):111–120.

11. Salter, R.B. *The Biological Concept of Continuous Passive Motion of Synovial Joints. The First Eighteen Years of Basic Research and its Clinical Implications.* Clin Orthop 1989;242:12–24.

12. Culav, E.M., Clark, C.H., Merrilees, M.J. *Connective Tissues: Matrix Composition and Its Relevance to Physical Therapy.* Phys Ther 1999;79:308–319.

13. Sapega, A.A., Quedenfeld, T.C., Moyer, R.A., Butler, R.A. *Biophysical Factors in Range-of-motion Exercise.* Physician Sports Med 1981;9(12):57–61.

14. De Deyne, P.G. Application of Passive Stretch and its Implications for Muscle Fibers. Phys Ther 2001;81:821–822.

15. Laulan, J., Bismuth, J.P., Sicre, G. *The Different Types of Algodystrophy after Fractures of the Distal Radius: Predictive Criteria after 1 Year.* J Hand Surg 1997;22B:441.

16. Ahn, S.T., Monafo, W.W., Mustoe, T.A. *Topical Silicone Gel for the Prevention and Treatment of Hypertrophic Scars.* Arch Surg 1991;126:499–504.

17. Ahn, S.T., Monafo, W.W., Mustoe, T.A. *Topical Silicone Gel: A New Treatment for Hypertrophic Scars.* Surgery 1989;106:781–787.

18. Quinn, K.J. *Silicone Gel in Scar Treatment.* Burns 1987;13:S33–S40.

19. Gibbons, M., Zuker, R., Brown, M., Candlish, S., Snider, L., Zimmer, P. *Experience with Silastic Gel Sheeting in Pediatric Scarring.* J Burn Care Rehabil 1994;15(1):69–73.

20. Carney, S.A., Cason, C.G., Gowar, J.P., Stevenson, J.H., McNee, J., Groves, A.R., Thomas, S.S., Hart, N.B., Auclair, P. *Cica-Care Gel Sheeting in the Management of Hypertrophic Scarring.* Burns 1994;20(2):163–167.

21. Sherris, D.A., Larrabee, W.F. Jr., Murakami, C.S. *Management of Scar Contractures, Hypertrophic Scars, and Keloid.* Otolaryngol Clin North Am 1995;28(5):1057–1068.

22. Tilkorn, H., Ernst, K., Osterhaus, A., Schubert, A., Schwipper, V. *The Protruding Scars: Keloids and Hypertrophic Diagnosis and Treatment with Silicon-gel-sheeting.* Polym Med 1994;24(1–2):31–44.

23. Fulton, J.E. Jr. *Silicone Gel Sheeting for the Prevention and Management of Evolving Hypertrophic and Keloid Scars.* Dermatol Surg 1995;21:947–951.

24. Shaffer, J.J., Taylor, S.C., Cook-Bolden, F. *Keloidal Scars: A Review with a Critical Look at Therapeutic Options.* J Am Acad Dermatol 2002;46(2):S63–S97.

25. Palmer, A.K., Werner, F.W., Murphy, D., Glisson, R. *Functional Wrist Motion: A Biomechanical Study.* J Hand Surg 1985;10A(1):39–46.

26. Ryu, J., Cooney, W.P., Askew, L.J., An, K.N., Chao, E.Y. *Functional Ranges of Motion and the Wrist Joint.* J Hand Surg 1991;16A(3):409–419.

27. Gartland, J.J., Werley, C.W. *Evaluation of Healed Colles' Fracture.* J Bone Joint Surg 1951;33A:895.

28. Hume, M.C., Gellman, H., McKellop, H., Brumfield, R.H. *Functional Range of Motion of the Joints of the Hand.* J Hand Surg 1990;15A:240.

29. Mullen, T.M. *Static Progressive Splint to Increase Wrist Extension or Flexion.* J Hand Ther 2000;13:313–314.

30. Lucas, S. Splinting the Stiff Wrist. In Skirven, T., Raphael, J. (Eds). *Contractures and Splinting. Atlas of the Hand Clinics.* WB Saunders, Philadelphia, 2001.

31. Schindeler-Grasse, P., Paynter, P. Splinting for Thumb Contractures. In Skirven, T., Raphael, J. (Eds). *Contractures and Splinting. Atlas of the Hand Clinics.* WB Saunders, Philadelphia, 2001.

12

Scaphoid Fractures

COLEEN T. GATELY, PT, DPT, MS

Of the eight carpal bones, the scaphoid is the most frequently fractured[1-3] (Figure 12-1). Seventy-nine percent of all carpal fractures are scaphoid fractures.[4] The mechanism of injury involves a high impact fall on an outstretched hand (FOOSH), with the wrist hyperextended and radially deviated.[5] Scaphoid fractures are more common in young or active individuals and frequently result from contact sports.

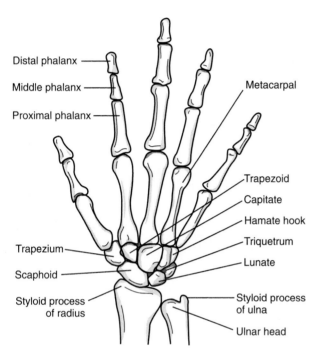

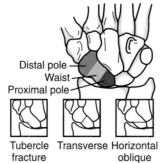

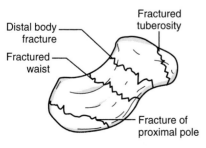

FIGURE **12-1** The scaphoid is the most commonly injured of the carpal bones. *(From Thibodeau, G.A., Patton, K.T. Anatomy & Physiology, 5th ed. Mosby, St. Louis, 2003, p. 240.)*

SURGICAL OVERVIEW

The scaphoid is divided anatomically into four parts: the proximal pole, waist, distal pole, and tuberosity (Figure 12-2). The majority of scaphoid fractures occur through the waist (70%), followed by the proximal pole (20%), with the least occurring at the distal pole (10%).[6,7] Although 90% to 95% of scaphoid fractures will heal if treated adequately with immobilization, 5% to 10% result in a nonunion.[6,8]

Reduction of scaphoid fractures can be accomplished via several means, depending on the nature of the fracture. Immobilization in a cast is appropriate for a nondisplaced fracture. Fractures that are minimally displaced may be treated with closed reduction and percutaneous pinning (CRPP). Open reduction with internal fixation (ORIF) is performed for displaced fractures.[6,8] Internal fixation options include Kirschner's wires, cannulated screws, or plating.

The distal pole of the scaphoid has a rich blood supply in comparison to the proximal pole (Figure 12-3). Fractures at the scaphoid waist can disrupt the blood supply to the proximal pole and contribute to avascular necrosis, delayed union, or nonunion.[3,9-13] Because of the poor blood supply, proximal pole scaphoid fractures take between 12 and 14 weeks to heal and require prolonged immobilization. Therefore, ORIF with a cannulated screw is commonly used to allow for early mobilization even when adequate reduction can be achieved with a closed manipulation.[9,14-16] Surgery may take place through a volar or dorsal approach.[17-19] A cannulated screw inserted into a threaded washer provides compression across the fracture site to provide stability as it heals (Figure 12-4). A nonvascularized or vascularized bone graft may be used for complex fractures to accelerate bone healing. Bone healing may also be facilitated by using an electrical bone growth stimulator.[20-22] The following guidelines have been developed for scaphoid fractures that have been reduced through ORIF.

REHABILITATION OVERVIEW

The amount of surgical stability achieved, as well as the location of the scaphoid fracture, determine the rate of progression of therapy in each phase of healing. Direct communication with the doctor is essential to determine the location and stability of the fracture for appropriate therapeutic progression.

FIGURE **12-2** The scaphoid is commonly divided into four parts: proximal pole, waist, distal pole, and tuberosity.

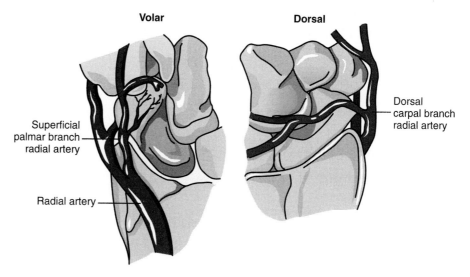

FIGURE **12-3** The distal pole of the scaphoid has a rich blood supply in comparison to its proximal pole. *(From Green, D.P., Hotchkiss, R.N., Pederson, W.C. Green's Operative Hand Surgery, 4th ed. Churchill Livingstone, New York, 1999, p. 810.)*

Volar

Dorsal

Superficial palmar branch radial artery

Radial artery

Dorsal carpal branch radial artery

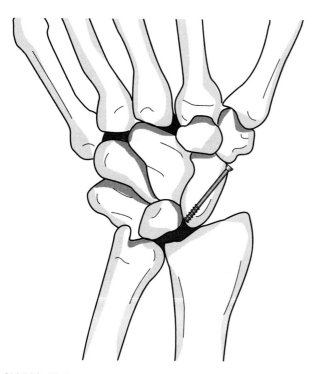

FIGURE **12-4** A cannulated screw may be used to fixate the fractured scaphoid.

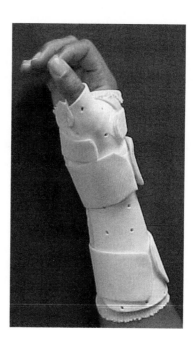

FIGURE **12-5** A forearm thumb spica splint with 0- to 20-degree wrist extension, with the thumb immobilized and the IP joint free.

POSTOPERATIVE PHASE I: PROTECTIVE (WEEKS 0 TO 4)

While maintaining correct protective immobilization, the goals of phase I include minimizing edema and pain and maintaining full range of motion (ROM) of uninvolved joints. When the postoperative dressing is removed within 2 to 4 weeks, a custom thermoplastic volar or bivalve forearm thumb spica splint is molded

with the wrist in 0 to 20 degrees of extension and the thumb in functional opposition. The interphalangeal (IP) joint of the thumb is free (Figure 12-5). At the first therapy visit, the patient is instructed in edema control. Edema control and wound care follow standard procedures, as described previously in this book. Active range of motion (AROM) to the uninvolved joints of the fingers, elbow, forearm, and shoulder begins immediately post-surgery. Forearm ROM is

Postoperative Phase I: Protective (Weeks 0 to 4)

GOALS
- Correct protective immobilization
- Edema and pain control
- Full ROM of uninvolved joints

PRECAUTIONS
- Early motion of the shoulder is critical to prevent adhesive capsulitis.

TREATMENT STRATEGIES
Protective Immobilization
- Custom thermoplastic volar or bivalve forearm thumb spica splint: 0- to 20-degree wrist extension and thumb immobilized with IP joint free

Wound Care
- Standard wound care procedures are followed for ORIF.

Edema/Pain Management
- Elevation, rest, ice/cold
- Light, compressive garment or wrap, that is, Coban, Isotoner gloves, and Tubigrip stockinette

ROM of Uninvolved Joints
- Differential tendon gliding exercises, that is, FPL, EDC, FDS, FDP
- Hand intrinsic muscle exercises, that is, interossei
- Elbow, forearm, and shoulder ROM exercises initiated postoperative day 1

CRITERIA FOR ADVANCEMENT
- Clinical union at fracture site or stability via surgical fixation

emphasized to prevent stiffness in forearm rotation. Patients are encouraged to use their uninvolved joints for light, functional activities within the limits of the forearm based thumb spica splint. Resistive activities are avoided.

Troubleshooting

Stiffness of the uninvolved digits is a common occurrence post-surgery. This is partially the result of edema and immobilization and partially the result of the development of tendon adhesions beneath the incision. It is not uncommon to see index flexor digitorum profundus (FDP) and thumb flexor pollicis longus (FPL) adherence following a volar approach. Likewise, index extensor digitorum communis (EDC) adhesions are common with a dorsal approach. To minimize adhesion formation, differential tendon gliding exercises are performed.

POSTOPERATIVE PHASE II: STABILITY (WEEKS 4 TO 16)

Clinical union at the fracture site or stability through surgical fixation will dictate when phase II in the reha-

bilitation program can begin. This may be as early as 4 to 6 weeks post-surgery or as late as 16 weeks. Goals from the previous phase continue to be addressed. Initiation of AROM to the wrist and thumb is physician-directed. Active-assisted range of motion (AAROM) and passive range of motion (PROM) begin a week after the initiation of AROM. Graded strengthening exercises are introduced 3 to 4 weeks later.[23] Patients are instructed to remove their protective splint throughout the day to perform ROM exercises. If swelling persists, contrast baths are added at this time. Scar management for the incision follows standard procedure, as described elsewhere in this book.

Troubleshooting

Limited wrist and thumb ROM is a common complication during this phase. Heat has been shown to promote muscle relaxation and is used before exercise.[24] Appropriate heat modalities include fluidotherapy, paraffin, and moist hot packs. Application of heat is followed by gentle passive stretching. As the fracture heals and becomes stable, prolonged stretching is introduced. See later section on troubleshooting in phase III.

Postoperative Phase II: Stability (Weeks 4 to 16)

GOALS

- Maximize ROM of the forearm, wrist, and hand in a pain-free range
- Restore light, functional use of the involved extremity
- Continue phase I goals as needed

PRECAUTIONS

- Fracture stability must be obtained through bony healing or surgical fixation before initiating wrist ROM or gentle joint mobilization techniques.

TREATMENT STRATEGIES

Protection Options

- Thumb spica forearm splint is continued.

Scar Management

- Scar massage and silicone gel sheeting is initiated once the wound is fully healed (to avoid infection).

Edema/Pain Management

- Cold pack
- Retrograde massage
- Gentle heat or contrast baths may be used if edema becomes brawny.

AROM Wrist

- Initiation of thumb ROM: opposition, MP flexion, abduction
- Initiation of wrist and forearm AROM: wrist flexion/extension, radial/ulnar deviation
- Progression to AAROM and gentle PROM
- To promote a more functional grip, isolated wrist extension exercises are begun early to prevent assistance of the long finger extensors in wrist extension.

Light, Functional Activities

- Fine motor coordination activities to promote thumb opposition: small object manipulation, writing, typing
- Restoration of normal movement patterns and return to ADL: eating, dressing, hygiene

CRITERIA FOR ADVANCEMENT

- Evidence of radiographic union or determination by MD of ability of fracture to withstand resistance/stress

POSTOPERATIVE PHASE III: FRACTURE CONSOLIDATION (WEEKS 8 TO 21)

The ability of the fracture to withstand stress and resistance marks the beginning of phase III. This may begin as early as 8 weeks or as late as 21 weeks. The physician will clear the patient for progression in therapy, based upon radiographic union. If the treating physician is confident in fracture consolidation, gentle grade I and II mobilizations are performed to facilitate the desired motion. To achieve end ROM, mobilization is progressed to grades III and IV.[25] Progressive strengthening begins to prepare the patient to return to function, work, and sports. Pinch strength is particularly weak and requires attention. Graded pinching exercises are performed in treatment and added to the home program. Activities, such as putty pinching, clothespins, and a Thumbicizer™, are used to strengthen lateral and the three-point pinch. Patients returning to sports or high levels of physical activity are provided with a transitional protective splint. A wrist guard or a small thumb splint ("cone splint") (Figure 12-6) is used upon initial return to high impact sports.

Troubleshooting

Joint limitations that persist are treated with serial static or static progressive splints that use "low load prolonged stretch" principles.[26-28] Static progressive thumb flexion/opposition splinting and serial static wrist splinting may be necessary to achieve ROM. The continuous passive motion (CPM) mode of the BTE PRIMUS is a useful tool to achieve wrist ROM.

Postoperative Phase III: Fracture Consolidation (Weeks 8 to 21)

GOALS

- Restore strength for return to functional activities and work
- Continue phase II goals as needed

PRECAUTIONS

- Progress strengthening exercises gradually, avoiding pain and compensatory motion

TREATMENT STRATEGIES

PROM and Splinting

- PROM, stretching, and joint mobilization to achieve end range potential
- Serial static and static progressive splints to achieve end range potential
- Examples: static progressive wrist flexion or extension splint

Strengthening

- Isometric and dynamic grip and pinch strengthening: putty, hand-helper, BTE PRIMUS, and Biometrics Ltd. ULE
- Wrist and forearm PREs: dumbbells, weight well, Thera-Band
- Work conditioning: activity-specific training and BTE PRIMUS

CRITERIA FOR DISCHARGE

- Restoration of functional AROM and strength and return to prior level of function
- Independence in home exercise program

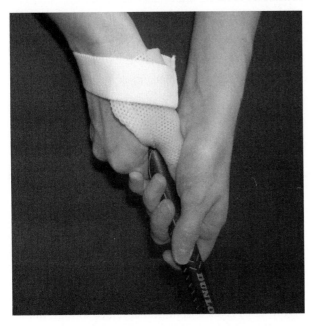

FIGURE **12-6** A thumb splint ("cone splint").

REFERENCES

1. Dunn, A.W. *Fractures and Dislocations of the Carpus.* Surg Clin North Am 1972;52:1513–1538.
2. Lichtman, D.M., Alexander, C.E. *Decision Making in Scaphoid Nonunion.* Orthop Rev 1982;11:55–67.
3. Osterman, A.L., Mikulics, M. *Scaphoid Nonunion.* Hand Clin 1988;14:437–455.
4. Amadio, P.C. *Scaphoid Fractures.* Clin Orthop North Am 1992;23:7–17.
5. Weber, E.R., Chao, E.Y. *An Experimental Approach to the Mechanism of Scaphoid Waist Fractures.* J Hand Surg 1978; 3A:142.
6. Herndon, J.H. *Scaphoid Fractures and Complications.* American Academy of Orthopaedic Surgeons, Rosemont, IL, 1994.
7. Schaefer, M., Siebert, H.R. *Fractures of the Semilunar Bone.* Unfallchirurg 2002;105:540–552.
8. Taleisnik, J. Fracture of the Carpal Bones. In Green, D.P. (Ed). *Operative Hand Surgery,* 2nd ed. Churchill Livingstone, New York, 1988.
9. Weber, E.R. *Biomechanical Implications of Scaphoid Waist Fractures.* Clin Orthop Relat Res 1980;149:83–89.
10. Obletz, B.E., Halbstein, B.M. *Non-union of Fractures of the Carpal Navicular.* J Bone Joint Surg 1938;20:424–428.
11. Gelberman, R.H., Menon, J. *The Vascularity of the Scaphoid Bone.* J Hand Surg 1980;5:508–513.
12. Gelberman, R.H., Gross, M.S. *The Vascularity of the Wrist. Identification of Arterial Patterns at Risk.* Clin Orthop Relat Res 1986;202:40–49.
13. Melone, C.P. *Scaphoid Fractures: Concepts of Management.* Clin Plast Surg 1981;8:83–94.
14. dos Reis, F.B., Koeberle, G., Leite, N.M., Katchburian, M.V. *Internal Fixation of Scaphoid Injuries Using the Herbert Screw Through a Dorsal Approach.* J Hand Surg 1993;8A: 792–797.
15. O'Brien, L., Herbert, T. *Internal Fixation of Acute Scaphoid Fracture: A New Approach to Treatment.* Aust N Z J Surg 1985; 55:387–389.
16. Rettig, M.E., Raskin, K.B. *Retrograde Compression Screw Fixation of Acute Proximal Pole Scaphoid Fractures.* J Hand Ther 1999;24A:1206–1210.

17. Watson, H.K., Pitts, E.C., Ashmead, D. IV, Makhlouf, M.V., Kauer, J. *Dorsal Approach to Scaphoid Nonunion.* J Hand Surg 1993;18(2):359–365.

18. Herbert, T.J. *Open Volar Repair of Acute Scaphoid Fractures.* Hand Clin 2001;17(4):589–599.

19. Herbert, T.J., Fisher, W.E. *Management of the Fractured Scaphoid Using a New Bone Screw.* J Bone Joint Surg 1984;66(1):114–123.

20. Albert, S.F. *Electrical Stimulation of Bone Repair.* Clin Podiatr Med Surg 1981;8(4):923–935.

21. Bora, F.W. Jr. *Treatment of Nonunion of the Scaphoid by Direct Current.* Orthop Clin North Am 1984;15(1):107–112.

22. Dunn, A.W. *Electrical Stimulation in Treatment of Delayed Union and Nonunion of Fractures and Osteotomies.* South Med J 1984;77(12):1530–1534.

23. "Diagnosis and Treatment Manual for Physicians and Therapists." CD-ROM. The Hand Rehabilitation Center of Indiana, Indiana, 2001.

24. Hayes, K.W. *Manual for Physical Agents.* Appleton & Lange, Norwalk, CT, 1993.

25. Maitland, G.D. *Peripheral Manipulation,* 2nd ed. Butterworth, Boston, 1977.

26. Mullen, T.M. *Static Progressive Splint to Increase Wrist Extension or Flexion.* J Hand Ther 2000;13:313–314.

27. Lucas, S. Splinting the Stiff Wrist. In Skirven, T., Raphael, J. (Eds). *Contractures and Splinting. Atlas of the Hand Clinics.* WB Saunders, Philadelphia, 2001;6(1):77–106.

28. Schindeler-Grasse, P., Paynter, P. Splinting for Thumb Contractures. In Skirven, T., Raphael, J. (Eds). *Contractures and Splinting. Atlas of the Hand Clinics.* WB Saunders, Philadelphia, 2001;6(1):165–188.

13

Phalangeal and Metacarpal Fractures

CAROL PAGE, PT, DPT, CHT

Phalangeal and metacarpal fractures are among the most common fractures of the upper extremity. Chung[1] reported that of all hand and forearm fractures reported in the United States in 1998, 23% were phalangeal and 18% were metacarpal. The highest rate of phalangeal fractures was in individuals age 85 and older. The highest rate of metacarpal fractures was found in 15- to 24-year-olds.

ANATOMICAL AND SURGICAL OVERVIEW

The method of fracture management indicated depends on several variables, including fracture location, configuration, stability, whether the fracture is open or closed, and whether there are associated injuries. The primary goal is proper bony alignment with adequate stability for safe, early motion, and restoration of hand function. Many phalangeal and metacarpal fractures are stable and can be treated with protective splinting and early mobilization.[2] Unstable shaft fractures and many articular fractures require fixation to restore stability.[3] Options for surgical fixation of unstable fractures include percutaneous pinning or open reduction with Kirschner's pin fixation, circumferential wiring, intramedullary fixation, compression screws, plate fixation, and external fixation.

Distal phalanx fractures are the most common fractures in the hand.[4] Tuft fractures and nondisplaced, stable fractures of the shaft are managed with extension splinting of the distal interphalangeal (DIP) joint for 3 weeks.[5] Displaced, transverse shaft fractures require fixation with a Kirschner's pin or screw. Injury to the nail matrix often occurs with open, displaced, transverse shaft fractures and with tuft fractures associated with crush injury. Intra-articular fractures of the distal phalanx usually include avulsion of the extensor tendon insertion at the dorsal base (mallet injury), or of the flexor digitorum profundus (FDP) insertion at the volar base.[3] FDP avulsion injuries require surgical fixation, whereas mallet injuries do not, unless there is evidence of volar subluxation of the distal phalanx.[6]

Metacarpal neck fractures most frequently occur in the ring and small fingers. This common fracture, known as a boxer's fracture, occurs from striking a solid object with a closed fist. Metacarpal shaft fractures result from direct impact or axial loading through the metacarpal head. Metacarpal neck and shaft fractures that are stable are treated with closed reduction and immobilization. Fractures that are unstable, angulated, malrotated, open, or involve multiple metacarpals require surgical fixation.[3]

Phalangeal fractures of the thumb are treated similarly to those of the fingers. Surgery to restore stability is indicated for avulsion fractures with disruption of the ulnar collateral ligament (UCL) at the base of the proximal phalanx. Extra-articular and intra-articular fractures of the base of the thumb proximal phalanx are more common than metacarpal shaft fractures. Extra-articular base fractures are treated with closed reduction, with the addition of percutaneous pinning, if required to maintain the reduction. Fracture subluxation of the thumb metacarpal base, known as a Bennett's fracture, occurs with axial loading of the partially flexed thumb metacarpal.[7] Treatment ranges from nonoperative management to closed or open surgical fixation.[3]

REHABILITATION OVERVIEW

The primary goal of rehabilitation of metacarpal and phalangeal fractures is to restore motion, strength, and functional use of the hand. For therapy to be progressed in a safe and timely manner, ongoing communication between the surgeon and therapist regarding the degree of stability and fracture healing is essential. Awareness of common complications facilitates early recognition and intervention. Complications of phalangeal and metacarpal fractures include malunion, nonunion, tendon adhesions, capsular contracture, and infection.[3]

The treatment guidelines that follow specifically address the postoperative management of fractures of the proximal and middle phalangeal shaft, metacarpal neck and shaft, and thumb metacarpal base. These guidelines may be used for fractures managed nonoperatively, with the time frames extended to allow for adequate stability via bony healing.

Treatment of distal phalanx fractures that involve the disruption of the flexor or extensor tendons follows tendon management guidelines (see Chapters 14 and 15). Postoperative management of proximal interphalangeal (PIP) joint injuries, PIP joint arthroplasty, boutonniere reconstruction, and thumb UCL injuries are discussed elsewhere in this book.

POSTOPERATIVE PHASE I: INFLAMMATION/ PROTECTION (WEEK 1)

Following surgical fixation of phalangeal and metacarpal fractures, acute postoperative inflammation is managed with strict elevation and immobilization in a bulky splint. Referral to outpatient therapy occurs on postoperative day 5, or as soon as the acute inflammation begins to subside. The patient is evaluated, fitted with a custom-molded splint, and instructed in a home program of edema control, pin and wound care, and motion exercises of the uninvolved joints.

A custom-molded, thermoplastic splint is fabricated to immobilize the joint below and above the fracture. The adjoining digit or digits are included. Splints are designed to accommodate and protect pins or external fixation devices. Middle and proximal phalanx shaft

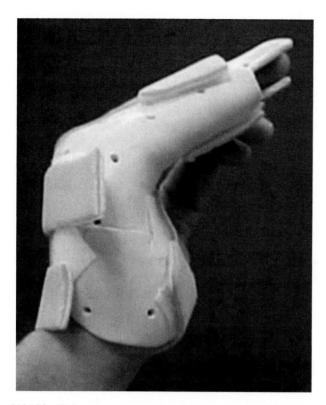

FIGURE **13-1** Hand-based ulnar gutter splint for protective immobilization following fractures of the middle, ring, and small proximal and middle phalanges.

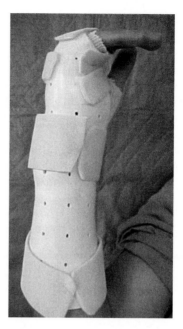

FIGURE **13-2** Forearm-based ulnar gutter splint for protective immobilization following fractures of the middle, ring, and small metacarpals.

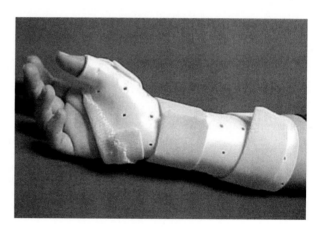

FIGURE **13-3** Forearm volar-based thumb spica for protective immobilization following fracture of the thumb metacarpal base.

fractures are immobilized in a hand-based splint, with the metacarpophalangeal (MP) joint flexed 70 to 80 degrees and the interphalangeal (IP) joints fully extended. An ulnar gutter splint is used for the long, ring, or small finger (Figure 13-1), and a radial gutter splint is used for the index finger. An alternative is a volar-based splint, with or without an additional protective dorsal component.

Metacarpal neck and shaft fractures are splinted following the same principles, with the addition of the wrist in 20-degree extension and the IP joints free, unless extra protection is required (Figure 13-2). Thumb metacarpal base fractures are immobilized in a forearm volar-based thumb spica splint with the wrist in 20-degree extension (Figure 13-3). The thumb IP may or may not be included in the splint, depending on the degree of fracture stability.

Pins are left dry or cleaned following the referring surgeon's instructions. Wounds and incisions are covered with sterile dressings. Edema is managed in phase I primarily through elevation. For stable fractures, cold packs, light retrograde massage, and light compressive wraps are used with caution, avoiding pressure or torque at the fracture site. Active motion of the IP joints in metacarpal fractures reduces IP joint stiffness and dorsal hand edema. Instruction is provided for

active motion of the uninvolved joints of the upper extremity to prevent stiffness.

The indications for progression to phase II are fracture stability through surgical fixation or bony healing and the diminishing of acute postoperative inflammation. Phase II may begin as early as 5 days after surgery. However, if the fracture remains unstable after surgical fixation, active motion of the adjacent joints is delayed until clinical union is achieved. Prolonged immobilization is avoided whenever possible, because immobilization for longer than 4 weeks has been shown to result in stiffness.[8]

Troubleshooting

Open injuries known as "fight bites" are seen in association with metacarpal neck fractures sustained in altercations.[9] These bite wounds are monitored, and signs of infection are reported promptly to the referring physician. Percutaneous pins, external fixation devices, incisions, and other wounds are also monitored.

Edema control is crucial in phase I for prevention of complications, such as joint stiffness and tendon adherence. As edema diminishes, the protective splint is modified and adjusted to maintain correct fit and positioning. Care is taken to ensure that the IP joints remain in full extension as the edema subsides.

POSTOPERATIVE PHASE II: STABILITY (WEEKS 2 TO 6)

Once the fracture is deemed stable by the referring surgeon, and acute, postoperative inflammation has diminished, therapy progresses to phase II. Active and active-assisted motion of the joints directly proximal and distal to the fracture is commenced.

During phase II, the protective splint is removed for hygiene and exercises. Scar management is initiated once the wounds are fully closed. Daily scar massage, avoiding excessive force over the fracture, and application of a silicone scar pad at night are recommended.

Postoperative Phase I: Inflammation/Protection (Week 1)

GOALS
- Protective immobilization
- Edema control
- Wound healing
- Full motion of uninvolved upper extremity joints

PRECAUTIONS
- Remold splints as edema diminishes for correct fit and positioning
- Accommodate and protect pins
- Avoid compressive gloves that apply uncontrolled forces to fracture during donning and doffing
- No motion of joints adjacent to fracture until stability is achieved through surgical fixation or clinical union

TREATMENT STRATEGIES
Protective Custom Thermoplastic Splint
- Middle and proximal phalanx fractures: hand-based ulnar gutter for middle, long, and small fingers, radial gutter for index finger (MP joints flexed 70 to 80 degrees, IP joints fully extended); include adjacent finger(s)
- Metacarpal neck and shaft fractures: forearm-based ulnar gutter for middle, long, and small fingers, radial gutter for index metacarpal (wrist extended 20 degrees, MP joints flexed 70 to 80 degrees, IP joints free unless inclusion is specified); include adjacent finger(s)
- Alternative to gutter splints: volar-based splints with or without dorsal protective component
- Thumb metacarpal base fracture: forearm volar-based thumb spica (wrist extended 20 degrees, IP included or free, depending on fracture stability)

Edema Control
- Elevation
- Cold packs, light retrograde massage, and light compressive wraps if fracture is stable
- Active motion of uninvolved joints

Pin and Wound Care
- Pin care as per referring physician's instructions (keep dry, or daily cleaning with solution of 50% hydrogen peroxide and 50% sterile water)
- Sterile dressings to wounds and incisions

A/AAROM of Uninvolved Joints
- Motion of all upper extremity joints, except joints adjacent to the fracture

CRITERIA FOR ADVANCEMENT
- Fracture stability through surgical fixation or clinical union
- Diminished acute, postoperative inflammation

The edema control measures initiated in phase I are continued as needed. Contrast baths and an elastic compression glove may be added as soon as the wounds are closed and the fracture is sufficiently stable. As edema diminishes further, the splint is modified and adjusted as needed to maintain correct fit and positioning.

Active and active-assisted motion exercises for the joints adjacent to the fracture are typically performed four times daily. Flexor and extensor tendon gliding and blocking exercises are performed to glide the tendons along the fracture site to prevent adherence to the fracture callus.[10] Patients are instructed in hook, straight, and composite fist, and isolated DIP and PIP joint motion to glide the flexor tendons differentially,[11] as well as in IP and MP joint extension exercises (Figure 13-4). MP joint abduction-adduction is performed with the hand supported on a table. Wrist motion in all planes is added for metacarpal fractures. Heat modalities are used to prepare the soft tissues for joint motion and scar mobilization techniques.

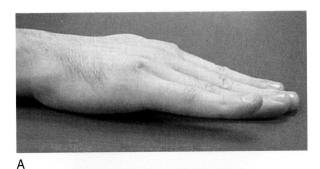

A

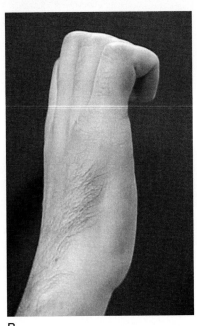

B

FIGURE **13-4** Metacarpophalangeal joint extension exercises for gliding the extensor tendons. *A.* Isolated digit extension. *B.* Extensor digitorum communis (EDC) glide.

Light, functional activities are performed within the constraints of the splint. During therapy sessions, gradual progression to supervised light, functional activities without the splint is useful to increase range of motion (ROM). Resistive activities, such as lifting objects weighing greater than a pound and weight-bearing on the hand, are avoided even with the protection of the splint. To protect thumb metacarpal base fractures from excessive force, strong pinching activities are also avoided.

Progression to phase III is indicated as soon as the physician determines that the fracture has consolidated sufficiently to tolerate passive stress and resistance. This determination is based on clinical examination and radiographic evidence of union.

Troubleshooting

Adhesions may form between the fracture and overlying flexor or extensor tendons. When this occurs, tendon excursion is limited, resulting in impaired active PIP or MP joint flexion or extension (extensor lag). After plate fixation of phalangeal and metacarpal fractures, extensor lag has been found to be one of the most common complications.[12] Extensor lag at the PIP joint is addressed with active extensor tendon gliding exercises, such as PIP extension with the MP joints blocked in flexion. For extensor lag at the MP joint, MP joint extension with the IP joints flexion is emphasized. Scar mobilization is crucial in prevention and treatment of both flexor and extensor tendon adherence (Figure 13-5).

Intrinsic muscle tightness may occur if immobilization with the intrinsic muscles in their shortened position is prolonged. In this case, active and active-assisted IP joint flexion with the MP joints blocked in extension is emphasized.

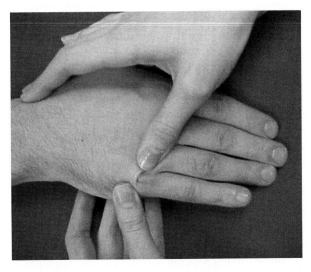

FIGURE **13-5** Scar mobilization for extensor tendon adherence following pinning of a metacarpal neck fracture.

Postoperative Phase II: Stability (Weeks 2 to 6)

GOALS

- Edema control
- Nonadherent scar
- Freely gliding flexor and extensor tendons
- Functional motion of joints adjacent to fracture

PRECAUTIONS

- No resistive exercises or activities
- Avoid excessive passive stress to fracture site
- Avoid strong pinching to protect thumb metacarpal base fractures
- Continue protective splinting, except for hygiene and exercises

TREATMENT STRATEGIES

- Edema control: may add contrast baths and compression glove when wounds have healed and fracture is stable
- Scar management: scar massage, silicone scar pad
- Heat modalities to prepare soft tissue for ROM and scar management
- A/AAROM of joints adjacent to fracture
- Flexor and extensor tendon gliding and blocking exercises
- Light, functional use of hand in splint, progressed to supervised light activities without splint

CRITERIA FOR ADVANCEMENT

- Fracture consolidation as evidenced by radiographic union or MD clinical examination, indicating ability of fracture to tolerate resistance and stress

POSTOPERATIVE PHASE III: FRACTURE CONSOLIDATION (WEEKS 7 TO 10)

Once the fracture has consolidated sufficiently to tolerate resistance and passive stress, the goals of therapy are to maximize ROM, increase strength, and facilitate return to the pre-injury level of activity.

During phase III, the protective splint is worn only during travel and sleep then discontinued when permitted by the surgeon. Scar and edema management techniques are continued until the scar is flat, pale, and nonadherent, the tendons glide freely, and the edema has resolved. Heat modalities, including paraffin wax and ultrasound, are used to prepare soft tissues for joint motion and scar mobilization techniques.

Active flexor and extensor gliding and blocking exercises are continued. If active motion and tendon gliding remain impaired, blocking splints are used to immobilize a joint to facilitate active motion at the adjacent joint or joints. For example, an MP blocking splint holds the MP joints in extension, allowing active flexion to be concentrated at the IP joints (Figure 13-6). Passive motion, stretching, and joint mobilization are added to address joint stiffness. For persistent stiffness, serial static and static progressive splints are used to provide a prolonged, low load force. Passive, as well as active, motion are often limited by scar adherence. For example, if the extensor tendons adhere to the dorsum of the

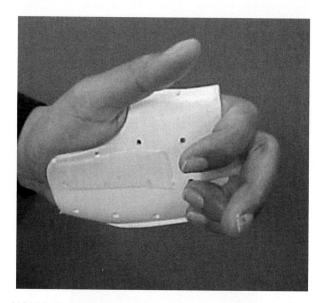

FIGURE **13-6** Metacarpal joint blocking splint for active blocking exercises to glide the flexor tendons and promote IP joint flexion.

metacarpal after plating or pinning of a metacarpal fracture, passive MP joint flexion will be limited. Scar mobilization and a balance of extension and flexion exercises are implemented to glide the tendons, increase passive MP joint flexion, and address extensor lag. Aggressive stretching is avoided because it may attenuate the adherent tendons and increase extensor lag.

In phase III, strengthening exercises for the intrinsic and extrinsic digit musculature are introduced and gradually progressed. Flexion exercises include isometric putty stamping with dowels of various sizes, progressing to isotonic putty grasping or use of a hand gripper with graded rubber band resistance. Flexion exercises are balanced with extension exercises, such as resistive dowel rolling and extension against putty loops. Resistive extension exercises are particularly helpful for gliding the extensor tendons and reducing extensor lag. Strengthening exercises for lateral pinch, palmar pinch, and lumbrical grasp are performed with putty and graded clothespins. If wrist strength is impaired, resistive exercises in all planes of wrist motion are added. Functional activities and conditioning exercises facilitate gradual return to the pre-injury level of function.

Discharge from therapy is considered when the patient has maximized motion, has developed enough strength and endurance to resume functional activities, and is independent in a home exercise program to address any residual deficits.

Troubleshooting

Flexion and extension contractures of the MP and PIP joints are among the most common complications following phalangeal and metacarpal fractures.[12] Static progressive and serial static splints are used to treat persistent joint stiffness. The splints are worn at night, or three to five times daily for 20-minute intervals. Wearing time is adjusted based on each individual's response to splinting. To address limited MP joint flexion, a forearm-based static progressive MP joint flexion splint is fabricated (Figure 13-7). For a PIP joint flexion contracture of 30 degrees or less, a PIP joint extension splint is fabricated for night use and serially remolded as extension increases (Figure 13-8). A prefabricated dynamic PIP joint extension splint is used for short intermittent periods during the day. Serial casting in PIP joint extension is considered for PIP flexion contractures of greater than 30 degrees. If extension casting is used, flexion must be closely monitored to assure that it does not become significantly impaired. Joint stiffness that is unresponsive to splinting or serial casting may require surgical treatment with capsulotomy.

Active motion that is significantly more limited than passive motion indicates tendon adherence. Extensor tendon lag and poor flexor tendon gliding should be noted in phase II and addressed early with active motion and scar management. If tendon adherence does not respond to a full course of therapy, tenolysis may ultimately be required.

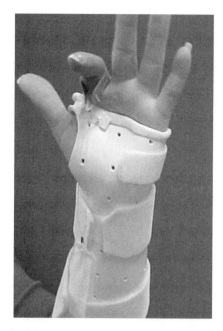

FIGURE **13-7** Static, progressive MP joint flexion splint for MP joint stiffness.

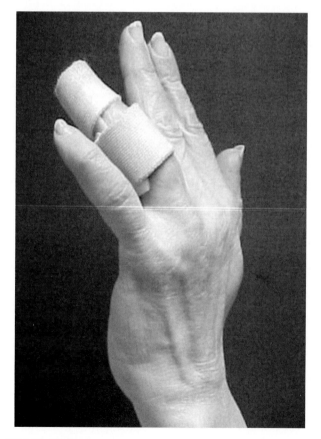

FIGURE **13-8** Serial static PIP joint extension splint (finger gutter) for PIP joint flexion contractures of 30 degrees or less.

Postoperative Phase III: Fracture Consolidation (Weeks 7 to 10)

GOALS

- Full or maximum motion with freely gliding tendons
- Functional strength and endurance
- Independence in activities of daily living (ADL)

PRECAUTIONS

- No resistance, stretching, or static progressive splints until fracture has consolidated
- Avoid overstretching vs gliding of adherent tendons.

TREATMENT STRATEGIES

- Wean from protective custom splint under direction of surgeon.
- Continue edema and scar management.
- Heat modalities, including paraffin and ultrasound, to prepare soft tissues for ROM, joint mobilization, and scar mobilization
- AROM, including flexor and extensor, tendon gliding, and blocking exercises; add blocking splints as needed.
- PROM, stretching, joint mobilization to address joint stiffness
- Serial static or static progressive splinting to address persistent joint stiffness
- Resistive exercises for intrinsic and extrinsic digit musculature and wrist
- Functional activities and conditioning for restoration of independent ADL

CRITERIA FOR DISCHARGE

- Full or maximum digit and wrist AROM with freely gliding tendons
- Functional strength and endurance
- Independence in ADL
- Independence in home program to address any residual impairments

REFERENCES

1. Chung, K.C., Spilson, S.V. *The Frequency and Epidemiology of Hand and Forearm Fractures in the United States.* J Hand Surg 2001;26A:908–915.

2. Pun, W.K., Chow, S.P., Luk, K.D., Ip, F.K, Chan, K.C., Ngai, W.K., Crosby, C., Ng, C. *A Prospective Study on 284 Digital Fractures of the Hand.* J Hand Surg 1989;14A:474–481.

3. Stern, P.J. Fractures of the Metacarpals and Phalanges. In Green, D.P., Hotchkiss, R.N., Pederson, W.C. (Eds). *Green's Operative Hand Surgery,* 4th ed. Churchill Livingstone, New York, 1999, pp. 711–771.

4. Schneider, L.H. *Fractures of the Distal Phalanx.* Hand Clin 1988;4:537–547.

5. Campbell, P.J., Wilson, R.L. Management of Joint Injuries and Intra-articular Fractures. In Hunter, J.M., Mackin, E.J., Callahan, A.D. (Eds). *Rehabilitation of the Hand: Surgery and Therapy,* 5th ed. Mosby, St. Louis, 2002, pp. 396–411.

6. Doyle, J.R. Extensor Tendons—Acute Injuries. In Green, D.P., Hotchkiss, R.N., Pederson, W.C. (Eds). *Green's Operative Hand Surgery,* 4th ed. Churchill Livingstone, New York, 1999, pp. 1950–1987.

7. Pellegrini, V.D. *Fractures at the Base of the Thumb.* Hand Clin 1988;4:87–102.

8. Strickland, J.W., Steichen, J.B., Kleinman, W.B., Hastings II, H., Flynn, N. *Phalangeal Fractures: Factors Influencing Digital Performance.* Orthop Rev 1982;11:39–50.

9. McNemar, T.B., Howell, J.W., Chang, E. *Management of Metacarpal Fractures.* J Hand Ther 2003;16:143–151.

10. Agee, J. *Treatment Principles for Proximal and Middle Phalangeal Fractures.* Orthop Clin North Am 1992;23:35–40.

11. Wehbe, M.A., Hunter, J.M. *Flexor Tendon Gliding in the Hand. Part II: Differential Gliding.* J Hand Surg 1985;10A:575–579.

12. Page, S.M., Stern, P.J. *Complications and Range of Motion Following Plate Fixation of Metacarpal and Phalangeal Fractures.* J Hand Surg 1998;23A:827–832.

14

Flexor Tendon Repairs

KARA GAFFNEY GALLAGHER, MS, OTR/L, CHT

Flexor tendon injuries in the forearm or hand occur when tendon continuity is disrupted by a laceration, crush, avulsion, or contusion. Flexor tendons are surgically corrected via a primary or secondary repair. Whether a repair is primary or secondary depends on how soon after injury that surgery occurs and the quality of the tendon. In a primary repair the loose ends of the injured tendon are approximated with sutures. An immediate primary repair is performed within 24 hours of injury, whereas a delayed primary repair is performed between 24 hours and 3 weeks after injury.[1] Primary end-to-end tendon repair performed within the first few days following injury is ideal and guarantees the best outcome.[1] Studies performed on canine and chicken tendons demonstrate that repairs performed within the first few days resulted in improved tendon excursion.[2] It is important to be aware that delayed tendon repair increases the possibility of rupture, tendon elongation, muscle shortening, and joint contractures.[3] A tendon injury that involves bone or neurovascular damage will complicate the rehabilitation process and possibly the outcome but does not contraindicate a primary repair.[4]

A secondary repair is considered 3 weeks post-injury, or in situations where the quality of the tendon is beyond surgical correction. After 3 weeks, flexor tendon repair becomes more complicated because of scarring, muscle contracture, and tendon retraction.[3] At this point, available options include a tendon graft, transfer, or two-stage tendon graft. Other situations that require a secondary repair include loss of palmar skin overlying the flexor system, flexor retinacular damage, and pulley destruction.[4]

In a secondary repair, a tendon graft from a noninvolved tendon (often palmaris longus [PL]) is harvested to approximate the free ends of the injured tendon. If scarring or damage to adjacent tissues is severe, a conventional tendon graft is unlikely to resume adequate gliding, and staged tendon grafts are performed. Transformation of the scarred, post-injury flexor tendon and surrounding tissues to a gliding, pliable, effective system is accomplished using a two-stage tendon graft method with a silicone implant.[1] In the first stage, a silicone implant is placed between the free ends, allowing the scar to envelope it and recreate a fibrous sheath to promote healing of the second-stage tendon graft.[1] Tendon injuries may occur in isolation or along with fractures and neurovascular injuries.

This chapter reviews the anatomy, surgery, and rehabilitation related to a flexor tendon injury, specifically an early active mobilization protocol that is appropriate for primary tendon repairs completed with a four-strand core suture and an additional epitendinous suture augmentation crossing the repair site.[4,5]

ANATOMICAL OVERVIEW

In the distal third of the volar forearm, the flexor tendons arise from the flexor muscles. The superficial group includes the wrist flexors: flexor carpi radialis (FCR), flexor carpi ulnaris (FCU), and PL. The middle group consists of the four tendons of the flexor digitorum superficialis (FDS) that originate from individual muscle bundles.[2] This allows for isolated individual flexion of each digit. The deep group includes the flexor digitorum profundus (FDP) and flexor pollicis longus (FPL). The FDP tendons originate from a common muscle belly and therefore act as a group.[2] Several surrounding anatomical structures are significant in flexor tendon injury. Flexor tendon injuries are categorized into five zones on the premises of anatomical features to systematically highlight these structures (Figure 14-1).[2]

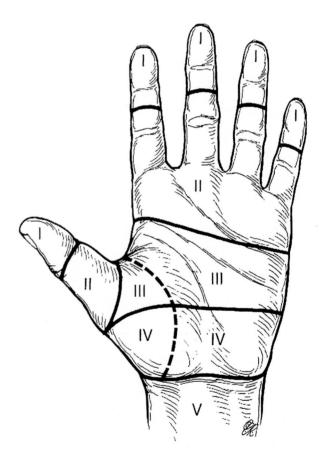

FIGURE **14-1** Flexor zones. *(From Strickland, J.W. Flexor Tendons—Acute Injuries. In Green, D.P., Hotchkiss, R.N., Pederson, W.C. [Eds]. Green's Operative Hand Surgery, 4th ed. Churchill Livingstone, New York, 1999, p. 1857, with permission.)*

ZONE V

Zone V spans the distal third of the forearm to the level of the wrist and contains the musculotendinous junction of the superficial and deep flexors. Median and ulnar nerves, as well as the radial and ulnar arteries, course through zone V and are often associated with injury to the tendons.[3] The vascular and neural structures must be protected in the early phases of rehabilitation. Early repair is especially recommended for tendons in this zone because of the high probability of tendon retraction with muscle contraction. The tendons lie deep in the skin and subcutaneous tissue and are particularly vulnerable to adhesions. Contracture and shortening of the tendons in this zone are common. Both adhesions and contracture can be reduced with a strong focus on differential tendon gliding during rehabilitation.

ZONE IV

In zone IV the flexor tendons are enclosed in synovial sheaths as they course through the carpal tunnel. Injuries in this zone often include more than one tendon, blood vessels, and nerves because of the close proximity of the structures to one another.[3] Adhesions between the tendons are common in the postoperative phase, and differential gliding of the tendons is effective in controlling adhesion formation.

ZONE III

The lumbrical muscles originate from the flexor digitorum profundus tendon at the point where the tendons emerge from the carpal tunnel in zone III.[2] Protective positioning in the lumbrical plus position (MP flexion with IP extension) can lead to adhesions and contracture of the intrinsic muscles in the early weeks. Therefore, gentle, passive metacarpophalangeal (MP) joint motion and gentle, passive intrinsic minus or hook fist (MP extension with interphalangeal [IP] flexion) early in rehabilitation are recommended for injuries in zone II.[3]

ZONE II

Zone II begins at the distal palmar crease and includes the origin of the flexor tendon sheath. Zone II extends to the middle of the middle phalanx, just distal to where the FDP emerges from the two slips of the FDS insertion (Camper's chiasm). In zone II the flexor tendons are supported by an intricate pulley system that tethers the tendons to the bones for increased mechanical advantage during flexion (Figure 14-2). Injured and repaired pulleys are potential sites of adhesion formation. Alternatively, unrepaired pulleys may cause "bowstringing" as the tendon pulls away from the bone in the palmar direction under muscle contraction. Zone II also

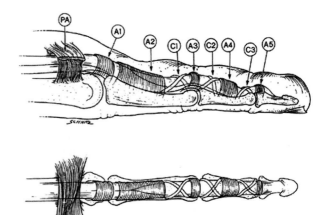
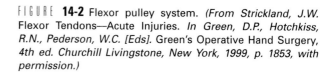

FIGURE **14-2** Flexor pulley system. *(From Strickland, J.W. Flexor Tendons—Acute Injuries. In Green, D.P., Hotchkiss, R.N., Pederson, W.C. [Eds].* Green's Operative Hand Surgery, *4th ed. Churchill Livingstone, New York, 1999, p. 1853, with permission.)*

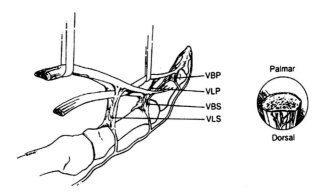

FIGURE **14-3** Viniculae. *(From Strickland, J.W. Flexor Tendons—Acute Injuries. In Green, D.P., Hotchkiss, R.N., Pederson, W.C. [Eds].* Green's Operative Hand Surgery, *4th ed. Churchill Livingstone, New York, 1999, p. 1853, with permission.)*

includes the viniculae, which provide vascularity and nutrition to the tendons (Figure 14-3).

Laceration in zone II often involves both FDS and FDP, in addition to the supporting structures. Historically, this region has been referred to as "no man's land" because of the complicated system of synovial sheaths, pulleys, and viniculae supporting the flexor tendons. In the past, poor results were expected with tendon injury in zone II because of the combination of intertendinous adhesions as well as the effects of injury to the sheath, viniculae, pulleys, and other surrounding structures.[3] During the last 10 years, advances in suture technique, strength, and early postoperative active mobilization protocols have improved the ability to obtain better results.

ZONE I

Zone I, the most distal zone, spans from the insertion of the FDS on the middle phalanx to the insertion of the FDP on the distal phalanx. Zone I includes only the FDP tendon as it emerges from the flexor sheath. This is a common site for FDP rupture, where the terminal tendon is avulsed with or without a bony component, at its insertion on the distal phalanx. Complications following tendon repair in zone I include development of distal interphalangeal (DIP) joint flexion contracture or poor gliding through the A-4 and A-5 pulleys.[3]

SURGICAL OVERVIEW

Surgical repair of flexor tendons has evolved over the years. For many years, two-strand repairs were performed. In the past decade, four-strand repairs have become more common. The number of strands in a repair refers to the number of times the suture material crosses the repair site. The strength of a tendon repair is roughly proportional to the number of strands that cross the repair.[6–18] Today, the most common primary repair is accomplished with a four-strand core suture plus an epitendinous suture crossing the repair site to strengthen the procedure.[4] Many core suture designs have been described in the literature, ranging from four to eight strands. These designs include the Bunnell, modified Kessler, Tajima, locking running epitendinous, and double-grasping techniques.[4] The surgeons at the Hospital for Special Surgery (HSS) typically use a four-strand modified Kessler core suture with a reinforcing epitendinous suture. Like other early active mobilization programs, this guideline requires a four-strand core repair and an epitendinous suture at the repair site. Therefore, motion can be initiated within the first 3 days post-surgery.[2] Early active mobilization requires adequate tensile strength of the suture material and appropriate design of the suture so that the tendon can withstand active muscle pull without rupture or gapping.*

REHABILITATION OVERVIEW

There are three approaches to rehabilitating a flexor tendon after surgical repair. They include immobilization, early passive mobilization,[22–24] and early active mobilization.† Passive mobilization programs, such as those described by Kleinert et al.[21,22] and Duran and Houser,[23,24] involve gentle passive flexion and active extension exercises that are performed in a dorsal block splint, with or without rubber band traction that assists the digits into flexion.‡ Early active mobilization consists of active hold or active place-hold programs. *Active*

---

*References 4, 6, 7, 10–17, 19, 20.
†References 6, 17, 22, 25–32.
‡References 6, 17, 26–29.

place-hold indicates that the therapist passively places the digits into flexion and then directs the patient to actively maintain the position with a gentle muscle contraction.[5] This guideline details an active hold/place-hold mobilization program that the authors have found to be most successful. Their version has been modified from protocols designed by Strickland,[30,31] Cannon,[32] and Silfverskiold and May.[33]

The goal of rehabilitation following flexor tendon repair is to promote an opportune environment for a strong repair to support normal forces acting on the tendon in everyday functional use.[5] Research demonstrates that stressing a repaired tendon with early mobilization facilitates healing, tensile strength, excursion, and minimizes adhesion formation.[8,34–36] This protocol offers a method to encourage a durable tendon repair that glides freely. Passive mobilization techniques based on principles from the Controlled Passive Mobilization Technique by Duran and Houser[23,24] and the method by Kleinert et al.[22] are also incorporated into this guideline. The passive mobilization techniques are included to preserve joint motion. Like most early active mobilization protocols, this guideline was developed for flexor tendon injuries in zone II. However, the principles can be applied to injuries in all zones.

ACTIVE MOBILIZATION

The active mobilization protocol must begin within 1 to 2 days of surgery, when the repair is physiologically strong. The tensile strength of the immobilized tendon diminishes 3 to 5 days postoperatively because of softening of the tendon ends.[37,38] A study by Hitchcock et al.[38] determined that the ends of flexor profundus tendons in chickens softened during the inflammatory phase of wound healing. The same study compared the immobilized group to a group that was mobilized 1 to 2 days after repair. The study found that the mobilized group did not encounter a notable inflammatory phase, and rather the repair gained strength, appearing to heal through intrinsic means, with less adhesion formation.

Active mobilization of the repaired tendon begins with place-hold positions protected by tenodesis (wrist extension with digit flexion/wrist flexion with digit extension). Active mobilization progresses toward active flexion along the following ladder: place-hold tenodesis, active tenodesis, differential tendon gliding, blocking, and strengthening. Strengthening begins with blocking with resistance, progressing toward isometric grip, and, finally, isotonic strengthening of grip and pinch.

CRITERIA FOR ADVANCEMENT

Rehabilitation of the repaired flexor tendon progresses through four phases of therapy that can last up to 16 weeks postoperatively. The phases of this protocol reflect the three stages of wound healing: inflammation, fibroplasia, and scar maturation. Advancement of the patient depends upon the stage of wound healing, excursion of the flexor tendon, and opinions of the surgeon and therapist. Ultimately, the surgeon prescribes an early active motion protocol and determines points of advancement based on examination of the patient, tendon excursion, and clinical feedback from the therapist. Each phase includes a new set of goals, precautions, splints, treatment strategies, and criteria for advancement.

STAGES OF WOUND HEALING

As the patient is advanced through a regimented rehabilitation program, internal forces applied through the tendon repair site increase. Traditionally, therapists have used a timeline based on the stages of wound healing to guide them through the progression of treatment.[5,39,40] The first phase of therapy includes both the inflammatory (0 to 5 days) and fibroplasia stages (5 to 21 days) of wound healing. The second, third, and fourth phases of therapy occur during the scar maturation or remodeling phase (3 weeks to 2 years) of wound healing. Phase II of therapy typically commences 4 weeks postoperatively, leading into phase III in the sixth postoperative week, and, finally, phase IV in the eighth week after surgery.

THREE-POINT ADHESION GRADING SYSTEM

A more clinical approach to the progression of treatment has been described recently.[39] This approach uses flexor tendon excursion as a guide in selecting the appropriate amount of force to apply across the tendon junction.[39] Tendon excursion is monitored by determining flexion lag. Flexion lag is measured as total passive flexion (sum of passive MP, PIP, and DIP flexion) minus total active flexion (sum of active MP, PIP, and DIP flexion).[39]

Groth[39] recently developed a model, known as the three-point adhesion grading system, to quantify how adhesions influence flexion lag. The model is used as an indicator for flexor tendon excursion, providing a clinical method for progressing the patient through the phases of therapy. Tendon lag is defined as absent, responsive, or unresponsive in Groth's three-point adhesion grading system.[39] Absent tendon lag is indicated by less than or equal to 5 degrees of difference between active and passive flexion. Responsive and unresponsive tendon lags are determined by measures taken between therapy sessions. A responsive tendon lag improves between sessions. Responsive flexion lag is concluded by greater than or equal to 10% improvement of lag between therapy sessions. Unresponsive flexion lag indicates less than or equal to 10% improvement of lag

between therapy sessions. Change in flexion lag between sessions is determined using the following formula:

$$a = \text{previous session flexion lag}$$
$$b = \text{present session flexion lag}$$
$$c = \text{percent of improvement}$$
$$c = (a - b)/a \times 100\%$$

HSS CRITERIA FOR ADVANCEMENT

The HSS guideline for progressing patients following flexor tendon repair relies on both wound healing principles and flexor tendon excursion. Groth's three-point adhesion grading system can assist in knowing when to progress or delay the therapy program.[39] In this guideline *absent* flexion lag indicates excellent tendon glide, and the patient should be progressed slower than the timeline that correlates with wound healing. *Responsive* flexion lag suggests that the phase and exercises are appropriate for the strength of the tendon repair and adhesion formation. Flexion lag must be monitored closely for unresponsiveness. *If the lag becomes unresponsive, advancement to the next level occurs sooner than the phase of wound healing indicates. Unresponsive* flexion lag reflects adhesion formation.[39] An unresponsive lag indicates advancement through the suggested timeline at a faster pace until the tendon lag resolves. Load application can increase per rehabilitation session until the lag becomes responsive. Once the lag becomes responsive, the patient continues at that level and progresses according to the suggested timeline in accordance with wound healing. The rehabilitation overview contains specific guidelines for applying the adhesion grading system to the standard timeline that is based on the principles of wound healing.

CONTRAINDICATIONS

Several factors contraindicate the use of early active motion. First, a tendon held together with less than a four-strand core repair or lacking the reinforcing epitendinous suture at the repair site cannot withstand such a program. Anything less than the recommended repair parameters may gap or rupture under active forces. Second, because of the postoperative change in tendon strength, the program should be avoided if the patient is more than 3 days post-surgery. Third, poor tendon quality or multiple associated injuries may contradict using this program. In such cases, the surgeon should dictate the appropriate postoperative approach. Last, this program requires active participation, compliance, and commitment from the patient. The patient must have a thorough understanding of the exercises and precautions. Children under age 10 and individuals who lack the ability or desire to commit to this program may not be appropriate candidates. It is worth noting that the authors have used this early active mobilization protocol successfully with a 5-year-old child, who demonstrated the ability and desire to follow through.

REHABILITATION OVERVIEW

POSTOPERATIVE PHASE I (24 HOURS TO 3–4 WEEKS)

Phase I of therapy includes protective immobilization, edema and scar management, protected motion, and instruction in a home exercise program (HEP). The following box includes specific information for each area of intervention. Therapy fosters a delicate balance between mobilizing the repaired tendon and protecting the tendon from rupture, attenuation, or excessive adhesion formation. In phase I, the inflammatory period slows as fibroplasia dominates the healing process during the first 5 days after injury.[4] Active motion during the fibroblastic period is essential to promote collagen formation that allows for normal movement.[4] At the same time, active motion must be guided and protected at all times for the first 6 weeks.[5] The home program in phase I includes passive range of motion (PROM) within the confines of the splint for protected

motion, and active place-hold tenodesis exercises once the patient correctly demonstrates competence with these exercises during therapy.

Splint

The repaired tendon is protected in a dorsal block splint that includes the distal two thirds of the forearm, wrist, MP, and IP joints of all the digits. If the thumb is uninjured, it remains free from the splint. Splint designs may vary slightly, based on the surgeon's preference and adjacent injured structures. The position of immobilization places the flexor tendons on slack, preventing tension on the repair site. The wrist is immobilized in 15 to 30 degrees of flexion. The MP joints are positioned in 50 to 60 degrees of flexion, and the IP joints are maintained in 0 degrees of extension.[5] If full IP extension is not achieved with strapping to the dorsal hood, a gutter splint can be used to avoid development of a PIP flexion contracture. The IP joints are positioned in slight flexion for tendon repairs that are accompanied by a digital nerve repair to avoid stress to the digital nerve. The splint is worn at all times, only to be removed for therapy and hygiene (Figure 14-4).

Postoperative Phase I (24 Hours to 3–4 Weeks)

GOALS
- Fabrication of custom immobilization splint
- Instruction in PROM and protected AROM
- Increased tendon excursion
- Edema control and scar management
- Independence in HEP

PRECAUTIONS
- Wear splint at all times—remove for hygiene and specific exercises
- No simultaneous wrist and digital extension
- Digital nerve injuries: IP position as per surgeon (slight flexion)

TREATMENT STRATEGIES
- *Splint: Static, dorsal, forearm based*
  - DBS
  - Wrist 15- to 30-degree flexion
  - MCPs 60- to 70-degree flexion
  - IP joints strapped into extension against DBS, unless digital nerves were repaired
  - PIP extension splint if needed to achieve full PIP extension
- *PROM*
  - Passive PIP/DIP flexion in splint followed by active extension to roof of splint
  - Composite passive flexion followed by active extension to roof of splint
  - 10 times each, every 2 hours
- *AROM (protected, supervised in therapy)*
  - Tenodesis: Place and hold composite and straight fist
  - 10 times each, every 2 hours
  - AROM
    - Active digital extension with wrist flexed
    - FDS blocking to *uninvolved* digits and tendons
    - FDP blocking to *uninvolved* digits, if FDP is *not* involved
    - 10 times each, every 2 hours

Postoperative Phase I (24 Hours to 3–4 Weeks)—cont'd

- *Scar management: to prevent tendon adhesions*
  - Silicone scar pads
  - Cross-frictional massage
- *Edema control*
  - Coban—light, pinch method; remove for AROM exercises
  - Retrograde massage
- *HEP*
  - PROM exercises every 2 hours
  - Tenodesis and AROM added when 100% competent in therapy
    - ○ Scar management as previous, 2 times a day
    - ○ Edema management as previous, as needed

CRITERIA FOR ADVANCEMENT

- Per surgeon
- Based on stage of wound healing
- Contingent upon tendon excursion measured 3 weeks postoperative and weekly thereafter
  - Determine flexion lag
    - ○ Absent: Prolong phase I until 6 weeks postoperative
    - ○ Responsive: Progress to phase II at 4 weeks postoperative
    - ○ Unresponsive: Progress to phase II at 3 weeks postoperative, continuing to increase load to tendon until lag becomes responsive

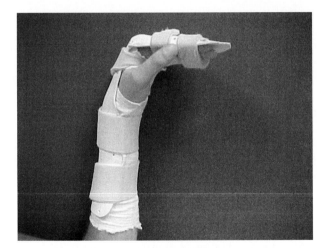

FIGURE **14-4** Dorsal block splint.

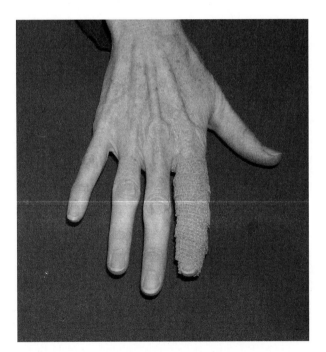

FIGURE **14-5** Coban wrap.

Edema Control and Scar Management

Edema control and scar management follow standard procedures. Emphasis on early edema control is crucial, because edema increases the drag and resistance on the tendon during active motion exercises.[42] Edema can be controlled during exercise sessions by wrapping the individual digits with 2-inch Coban (3M Health Care, St. Paul, MN), using the pinch technique (Figure 14-5). Retrograde massage from the digit to medial elbow area, elevation, and cold compresses assist in reducing edema and preparing the digit for motion. Scar management with cross-frictional massage and silicone gel pads is initiated as soon as the wound site has healed. The patient is instructed to wear the scar product at all times during protective

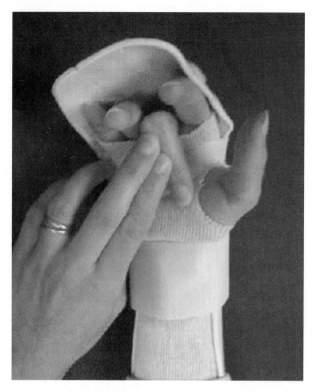

FIGURE **14-6** Passive PIP flexion within splint.

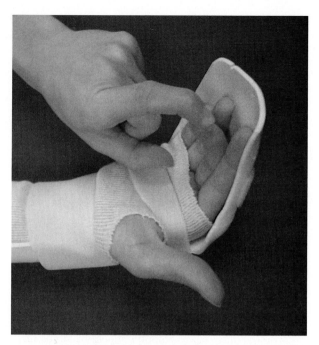

FIGURE **14-7** Passive DIP flexion within splint.

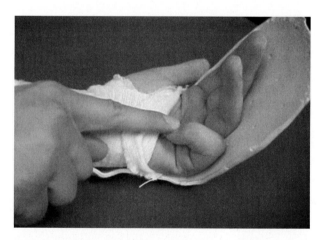

FIGURE **14-8** Passive composite flexion within splint.

splinting and then at night only once the splint has been discharged.

Motion

The repaired tendon is prepared for active motion through the following sequence: edema management, passive joint flexion, passive tenodesis, and, finally, controlled active flexion in the protected position. This sequence assists in minimizing the drag and work for the tendon caused by edema and joint stiffness. Passive motion is performed with passive IP joint flexion followed by protected active extension. Passive motion is performed in the splint by removing the distal straps. The PIP joint is passively flexed to end range followed by active extension within the confines of the splint (Figure 14-6). Next the DIP joint is passively flexed, with the PIP joint held in extension and the MP joint held in flexion, to stretch the terminal extensor tendon and oblique retinacular ligament (ORL) (Figure 14-7). The PIP and DIP joints are then passively flexed together to end range followed by active extension to 0 degrees with the MP joints blocked in flexion (Figure 14-8). Protected passive PIP and DIP extension is performed with the wrist and MPs flexed at 2 weeks post-surgery.

The splint is removed for therapist-assisted passive tenodesis of the wrist and digits. The therapist passively extends the wrist while flexing the digits into a gentle composite fist (Figure 14-9), followed by passive wrist flexion with MP and IP extension (Figure 14-10). This is repeated until the hand and wrist can be passively moved from one position to the next with minimal effort.

Once passive motion feels fluid and unrestricted, the repaired tendon is mobilized through carefully controlled active flexion. The therapist passively places the wrist in 20 degrees extension while simultaneously, passively flexing the digits into a modified full fist with the MP joints at 75 degrees of flexion, the PIP joints flexed 70 degrees, and the DIP joints flexed 40 degrees (Figure 14-11). After the wrist and digits have been placed in this position, the patient is asked to actively hold the position with just enough force to

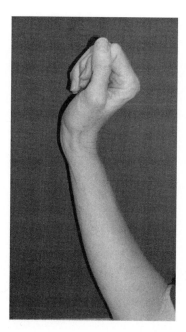

FIGURE **14-9** Tenodesis: wrist extension with digital flexion.

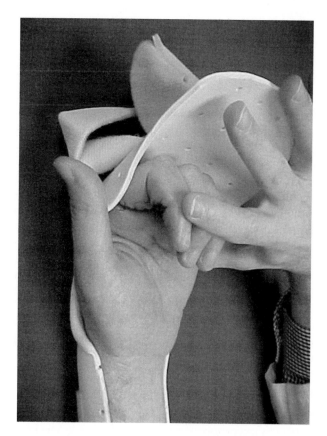

FIGURE **14-11** Place-hold composite fist.

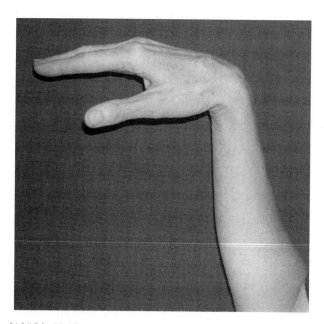

FIGURE **14-10** Tenodesis: wrist flexion with digital extension.

maintain the position. The therapist then passively flexes the wrist, and the patient actively extends the IP joints while the therapist blocks the MP joints at 75 degrees. Following approximately 10 repetitions, the therapist passively extends the wrist 20 degrees and passively places the hand into a modified straight fist with MPs at 75 degrees and PIPs at 70 degrees (Figure 14-12). The patient then actively holds this position. Last, the therapist places the wrist in flexion, and the patient actively extends the IP joints while the MP

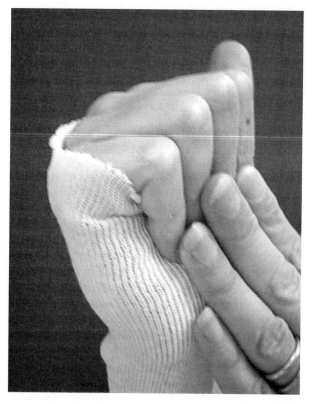

FIGURE **14-12** Place-hold straight fist.

joints are blocked in 75 degrees of flexion. When the patient demonstrates competence with controlled active flexion and extension, he or she is added to the home program.

Criteria for Advancement

The patient is advanced to phase II in the third or fourth postoperative week, based upon the surgeon's examination and the nature of tendon excursion. The three-point adhesion grading system is used in the third postoperative week. If the tendon shows excellent gliding with absent lag, phase I is continued through the sixth postoperative week. In a tendon that demonstrates a responsive lag between sessions (increased total active motion), treatment progresses to phase II at the end of the fourth postoperative week. An unresponsive tendon lag, with no change in composite flexion in the third week, indicates heavy adhesion formation and immediate progression to phase II. An unresponsive tendon is progressed through the sequence of active motion until the lag begins to respond.

POSTOPERATIVE PHASE II (3 TO 6 WEEKS)

Phase II may begin as early as 3 weeks post-surgery, if tendon excursion is poor, or as late as 6 weeks if tendon excursion is excellent. Phase II focuses on gently increasing the stress placed on the repaired tendon by adding a place-hold hook fist (Figure 14-13). Edema and scar management techniques continue through this phase.

Splint

The dorsal block splint is modified to a neutral wrist position and MP flexion position of 45 degrees. If the patient is not progressing (presents with an unresponsive flexion lag), the splint is weaned at 4 weeks. PIP joint flexion contractures are addressed with either an LMB (DeRoyal, Powell, TN) extension splint or a serial static splint within the dorsal block splint. The splint is removed for therapy and home program.

Motion

Place and hold hook fisting is added to the passive tenodesis sequence (see Figure 14-13). Hook fisting places the most tension on the repair site because it demands the maximum differential glide between the FDS and FDP tendons. Place and hold tenodesis exercises are progressed to active tenodesis for gentle tabletop, straight, hook, and composite fisting. In active tenodesis motion, the patient actively extends the wrist while actively making a composite or straight fist. Repetition of exercises is increased to improve tendon glide. An

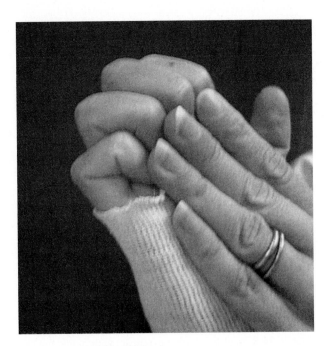

FIGURE **14-13** Place-hold hook fist.

unresponsive flexor lag requires upgrading to phase II, including isolated FDS gliding (Figure 14-14), unprotected tendon gliding, and gentle PIP and DIP blocking (Figures 14-15 and 14-16).

Joint stiffness requires mobilization. Joint mobilization is performed with the adjacent joints in flexion to limit tension on the repair site. The home program is upgraded to include active tenodesis of composite, straight, and hook fist. The frequency of exercises is reduced from hourly to three to five times daily.

Criteria for Advancement

Phase III may begin as early as 4 to 5 weeks post-surgery, if tendon excursion is poor, or as late as 8 weeks if tendon excursion is excellent. By this stage of wound healing, the tendon has entered the scar maturation phase. Scar tissue will continue to remodel and mature for up to 1 year postoperatively. If the patient does not demonstrate a flexion lag, phase III commences in the eighth week because excellent tendon glide may indicate limited scar adhesions or maturation. A flexion lag that improves from one treatment session to the next indicates progression to phase III in the sixth postoperative week. In the case of a stubborn flexion lag that does not improve between sessions, progression to phase III can be as early as 4 weeks after surgery, increasing load to the tendon, as appropriate to decrease the lag.

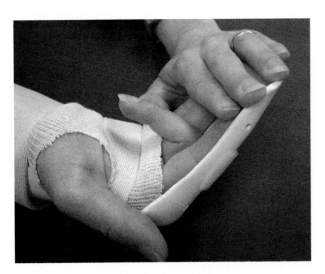

FIGURE **14-14** FDS glide.

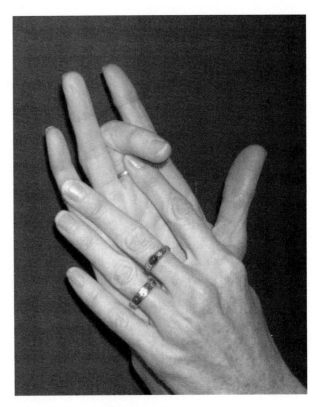

FIGURE **14-15** PIP blocking.

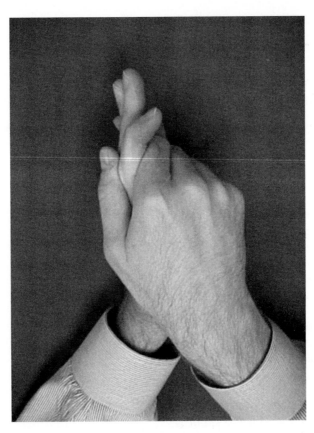

FIGURE **14-16** DIP blocking.

Postoperative Phase II (3 to 6 Weeks)

GOALS

- Increased tendon excursion
- Decreased adhesion formation
- Increased active flexion of the involved digit

PRECAUTIONS

- Continue DBS, unless patient shows unresponsive flexion lag
- Watch for PIP flexion contracture; initiate extension splinting if needed
- No active or passive simultaneous wrist and digital extension

TREATMENT STRATEGIES

- *Splint*
  - Continue with DBS, if absent flexor lag
  - Modify DBS, if responsive flexor lag
    - ◦ Wrist extension to neutral and MP extension to 30 to 45 degrees
  - Discontinue DBS, if unresponsive flexor lag at 4 weeks postoperative
- *PROM*
  - Continue as in phase I
  - Begin joint mobilization for joint stiffness
- *AROM*
  - Begin place and hold hook fist tenodesis
  - Progress to active tenodesis for composite, straight, and hook fists
  - Increase repetition of exercises
- *HEP*
  - Add active tenodesis for tabletop, composite, straight, and hook fists
  - Increase repetition of each exercise
  - Reduce frequency of sessions at home to three times per day

CRITERIA FOR ADVANCEMENT

- Tendon integrity determined by surgeon
- Based on stage of wound healing
- Contingent upon tendon excursion
  - Determine flexion lag
    - ◦ Absent: Prolong phase II until 8 weeks postoperative
    - ◦ Responsive: Progress to phase III at 6 weeks postoperative
    - ◦ Unresponsive: Progress to phase III as early as 4 weeks postoperative, continuing to increase load to tendon until lag becomes responsive

POSTOPERATIVE PHASE III (6 TO 8 WEEKS)

Phase III focuses on increasing the stress placed on the repaired tendon by adding active tendon gliding and blocking exercises. Nighttime splinting for flexion tightness or contractures is added at this point. Edema and scar management techniques continue through this phase.

Splint

With approval from the surgeon, the dorsal block splint is discharged at 6 weeks postoperatively. The surgeon may opt to continue splint protection for up to 8 weeks, if the patient shows excellent tendon excursion, which is indicated by an absent flexion lag. Good tendon gliding and normal excursion suggest minimal scar tissue and weaker tendon. A flexor stretcher splint is considered to decrease extrinsic flexor tightness. The flexor stretcher resembles a resting pan splint. The wrist is positioned in neutral, and the MP and IP joints are placed in maximum possible extension (Figure 14-17). This splint is modified by increasing wrist extension while maintaining MP and IP joints in full extension. Extension splinting for PIP joint stiffness or contracture continues. Removable splints vs serial casting are preferred so that the patient can perform active flexion exercises. Some examples include, but are not limited to, the following: LMB (DeRoyal, Powell, TN), a three-point-wire extension splint, and a belly gutter PIP extension splint.

Motion

Passive motion is upgraded to include simultaneous passive MP and IP extension with the wrist flexed. At 8 weeks postoperative, this stretch is performed with the

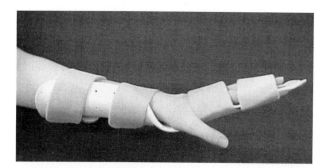

FIGURE **14-17** Flexor stretcher.

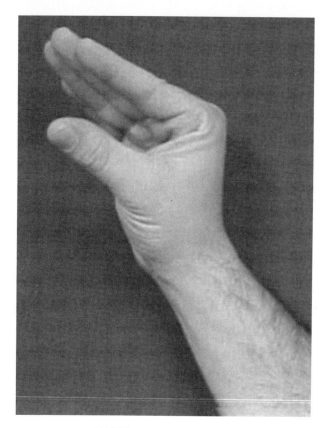

FIGURE **14-18** Tabletop fist.

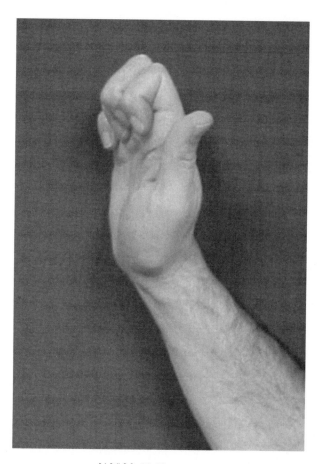

FIGURE **14-19** Hook fist.

that is limited by adhesions and can be performed along with active motion exercises and functional isometric grasp and pinch activities.

Functional Activities

The patient is encouraged to use the hand for light activity and is instructed to avoid activities that require resistance. Light activity includes basic activities of daily living (ADL) and tabletop or desktop activities. Resistive activity includes anything that involves gripping, lifting, pulling, or pushing. Examples of heavier ADL include using the involved hand for cooking a full meal, carrying a grocery bag, and using the involved hand in racquet sports.

Criteria for Advancement

Assessing flexor lag at this point continues to be important in deciding whether to progress the patient along the recommended timeline. If good tendon excursion is present with an absent lag, phase III is prolonged until 10 to 12 weeks postoperatively. A responsive flexor tendon lag that improves between sessions will begin phase IV in the eighth postoperative week. A digit that shows a persistent, nonimproving flexion lag can be progressed to phase IV as early as 6 weeks after surgery.

wrist in neutral. Joint mobilization for stiff joints continues. Active motion for an absent or responsive tendon lag continues to include active tenodesis and is gently progressed to active tendon gliding, including full fist (Figures 14-18 to 14-21). Isolated FDS and FDP gliding is initiated at 7 weeks (see Figure 14-14). Blocking exercises are introduced at 8 weeks (see Figures 14-15 and 14-16). If flexion lag is nonresponsive, gentle PIP and DIP blocking exercises begin as early as 6 weeks after surgery to increase the load on the repaired tendon. Neuromuscular electric stimulation (NMES) is considered for muscle reeducation in cases of poor tendon excursion. NMES facilitates maximal tendon excursion

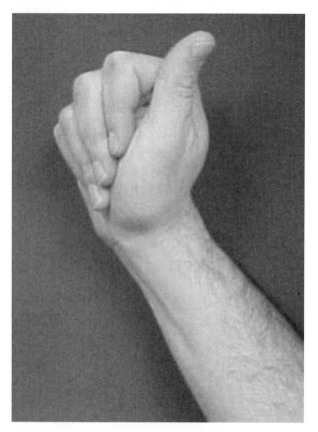

FIGURE **14-20** Straight fist.

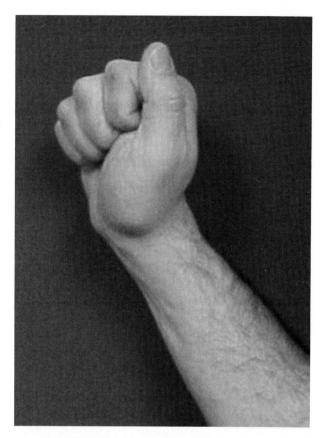

FIGURE **14-21** Full fist.

Postoperative Phase III (6 to 8 Weeks)

GOALS

- Full passive motion by 8 weeks
- Increased tendon excursion and controlled adhesion formation
- Independence with ADL

PRECAUTIONS

- No strengthening with good tendon excursion (absent tendon lag)
- No grip and strength testing because this requires maximal effort

TREATMENT STRATEGIES

- *Splints*
  - Discontinue DBS
  - Continue PIP and/or DIP extension splint
  - Consider flexor stretcher for night
    - Wrist neutral, digits at comfortable end range
    - Wear at night
    - Continue to modify flexor stretcher to position flexor tendons at end of available range
- *Passive Motion*
  - Upgrade PROM as needed
  - In therapy *only:*
    - Passive digit extension, with wrist in flexion advancing to neutral
  - Joint mobilization for stiff joints

Postoperative Phase III (6 to 8 Weeks)—cont'd

- *Active Motion*
  - Active tenodesis for composite, straight, and hook fists
  - Progression toward active tendon glides
  - Isolated FDS and FDP glide of repaired tendon
  - NMES for muscle reeducation may be necessary
  - Gentle blocking FDS and FDP at 6 weeks, if unresponsive flexion lag
- *Functional Activities*
  - Resistive exercises with isometric pinch and grip
  - NMES with functional activities
- *HEP*
  - Tendon gliding
  - Education for light activity—use of newly splint-free hand

CRITERIA FOR ADVANCEMENT
- Absent flexor lag: Prolong phase III until 10 to 12 weeks postoperatively
- Responsive flexor lag: Progress to phase IV by week 8
- Unresponsive flexor lag: Progress to phase IV by week 6

POSTOPERATIVE PHASE IV (8 TO 16 WEEKS)

Splint

The flexor stretcher and PIP extension splints are continued as needed to achieve full extension of the MP, PIP, and DIP joints. The splints are modified as needed for maximal stretch. MP and DIP blocking splints are fabricated for differential glide exercises.

Motion

Passive motion and joint mobilization are added to achieve full range of motion (ROM). Active motion continues with the addition of resistive blocking for differential tendon glide. Resistive blocking is accomplished using blocking splints.

Functional Activities

Functional activities focus on isometric grip and pinch activities. By week 12, isotonic grip and pinch strengthening are added to the program. Fine motor control activities are added to increase individual finger control.

Criteria for Discharge

The patient is expected to achieve full active flexion and extension of the involved digits, with no more than 5 degrees of flexion lag. Strength of the involved hand should be 75% of the noninjured hand as measured with the Jamar dynamometer (Preston, Jackson, MI). Last, the patient should return to full duty work, homemaking, or other necessary life roles.

Postoperative Phase IV (8 to 16 Weeks)

GOALS
- Full active motion (absent flexor lag)
- Functional grip strength (75% of noninjured hand)
- Independence with self-care, homemaking, work, school, leisure
- Independent knowledge of precautions

PRECAUTIONS
- Do not measure grip and pinch with excellent tendon excursion
- Extreme uncontrolled force against the tendon may cause tendon rupture up to 12 weeks
- No lifting until 12 weeks with good tendon glide
- No sports or heavy labor until 16 weeks

Continued

Postoperative Phase IV (8 to 16 Weeks)—cont'd

TREATMENT STRATEGIES
- Splints
  - Continue flexor stretcher as needed
  - Continue PIP extension splinting as needed
  - Blocking splints
    - MP block for hook fisting
    - PIP block for DIP flexion
- Passive Motion
  - Full PROM
- Joint mobilization active motion
  - Tendon gliding
  - Blocking with resistance
  - NMES
- Functional activity
  - Full participation in ADL by 12 weeks
  - Grip and pinch strengthening
    - Progress from isometrics to sponge to putty to hand helper
    - Avoid specific strengthening if excellent tendon excursion
- HEP
  - Blocking exercises
  - Progress to full use of involved hand in all ADL

CRITERIA FOR DISCHARGE
- Functional active motion (less than 5 degree flexor lag)
- Functional strength (involved 75% of noninjured hand)
- Able to return to full duty work, homemaking, sports by 16 weeks post operatively

EXPECTED OUTCOME

The American Society for Surgery of the Hand (ASSH) rates post-surgical outcomes according to the percent of total active motion (TAM) achieved.[1,41] The ASSH also accepts TAM comparison with the individual's contralateral finger for a percentage of that person's norm. An excellent result indicates 100% TAM, a good result equals 75% to 99% TAM, a fair result ranges from 50% to 74% TAM, and a poor result denotes less than 50% TAM. A good result is expected, and an excellent result is preferred. Most importantly, the patient should be able to resume premorbid roles and ADL.

Formula Percent of TAM:

$$TAM = [(\text{Sum of MP/PIP/DIP flexion}) - (\text{Sum of MP/PIP/DIP extension deficit})]/260 \times 100$$

REFERENCES

1. Mackin, E., Callahan, A.D., Skirven, T.M., Schneider, L.H., Osterman, A.L., Hunter, J.M. Staged Flexor Tendon Reconstruction. In Mackin, E.J. (Eds). *Rehabilitation of the Hand and Upper Extremity.* Mosby, St. Louis, 2002, pp. 469–497.
2. Strickland, J.W. Flexor Tendons—Acute Injuries. In Green, D.P., Hotchkiss, R.N., Pederson, W.C. (Eds). *Green's Operative Hand Surgery,* 4th ed. Churchill Livingstone, New York, 1999, pp. 1851–1897.
3. Stewart, K.M. Tendon Injuries. In Stanley, B.J., Tribuzzi, S.M. (Eds). *Concepts in Hand Rehabilitation.* FA Davis Company, Philadelphia, 1992, pp. 353–392.
4. Culp, R.W., Taras, J.S. Primary Care of Flexor Tendon Injuries. In Mackin, E.J., Callahan, A.D., Skirven, T.M., Schneider, L.H., Osterman, A.L., Hunter, J.M. (Eds). *Rehabilitation of the Hand and Upper Extremity.* Mosby, St. Louis, 2002, pp. 415–430.
5. Pettengill, K.M., Van Strien, G. Postoperative Management of Flexor Tendon Injuries. In Mackin, E.J., Callahan, A.D., Skirven, T.M., Schneider, L.H., Osterman, A.L., Hunter, J.M. (Eds). *Rehabilitation of the Hand and Upper Extremity.* Mosby, St. Louis, 2002, pp. 431–456.
6. Cullen, K.W., Tolhurst, P., Lang, D., Page, R.E. *Flexor Tendon Repair Zone 2 Followed by Controlled Active Mobilisation.* J Hand Surg 1989;14B:392.
7. Gelberman, R.H., Botte, M.J., Spiegelman, J.J., Akeson, W.H. *The Excursion and Deformation of Repaired Flexor Tendons Treated with Protected Early Motion.* J Hand Surg 1986;11A:106.
8. Gelberman, R.H., Nunley, J.A. II, Osterman, A.L., Breen, T.F., Dimick, M.P., Woo, S.L. *Influences of the Protected Passive Mobilization Interval on Flexor Tendon Healing.* Clin Orthop 1991;264:189.
9. Lee, H. Double Loop Locking Suture: *A Technique of Tendon Repair for Early Active Mobilization. Part II.* J Hand Surg 1990;15A:953.
10. Lee, H. *Double Locking Suture: A Technique of Tendon Repair for Early Active Mobilization. Part I.* J Hand Surg 1990;15A:945.
11. Matthews, J.P. *Early Mobilisation after Flexor Tendon Repair.* J Hand Surg 1993;14B:363.

12. Pruitt, D.L. *Cyclic Stress Analysis of Flexor Tendon Repair.* J Hand Surg 1991;16A:701.

13. Riaz, M. *Long Term Outcome of Early Active Mobilization Following Flexor Tendon Repair in Zone II.* J Hand Surg 1999; 24B:157.

14. Robertson, G.A., Al-Qattan, N.M. *A Biomechanical Analysis of a New Interlock Suture Technique for Flexor Tendon Repair.* J Hand Surg 1992;17B:92.

15. Savage, R. *The Influence of Wrist Position on the Minimum Force Required for Active Movement of the Interphalangeal Joints.* J Hand Surg 1988;13B:262.

16. Savage, R. *Flexor Tendon Repair Using a "Six-strand" Method of Repair and Early Active Mobilization.* J Hand Surg 1989;14B: 396.

17. Small, J.O., Brennen, M.D., Colville, J. *Early Active Mobilisation Following Flexor Tendon Repair Zone 2.* J Hand Surg 1989;14B:383.

18. Trail, I.A., Powell, E.S., Noble, J. *The Mechanical Strength of Various Suture Techniques.* J Hand Surg 1992;17B:89.

19. Gelberman, R.H., Manske, P.R., Akeson, W.H., Woo, S.L., Lundborg, G., Amiel, D. *Flexor Tendon Repair.* J Orthop Res 1986;4:119.

20. Thurman, R.T., Trumble, T.E., Hanel, D.P., Tencer, A.F., Kiser, P.K. *Two-, Four-, and Six-strand Zone II Flexor Tendon Repairs: An In Situ Biomechanical Comparison Using a Cadaver Model.* J Hand Surg 1998;23A:261.

21. Kleinert, H.E., Kutz, J.E., Cohen, M.J. Primary Repair of Zone 2 Flexor Tendon Lacerations. In *AAOS Symposium on Tendon Surgery in the Hand.* Mosby, St. Louis, 1975, pp. 91–104.

22. Kleinert, H.E., Kutz, J.E., Cohen, M.J. *Primary Repair of Lacerated Flexor Tendons in No-man's-land.* J Bone Joint Surg 1967;49A:577.

23. Duran, R., Houser, R. Management of Flexor Tendon Lacerations in Zone 2 Using Controlled Passive Motion Postoperatively. In Hunter, J., Schneider, L., Mackin, E., Bell, J. (Eds). *Rehabilitation of the Hand.* Mosby, St. Louis, 1978, pp. 217–224.

24. Duran, R., Houser, R. Controlled Passive Motion Following Flexor Tendon Repair in Zones 2 and 3. In *AAOS Symposium on Tendon Surgery in the Hand.* Mosby, St. Louis, 1975, pp. 105–144.

25. Allen, B.N., Frykman, G.K., Unsell, R.S., Wood, V.E. *Ruptured Flexor Tendon Tenorrhaphies in Zone II: Repair and Rehabilitation.* J Hand Surg 1987;12A:18.

26. Bainbridge, L.C., Robertson, C., Gillies, D., Elliot, D. *A Comparison of Post-operative Mobilization of Flexor Tendon Repairs with "Passive Flexion-active Extension" and "Controlled Active Motion" Techniques.* J Hand Surg 1994;19B:517.

27. Elliot, D., Moiemen, N.S., Flemming, A.F., Harris, S.B., Foster, A.J. *The Rupture Rate of Acute Flexor Tendon Repairs Mobilized by the Controlled Active Motion Regimen.* J Hand Surg 1994;19B:607.

28. Gratton, P. *Early Active Mobilization after Flexor Tendon Repairs.* J Hand Ther 1993;6:285.

29. Yii, N., Urban, M., Elliot, D. *A Prospective Study of Flexor Tendon Repair in Zone 5.* J Hand Surg 1998;23B:642.

30. Strickland, J.W. *Flexor Tendon Injuries II: Operative Technique.* J Acad Orthop Surg 1995;3:55.

31. Strickland, J.W. *Flexor Tendon Injuries: Foundations of Treatment.* J Am Acad Orthop Surg 1995;3:44.

32. Cannon, N. *Post Flexor Tendon Repair Motion Protocol.* Indiana Hand Cent Newsl 1993;1:13.

33. Silfverskiold, K.L., May, E.J. *Flexor Tendon Repair in Zone II with a New Suture Technique and an Early Mobilization Program Combining Passive and Active Flexion.* J Hand Surg 1994;18A:654.

34. Woo, S.L., Gelberman, R.H., Cobb, N.G., Amiel, D., Lothringer, K., Akeson, W.H. *The Importance of Controlled Passive Mobilization on Flexor Tendon Healing.* Acta Orthop Scand 1981;52:615.

35. Gelberman, R.H., Woo, S.L., Lothringer, K., Akeson, W.H., Amiel, D. *Effects of Early Intermittent Passive Mobilization on Healing Canine Flexor Tendons.* J Hand Surg 1982;7:170.

36. Gelberman, R.H., Amifl, D., Gonsalves, M., Page, R.E. *The Influence of Protected Passive Mobilization on the Healing Flexor Tendons: A Biomechanical and Microangiographic Study.* Hand Clin 1981;13:120.

37. Mason, J., Allen, H. *The Rate of Healing Tendons: An Experimental Study of Tensile Strength.* Ann Surg 1941;113:424.

38. Hitchcock, T.F., Light, T.R., Bunch, W.H., Knight, G.W., Sartori, M.J., Patwardhan, A.G., Hollyfield, R.L. *The Effect of Immediate Constrained Digital Motion on the Strength of F lexor Tendon Repairs in Chickens.* J Hand Surg 1987;12A:590.

39. Groth, G.N. *Pyramid of Progressive Force Exercises to the Injured Flexor Tendon.* J Hand Ther 2004;17:31.

40. Stewart Pettengill, K. Postoperative Therapy Concepts in Management of Tendon Injuries: Early Mobilization. In Hunter, J., Schneider, L., Mackin, E. (Eds). *Tendon and Nerve Surgery in the Hand: A Third Decade.* Mosby, St. Louis, 1997, pp. 332–341.

41. American Society for Surgery of the Hand (ASSH): *Clinical Assessment Committee Report.* American Society for Surgery of the Hand, 1976.

42. Halikis, M.N., Manske, P.R., Kubota, H., Aoki, M. *Effect of Immobilization, Immediate Mobilization, and Delayed Mobilization on the Resistance to Digital Flexion Using a Tendon Injury Model.* J Hand Surg 1997;22A:464.

15

Extensor Tendon Repairs

KARA GAFFNEY GALLAGHER, MS, OTR/L, CHT

The extensor system is divided into eight zones that extend from the fingertips to the forearm (Figure 15-1). The thumb is divided into five zones (T-1 through T-5) (Figure 15-1). The extensor tendons in the hand are particularly susceptible to injury because of their unique anatomy and superficial location as the tendons course distally beyond the wrist. Research in human cadavers indicates that the thickness of the extensor tendons ranges from 1.7 mm in the forearm to 0.65 mm in the distal fingertip.[1] Limited subcutaneous tissue and elastic skin cover the extensor tendons on the dorsal wrist, hand, and digits, leaving the extensor tendons vulnerable to injury. Laceration, deep abrasion, crush, forceful rupture, and avulsion fracture are the major causes of extensor tendon injuries.[1] Systemic disease, such as rheumatoid arthritis, also affects the integrity of the extensor tendons, predisposing them to attenuation and rupture.

Extensor tendon injuries are treated conservatively via immobilization or with surgical repair. Immobilization is used to treat closed terminal tendon disruption in the digits and thumb, because injury to the terminal tendon does not result in retraction of the tendon ends because of soft tissue attachments and interconnections at multiple levels.[1-3] All other extensor tendon injuries are treated surgically. This allows for early mobilization to begin as early as 24 hours postoperatively. Suture techniques that have been used successfully for flexor tendon repair have been modified to accommodate the thinner extensor tendons in the fingers. Extensor tendons exhibit approximately 50% of the strength of repaired flexor tendons because of reduced tendon dimension and collagen cross linking.[4] Postoperative extensor tendons require protective splinting and carefully controlled mobilization following surgery.

REHABILITATION OVERVIEW

Historically, extensor tendon repairs have been immobilized in a splint, whether conservatively or surgically managed, for a minimum of 3 weeks. Studies over the last 20 years indicate that immobilization of tendons following surgical repair leads to a high percentage of fair to poor results[1,5,6] because of adhesion formation that limits tendon excursion and joint motion.[7-9] In the past several years, early mobilization, supported by evidence related to flexor tendon management, has been advocated in the care extensor tendon injuries. Studies on postoperative flexor and extensor management demonstrate that repaired tendons tolerate early active motion and have better outcomes.[7,8,10] Evans[7,11] has described the following principles for the therapeutic management of extensor tendons.

- Extensor tendons in all zones (with the exception of zones I and II) tolerate early controlled active motion.
- Wrist position affects tendon excursion by decreasing the resistive forces from the flexor system.
- Early therapeutic intervention, within 24 hours to 3 days postoperatively, is critical.[10]
- Accurate splint design and diligent postoperative control of force, excursion, and design prevent gapping and rupture.

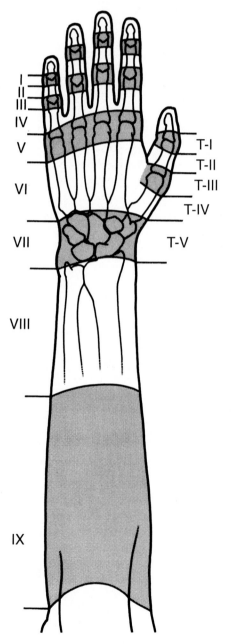

FIGURE 15-1 Zones of extensor tendon injuries in the digits and thumb. *(From Doyle, J. Extensor Tendons—Acute Injuries. In Green, D.P., Hotchkiss, R.N., Pederson, W.C. [Eds]. Green's Operative Hand Surgery, 4th ed. Churchill Livingstone, New York, 1999, p. 1956.)*

The decision to use an immobilization or early mobilization protocol depends on several factors. To withstand the force of early mobilization, a strong surgical repair and good tendon quality are required. Conservatively managed tendons, not surgically managed, require a period of immobilization to allow the gap between the interrupted tendons to heal sufficiently. In addition, the physiology of the tendons over the distal phalanges of the fingers and thumb prevents these tendons from being able to tolerate the stress of early mobilization. Therefore, tendons in zones I, II, and T-I, whether treated conservatively or surgically, benefit from an immobilization period. Tendons in zones III through VIII and T-II through V tolerate and benefit from early mobilization protocols.

At the Hospital for Special Surgery (HSS), the authors use an early mobilization program for postoperative care of extensor tendons in all zones, except zones I, II, and T-I, where active force is not tolerated by the flat, thin, and broad extensor tendon. Early mobilization refers to either controlled passive motion or early active motion. Early mobilization programs require a strong surgical repair, good tendon integrity, patient compliance, and referral to therapy within 24 hours to 3 days after surgery. The early active motion program is based on the scientific studies describing an immediate active short arc motion protocol by Evans[5,7,11–14] and studies regarding positive effects of active mobilization for flexor tendons.[10,15–19] The early mobilization guidelines for thumb zones T-II and T-IV are also based on Evans'[7] suggestions. Early active motion requires a strong repair to withstand active tension of the involved extensor tendon. In addition, early active motion must begin when the repaired tendon quality is at its best 24 hours to 3 days after surgery. Studies indicate that the projected tensile strength of an unstressed tendon repair may decrease as much as 25% to 50% at 5 to 51 days after surgery because of softening of the tendon ends.[7,10,20,21] The following guideline describes extensor tendon anatomy, injury, surgery, and rehabilitation by zone, expected outcome, and criteria for discharge from therapy.

Early active motion for zones III through VIII and zones T-IV and T-V in the thumb begins with passive wrist tenodesis exercises, followed by active place-hold extension, and protected active extension. A safe arc of motion is described for each zone to protect the repair site and promote healing. The arc of motion has been determined by calculations of tendon excursion measured in radians.[7] Protected joint motion allowing for 3 to 5 mm of tendon excursion has been defined as safe and effective in preventing rupture or gapping while promoting functional glide and cellular healing.[7,11,18,22]

CALCULATING EXTENSOR TENDON EXCURSION

To theoretically determine how much joint motion provides 3 to 5 mm of tendon excursion, Evans[7] synthesized information from excursion studies in the literature, mathematical calculations by radians,[11,22–24] and intraoperative measurements.[11,22] In zones III and IV, 30 degrees of proximal interphalangeal (PIP) flexion creates 4 mm of extensor digitorum communis (EDC) excursion.[11,13] In zones V through VIII, 30 to 40 degrees of metacarpophalangeal (MP) flexion offers 4 to 5 mm of EDC excursion.[11,22] In zones T-III through T-V, 60 degrees of interphalangeal (IP) flexion allows 5 mm of extensor pollicis longus (EPL) excursion.[7]

CONTRAINDICATIONS FOR EARLY ACTIVE MOTION

As described previously, closed zone I and II tendon injuries in the digits and zone I in the thumb are treated via immobilization. Children under age 10 and noncompliant or incompetent adult patients are better managed with immobilization protocols. Patients referred to therapy more than 3 days postoperatively cannot begin early mobilization because of decreased tensile strength of the repair. In this case, immobilization for 3 weeks is indicated to allow for healing to occur.

SPLINTING

Various splint designs are described and pictured in this guideline. Splint design varies by zone of injury and associated structures involved in the injury. The basic splints included in this guideline are static finger or forearm-based splints that include only the joints crossed by the affected tendon. Static progressive and dynamic splints to affect tendon extensibility or joint stiffness may or may not be incorporated into the rehabilitation process, depending on progress and functional gains. These splints will be mentioned in considerations for each zone.

EDEMA CONTROL

Edema control is mandatory in treating the postoperative extensor tendon. Postoperative edema relates directly to the fibroblastic response and collagen production at the injury site.[7] Digital edema is minimized with a single layer of Coban (3M Health Care, St. Paul, MN) for as long as any excessive volume is present around the PIP joint (up to 8 to 12 weeks postoperatively). Dorsal hand edema is controlled with bulky, compressive dressing between exercises and therapy sessions. Elevation, motion of the uninvolved joints, and controlled motion of the involved joints assist in decreasing edema.

SCAR MANAGEMENT

Superficial finger digital scars are managed with a silicone gel pad. Dorsal hand and forearm scars often require custom silicone scar pads for improved fit and effectiveness. Cross-friction scar massage helps soften adhesions and increase the pliability of the skin and underlying structures.

HOME EXERCISE PROGRAM

The patient is instructed in a specific home exercise program (HEP) that is appropriate for the repaired zone. The HEP also includes education for safe splint donning/doffing techniques. Exercises are performed in the confines of the splint until the patient demonstrates competence. The therapist determines the frequency of exercise based on the quality of tendon glide. Each zone in this guideline recommends a specific HEP with suggested frequency.

CRITERIA FOR ADVANCEMENT

The criterion for advancement in all zones is the presence of an extensor lag. *Extensor lag* is defined as passive extension that exceeds active extension. When full active extension is present, there is no lag, and treatment is progressed according to the phases in the guideline. When an extension lag of 10 degrees or more is present, active flexion is curtailed and the focus is aimed at obtaining full active extension before advancement to the next phase. It is important to concentrate on the extension exercises and avoid emphasizing flexion at the expense of extension. Increases in passive and active flexion are avoided unless full active extension has been achieved.[7]

REHABILITATION BY EXTENSOR TENDON ZONE: ZONES I AND II

ANATOMY, INJURY, AND TREATMENT

Zone I includes the distal interphalangeal (DIP) joint, and zone II encompasses the middle phalanx proximal to the DIP joint. The terminal extensor tendon in zone I is composed of the merged lateral bands arising from the lumbricals and interossei and inserts on the dorsal base of the distal phalanx. The oblique retinacular ligament (ORL) borders the terminal tendon, inserting on the lateral base of the distal phalanx. Treatment of the central fibers of the terminal extensor tendon includes the ORL as a result of the merging of adjacent tendon and ligament fibers as they approach insertion on the distal phalanx.[4] Zones I and II extensor tendon injuries

are referred to as *mallet finger, baseball finger,* or *drop finger.* Mallet finger, the most frequently used description, indicates interruption in the continuity of the terminal extensor tendon over the DIP joint and/or lateral bands on either side of the DIP joint.[1,4,25,26] The DIP joint postures in varying degrees of flexion; full passive extension is usually available, but the patient cannot actively extend the joint. PIP joint hyperextension may occur because of an unopposed central slip and joint laxity.[1,27]

Mallet finger results from open or closed injury caused by sports or occupational activities.[1,25] Closed injuries are more common and are caused by sudden acute, forceful flexion of the extended digit, leading to a rupture of the terminal extensor tendon or fracture of the distal phalanx, with avulsion of the tendon insertion with or without a small bony fragment.[1] Closed mallet finger can also occur secondary to an intra-articular fracture in the base of the distal phalanx involving one third more bone.[1,25] This fracture differs from an avulsion fracture involving the terminal tendon and requires treatment separate from the protocol described here (see Chapter 13). Open mallet finger injuries can be the result of direct sharp or crushing lacerations to the tendon and often require surgical repair of the skin and tendon.[1] Untreated mallet fingers or poorly managed cases may progress into swan-neck deformity because of the imbalance of forces that causes the finger to posture in PIP hyperextension with DIP flexion.

Closed mallet fingers, including avulsion fractures, are treated with nonsurgical immobilization of the DIP joint in extension to slight hyperextension.[1,4] The PIP joint is included at 30 to 45 degrees of flexion if it presents in slight hyperextension.[1] Immobilization continues for 6 weeks. Mallet finger injury is treated surgically with K-wire fixation of the DIP joint in the case of nonreducible or complex fractures to compress the fracture site and prevent proximal retraction of the terminal tendon.[4] K-wire fixation is also used with chronic/recurrent deformity and noncompliant or pediatric patients.[4,7] In a complex open mallet finger injury, surgery may be needed to reapproximate the skin and tendon as well as to treat an associated fracture.[4,28] Direct repair of the terminal extensor tendon is not advised because sutures in the thin extensor tendon over the distal phalanx almost always rupture.[1] Terminal tendon ends can be approximated with intramedullary K-wire pinning of the DIP joint in slight hyperextension without the need for sutures in the tendon.[4] However, it may be necessary to both pin and reconnect the tendon ends with either a horizontal or interrupted suture repair to achieve optimum results.[4]

POSTOPERATIVE MANAGEMENT

Motion

Postoperative extensor tendon injuries in zones I and II are treated with immobilization for 6 weeks. Immobilization continues for 6 weeks when gentle active flexion and extension exercises commence. If an extension lag is present, immobilization continues and mobilization is delayed for an additional 2 weeks. During the first week of mobilization, the patient actively flexes the DIP joint no more than 20 to 25 degrees. The flexion angle is increased to 35 degrees in the second week, as long as full active extension is maintained. DIP flexion is gradually increased with close monitoring of active extension. If an extension lag develops, active flexion is halted and therapy refocuses on achieving full active extension. Gentle tendon gliding (with the exception of composite fisting) and ORL stretch begin during the second to third week of mobilization. The ORL is passively stretched by manually extending the PIP joint and gently flexing the DIP joint. Active composite fisting begins 9 weeks after the start of immobilization. Full active flexion and extension should be achieved within 12 weeks of immobilization.

Splints

The DIP joint is splinted in extension in approximately 0 to 10 degrees of hyperextension for 6 weeks, regardless of whether the injury was treated with conservative or operative management (Figure 15-2). Hyperextension greater than 10 degrees is avoided because it compromises circulation to the dorsal skin by stretching the volar vessels. Placing extreme stretch on the volar vasculature hinders nutrition to the area distal to the end of the termination of the dorsal vasculature, thereby creating skin necrosis.[7,29] Skin blanching precedes skin necrosis and can be used as a guide in setting the DIP joint in a safe position of hyperextension.[7,30] The DIP

joint is positioned at an angle of hyperextension less than the angle that causes blanching of the volar skin.[7,30]

Custom thermoplastic splints best support the DIP joint in extension to hyperextension and allow for adjustments as swelling subsides. A dorsal splint with the volar component supporting the distal phalanx and the dorsal component crossing the DIP joint and extending just distal to the PIP joint applies two points of counterpressure to hold the DIP joint in a safe position for healing. The splint can be taped into position or secured with Velcro over the middle phalanx, and the PIP joint is free to move.

The splint design must support the DIP joint in extension in 0 to 10 degrees of hyperextension. A position of slight flexion will result in an extensor lag because the terminal tendon will heal in an elongated position.[7,31] If the PIP joint assumes or develops slight hyperextension, the joint should be splinted at 30 to 45 degrees of flexion with DIP joint in 0 to 10 degrees of hyperextension in a figure-eight design (Figure 15-3). This position will advance the lateral bands dorsally and promote closer approximation of the injured extensor tendon ends.[7,31] The patient is monitored weekly during the immobilization phase for splint adjustments as needed, wound care, and maintenance of motion in the uninvolved joints. Weekly visits are particularly important for splint adjustments to accommodate changes in edema. Typically, edema will decrease in the digit within the first week or two. A splint that is too large will allow for DIP flexion and defeat the purpose of extension splinting if left unchanged.

Patient education regarding donning and doffing the splint, as well as skin care, are essential components to promote speedy recovery. Skin maceration is a concern

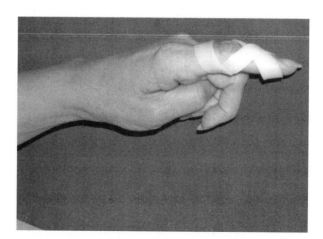

FIGURE 15-3 Figure-eight splint for mallet finger injury when PIP hyperextends with attempted DIP extension: PIP joint in 30 to 45 degrees flexion, DIP joint in 0 to 10 degrees hyperextension.

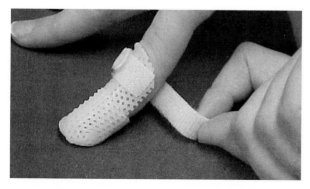

FIGURE 15-2 Splint for mallet finger injury: DIP joint in 0 to 10 degrees hyperextension.

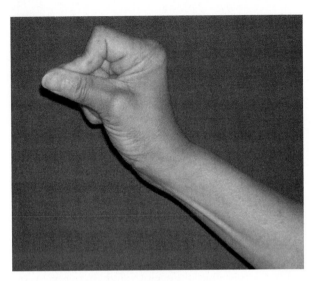

FIGURE **15-4** Safe position to maintain DIP joint in hyperextension when donning/doffing splint.

when continuously wearing the plastic splint. Therefore, the patient is instructed to change to a dry splint when the finger has become wet or damp. During the change of splints, the DIP joint is supported in hyperextension to preserve any healing that has occurred. This is achieved by using the ipsilateral thumb to hold the DIP joint in hyperextension while using the noninvolved hand to cleanse and apply the dry splint[7] (Figure 15-4). Two splints are made for the patient to ensure constant splinting throughout the 6 weeks; one splint is always ready to go if the patient needs to change splints for any reason.

Once the mobilization phase begins at 6 weeks, the patient is gradually weaned from the splint, unless an extensor lag develops. If an extensor lag develops, splinting continues until the lag resolves. During week 7, the splint is removed for exercises only. In week 8, the splint is removed intermittently during the day and continues to be worn at night. During week 9, splinting continues at night only. By week 10, the splint is discontinued.

Functional Activity

During the 6 weeks of immobilization, the patient may use the digit for light to moderate activities, ensuring that the splint stays in place. Heavy occupational or athletic activities are avoided during the 6 weeks. Prehension and coordination activities are gradually introduced to complement range of motion (ROM) exercises by the second week of mobilization. Once the splint has been discharged during the day, by 8 weeks, the affected digit is gradually incorporated into functional activity. Unrestricted hand use is encouraged by week 12. A return to heavy labor and sports is permitted by 16 weeks.

HOME EXERCISE PROGRAM

During the period of immobilization, the patient performs a HEP of active and passive MP and PIP flexion and extension to maintain joint mobility. Once active motion commences at 6 weeks, active DIP flexion/extension exercises are added to the program. DIP flexion is graded as described previously. Passive DIP flexion and composite fisting begin at 9 weeks. The home program includes standard techniques for edema and scar management. In addition, active ROM of uninvolved joints is recommended three times per day.

TROUBLESHOOTING

If the patient presents with a hypermobile PIP joint that hyperextends with attempted DIP extension, a figure-eight splint is worn while exercising. In this case, the DIP extensor lag is monitored because it can lead to a swan-neck deformity.

Zones I and II: Immobilization

GOALS

- 0 to 6 weeks
  - Splint to prevent DIP extensor lag and educate patient for proper donning/doffing of splint to protect healing extensor tendon
  - Weekly check splint fit to ensure DIP joint is held in full to slight hyperextension
- 6 to 12 weeks
  - Maintain 0 degrees of active DIP extension
  - Attain 70 degrees of active DIP flexion

PRECAUTIONS

- Do not splint DIP joint in so much hyperextension that beginning signs of ischemia develop (volar distal phalange blanches).
- No active or passive DIP motion until week 6 (if no surgery)
- No active or passive DIP motion until week 5 (if surgery)
- Avoid moderate to heavy ADL until week 12.

TREATMENT STRATEGIES
Splints

- Static DIP extension splint with two points of counterpressure
  - Include volar and dorsal distal phalanx
  - Cross the dorsal DIP joint, covering the dorsal middle phalanx distal to the PIP joint
  - 0 to 10 degrees of DIP joint hyperextension
  - Continuous splinting for at least 6 weeks (if no surgery)
  - Continuous splinting for at least 5 weeks (if surgery)
  - Possibly continue splinting between exercise sessions and at night if extensor lag present
- Static DIP extension and PIP flexion (figure-eight design)
  - If patient develops PIP hyperextension in addition to mallet finger
  - DIP 0 to 10 degrees extension, PIP 30 to 45 degrees of flexion
- Blocking splints: 6 weeks+
  - Static palm-based MP extension blocker for hook fisting
  - Static palm-based MP and PIP extension blockers for isolated DIP flexion

Motion

- 0 to 6 weeks
  - No active or passive DIP joint motion
  - Active motion of uninvolved joints
- 6+ weeks
  - 6 to 7 weeks
    - Active DIP flexion/extension 0 to 25 degrees
  - 7 to 8 weeks
    - Active/passive DIP flexion/extension 0 to 35 degrees
    - Gentle tendon gliding—tabletop, straight, hook, full fists
    - ORL stretch
  - 8 to 12 weeks
    - Gradually increase DIP extension/flexion to 0 to 70 degrees
    - Add composite fist to tendon gliding

Functional Activity

- 0 to 6 weeks
  - Light ADL with splint donned at all times, including bathing/showering
- 6 to 12 weeks
  - Incorporate prehension and fine motor coordination activities into therapy session.
  - Light ADL without splint (if no extensor lag)
  - Light ADL with splint until extensor lag resolves
- 12 weeks
  - Resume all ADL without splint
- 16 weeks
  - Return to heavy labor and sports

HOME EXERCISE PROGRAM

- 0 to 6 weeks: patient educated for safe donning/doffing of splint
- 6+ weeks: incorporate exercises from therapy (10 times each, 3 times/day)

CRITERIA FOR DISCONTINUING SPLINT

- No extensor lag at 6 weeks indicates initiation of active DIP motion.
- Extensor lag at 6 weeks indicates 2 additional weeks of splinting full time.

ZONES III AND IV

ANATOMY

Zone III encompasses the PIP joint, and zone IV extends beyond the proximal phalanx to the MP joint. The central slip from EDC, which primarily extends the PIP joint, courses distally through zone IV to insert on the middle phalanx in zone III. The EDC also gives off lateral slips that join medial slips from the interossei and lumbricals to form the lateral bands in zone IV. With PIP flexion, the lateral bands migrate palmarly. As the central slip extends the PIP joint, the lateral bands glide dorsally and increase tension to assist PIP extension.[1] The transverse retinacular ligaments connect the lateral bands and also contribute to the extension of the PIP joint.[1] Hyperextension of the PIP joint is prevented by the palmar plate and flexor digitorum superficialis (FDS) tendon.[1]

INJURY AND TREATMENT

Injury in zones III and IV results from closed trauma, laceration, burns, rheumatoid synovitis, or tightly placed casts or splints.[1] Interruption of the central slip and retinacular ligaments affects the muscle balance at the PIP joint. The PIP joint assumes a flexed position after injury, and attempted active extension transmits force only to the DIP joint through the intact lateral bands. Interruption to the central slip and triangular ligament is easily corrected in the acute phase, but over time unopposed PIP flexion increasingly resists correction as the extensor mechanism migrates proximally, ligaments shorten, flexor tendons contract, and the lateral bands assume a more palmar position.[1] If left untreated, the finger will develop a boutonniere deformity of PIP flexion with DIP hyperextension that negatively affects prognosis for treatment (Figure 15-5). The lateral bands may be involved in the injury, but they are often spared because of their ulnar or radial location.[1,32,33] Injuries to zones T-III and T-IV in the thumb may involve the extensor pollicis longus (EPL) and/or extensor pollicis brevis (EPB). EPL injury results in loss of thumb IP extension, and EPB disruption leads to some loss of MP extension.[1]

Depending on the severity of injury to the central slip and/or lateral bands, surgery may be required to achieve functional extension of the PIP joint. For a mild extension lag (loss of active extension with full passive extension), immobilization of the PIP joint at 0 degrees is recommended. PIP motion is reassessed after 1 week; if the PIP joint can actively extend, splinting continues for 2 more weeks.[1] However, if the extension lag persists, immobilization in extension is continued for an additional 6 weeks. Surgical repair is indicated when the finger presents with active and passive extension loss, joint instability, and/or fracture.[1] Severe tendon and soft

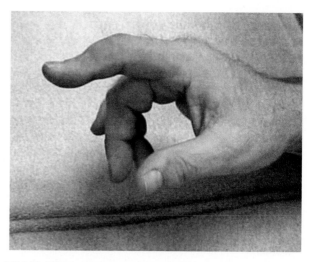

FIGURE **15-5** Boutonniere deformity. *(Courtesy of Aviva Wolff, OTR/L, CHT, New York.)*

tissue injuries combined with a fracture may require staged tendon reconstruction.[1] A modified version of sutures used for the flexor tendons is used to repair the tendon.

POSTOPERATIVE MANAGEMENT

Motion

Postoperative extensor tendon injuries in zones III and IV are managed with immobilization or early active motion. Extensor tendons that are repaired surgically can be treated with an early active motion protocol. An immobilization protocol is used for extensor tendons in zones III and IV, which are managed conservatively. This guideline describes the early active motion approach that is initiated within the first 3 days post-surgery.

The early active motion guideline for zones III and IV are based on Evans'[7] short arc motion for the repaired central slip. Positioning of the wrist and MP joints is critical to avoid stress on the repair site. For active exercises, the wrist is positioned at 30 degrees of flexion and the MP joint in 0 degrees for the first 6 weeks. This position uses the tenodesis effect to place slight tension on the involved extensor tendon, thereby assisting active extension and reducing the antagonistic resistance of the flexors.[7] The PIP and DIP joints move in a controlled range that is limited by the template splints. MP joint and wrist active motion begins immediately without restrictions with the digit splint in place.

In the first week after surgery, two template splints are fabricated (Figures 15-6 and 15-7). The PIP joint is actively flexed and extended 30 degrees, and the DIP joint is actively flexed and extended 25 degrees within template splint *A* (see Figure 15-6). The DIP joint is flexed and extended using template splint *B*, which

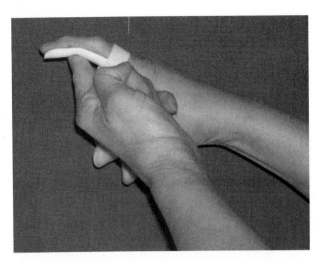

FIGURE **15-6** Short arc motion protocol for zones III and IV: Template splint *A* blocks PIP flexion at 30 degrees and DIP flexion at 25 degrees.

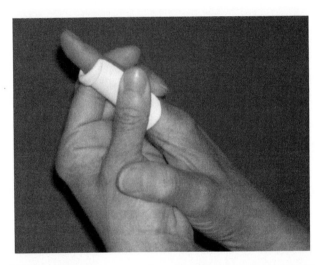

FIGURE **15-7** Short arc motion protocol for zones III and IV: Template splint *B* blocks PIP in 0 degrees extension and allows full DIP flexion.

blocks the PIP joint in 0 degrees extension (see Figure 15-7). If the lateral bands were not involved, full active DIP flexion and extension is allowed, using template splint *B*. If the lateral bands were repaired, then DIP flexion is limited to 30 to 35 degrees, using a modified version of template splint *B*[7] (Figure 15-8). Both splints are manually held in place by the patient. Each exercise is performed slowly, with a brief hold period in the fully extended position. Twenty repetitions of each exercise are recommended.

At 2 weeks post-surgery, the flexion angle of the PIP template splint is increased to allow 40 degrees of PIP motion, as long as an extensor lag has not developed.[7] PIP flexion increases by 10 degrees per week, as long as no extensor lag develops.[7] At 5 weeks post-surgery, the template splints are discontinued, and isolated DIP and

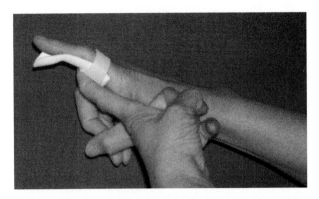

FIGURE **15-8** Short arc motion protocol for zones III and IV: Modified template splint *B* blocks PIP in 0 degrees extension and blocks DIP flexion at 30 to 35 degrees because of lateral band involvement.

PIP flexion and extension exercises with the MP joint in extension are added. This is followed by combined IP flexion and extension with the MP joint blocked in extension and flexion. Passive range of motion (PROM) to increase PIP flexion and extension is also added at this time. During mobilization techniques, the MP joint and wrist is held in extension to avoid tension on the repaired extensor tendon. At 6 weeks, tendon gliding exercises are added in the following sequence—tabletop, straight fist, composite fist, and hook fist—to encourage EDC gliding (Figure 15-9, *A* and *B*). Strengthening begins at 8 to 10 weeks post-surgery, as long as the PIP joint can actively extend to 0 degrees.

Splints

The early active motion program for zones III and IV requires immobilization of the repaired structures at all times, except during exercise. Immobilization with a static splint continues for 5 to 6 weeks after surgery. A custom volar or circumferential splint that supports the PIP and DIP joints in extension is fabricated (Figure 15-10).

If the patient presents with a stiff PIP joint and limited flexion 4 weeks postoperatively, an intermittent PIP flexion splint may be needed (Figure 15-11). The static extension splint continues at other times and in between exercise sessions until week 6, when weaning from the splint during the day begins. Nighttime wear continues until week 8.

Functional Activity

During the first 6 weeks post-surgery, the patient may use the hand for light to moderate activities while wearing the splint. Heavy occupational or athletic activities are avoided during the 6 weeks. Prehension and coordination activities are gradually introduced during therapy to complement ROM exercises by week 7, when weaning from the splint during the day begins.

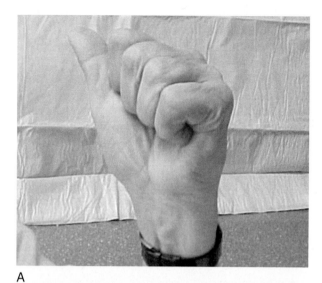

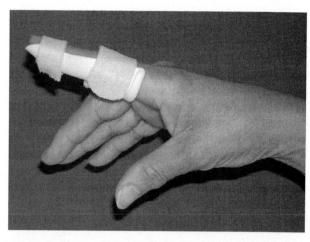

FIGURE **15-10** Custom volar digital splint supporting PIP and DIP joints in 0 degrees extension.

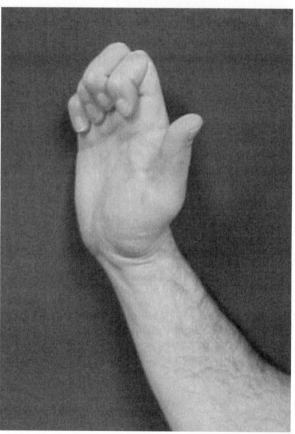

FIGURE **15-9** EDC glides: active extension from composite fist to hook fist. *A.* Composite fist. *B.* Hook fist.

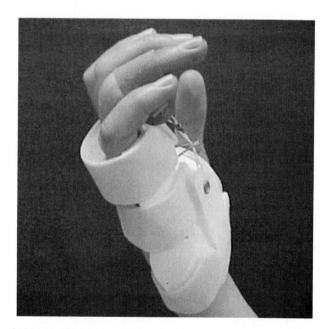

FIGURE **15-11** Static progressive PIP joint flexion splint. *(Courtesy of Amy Barenholtz, OTR/L, CHT, New York.)*

TROUBLESHOOTING

A weekly assessment of extensor lag is required to determine when to advance to the next exercise. If an extensor lag of greater than 10 degrees is present, the angle of the splint is altered (increased extension) to minimize the effort in returning to full extension. Place-hold exercises at various angles of extension provide another way to emphasize extension over flexion. Conversely, if PIP or DIP flexion is limited, then static progressive splinting may be necessary to increase joint mobility and tendon extensibility.

Once the splint has been discharged during the day, by 8 weeks, the affected hand is gradually incorporated into functional activities. Unrestricted hand use for ADL and light occupations is expected by week 12. A return to sports and heavy labor is permitted 16 weeks postoperatively.

Zones III and IV: Early Active Motion (Short Arc Motion)

GOALS

- Full active DIP and PIP extension and flexion
- Incorporate injured digit into ADL
- Independence with premorbid ADL

PRECAUTIONS

- *Do not* use this protocol unless involved tendons were surgically repaired.
- Avoid emphasizing flexion gains over extension.
- Position wrist in 30 degrees flexion/MP joints in 0 degrees during active IP motion during first 6 weeks.

TREATMENT STRATEGIES
Splints

- Immobilization splint
  - Static volar gutter extension splint with DIP and PIP in 0 degrees extension
  - Immobilization straps placed over joints to ensure full extension
  - Continue 5 to 6 weeks postoperatively
- Exercise splints
  - Splint A: DIP allowed 25 degrees of flexion; PIP allowed 30 degrees of flexion
  - Splint B: PIP extension blocking splint for active DIP flexion
- Static progressive or dynamic PIP flexion splint
  - Not until week 4
  - Intermittent use to decrease joint stiffness

Motion

- Early active short arc motion
  - 0 to 1 week
    - Splint A: active flexion to splint limits followed by active extension to 0 degrees
    - Splint B: full active DIP flexion, if lateral bands are not involved
    - Splint B: limit active DIP flexion to 30 to 35 degrees, if lateral bands are repaired
    - Repeat each exercise 20 times, with a hold for three counts
  - 2 to 3 weeks
    - Splint A: increase flexion angle to allow 40 degrees of active flexion/extension
    - Splint B: continue with unlimited active DIP flexion; if lateral bands were repaired, increase angle to 45 degrees
  - 4 to 5 weeks
    - Splint A: increase flexion angle to 50 degrees in beginning of week 4; continue to increase angle up to 80 degrees by end of week 5
    - Splint B: allow full DIP flexion
    - Gentle passive ROM of all joints on individual basis with others held in protected position
  - 5+ weeks
    - Discontinue exercise splints
    - Unrestricted isolated and composite DIP and PIP active motion (hold MP joints in 0 degrees extension)
    - Initiate tendon glides (hook, tabletop at 5 weeks; straight, composite at 6 weeks)
    - Manual mobilization to increase PIP flexion
    - Isometric, then isotonic grip strengthening
- MP joint and wrist AROM
  - Begin immediately with static extension splint in place.

Functional Activity

- 0 to 6 weeks: light ADL with immobilization splint donned
- 6 to 8 weeks:
  - Light ADL without splint (unless extensor lag)
  - Incorporate static prehension and coordination activities into therapy sessions (dowel putty stamping, BTE Work Simulator, MULE)
- 8 to 12 weeks
  - Moderate ADL without splint (unless extensor lag)
  - Incorporate dynamic prehension and grip activities into therapy sessions
- 12 weeks: resume full participation in all ADL
- 16 weeks: heavy labor and sports permitted

HOME EXERCISE PROGRAM

- 0 to 6 weeks: add template splint exercises when patient becomes competent (10 times each, 3 times/day)
- 6+ weeks: tendon gliding, fine motor coordination activities, static grip strengthening

ZONES V AND VI

ANATOMY

Zone V includes the dorsal surface of the MP joint, the dorsal extensor hood, and the sagittal bands that are derived from the extrinsic extensor system. The sagittal bands stabilize the EDC in the center of the MP joint. Zone V in the thumb, the last of the thumb zones, includes the carpometacarpal (CMC) joint, over which the EPB and abductor pollicis longus (APL) run.[1,7] Zone VI extends proximally over the dorsum of the hand from the MP joints to the wrist and includes the EDC, extensor indicis proprius (EIP), extensor digiti quinti (EDQ) tendons, and juncturae tendinum. The juncturae tendinum are broad intertendinous connections proximal to the MP joints that extend from the extensor tendon of the ring finger to connect with EDC tendons of the long and small, and sometimes the index, fingers.[4] These bands assist with extension by transmitting force to associated fingers.[4] Extensor tendon injury proximal to zone VI may be overlooked by the contribution of intact juncturae tendinum.[4]

INJURIES AND TREATMENT

Injuries in zone V are frequently associated with open wounds and subsequent laceration of the extensor tendon and/or sagittal bands at the MP joint. Injury to the sagittal bands can result in radial or ulnar subluxation of the EDC tendon over the MP joint.[4] Open lacerations of the sagittal bands in zone V are surgically repaired to stabilize the extensor tendon over the center of the MP joint.[1] If the sagittal band is not repaired, the extensor tendon may sublux, thereby impairing extension of the associated finger and leading to deviation and flexion at the MP level.[1,4] Closed rupture of the sagittal band and oblique fibers of the extensor hood as a result of forceful MP flexion is treated with 6 weeks of immobilization splinting.[1] Delayed treatment of a closed rupture (longer than 2 weeks) may require surgical repair to centralize the extensor tendon.[1]

POSTOPERATIVE MANAGEMENT

Postoperative care of zones V and VI includes immobilization, early passive mobilization, and early active mobilization protocols. The choice of protocol is determined by the method of intervention (surgical repair or immobilization), the quality of the tendon, the strength of the repair, associated injuries, and compliance of the patient. When possible, early active mobilization is the preferred treatment protocol for surgically repaired injuries in this zone. The following guideline describes early active mobilization following surgical management.

Motion

Phase I: Days 0 to 21. Therapy begins with passive wrist tenodesis exercises to improve controlled movement of the repair site.[7,34,35] The wrist is passively moved to full extension, and the MPs are passively flexed to 40 degrees. Next, the wrist is passively flexed to 20 degrees as the MP and IP joints are passively extended to 0 degrees. Following passive tenodesis, the place and active place-hold exercise is performed with the wrist passively held in 20 degrees of flexion to reduce antagonistic tension from the flexors. The MP and IP joints are then passively placed in extension, and the patient actively holds the position to create some minimal active tension across the repair site (Figure 15-12). Last, the active component includes active extension from a placed position of flexion. The MP joint is passively placed in 30 degrees of flexion from which the patient actively extends the joint to 0 degrees while the wrist is passively held in 20 degrees of flexion (Figure 15-13, *A* and *B*). Active PIP and DIP flexion/extension (hook fist) are performed within the confines of the splint 10 times per hour.

Phase II: Week 3. At 3 weeks, if no extension lag is noted, the position of passively placed MP flexion increases to 40 to 60 degrees. This is followed by active or active-assisted MP extension to 0 degrees. The wrist is supported in neutral throughout this exercise. Active IP flexion in a hook fist continues, and active IP extension is performed with the wrist in neutral and the MP joints at 0 degrees.

At 4 weeks after surgery, passive wrist tenodesis is replaced with active wrist tenodesis. Graded composite MP and IP flexion, with the wrist extended, is added to the exercise regimen, with the wrist in neutral. Graded dowels can be used to achieve this motion.[7] EDC glides are added to the program. The MP joints are actively

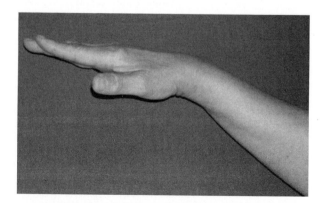

FIGURE **15-12** Protected place-hold digital extension: Wrist is placed in 20 degrees flexion and MP and IP joints in 0 degrees extension followed by active hold of this position.

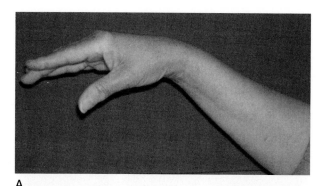

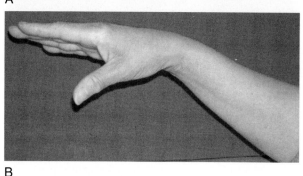

FIGURE **15-13** Protected active MP joint extension. *A.* Wrist is placed in 20 degrees flexion, and MP joints are placed in 30 degrees flexion. *B.* Active MP extension to 0 degrees from placed position of 30 degrees flexion (maintaining 20 degrees of wrist flexion).

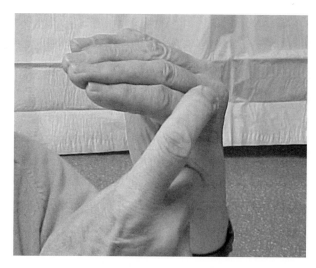

FIGURE **15-14** Active intrinsic extension: MP joints are blocked in flexion and followed by active extension of IP joints from either straight or composite fist.

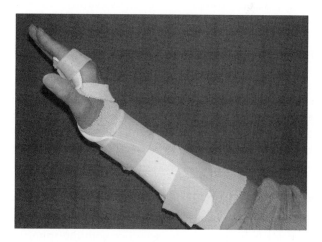

FIGURE **15-15** Custom volar forearm-based splint supporting wrist in 40- to 45-degree extension and MP joints in 15- to 20-degree flexion.

extended from a composite fist while maintaining the IP joints in flexion (see Figure 15-9, *A* and *B*). To encourage intrinsic function in extension, the MP joints are placed in flexion, and the IP joints are actively extended from a straight fist and full fist (Figure 15-14). At week 5, passive flexion of the wrist and individual finger joints is added. Extensor lag must be monitored closely once PROM begins. In the presence of a lag, passive flexion is delayed to avoid attenuation of the extensor tendon.

Phase III: Weeks 6 to 12. Active and passive composite finger flexion and wrist flexion exercises are added at 6 weeks. Graded functional grip-and-pinch activities begin at week 7. At 8 weeks, extensor strengthening begins. Evans[7] recommends using a 1-pound weight to strengthen wrist extension/flexion and forearm pronation/supination. Grip strengthening is added in week 8.

Splints

A volar static immobilization splint is used to protect repairs in zones V and VI for 5 to 6 weeks following surgery. The splint holds the wrist in 40 to 45 degrees of extension, the MP joints in 15 to 20 degrees of

flexion, and the IP joints and thumb free (Figure 15-15). A removable volar IP extension component is added for night use to prevent PIP volar plate tightness, extensor lag, and digital flexor tightness. During the first 5 to 6 weeks, the splint is worn at all times and removed for therapy and the home exercise program. During week 7, the splint is gradually weaned during the day and continued to be worn at nighttime. By week 8, the splint is discontinued. If the laceration is distal to or includes the juncturae tendinum, the two adjacent fingers are included in the splint. Corrective splinting, such as static progressive flexion splinting, begins at 4 weeks postoperatively, if passive MP or PIP flexion is

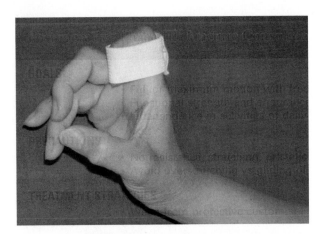

FIGURE **15-16** PIP/DIP flexion strap.

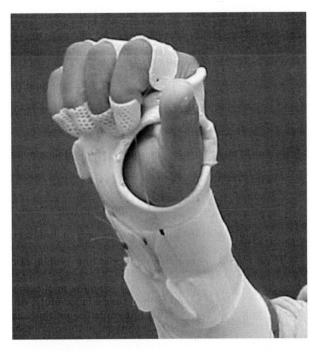

FIGURE **15-17** Static progressive composite MP and IP flexion splint. *(Courtesy of Aviva Wolff, OTR/L, CHT, New York.)*

limited at 30 to 40 degrees with a hard end-feel. MP or PIP joint stiffness will require individual splints because composite MP and PIP flexion is not permitted until 6 weeks postoperatively. If passive MP and PIP flexion is limited at 50 to 60 degrees at 6 weeks postoperatively, then composite flexion splinting begins at this point.

Stiff PIP and DIP joints with resolving MP and wrist extensor tightness are treated with PIP/DIP flexion straps (Figure 15-16). Static progressive splinting for extrinsic extensor tightness begins with the wrist in neutral (Figure 15-17). Once composite digital flexion is achieved, wrist flexion is added for a composite stretch.

Functional Activity

During the first 6 weeks postoperatively, the hand is used for light to moderate activities with the splint in place. Heavy occupational and athletic activities are avoided during this time. Prehension and coordination activities are gradually added during therapy to complement ROM exercises by week 7, when weaning from the splint during the day begins. Once the splint has been discharged by 8 weeks postoperatively, the affected hand is gradually incorporated

into functional activity. Unrestricted hand use for light activities is permitted by week 12, and the return to heavy labor and/or sports is allowed at 16 weeks postoperatively.

TROUBLESHOOTING

Weekly assessment of extensor lag is required to determine when therapy can be advanced to the next level. If an extensor lag of greater than 10 degrees exists, progression is halted, and active extension is emphasized over flexion. Decreasing the MP flexion angle minimizes the effort in returning to full extension. Place-hold exercises at varying angles of MP extension encourage gliding of the extensor mechanism. When PIP, DIP, or MP joint flexion is limited, static progressive splinting is initiated to increase joint mobility and extensor tendon extensibility.

Zones V and VI: Early Active Mobilization

GOALS

- Full active DIP and PIP extension and flexion
- Incorporate injured digit into ADL
- Independence with premorbid ADL

PRECAUTIONS

- *Do not* use this protocol unless involved tendons were surgically repaired
- Avoid emphasizing flexion gains over extension
- Progress slowly if MP joint extension lag develops at any point

TREATMENT STRATEGIES

Splints

- Static volar forearm-based splint with wrist and MP joints included
  - Wrist in 40 to 45 degrees of extension; MP joints in 15 to 20 degrees of flexion; IP joints and thumb free
  - Full time 0 to 6 weeks; nighttime 6 to 8 weeks; discontinue at 8 weeks
- Nighttime removable volar IP extension splint with IP joints in 0 degrees of extension
- Static progressive MP flexion splints
  - 4 weeks postoperative *if* active MP and/or PIP flexion is limited at 30 to 40 degrees with hard end-feel
    - Note: separate splints for MP and PIP flexion; no composite flexion at this point
  - 6 weeks postoperative *if* active MP and /or PIP flexion is limited at 50 to 60 degrees with hard end-feel
    - Note: can treat MP and PIP flexion tightness with one splint; composite flexion permitted

Motion

- Phase I: 0 to 21 days postoperatively
  - Passive wrist tenodesis by therapist
    - Passive full wrist extension with passive MP flexion to 40 degrees
    - Passive wrist flexion to 20 degrees with passive MP extension to 0 degrees
  - Active place-hold MP and IP extension at 0 degrees with wrist in 20 degrees of flexion
  - Protected active MP extension
    - Wrist placed in 20 degrees of flexion
    - MP joints placed in 30 degrees of flexion
    - Active MP extension to 0 degrees from start position
  - Active hook fisting with MP and wrist supported in splint
- Phase II: 3 weeks postoperatively
  - Discontinue place-hold if patient extends to 0 degrees from a position of 60 degrees of flexion
  - Continue passive wrist tenodesis
  - Continue protected active extension, but increase the arc of motion 10 to 20 degrees
- 4 weeks
  - Transition to active tenodesis
  - Add graded composite MP and IP flexion with neutral wrist
  - Add tendon gliding with the wrist extended
  - Add EDC glides and digital abduction/adduction with neutral wrist
- 5 weeks
  - Add passive flexion of individual finger joints and wrist
- Phase III: 6+ weeks postoperatively
  - Add graded composite MP, IP, and wrist flexion
  - Add graded strengthening for wrist extension/flexion and forearm supination/pronation

Functional Activity

- 0 to 6 weeks postoperatively
  - Light ADL with splint protection
- 6 to 8 weeks postoperatively
  - Static grip and prehension activities in therapy
  - Light ADL without splint protection unless MP joint extensor lag; if lag use splint until 8 weeks

Continued

Zones V and VI: Early Active Mobilization—cont'd

- 8 to 12 weeks postoperatively
  - Dynamic grip and prehension activities in therapy
  - Moderate ADL without splint
- 12 weeks postoperatively: Resume full participation in ADL without restriction
- 16 weeks postoperatively: Heavy labor and sports permitted

HOME EXERCISE PROGRAM
- 0 to 4 weeks
  - Active hook fisting in the splint
  - Active place-hold MP extension
- 4 weeks: Add active tenodesis, tendon gliding with wrist extended, and EDC gliding with wrist neutral
- 8 weeks: Add strengthening for digital extension, wrist extension/flexion, forearm supination/pronation

ZONES VII AND VIII

ANATOMY

Zones VII through VIII contain the finger and wrist extensor tendons and musculature proximal to the wrist into the dorsal forearm. Zone VII encompasses the dorsal wrist where the extensor tendons of the fingers and wrist pass under the dorsal retinaculum. Zone VIII includes the musculotendinous junction of the wrist and finger extensors in the distal forearm.

INJURY AND TREATMENT

The wrist and finger extensors in zones VII and VIII are subject to laceration or rupture by distal radius and ulnar fractures and dislocations. In addition, tendon attrition with delayed rupture has been described with fixation screw use,[4,36] in rheumatoid tenosynovitis,[4,37] distal ulnar instability after excessive surgical excision,[4,38] scaphoid nonunion,[4,37] and Kienbock's disease.[4,36]

POSTOPERATIVE MANAGEMENT

Surgical repair of extensor tendon injuries in zones VII and VIII are treated postoperatively via immobilization or early active motion. The decision to use one protocol over the other is determined by the surgeon based upon factors similar to those discussed previously in the treatment of zones V and VI tendon injuries. At HSS, the authors prefer the early active motion protocol for zones VII and VIII when possible. Immediate active and passive IP motion is permitted with either protocol. The immobilization plan restricts active motion at the MP and wrist level until 3 weeks post-surgery, whereas the early active motion program allows active place-hold

extension at both the MP joints and wrist. This guideline describes the early active motion protocol.

Motion

Exercises follow the recommended sequence for zones V and VI (passive wrist tenodesis, place and hold MP extension, and protected active MP extension). The position of the wrist during early active exercises depends upon whether the digital extensors or wrist extensors are repaired.[7] Increased wrist extension increases resistance from the flexor tendons, requiring more work from the extensor tendons with active extension. This can cause increased tension on the repair. Proper wrist position protects the repair site and allows for safe early motion of the involved tendons.

Wrist position is particularly important with the place and hold exercises from 0 to 21 days postoperatively. For digital extensor tendon repairs, the wrist is passively placed in 20 degrees of flexion with the MP and IP joints in 0 degrees of extension[7] and actively held for 3 seconds (Figure 15-12). For wrist extensor tendon repairs, the wrist is positioned in 0 to 20 degrees of extension, and a gentle active hold is attempted for 3 seconds. The rule described for protected active MP and IP extension exercises and passive wrist tenodesis for zones V and VI is applied to zones VII and VIII. Repaired wrist extensor tendons regain 25% to 30% of their tensile strength by the third to fourth postoperative week.[7,21] Therefore, it is safe to begin active wrist extension from 0 degrees to full range in the gravity eliminated position during the third postoperative week. In the first week of active wrist extension, it is acceptable for the EDC tendons to assist the wrist extensors. After that point, placing a dowel in the patient's hand relaxes the EDC, thus isolating the wrist extensor tendons (Figure 15-18). In the

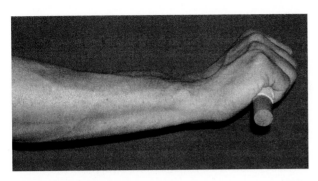

FIGURE **15-18** Isolated wrist extension, using a dowel to quiet the digital extensors.

fifth to eighth postoperative week, active wrist flexion is added in increments of 10 to 15 degrees weekly. Ulnar and radial deviation exercises are incorporated to maximize extensor carpi ulnaris (ECU) tendon excursion.

Splint

Tendon repairs to the digital and/or wrist extensor tendons are protected in a volar static forearm-based splint with the wrist positioned in 40 degrees of wrist extension, the MP joints in 30 degrees of flexion, and the IP joints are free (see Figure 15-15). Typically protective immobilization is required between exercise sessions for 5 to 6 weeks following digital extensor tendon repair (EDC, EIP, EDQ). Because the demand and force requirements for the wrist extensors are high with functional activity, 8 weeks of protective splinting is suggested following repair of extensor carpi radialis longus (ECRL), extensor carpi radialis brevis (ECRB), or ECU.[7,24]

Functional Activity

During the first 6 postoperative weeks, the hand may be used for light to moderate activities with the splint. Heavy occupational and athletic activities are avoided during the 6 weeks. Prehension and coordination activities are added during therapy to complement ROM

exercises by week 7, when weaning from the splint during the day begins. Once the splint has been discharged by 8 weeks postoperatively, the affected hand is incorporated into functional activity. Unrestricted hand use for ADL and light activity is permitted by week 12, and the return to heavy labor and/or sports is recommended at 16 weeks postoperatively.

HOME EXERCISE PROGRAM

The home program includes edema and scar management techniques beginning in the first week and continuing through week 12. Active PIP and DIP flexion/extension exercises are performed 10 times per hour with the splint. Once the patient demonstrates competence, exercises performed in therapy are added to the home program. Active range of motion (AROM) of uninvolved joints is performed three times per day. Coban wrap is removed for exercises because it adds resistance to exercise. The splint is gradually weaned (refer to schedule for weaning splint).

TROUBLESHOOTING

A weekly assessment of extensor lag determines when advancement to the next level is appropriate. If there is an extensor lag of greater than 10 degrees at the MP or wrist level, the position of the MP and wrist is adjusted into more extension to minimize the effort in returning to full extension. Place-hold exercises at various angles of MP and wrist extension are also used to emphasize extension over flexion. If finger and/or wrist flexion is limited, static progressive splinting is required to increase joint mobility and extensor tendon extensibility. If flexion is limited by joint stiffness, static progressive splinting is applied to the stiff joint to resolve the problem. When flexion is limited by soft tissue tightness of the extensor tendons, static progressive splinting is first applied to restore MP flexion, and then followed by IP flexion. A composite static progressive flexion splint is used to achieve this goal (see Figure 15-17).

Zones VII and VIII: Early Active Mobilization

GOALS

- Full active DIP and PIP extension and flexion
- Incorporate injured digit into ADL
- Independence with premorbid ADL

PRECAUTIONS

- *Do not* use this protocol unless involved tendons were surgically repaired
- *Do not* flex the wrist past neutral until 3 to 4 weeks after wrist extensor tendon repair
- Avoid emphasizing flexion gains over extension
- Progress more slowly if MP joint or wrist extension lag develops at any point
- Wrist position with active MP motion from 0 to 21 days postoperatively depends on whether digital extensor tendons or wrist extensor tendons were repaired

TREATMENT STRATEGIES

Splint

- Static volar forearm-based splint with MP joints included
  - Wrist extended 40 degrees
  - MP joints flexed 30 degrees
  - Continuous wear except for exercises
    - Digital extensor tendon repair: 5 to 6 weeks
    - Wrist extensor repair: 8 weeks

Motion

- 0 to 21 days
  - Passive wrist tenodesis:
    - Passive full wrist extension with passive MP flexion to 40 degrees
    - Passive wrist flexion to 20 degrees with passive MP extension to 0 degrees
  - Active place-hold MP extension with digital extensor tendon repair
    - *Wrist placed in 20 degrees of *flexion*
    - MP and IP joints placed in 0 degrees of extension for active hold
  - Active place-hold MP extension with wrist extensor tendon repair
    - *Wrist placed and supported in 0 to 20 degrees of *extension*
    - MP and IP joints placed in 0 degrees of extension for active hold
  - Protected active MP extension with digital extensor tendon repair
    - *Wrist placed and supported in 20 degrees of *flexion*
    - MP joints placed in 30 degrees of flexion
    - Active extension to 0 degrees from start position
  - Protected active MP extension with wrist extensor tendon repair
    - *Wrist placed and supported in 20 degrees of *extension*
    - MP joints placed in 30 degrees of flexion
    - Active extension to 0 degrees from start position
- 3 weeks
  - Add placed MP flexion to 40 to 60 degrees, followed by active-assisted MP extension to 0 degrees (all with wrist held in full extension)
  - Add active wrist extension and ulnar deviation with gravity eliminated (0 degrees to end range)
  - Add EDC gliding and digital abduction/adduction
  - Discontinue active place-hold
- 5 to 8+ weeks
  - Begin active wrist flexion to 15 degrees maximum
  - Increase wrist flexion arc by 10 to 15 degrees/week
  - Begin active wrist extension and ulnar/radial deviation against gravity

Functional Activity

See recommendations for zones V and VI.

HOME EXERCISE PROGRAM

See recommendations for zones V and VI.

Note: Position of wrist with active place-hold MP extension depends upon whether the digital or wrist extensor tendons were repaired.

THUMB

Postoperative protocols for thumb extensor tendon injuries follow the same principles as those for the digits. The appropriate protocol is chosen based on the level of injury. Zone T-I is treated via an immobilization protocol regardless of surgical or conservative management, zones T-III and T-IV are treated with controlled passive motion, and zones T-II and T-V with early active motion program if the tendons have been surgically repaired. Passive range of motion of individual joints begins 6 weeks post surgery in all zones.

All thumb extensor tendon injuries are splinted with the IP and MP joints in 0 degrees of extension, the CMC joint midway between palmar and radial abduction, and the wrist in 30 to 45 degrees of extension. The immobilization period varies in each zone. If an extensor lag exists at the IP or MP level the splint continues to be used for an additional two weeks.

THUMB ZONES T-I AND T-II
ANATOMY, INJURY, AND TREATMENT

Zone T-I in the thumb includes the IP joint and EPL insertion. Zone T-II extends from the IP joint to the proximal phalanx and includes the EPL tendon. Thumb mallet finger injuries in zone T-I are treated either surgically or conservatively. A closed mallet thumb is treated conservatively with immobilization of the IP joint in extension for 8 weeks.[7] Open mallet thumb injuries caused by lacerations or crush injuries often require surgical repair and are immobilized for 5 to 6 weeks.[1,7] Zone T-II injuries to the EPL are treated surgically and are completely immobilized for 2 weeks. Early active motion begins in the third postoperative week.[1,7]

Motion

For zone T-I injuries, motion begins at 5 to 6 weeks postoperatively. Active, isolated thumb IP and MP flexion begins slowly, with gradual increases of up to 20 degrees per week. Graded flexion continues weekly. If an extensor lag develops in the IP joint, the flexion arc is decreased and splinting time is increased. Active wrist and MP extension and flexion begin immediately. Composite IP and MP flexion begins at week 6. Gentle passive flexion is permitted at 8 weeks, with care taken to avoid tendon attenuation and creation of an extensor lag. Light grip and prehension activities may begin at 10 weeks post-surgery, as long as an extensor lag has not developed. Protective splinting between exercise and therapeutic activities continues until 8 weeks after surgery.

For zone T-II surgical repairs, early active motion is preferred. In the early active mobilization protocol, the thumb is immobilized for the first 2 postoperative weeks, with a short arc motion program beginning by the third week.[7] Protective splinting between exercise sessions continues for 6 weeks. Active thumb IP flexion and extension is initiated in a short arc of 30 degrees, increasing to 60 degrees over the following 3 weeks.[7] If necessary, a template splint is used to control motion. At 3 postoperative weeks, the splint is modified to allow active IP flexion and extension. Active isolated MP joint, CMC joint, and wrist motion are introduced at 4 weeks postoperatively. Composite active flexion, opposition, and radial/palmar abduction are introduced by 4 and 6 weeks, and passive motion for individual joint and composite flexion begins at 6 weeks. Light prehension and coordination activities are added at 6 weeks post-surgery, and the splint is discontinued if no extensor lag is present.

Thumb Zones T-I and T-II: Immobilization

GOALS

- Full active thumb IP extension and flexion
- Incorporate injured digit into ADL
- Independence with premorbid ADL

PRECAUTIONS

- No early active motion
- Avoid emphasizing flexion gains over extension
- Progress more slowly, if thumb IP joint extension lag develops at any point

TREATMENT STRATEGIES

Splint

- Thumb in 0 degrees
- Continuous splint for 6 weeks
- At 6 weeks, discharge splint if no lag

Motion

- 0 to 6 weeks
  - AROM: MP extension/flexion 0 to 70 degrees
  - AROM: Wrist extension/flexion
- 6 weeks
  - AROM: IP flexion/extension
  - AROM: Composite IP and MP flexion
- 8 weeks
  - PROM: for each thumb joint and composite thumb flexion
  - Graded grip and prehension activities

Functional Activity

- 0 to 6 weeks
  - Light ADL with splint donned
- 6 to 8 weeks
  - Light prehension activities without splint in therapy
  - Light ADL with splint donned
- 8 to 12 weeks
  - Light to moderate ADL without splint
- 12 weeks
  - Resume full participation in all ADL without splint; sports/heavy labor at 16 weeks

HOME EXERCISE PROGRAM

- 0 to 6 weeks: Patient is educated for safe donning/doffing of splint and incorporates exercises from therapy.
- 6+ weeks: Incorporate exercises from therapy, 10 times each, 3 times/day

THUMB ZONES T-III AND T-IV

ANATOMY, INJURY, AND TREATMENT

Zone T-III includes the EPL and EPB tendons. Lacerations of the tendons in zones T-III and T-IV are repaired with four-strand repairs like the Bunnell, Kleinert, or Kessler because of the thickness of the tendons.[1] Zones T-III and T-IV injuries are treated similarly to digital extensor zones III and IV injuries. The thumb extensor tendons are substantially thicker than the digital extensor tendons and can tolerate a standard core suture and cross-stitch.[1] Postoperative protective splinting is necessary for at least 6 weeks post-surgery.

Motion

Either an immobilization program or controlled passive motion program is used for zones T-III and T-IV. Our preference is to use a controlled passive mobilization program that begins within 24 hours of surgery. Passive wrist tenodesis exercises with the thumb supported in extension are performed in therapy. Following passive tenodesis, controlled passive thumb MP flexion and extension in a 30-degree arc with the IP joint and wrist held in maximal extension are performed by the therapist. The wrist is passively ranged to full extension with the thumb relaxed, to neutral with the thumb ray held

Thumb Zones T-III and T-IV: Controlled Passive Motion

GOALS

- Full active thumb IP and MP extension and flexion
- Incorporate injured digit into ADL
- Independence with premorbid ADL

PRECAUTIONS

- Avoid emphasizing flexion gains over extension
- Progress more slowly if thumb MP joint extension lag develops at any point

TREATMENT STRATEGIES

Splint

- Thumb IP and MP extension to 0 degrees, CMC midway between palmar and radial abduction, wrist 30 to 45 degrees of extension
  - 0 to 6 weeks: At all times except exercises
  - 3 weeks: Modify to allow active IP extension/flexion
  - 6 weeks: Discontinue splint as long as no extensor lag
- Static progressive MP flexion splint
  - Begin at week 7 if MP flexion proves difficult to recover
  - Wear intermittently throughout the day

Motion

- 0 to 4 weeks
  - Passive wrist tenodesis in therapy (20 times)
    - Wrist passively moved to full extension with relaxed thumb
    - Wrist passively flexed to neutral with the thumb held in full extension
  - Controlled passive thumb MP extension/flexion during therapy only
    - Passive MP extension/flexion in a 30-degree arc (20 times)
    - Thumb IP and wrist held in maximum extension during passive motion
- 4 weeks
  - Begin active MP extension and flexion
  - Okay to use joint mobilization to increase extension/flexion
- 6 weeks
  - PROM: Individual and composite joint flexion
  - Grip and prehension activities
- 8 weeks
  - Strengthening: Grip, pinch, wrist

Functional Activity

- 0 to 4 weeks: Light ADL within the splint
- 4 to 8 weeks: Light ADL without splint
- 8 to 12 weeks: Moderate ADL without splint
- 12 weeks: Resume full participation in ADL
- 16 weeks: Heavy labor and sports permitted

HOME EXERCISE PROGRAM

- Integrate above functional activity and exercises into daily home program 3 times/day, 10 repetitions each.

---

in total extension, then the thumb is relaxed, and the wrist is passively returned to full extension. At 3 weeks, the splint is modified to allow IP flexion and extension. At 4 weeks, active MP flexion and extension is introduced. Passive motion for individual and composite joint flexion begins at 6 weeks. If active MP flexion is difficult to regain, static progressive splinting and manual joint mobilization for the MP joint are added at 7 weeks.

THUMB ZONE T-V

ANATOMY, INJURY, AND TREATMENT

Thumb zone T-V injuries are associated with either EPB or APL and surgically managed with a modified Kessler and cross-stitch.[1] Postoperatively, the patient is placed in a volar static wrist and thumb extension splint, as described previously.[7] Protective splinting continues between exercises for 6 weeks.

Motion

Early active mobilization begins during the first post-operative week and is specifically outlined.[7] As suggested by Evans,[7] the thumb is prepared for active place-hold exercises with the controlled, passive thumb MP motion and wrist tenodesis exercises described previously for zone T-IV. This helps reduce resistance caused by edema and joint stiffness.[7] Following the passive exercises, active place-hold is attempted by placing the wrist in 20 degrees of flexion with the CMC, MP, and IP joints in 0 degrees of extension. This position is held for 3 seconds and repeated 20 times.

During the third to fourth weeks after surgery, active flexion exercises are performed individually for each joint, in graded increments. As one thumb joint

Thumb Zone T-V: Early Active Motion

GOALS

- Full active thumb IP and MP extension and flexion
- Incorporate injured digit into ADL
- Independence with premorbid ADL

PRECAUTIONS

- Avoid emphasizing flexion gains over extension
- Progress more slowly if thumb MP joint extension lag develops at any point

TREATMENT STRATEGIES

Splints

- Thumb IP and MP extension to 0 degrees, CMC midway between palmar and radial abduction, wrist 30 to 45 degrees of extension
  - 0 to 6 weeks: At all times except exercises
  - 3 weeks: Modify to allow active IP extension/flexion
  - 6 weeks: Discontinue splint as long as no extensor lag
- Static progressive MP flexion splint
  - Begin at week 7 if MP flexion proves difficult to recover
  - Wear intermittently throughout the day

Motion

- 0 to 3 weeks
  - Passive wrist tenodesis (20 times)
  - Controlled passive thumb MP extension/flexion (20 times)
  - Active place-hold thumb MP extension (20 times)
  - Active thumb IP flexion/extension in dynamic IP extension splint (10 times/hr)
- 3 weeks
  - Graded active flexion of thumb IP and MP joints
  - Graded active motion of thumb CMC joint (palmar abduction, radial abduction, extension)
  - Graded active wrist flexion/extension
  - *Note: Perform all above exercises with remaining joints in the kinetic chain of the thumb held in full extension*
- 5 weeks (AROM only)
  - Graded opposition
  - Composite thumb flexion across the palm
  - Radial and palmar abduction
- 6 weeks
  - PROM: Individual and composite joint flexion

Functional Activity

- 0 to 3 weeks: Light ADL within splint
- 3 to 6 weeks: Shower/bathe without splint, exercise without splint; otherwise, wear splint
- 6 to 12 weeks: Wean from splint, light ADL without splint
- 12 weeks: Resume full participation in ADL

HOME EXERCISE PROGRAM

- Integrate above functional activity and exercises into daily home program 3 times/day, 10 repetitions each.

actively flexes, the other joints in the kinetic chain of the thumb are held in full extension. For instance, as the patient actively flexes the thumb IP joint, the MP, CMC, and wrist are held in full extension to minimize tension on the repair site. At this time, the splint can be modified to allow unrestricted IP flexion and extension. Active composite thumb flexion, abduction, and opposition is initiated by the fifth postoperative week.[7] Passive motion for individual joint and composite flexion begins 6 weeks after surgery, and light, functional activity involving the thumb is introduced at 6 to 8 weeks.

EXPECTED OUTCOME

The American Society for Surgery of the Hand (ASSH) rates results according to the percent of total active motion (TAM) achieved.[39] The ASSH also compares TAM to the patient's contralateral finger for a percentage of the patient's norm. One hundred percent TAM is considered an excellent result, 75% to 99% TAM is considered a good result, and 50% to 74% TAM is considered a fair result. A poor result is considered an achievement of less than 50% TAM. It is expected that the patient will have at least a good result, with a goal of an excellent result. Most importantly, the patient should be able to resume premorbid roles and ADL.

CRITERIA FOR DISCHARGE

The authors' criteria for discharge for all extensor tendon injuries are determined by the demonstration of functional active motion and strength, as well as the ability to return to full duty life roles (e.g., worker, homemaker, athlete). Functional active motion is defined as a less than 5-degree extension lag with full flexion. Grip strength that is 75% of noninjured hand is considered functional.

REFERENCES

1. Doyle, J. Extensor Tendons—Acute Injuries. In Green, D.P., Hotchkiss, R.N., Pederson, W.C. (Eds). *Green's Operative Hand Surgery*, 4th ed. Churchill Livingstone, New York, 1999, pp. 1950–1986.
2. Kaplan, E. *Anatomy, Injuries, and Treatment of the Extensor Apparatus of the Hand and Fingers.* Clin Orthop 1959;13:24–41.
3. McFarlane, R.M., Hampole, M.K. *Treatment of Extensor Tendon Injuries of the Hand.* Can J Surg 1973;16:366–375.
4. Rosenthal, E. The Extensor Tendons: Anatomy and Management. In Callahan, A., Mackin, E.J., Skirven, T.M., Shcneider, L.H., Osterman, A.L., Hunter, J.M. (Eds). *Rehabilitation of the Hand and Upper Extremity,* 5th ed. Mosby, Philadelphia, 2002, pp. 498–540.
5. Evans, R. *Early Active Short Arc Motion for the Repaired Central Slip.* J Hand Surg 1994;19A(6):991–997.
6. Saldana, M.J., Choban, S., Westerbeck, P., Schacherer, T.G. *Results of Acute Zone III Extensor Tendon Injuries Treated with Dynamic Extension Splinting.* J Hand Surg 1991;16A(6): 1145–1150.
7. Evans, R. Clinical Management of Extensor Tendon Injuries. In Callahan, A., Mackin, E.J., Skirven, T.M., Schneider, L.H., Osterman, A.L., Hunter, J.M. (Eds). *Rehabilitation of the Hand and Upper Extremity,* 5th ed. Mosby, Philadelphia, 2002, pp. 542–579.
8. Chang, J. *Molecular Studies in Flexor Tendon Wound Healing: The Role of Basic Fibroblastic Growth Factor Gene Expression.* J Hand Surg 1998;23A(6):1052–1058.
9. Khan, U., Occleston, N.L., Khaw, P.T., McGrouther, D.A. *Differences in Proliferative Rate and Collagen Lattice Contraction Between Endotenon and Synovial Fibroblasts.* J Hand Surg 1998; 23A:266.
10. Hitchcock, T.F., Light, T.R., Bunch, W.H., Knight, G.W., Sartori, M.J., Patwardhan, A.G., Hollyfield, R.L. *The Effect of Immediate Constrained Digital Motion on the Strength of Flexor Tendon Repairs in Chickens.* J Hand Surg 1987;12A(4):590–595.
11. Evans, R.B. *Immediate Short Arc Motion Following Extensor Tendon Repair.* Hand Clin 1995;11(3):483–512.
12. Evans, R.B. *Rehabilitation Techniques for Applying Immediate Active Tension to the Repaired Extensor System.* Tech Hand Up Extrem Surg 1999;3:139.
13. Evans, R.B., Thompson, D.E. *An Analysis of Factors that Support Early Active Short Arc Motion of the Repaired Central Slip.* J Hand Ther 1992;5:187–201.
14. Evans, R.B., Thompson, D.E. *The Application of Stress to the Healing Tendon.* J Hand Ther 1993;6(4):262–284.
15. Gelberman, R.H., Gonsawes, M., Woo, S., Akeson, W.H. *The Influence of Protected Passive Mobilization on the Healing Flexor Tendons: A Biomechanical and Microangiographic Study.* Hand 1981;13(2):120.
16. Gelberman, R.H., Woo, S.L., Lothringer, K., Akeson, W.H., Amiel, D. *Effects of Early Intermittent Passive Mobilization on Healing Canine Flexor Tendons.* J Hand Surg 1982;7(2):170.
17. Gelberman, R.H., Nunley, J.A. II, Osterman, A.L., Breen, T.F., Dimick, M.P., Woo, S.L. *Influences of the Protected Passive Mobilization Interval on Flexor Tendon Healing.* Clin Orthop 1991; 264:189–196.
18. Gelberman, R.H., Botte, M.J., Spiegelman, J.J., Akeson, W.H. *The Excursion and Deformation of Repaired Flexor Tendons Treated with Protected Early Motion.* J Hand Surg 1986;11A: 106–110.
19. Gratton, P. *Early Active Mobilization after Flexor Tendon Repairs.* J Hand Ther 1993;6(4):285–289.
20. Crosby, C.A., Wehbe, M.A. *Early Protected Motion after Extensor Tendon Repair.* J Hand Surg 1999;24A(5):1061–1070.
21. Mason, M.L., Allen, H.S. *The Rate of Healing Tendons: An Experimental Study of Tensile Strength.* Ann Surg 1941;113:424.
22. Evans, R.B., Buckhalter, W.E. *A Study of the Dynamic Anatomy of Extensor Tendons and Implications for Treatment.* J Hand Surg 1986;11A(5):774–779.
23. Brand, P.W. *Biomechanics of the Hand.* Mosby, St. Louis, 1985.
24. Brand, P.W., Hollister, A. *Clinical Mechanics of the Hand,* 2nd ed. Mosby, St. Louis, 1993.
25. Abouna, J.M., Brown, H. *The Treatment of Mallet Finger: The Results of a Series of 148 Consecutive Cases and a Review of the Literature.* Br J Hand Surg 1968;55B:653–667.
26. Stark, H.H., Boyes, J.H., Wilson, J.N. *Mallet Finger.* J Bone Joint Surg 1962;44A:1061–1068.
27. Evans, D., Weightman, B. *The Pipflex Splint for Treatment of Mallet Finger.* J Hand Surg 1988;13B:156–158.
28. Cullen, K.W., Tolhurst, P., Lang, D., Page, R.E. *Flexor Tendon Repair Zone 2 Followed by Controlled Active Mobilisation.* J Hand Surg 1989;14B:392.

29. Burkhalter, W.E. Wound Classification and Management. In Mackin, E., Hunter, J.M. (Eds). *Rehabilitation of the Hand.* Mosby, St. Louis, 1990.

30. Rayan, G.M., Mullin, P.T. *Skin Necrosis Complicating Mallet Finger Splinting and Vascularity of the Distal Interphalangeal Joint Overlying Skin.* J Hand Surg 1987;12A(4):548–552.

31. Iselin, F., Lerame, J., Godoy, J. *A Simplified Method for Treating Mallet Fingers: Tenodermodesis.* J Hand Surg 1977;2(2):118–121.

32. Nichols, H. *Manual of Hand Injuries.* Year Book Medical Publishers, Chicago, 1960, pp. 180–181.

33. Verdan, C.E. Primary and Secondary Repair of Flexor and Extensor Tendon Injuries. In Flynn, J.E. (Ed). *Hand Surgery.* Williams & Wilkins, Baltimore, 1975, p. 149.

34. Horii, E., Lin, G.T., Cooney, W.P., Linscheid, R.L., Chao, E.Y. *Comparative Flexor Tendon Excursions after Passive Mobilization: An In Vitro Study.* J Hand Surg 1992;17A(2):559–566.

35. Cooney, W.P., Lin, G.T., An, K.N. *Improved Tendon Excursion Following Flexor Tendon Repair.* J Hand Ther 1989;2:102.

36. Miki, T., Yamamuro, T., Kotoura, Y., Tsuji, T., Shimizu, K., Itakura, H. *Rupture of the Extensor Tendons of the Fingers: A Report of Three Unusual Cases.* J Bone Joint Surg 1986;68A(4): 610–614.

37. Harvey, F.J., Harvey, P.M. *Three Rare Causes of Extensor Tendon Rupture.* J Hand Surg 1989;14(6):957–962.

38. Newmeyer, W.L., Green, D.P. *Rupture of Digital Extensor Tendons Following Distal Ulnar Resection.* J Bone Joint Surg 1982;64A(2):178–182.

39. American Society for Surgery of the Hand, *Clinical Assessment Committee Report.* American Society for Surgery of the Hand, 1976.

16

Flexor Tenolysis

AMY BARENHOLTZ-MARSHALL, OTR, CHT

Tenolysis is a surgical release of nongliding adhesions that form along the surface of a tendon after injury or repair.[1-3] It is an elective surgical procedure that is performed in an effort to salvage tendon function after all therapy techniques have failed. If the patient has been compliant with a continuous therapy program for a minimum of 3 to 6 months with no significant improvement in active range of motion (AROM), a tenolysis is considered.[1,3] Prerequisites for this procedure include full fracture and wound healing and resolution of joint contractures with normal or nearly normal passive range of motion (PROM).[1,4] To improve the likelihood of successful results, the patient must be motivated, committed, and able to follow through with a postoperative therapy program. In addition, close communication among the therapist, surgeon, and patient is essential. A preoperative visit for patient education is strongly recommended to reinforce the commitment and expectations during the postoperative phase. Poor compliance with therapy following tenolysis leads to poor results.[2]

ANATOMICAL AND SURGICAL OVERVIEW

The tenolysis procedure is performed under local anesthesia that is supplemented with an intravenous sedative drug.[2,3,5] This allows for a thorough evaluation of AROM in which the patient is participatory. The involved flexor system is approached via a zigzag incision, long enough to expose the adhered tendon. The adhesions are excised with all efforts made to preserve the pulley systems, specifically the A2 and A4 pulleys.[1,4] These pulleys are critical in maintaining the correct moment arm for the tendons to function most efficiently and prevent tendon bowstringing. Without the pulleys, more force is required to generate tension to produce full digital flexion. When it is not possible to preserve the pulleys, they are reconstructed at this time. Joint contractures, if present, are released through a capsulectomy. During this procedure, the active motion is reevaluated frequently to confirm adequate tissue release. The tendon is assessed for gapping at the repair site. A tendon with a large gap that has filled in with scar tissue will be too long, inefficient, and prone to rupture. Staged flexor tendon reconstruction may be necessary, if an adequate pulley system cannot be preserved and/or the flexor mechanism cannot be salvaged[2] (Figures 16-1 through 16-4).

REHABILITATION OVERVIEW

Immediate initiation of a hand therapy program is crucial to the success of a tenolysis. Early and frequent therapy will reduce the opportunity for rescarring. Referral information should include the integrity of the

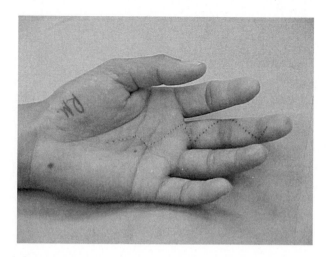

FIGURE **16-1** Zigzag incision along the flexor surface of the long finger.

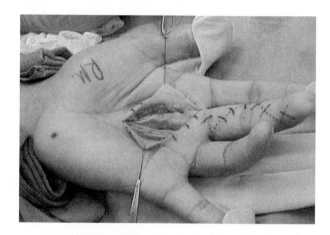

FIGURE **16-2** Peritendinous scar tissue.

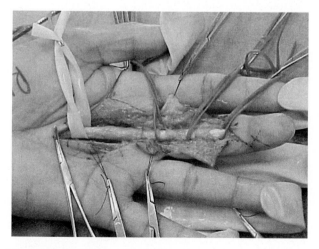

FIGURE **16-3** Excision and release of binding adhesions with preservation of annular pulleys.

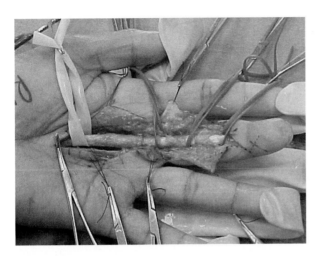

FIGURE **16-4** Assessing tendon excursion to confirm adequate release.

lysed tendon, intraoperative AROM and PROM measures, digit vascularity, prognosis for motion, and any concomitant procedures performed, such as a capsulectomy or pulley reconstruction. Additional corrective procedures complicate the patient's recovery.

A tendon of good quality, with intact pulleys, requires a more vigorous postoperative therapy program. When the quality is poor (also known as *frayed tendon*) and/or there is pulley reconstruction, a less aggressive approach is used to decrease the demands of the involved structures and reduce the risk of tendon rupture.[5] The protocol that follows is similar to that following a tendon repair (see Chapter 14).

General rehabilitation goals are to achieve and maintain intraoperative AROM/PROM, prevent adhesion formation, maximize tendon glide/excursion, and maximize strength for restoration of normal hand function.

POSTOPERATIVE PHASE I: INFLAMMATION (WEEK 1)

Phase I of therapy lasts 1 week and corresponds to the early inflammatory period. Initiation of an early range of motion (ROM) program is essential for a successful outcome. ROM exercises are initiated in the recovery area just following surgery. This first week is crucial in the postoperative management, and therapy is attended daily.

The first postoperative visit includes splint fabrication, assessment of the wound, edema, sensibility, ROM, and pain levels. A forearm-based, volar splint is fabricated with the wrist in 15-degree extension and all digits in maximum available end range extension to prevent flexion contractures. The splint is for night

use only, and the patient is encouraged active hand use. If a patient experiences significant pain and/or swelling, the splint may be used between exercise sessions to rest the "violated" tissue. Protective wound dressings vary according to the surgeon's preference. Restrictive dressings are avoided, and light, nonbulky dressings that are individualized to each digit are preferred. During the first visit, the patient is instructed in wound care and dressing changes. Treatment includes edema control, ROM, splinting regime, and a home exercise program. Edema reduction is emphasized. Edema is controlled early to avoid scarring, fibrosis, and increased demand on the tendon. Standard edema reduction techniques are implemented. Caution is advised when using any form of compression wraps to protect delicate vascularity and not to impede motion. Wraps may be worn full-time, if necessary, and removed for exercises and wound care. AROM includes isolated tendon gliding exercises, place-hold composite flexion in varied ranges, and isolated extension exercises. Tendon gliding exercises maximize differential gliding and are not recommended if the tendon quality is poor. Extension exercises are emphasized if flexion contractures were present before surgery. Passive flexion and extension is performed in gross and isolated joint fashion. The goal is to achieve or maintain the AROM/PROM obtained in surgery. If this is not possible, an outcome of 10 degrees within the range of intraoperative motion is acceptable. To reduce the risk of stiffness and increased inflammation, exercises are performed on an hourly basis. Consistency throughout the day is emphasized over intensity and repetition of exercises. Five to 10 repetitions of each exercise are performed in each session. The number of repetitions is upgraded or downgraded, according to tissue tolerance and reactivity.

Troubleshooting

Too much stress applied prematurely to the tendon can increase pain and inflammation and increase the risk of tendon rupture. All efforts are made to avoid factors that impede gliding and redevelopment of adherent scars. Such factors include significant pain, persistent edema, bleeding, infection, and an inability to tolerate postoperative therapy. Pain levels are continually monitored to measure patient's reactivity toward treatment. This is an indicator of how and when to progress treatment.

When the quality of a tendon is poor, tenodesis place-hold fisting is the only active exercise performed. As the wrist is placed into extension, the fingers are positioned in a full fist. This position is actively maintained for 5 seconds. The home program is less aggressive, and 10 to 15 repetitions are performed every 2 hours rather than hourly.

Postoperative Phase I: Inflammation (Week 1)

GOALS

- Control edema
- Achieve or maintain AROM/PROM obtained in surgery
- Decrease pain
- Promote wound healing
- Patient education
- Maintain ROM of uninvolved joints

PRECAUTIONS

- Avoid exacerbation of pain and inflammation
- Prevent flexion contractures
- Avoid neurovascular compromise

TREATMENT STRATEGIES

- Initiate therapy on the day of surgery
- Nighttime extension splinting
- Wound care: nonbulky, sterile protective dressing, as not to impede motion
- Elevated positioning at all times
- Compression wraps: Coban wrap, Ace wrap, or Isotoner glove applied with little to no tension
- Gentle PROM (all planes) to involved joints
- Active tendon gliding exercises
  - Tenodesis place-hold may be the only appropriate exercise if the tendon quality is poor
- Active isolated/composite extension exercises
- Cryotherapy
- Daily therapy with strong emphasis on home exercise program (HEP)

CRITERIA FOR ADVANCEMENT

- Evidence of wound healing
- Reduction in edema
- Minimal inflammatory responsiveness

POSTOPERATIVE PHASE II: FIBROPLASIA (WEEKS 2 AND 3)

Phase II begins 1 week postoperatively. During this phase there is an increase in collagen synthesis, which leads to a stronger wound and the formation of scar tissue. All efforts are made in therapy to model the scar in the desired direction and prevent restricting adhesions.[2] This is accomplished through AROM exercises and a splinting regime. AROM exercises are upgraded to include flexor digitorum superficialis (FDS) and flexor digitorum profundus (FDP) blocking exercises for localized excursion at specific joints. The splint continues to be used at night. If digit extension is limited, the splint is adjusted to lengthen the soft tissue. Splints are monitored at regular intervals to ensure that end range extension is maintained. Day splinting is used to improve flexion or extension in cases of joint stiffness and soft tissue tightness. Once the wound closes, scar management commences. The patient is instructed in deep friction scar massage, compression, and the use of silicone gel sheets. Other options are compressive finger sleeves and elastomer molds. Moist heat is used before exercise to increase tissue extensibility, decrease pain, and improve joint mobility.[2]

Although outpatient therapy visits are reduced to 3 times per week, the home program continues to be critical and is supplemented to include scar massage 4 to 5 times a day. Patients are encouraged to maintain compliance with routine exercises and use their hands functionally for light activities of daily living (ADL). For the frayed tendon, full AROM is initiated at 3 weeks post-surgery.

Troubleshooting

Problems that interfere with the progression of treatment include persistent edema, excessive scar formation, soft tissue shortening, minimal gains in ROM, and loss of motion. During this phase the tendon remains at risk for rupture. Exercises continue to be prescribed, on an individual basis, and monitored carefully. A continuous passive motion (CPM) hand unit can be used for the patient who demonstrates difficulty with active exercises. A CPM unit never replaces AROM exercises; it merely serves as an adjunct to treatment. This must be strongly emphasized with the patient to ensure that they continually strive to perform AROM exercises. The proximal interphalangeal (PIP) joints are monitored for

Postoperative Phase II: Fibroplasia (Weeks 2 to 3)

GOALS

- Facilitate wound healing
- Promote scar mobility and minimize adhesions
- Reduce edema
- Maximize AROM
- Maintain full PROM
- Encourage functional hand use in light ADL

PRECAUTIONS

- Same as phase I
- Monitor soft tissue responses to treatment and upgrade techniques accordingly
- Watch for signs of adhesions (i.e., discrepancy in ROM where PROM is significantly greater than AROM); if adhesions are significant, upgrade AROM/blocking exercises

TREATMENT STRATEGIES

- Discharge splint during the day, continue at night
  - May need to adjust splint to achieve greater extension if it has not already been achieved
- Retrograde massage
- Initiate scar management after sutures are removed and incision is fully closed
  - Scar massage
  - Silicone sheets
  - Compression wraps during day, at night if tolerated
- Tendon gliding exercises
- Blocking exercises to isolate FDS and FDP
  - Assistive blocking splints if needed
- PROM
- Light soft tissue stretching
- Day splinting (static-progressive) for joint stiffness or soft tissue tightness
- Dexterity exercises
- Functional activities
- Sensibility testing if indicated
- HEP

CRITERIA FOR ADVANCEMENT

- Evidence of soft tissue healing
- Complete wound closure
- AROM is close or equal to PROM.
- *AROM is WNL.*

early signs of flexion contractures. "Reverse blocking"[2] exercises are performed to encourage isolated PIP extension (see Chapter 21). This exercise is performed with the metacarpophalangeal (MP) joints manually blocked in hyperflexion to allow isolated extension at the PIP joints. Blocking splints are helpful in isolating joint motion and facilitating differential tendon gliding. Night splints are monitored closely to ensure end range positioning. If the tendon quality is good and excessive scarring continues to limit motion, treatment is progressed to the next level, despite differential tendon gliding exercises. Resistive flexion exercises are added to increase tendon pull-through (see next phase).

POSTOPERATIVE PHASE III: SCAR MATURATION (WEEKS 4 TO 10)

As the proliferative phase ends, scar maturation (remodeling) begins and collagen fibers gain strength.[2,5] Strong efforts are made to remodel scar and facilitate remodeling along the lines of tension (desired direction). This is accomplished by upgrading therapeutic exercise intensity and instruction in scar management techniques. Deep friction massage is commenced and includes mobilization techniques. Exercises are performed more frequently, with greater intensity, and include isometric gripping with a slow progression toward resistive gripping. Night splinting is continued

Postoperative Phase III: Scar Maturation (Weeks 4 to 10)

GOALS

- Maximize AROM to achieve intraoperative range
- Eliminate any residual edema
- Scar management
- Improve endurance
- Increase grip-and-pinch strength
- Return to full hand use

PRECAUTIONS

- Graded introduction of PREs

TREATMENT STRATEGIES

- Continue night splinting for 6 to 8 weeks (10 to 12 weeks for the frayed tendon).
- Continue with edema reduction as needed.
- Scar management
  - Scar mobilization techniques
  - Deep friction massage
- Upgrade AROM exercises
- Tendon gliding
- Passive stretching
- Joint mobilizations if joint stiffness is present
- Continue with day splinting (static or static-progressive) as needed.
- Dexterity exercises
- Functional activities
- If tendon integrity is good, sustained gripping exercises may be initiated at 3 to 4 weeks postoperatively.
  - Isometrics
  - Rubber dowel squeezes
  - Dowel stamping in firm putty
- Heavy resistance activities can begin at 8 weeks postoperatively (12 weeks for frayed tendon). If noted to have significant adhesions, patient can add resistive exercises sooner.

CRITERIA FOR DISCHARGE

- Elimination of edema
- AROM/PROM has plateaued for 4 weeks.
- Patient has resumed full use of hand in all ADL/vocational and recreational tasks.

for 6 to 8 weeks. For the frayed tendon, splinting should continue for approximately 10 to 12 weeks, dependent on the degree of tissue tightness or joint contractures. When full ROM has been achieved, the goals are aimed at improving strength, increasing endurance, and maximizing functional use of the hand. The home exercise program is upgraded to include progressive resistive exercise and grip-and-pinch strengthening.

Troubleshooting

If joint contractures exist, treatment addresses the stiff joints. Treatment includes PROM, joint mobilization, low-load prolonged stretching, and static-progressive splinting that is well described in other chapters of this book.

References

1. Strickland, J.W. (Ed). Flexor Tenolysis. In *Hand Clinics,* vol 1, no 1. WB Saunders, Philadelphia, 1985.
2. Feldshcer, S.B., Schneider, L.H. *Flexor Tenolysis.* Hand Surg 2002;7(1):61–74.
3. Schneider, L.H. Flexor Tendons—Late Reconstruction. In Green, D.P., Hotchkiss, R.N., Pederson, W.C. (Eds). *Green's Operative Hand Surgery,* 4th ed. Churchill Livingstone, New York, 1999, pp. 1921–1925.
4. Wehbe, M.A. *Flexor Tendon Injury—Late Solution.* Hand Clin 1986;1:133–137.
5. Schneider, L.H., Feldscher, S.B. Tenolysis: Dynamic Approach to Surgery and Therapy. In Mackin, E.J., Callahan, A.D., Skirven, T.M., Schneider, L.H., Hunter, J.M. (Eds). *Rehabilitation of the Hand,* 5th ed. Mosby, St. Louis, 2002, pp. 457–467.

17

Upper Extremity Surgical Intervention in Patients with Cerebral Palsy: Musculotendinous Procedures

KARA GAFFNEY GALLAGHER, MS, OTR/L, CHT

JENNIFER P. LEWIN, OTR/L

Cerebral palsy is a general term used to describe a condition characterized by irreversible brain damage and associated neuromotor dysfunction in the developing child.[1] Cerebral palsy results from an injury to the brain before birth, during birth, or during the first 2 to 3 years of childhood.[1,2] The extent of involvement of motor function, sensibility, and intelligence is highly variable.[3-5] Cerebral palsy occurs in an estimated 0.6 to 2.5 of 1000 live births. It occurs in an estimated 5.2 of 1000 live births in the United States and in approximately 1 of 7 children worldwide.[6,7] The number of cases is difficult to determine, because there is no system for monitoring the occurrence of cerebral palsy in the United States.[8]

Several systems are used to classify cerebral palsy. The most common systems use the number of involved extremities and type of muscle tone.[9] The main terms used to describe the extent of involved extremities include *monoplegia* (one limb), *hemiplegia* (one arm, one leg), *quadriplegia* (all limbs), and *diplegia* (quadriplegia with upper limb involvement milder than lower limbs). Terms used to describe muscle tone are *spasticity* (high tone), *flaccidity* (markedly low tone), *athetosis* (mixed tone), and *ataxia*. Ataxia is associated with primitive movement patterns and decreased coordination, such as dysmetria, dysdiadochokinesia, tremors at rest, and balance.[9] Spastic involvement of a muscle (i.e., agonist) often pairs with a weak antagonistic muscle, which leads to deformity in the direction of the agonist.

Cerebral palsy is a static, nonprogressive condition, although abnormal movement patterns and imbalanced muscle tone, combined with the effects of gravity and normal growth, may cause the child to develop contractures and deformities. As a result, function becomes increasingly impaired. Upper extremity reconstructive surgery in the patient with cerebral palsy improves function and prevents further deformity. The goals of surgery are to correct deformity, rebalance the muscles to increase functional use,[3,10-14] and improve hygiene and appearance. Rehabilitation following surgery is essential to facilitate active use of the muscles and integrate the upper extremity into functional activity. The following guideline describes common surgical reconstructive procedures and the preoperative and postoperative therapeutic interventions.

ANATOMICAL AND SURGICAL OVERVIEW

The typical pattern of deformity in the spastic upper extremity is shoulder adduction and internal rotation, elbow flexion, forearm pronation, wrist flexion, finger flexion, and thumb flexion.[3,10-12] The pattern of deformity is evident by the time the child reaches age 3.[11] The goals of upper extremity reconstructive surgery are to correct these patterns and prevent further impairment.

It is imperative that therapists, patients, and caregivers appreciate that surgery can augment function, yet rarely provides restoration of a normal arm.[3]

The surgeon establishes a realistic operative plan, based on a thorough physical examination, videotaped motion analysis,[3,16] and, occasionally, a dynamic electromyography (EMG) test,[3,12,17,18] to meet the patient's functional goals. To rebalance agonistic and antagonistic muscles, the agonist is released and the antagonist is augmented through muscle transfers. Muscular release can take several forms, including release of the origin of the muscle, release of the insertion of the muscle, and lengthening of the muscle.[3] A spastic muscle often provides a good choice for transfer to a weak muscle.[3] Box 17-1 is a summary of the common procedures performed to correct upper extremity deformities in the patient with cerebral palsy.

SHOULDER

The shoulder postures in adduction and internal rotation.[3,11] This position is caused by spasm or contracture of the subscapularis and pectoralis major. An adducted and internally rotated shoulder prevents the patient from reaching overhead and out to the side. With the arm in this position, tasks such as bathing and dressing are difficult to perform. Hygiene within the axilla may also be a problem in more severe cases. A lengthening or release of the subscapularis is performed to correct the adduction and internal rotation deformity.[3] Occasionally, a patient postures in external rotation and abduction of the shoulder. This position makes it difficult to perform activities in midline. A release of the supraspinatus, infraspinatus, and teres minor can place the shoulder joint in a more functional position, permitting midline activities.[3] Glenohumeral dislocation can occur in athetoid cerebral palsy and is treated surgically with a glenohumeral arthrodesis.[3]

ELBOW

The elbow typically postures at rest in some degree of flexion. The degree of flexion increases with associated reactions[3,11] caused by spastic contracture of any or all of the muscles of the elbow (biceps, brachialis, and brachioradialis [BR]). Long-standing deformities may result in soft tissue contractures and skin breakdown in the antecubital fossa. Elbow flexion contractures inhibit the patient's ability to reach forward for objects and effectively perform bimanual activities, such as placing an object on a table with two hands. Elbow flexion deformities, in a *functional* upper extremity, that are greater than 45 degrees at rest, with activity, or during ambulation benefit from surgical correction.[3] Elbow flexion deformities, in the *nonfunctional* upper extremity, that are greater than 100 degrees benefit from surgery to

BOX **17-1** Summary of Upper Extremity Surgical Reconstruction in the Patient with Cerebral Palsy

- Shoulder internal rotation
  - Release of subscapularis
- Shoulder external rotation
  - Release of supraspinatus, infraspinatus, and teres minor
- Elbow flexion
  - Release of biceps, brachialis, and brachioradialis
  - Flexor-pronator slide
- Forearm pronation
  - Release of PQ and flexor aponeurosis
  - PT rerouting
  - Flexor-pronator slide
- Wrist flexion
  - Wrist arthrodesis
  - Muscle transfers for wrist and digital extension
    - ECU to ECRB
    - FCU to ECRB
    - PT to ECRB
    - BR to ECRB
    - FCU to EDC
  - Wrist flexor tendon tightness
    - Tendon lengthening of FCR
    - Tendon lengthening of FCU
  - Volar wrist capsule contracture
    - Proximal row carpectomy
    - Wedge resection arthrodesis
- Digital flexion tightness
  - Flexor-pronator slide
  - Fractional lengthening of FDS and/or FDP
  - Z-lengthening of FDS and FDP
  - Transfer of FDS to FDP (superficialis to profundus or STP)
- Intrinsic muscle spasticity
  - Interosseous muscle origin slide
  - Ulnar motor neurectomy
  - Central slip tenotomy (for swan-neck deformity)
  - FDS tenodesis (for swan-neck deformity)
- Thumb-in-palm deformity
  - Web space release
  - Release or lengthening of first dorsal interosseous, AP, FPB, and/or FPL
  - EPL rerouting
  - Transfer of BR to EPB
  - Thumb MP joint capsulodesis

AP, adductor pollicis; *BR,* brachioradialis; *ECRB,* extensor carpi radialis brevis; *ECU,* extensor carpi ulnaris; *EDC,* extensor digitorum communis; *EPB,* extensor pollicis brevis; *EPL,* extensor pollicis longus; *FCR,* flexor carpi radialis; *FCU,* flexor carpi ulnaris; *FDP,* flexor digitorum profundus; *FDS,* flexor digitorum superficialis; *FPB,* flexor pollicis brevis; *FPL,* flexor pollicis longus; *MP,* metacarpophalangeal; *PQ,* pronator quadratus; *PT,* pronator teres.

improve functional transfers and hygiene.[3] Elbow flexion deformities between 45 and 100 degrees in the nonfunctional elbow may be surgically addressed only if cosmesis is a concern.[3]

Surgery to correct an elbow flexion deformity includes a musculocutaneous neurectomy, a flexor-pronator slide, or lengthening of the elbow flexor muscles. The most direct method to address an elbow flexion deformity is via fractional lengthening of the biceps, brachialis, and brachioradialis (BR).[3] The patient can anticipate a gain of 40 degrees of elbow extension with minimal loss of flexion or functional power.[3] Musculocutaneous neurectomy is contraindicated for a functional upper extremity because active control of the biceps and brachialis is required for elbow flexion. It is also contraindicated in situations where muscle contracture exists.

FOREARM

Spasticity in the pronator teres (PT) and pronator quadratus (PQ) creates a pronation deformity.[3] This prevents the patient from being able to bring the palms together for tasks requiring bimanual manipulation of objects. Furthermore, the pronated forearm cannot be used effectively to carry large objects because of the palm-down position of the hand. Procedures to correct pronation deformity include a flexor pronator slide, release of the pronator quadratus, pronator teres (PT) and flexor aponeurosis, and a pronator rerouting. A flexor-pronator slide involves the release of the PT at its origin, whereas a pronator tenotomy, or rerouting, involves the release of the PT at its insertion.[3] When active pronation is present in the absence of active supination, a PT rerouting provides active supination.[3] When both active supination and pronation are lacking, a pronator teres rerouting suspends the forearm in a neutral position, using a tenodesis effect.[3]

WRIST AND DIGITS: EXTRINSIC MUSCULATURE

The wrist often postures in flexion with fisted digits, which is a result of weak wrist and digital extensors, contracted or spastic wrist and digital flexor tendons, or a volar wrist capsular contracture.[3] The flexed position interferes with the normal tenodesis balance between the wrist and digital flexor and extensor muscles, thereby impairing grasp and release of everyday objects. The poor mechanical advantage of the digital flexors in wrist flexion impairs grip strength. Weak extensors and/or contracted flexors inhibit the release of objects.

Ulnar deviation is another common posture of the wrist, which is caused by spasticity or contracture of the flexor carpi ulnaris (FCU) or extensor carpi ulnaris (ECU). The FCU causes ulnar deviation with wrist flexion, whereas the ECU causes ulnar deviation with wrist extension. The flexor muscle causing the deformity often serves as the transfer muscle to the weak extensor group.[3] For example, if the FCU pulls the wrist into ulnar deviation with wrist flexion, then the FCU may be transferred to the extensor carpi radialis brevis (ECRB) to augment extension. An FCU to ECRB transfer improves wrist extension while eliminating the ulnar deviating force with wrist flexion.

Impaired wrist/digital extension caused by contracture or spasticity of the flexors requires release or lengthening of the involved flexor muscles. When wrist and digital extension is impaired without flexor contracture or spasticity, surgery involves muscle transfers to augment extension. A combination of flexor contractures (or spasticity) with extensor weakness requires both release and lengthening of the flexors, as well as a transfer to the extensors for increased power.

Wrist and Digital Extensor Weakness

One or more of the following procedures may be performed to improve wrist and digital extension, depending on the strength of donor muscles ECU to ECRB, FCU to ECRB, PT to ECRB, BR to ECRB, or FCU to extensor digitorum communis (EDC).[3] When the flexion deformity at the wrist is severe, and a joint contracture has developed, a proximal row carpectomy may be the only option to position the wrist in neutral.[3]

Wrist and Digital Flexor Tightness

Spasticity or contracture of the FCU tendon is the dominant cause of a wrist flexion deformity in patients with cerebral palsy.[3] Spasticity or contracture of flexor carpi radialis (FCR), palmaris longus, flexor digitorum superficialis (FDS), flexor digitorum profundus (FDP), and flexor pollicis longus (FPL) can also contribute to the deformity.[3] Procedures to lengthen the flexor tendons include flexor-pronator slide, fractional lengthening, Z-lengthening, superficialis to profundus transfer, and bony shortening at the wrist.[3] Digital flexor lengthening decreases the strength of the flexors, yet provides improved wrist extension, which enhances force.[3]

HAND: INTRINSIC MUSCULATURE

Spasticity or contracture of the intrinsic muscles of the hand (lumbricals and interossei) leads to flexion at the metacarpophalangeal (MP) joints and extension at the proximal interphalangeal (PIP) joints (Figure 17-1). The EDC can usually overpower intrinsic spasticity to extend the MP joints and open the hand.[3] A functional problem arises when the EDC cannot overcome the intrinsic spasticity to open the hand, thereby preventing effective grasp and release.[3] The imbalance created by spastic intrinsic muscles and weak flexor muscles can lead to a swan-neck deformity over time (Figure 17-2). In a swan-neck deformity, the PIP joint can lock in hyperextension, making flexion of this joint very difficult.

Surgical correction for intrinsic muscle spasticity includes interosseous muscle origin slide or ulnar motor

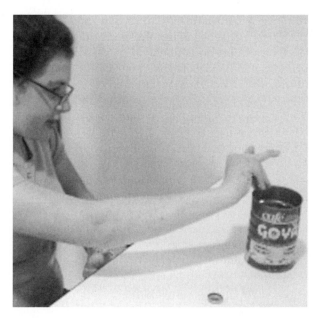

FIGURE **17-1** Hand intrinsic spasticity in patient with cerebral palsy.

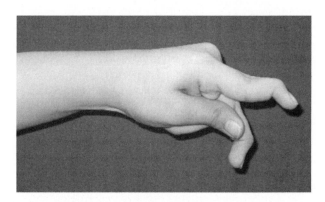

FIGURE **17-2** Swan-neck deformity and thumb-in-palm deformity in patient with cerebral palsy.

neurectomy.[3] The muscle origin slide adjusts the spasticity of the muscle, decreases the contracture, and permits some intrinsic function. Ulnar motor neurectomy releases the spasticity of the intrinsic muscles but does not address the joint contracture. A swan-neck deformity can be corrected with a central slip tenotomy or FDS tenodesis.[3]

THUMB

Flexion of the thumb into the palm greatly impairs hand function by preventing opposition and prehension grasp (see Figure 17-2). This deformity is caused by web space contracture; spasticity or contracture of the adductor pollicis (AP), flexor pollicis brevis (FPB), and first dorsal interosseous; spasticity of the FPL with the wrist extended and flexed; or a weak abductor pollicis longus (APL), extensor pollicis longus (EPL), or extensor pollicis brevis (EPB).[3] Hyperextension of greater than 20 degrees in the thumb MP joint is also a concern and may need to be addressed.[3]

Surgery is determined according to the cause of the deformity. Common reconstructive thumb procedures include release of the spastic muscles, augmentation of the impaired extensor and abductor muscles, stabilization of the thumb MP joint, and release of the web space contracture. Thumb abduction and extension can be improved by various tendon transfers, including BR, palmaris longus, FCR, FCU, ECRB, extensor carpi radialis longus (ECRL), and FDS.[3] FPL rerouting and abductorplasty also improve extension and abduction.[3] If the thumb MP joint actively extends more than 20 degrees past zero, MP joint arthrodesis or capsulodesis is performed to prevent hyperextension.[3]

REHABILITATION OVERVIEW

PREOPERATIVE CARE

The preoperative phase is critical in providing the surgeon with the information required to formulate and finalize the surgical plan. This phase focuses on completing a thorough upper extremity evaluation that includes a videotaped motion analysis,[3,16] functional performance tests, and, occasionally, a dynamic EMG study.[3,17,18] The preoperative evaluation is completed by an occupational or hand therapist and reviewed with the treating hand surgeon. The therapist, surgeon, and patient determine preoperative therapy goals once the evaluation has been reviewed. Preoperative therapy is not always necessary, depending on the needs of the patient. It is indicated to maximize range of motion (ROM) before surgery. For example, botulinum toxin A (BTX-A) injection is used preoperatively to temporarily relax a spastic muscle.[12,19-21] A serial cast or splint is then applied to elongate this spastic muscle in preparation for surgery.[3,11] BTX-A may also be used to determine whether a particular surgical procedure will enhance function in the hand.[22,23] The surgeon injects BTX-A into a specific muscle to determine whether its release will enhance function. The therapist then instructs the patient in exercises to test the effects of the BTX-A and the function of the antagonistic muscles.

POSTOPERATIVE CARE OVERVIEW

Rehabilitation focuses on the following goals: protection of the rebalanced length-tension relationship of the postoperative structures; neuromuscular reeducation of the transferred muscles; and integration of the arm into functional use. The postoperative upper extremity in a patient with cerebral palsy is subject to muscle spasms and spasticity following surgery. Therefore, despite the trend in rehabilitation toward early mobility, this patient is immobilized for 4 weeks following surgery during phase I. Immobilization is necessary to protect the rebal-

---

Preoperative Therapy

GOALS
- Complete upper extremity evaluation, motion analysis video, and functional performance testing
- Refer patient for EMG study, when necessary
- Maximize AROM/PROM

PRECAUTIONS
- None

TREATMENT STRATEGIES
- BTX-A injection into spastic muscle
- Apply serial cast or splint within 3 days of injection and continue until PROM stabilizes (6 weeks)
- Home exercise program for AROM/PROM of spastic and/or contracted muscle

CRITERIA FOR ADVANCEMENT
- PROM is stabilized.
- BTX-A demonstrates a positive effect on upper extremity function.
- Consider surgery to permanently recreate effects of BTX-A.

anced muscles at their resting lengths, despite postoperative, unpredictable spasms and increased tone.

Phase II begins 4 weeks after surgery, once the immobilization period has ended. This phase consists of protective splinting and intensive therapy to assist the patient in developing increased control over the rebalanced limb. During phase II the patient is splinted according to the surgical procedures and surgeon's orders. The splint remains in place at all times, except during therapy, the home exercise program (HEP), and bathing. Clinicians should use traditional therapeutic methods to improve ROM and strength, as well as neurorehabilitative techniques to facilitate movement out of the preoperative synergistic patterns.

Phase III begins 8 weeks after surgery. The clinician assists the patient in integrating the arm into functional use through activity practice. Therapeutic activities include both unilateral and bilateral tasks to integrate the upper extremity into function. The splint is removed during the day to complete activities of daily living (ADL). The splint continues to be worn at night, sometimes up to 16 weeks postoperatively, to prevent recurrence of the preoperative deformities.

This guideline delineates desired goals, precautions, and treatment strategies to facilitate motion, strength, motor control, and function in the upper extremity after reconstructive surgery in the patient with cerebral palsy. Criteria for advancement are included for each phase. In addition, the guideline includes splint designs applicable for phases II and III.

POSTOPERATIVE PHASE I (WEEKS 0 TO 4)

Phase I includes the inflammation and fibroblastic stages of wound healing. During this period, the patient's postoperative upper extremity is subject to an increase in muscle spasms and tone. The arm is immobilized in a postoperative dressing that consists of a bulky plaster half cast held in place with a wrap. Immobilization allows for collagen fiber continuity and increased tensile strength of the wound, despite postoperative muscle spasms and increased tone.[24] The postoperative cast remains in place for 4 weeks. The joints not affected by muscles involved in the surgery remain free from the cast. The HEP includes instructions for edema control and ROM of uninvolved joints. The following box outlines the goals, precautions, treatment strategies, criteria for advancement, and special considerations for phase I of postoperative therapy.

Postoperative Phase I (Weeks 0 to 4)

GOALS
- Immobilization of surgical areas
- Independence with HEP
- Independence with edema control techniques
- Preparation for phase II therapy

PRECAUTIONS
- Bulky postoperative dressing may not be removed.
- Loose dressing must be secured and the surgeon contacted.
- No heavy grasping or pinching; light self-care acceptable

TREATMENT STRATEGIES
- HEP
  - AROM/PROM of uninvolved joints
  - 3 times/day, 10 repetitions each, with 5-second hold
- Edema control
  - Ice, compression, elevation
  - Sleep with arm elevated

CRITERIA FOR ADVANCEMENT
- Immobilization period ends at 4 weeks with cast removal by surgeon.
- Surgeon's approval to proceed to phase II

SPECIAL CONSIDERATIONS
- If problems arise with the cast, surgeon may remove it and initiate splint earlier than 4 weeks postoperatively.

POSTOPERATIVE PHASE II (WEEKS 4 TO 8)

Phase II marks the transition from the fibroblastic stage to the scar maturation, or remodeling stage, which may last up to 2 years. The wounds strengthen as the collagen becomes structurally stronger.[24] The postoperative cast and dressing are removed, and a custom, thermoplastic splint is designed and fitted for the patient. Box 17-2 describes the most commonly used splints during phase II. The design of the splint depends on the surgical reconstruction. Some patients require more than one splint to meet their postoperative needs (Figures 17-3 through 17-6).

A therapeutic hands-on approach of manual therapy is critical to facilitate motion out of the synergistic flexor pattern (i.e., elbow extension, forearm supination, wrist extension, thumb abduction/extension, and digital extension). Manual stabilization of the joints proximal to the joint being addressed promotes isolated motion. The patient begins an intensive therapy program two to three times a week with a therapist who specializes in the upper extremity. Therapy concentrates on motion, neuromuscular reeducation, functional activities, scar management, and instruction in a home program. The patient is required to perform a daily home program

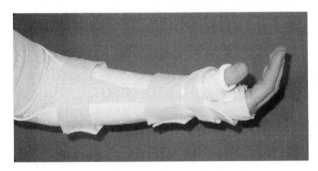

FIGURE **17-3** Modified sugar tong splint.

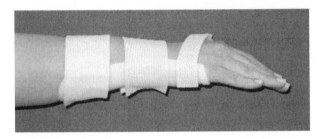

FIGURE **17-4** Ulnar-side block in the wrist or thumb spica splint to prevent ulnar deviation.

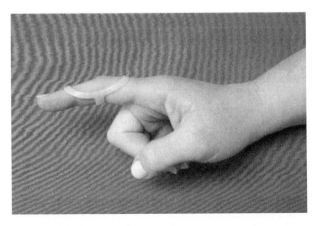

FIGURE **17-5** Figure-eight (modified Oval 8) digital splint with 10 degrees of flexion.

BOX 17-2   Postoperative Splints of Phase II

- **Modified sugar tong:** Forearm procedures (see Figure 17-3)
  Forearm position depends on procedure.
  - Flexor-pronator muscle slide
    - Forearm supinated to end range
    - Wrist extended 10 to 30 degrees
    - Thumb radially abducted 45 degrees
    - Fingers free
  - Pronator teres release
    - Forearm neutral
    - Wrist/thumb/forearm as above
  - Pronator teres rerouting
    - Forearm supinated 45 degrees
- **Thumb spica with ulnar build-up:** Wrist and thumb procedures (see Figure 17-4)
  - Wrist extended 0 to 30 degrees, as per doctor
  - Thumb radially abducted 45 degrees
- **Wrist splint with ulnar build-up:** Wrist procedures only (see Figure 17-4)
  - Wrist extended 0 to 30 degrees, as per doctor
- **Custom figure-eight digital splint:** Swan-neck correction (see Figure 17-5)
  - PIP joints flexed 10 degrees
- **Resting pan add-on:** Digital flexor lengthening (see Figure 17-6)
  - MP/PIP/DIP joints extended to 0 degrees

DIP, distal interphalangeal; *MP*, metacarpophalangeal; *PIP*, proximal interphalangneal.

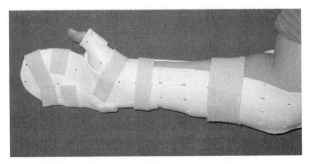

FIGURE **17-6** Resting pan add-on component to modified sugar tong for long flexor stretch.

Postoperative Phase II (Weeks 4 to 8)

GOALS
- Protective immobilization with custom splint
- Active firing of transferred and lengthened muscles
- Patient education

PRECAUTIONS
- Wear splint at all times, except during bath, exercise, and scar management.
- Protective splint must be worn during physical education classes and recess.
- No passive forearm pronation, wrist flexion, or heavy grasp/pinch

TREATMENT STRATEGIES
- Custom splint, as ordered by surgeon
- Isolated motion: AA/AROM/PROM progressing from a gravity-eliminated position to against-gravity position
  - Elbow extension/flexion: supine then standing
  - Forearm supination/pronation: seated, elbow by side
  - Wrist extension/flexion: seated, forearm supported
  - Digital extension/flexion: open/close fist
  - Thumb abduction and extension: hand on table, palm down, bring thumb out to side
- Neuromuscular reeducation
  - Facilitation of transferred muscle
  - Tapping, cold, or vibration to stimulate the transferred muscle
  - NDT and PNF techniques to facilitate movement out of synergy
- Functional activities (Week 6)
  - Grasping objects to encourage spherical or cylindrical patterns (see Figure 17-15)
  - Pinching light objects to promote tip-to-tip or 3-jaw chuck prehension (see Figure 17-16)
  - School, art, athletic, self-care activities of low demand on muscles
    - Examples: turning pages in book, finger painting, catching/rolling lightweight ball, finger foods
- Scar management
  - Scar massage (cross-frictional) 5 minutes each scar
  - Scar pressure: silicone pads at night only
- HEP
  - Place-hold and AROM/PROM of involved joints
  - Keep simple: one exercise per joint

CRITERIA FOR ADVANCEMENT
- Active control of muscle transfers
- Beginning to use hand for light activities
- Clearance from surgeon

SPECIAL CONSIDERATIONS
- Consider electric stimulation for transferred muscle in case of poor active initiation of movement.
- Focus therapy on new muscle patterns via neuromuscular reeducation and functional activities.
- Preference for adduction of thumb and initiation of movement from the tip may persist; splint thumb IP in 10 to 15 degrees of flexion to encourage radial abduction.

that includes scar management. The following box specifies the goals, precautions, treatment strategies, criteria for advancement, and special considerations for the second phase of postoperative therapy. For example, the shoulder is stabilized in neutral to prevent shoulder extension and internal rotation as active elbow extension is attempted. Neuromuscular facilitation techniques can be applied to encourage the transferred muscle to fire. The original motion of the muscle is resisted to encourage active contraction of the transferred muscle. In a BR to EPB transfer, elbow flexion is resisted as abduction and extension of the thumb are attempted. Performing the exercises in front of a mirror provides visual feedback regarding proper body position when attempting the new motion. Suggestions for body position are as follows:

Elbow: Extension is more easily achieved in supine, with the scapula and shoulder stabilized (Figure 17-7, *A*

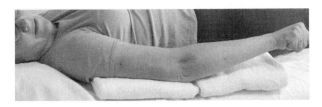

FIGURE **17-7** Active elbow extension in supine.

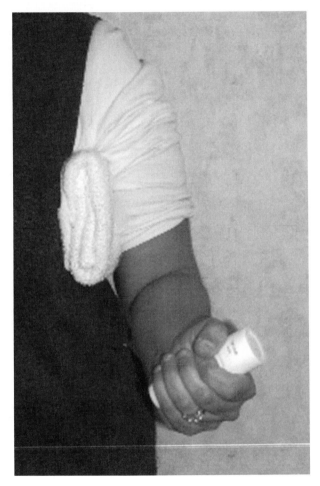

FIGURE **17-8** Active supination while seated: towel under arm to limit shoulder compensation and dowel in hand for target.

and *B*). A rolled towel is positioned under the arm to prevent simultaneous shoulder extension and internal rotation as elbow extension is attempted. Once control in the supine and seated positions is achieved, elbow extension is progressed to an overhead position and then to a standing position.

Forearm: Forearm supination is performed with the patient seated (Figure 17-8). A towel roll placed in the axilla provides cues to maintain neutral shoulder alignment and prevent compensatory motion. Once control of supination is achieved in the seated position, the same exercise is repeated in standing. Functional activities that facilitate supination are encouraged.

Wrist and digits: Wrist and digital extension is performed in sitting with the forearm supported. A dowel is placed in the patient's hand to isolate the wrist extensors and prevent the digital extensors from compensating (Figure 17-9, *A* and *B*). For isolated digital extension, the wrist is manually blocked in neutral (Figure 17-10).

Thumb: Radial abduction and extension is achieved in sitting with the hand supported palm-down on a tabletop (Figure 17-11). It is helpful to sprinkle talcum powder on the tabletop to limit the friction caused by thumb motion. The patient may attempt to initiate abduction and extension with the tip of the thumb, which leads to thumb IP extension and adduction. A dorsal thumb IP extension blocking splint is applied with the IP positioned in 10 to 15 degrees of flexion to prevent this compensatory movement (Figure 17-12).

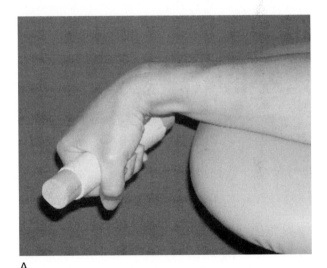

A

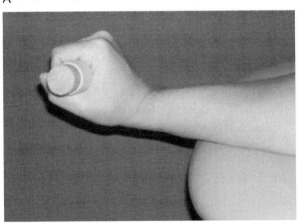

B

FIGURE **17-9** *A.* Start exercise with wrist flexion with forearm supported on a flat surface. *B.* Extend wrist from this position with dowel in hand to isolate wrist extensors.

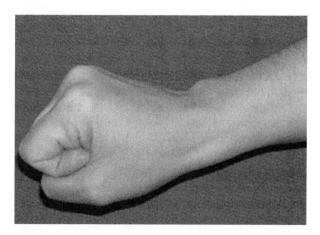

FIGURE **17-10** Active digital flexion.

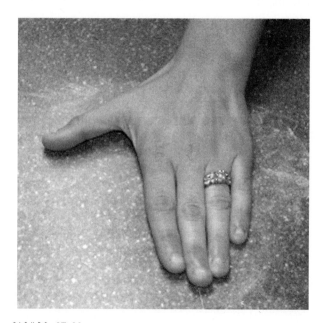

FIGURE **17-11** Active thumb radial abduction and extension with hand (palm-down) resting on tabletop.

Neuromuscular Electrical Stimulation. Neuromuscular electrical stimulation (NMES) can be used on the transferred muscle to help the patient identify and learn to control the desired motion. NMES is used as an adjunct to therapy to activate the muscle transfer and assist with neuromotor retraining. Studies demonstrate significant improvement in ROM as well as grasp, prehension, and release following use of either functional or NMES in children with hemiplegia and cerebral palsy.[22,25-27] The caregiver is trained to apply the NMES to the child so that it can become part of the daily HEP. A typical schedule consists of two sessions per day lasting 15 minutes each. Suggested parameters for the NMES unit are listed in Box 17-3.

Functional activities are performed with NMES once the transferred muscle fires actively. For example, when stimulating BR for thumb abduction and extension, a small object is picked up during the off cycle and released during the on cycle.

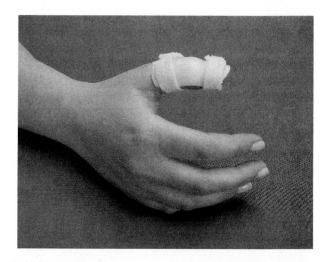

FIGURE **17-12** Thumb IP extension blocker with 10 to 15 degrees of flexion.

BOX 17-3   Parameters for Neuromuscular Electrical Stimulation (NMES)

Equipment
- Stimulator unit with current output that can be set from 0 to 100 mA
- Two electrodes
- Connecting wires

Waveform
- Biphasic
- Symmetrical, rectangular pulses
- 200 μsec duration

Pulse Rate
- Produces titanic muscle contraction
- 40 to 60 pulses per second

Stimulus Amplitude
- Produce tolerable stimulus
- 30 to 40 mA

Ramp
- 2-second ON
- 2-second OFF

Duty Cycle
- 1:1 ON/OFF ratio for rhythmic muscle contractions
- 10 seconds ON
- 10 seconds OFF

POSTOPERATIVE PHASE III (WEEK 8 TO 6 MONTHS)

The scar maturation process continues in phase III, and the surgical sites are well healed at this phase. Therapy between 8 to 12 weeks postoperatively is aimed at strengthening the new movement patterns and engaging the upper extremity in activities. Intensive therapy (two to three times per week) continues until week 12. The splint is worn at night until week 12 and can continue for up to 6 months. Intermittent therapy (weekly or bimonthly) from week 16 to 6 months postoperatively is continued to monitor skill acquisition and motor integration. Functional gains continue up to 1 year postoperatively. The preceding box outlines the goals, precautions, treatment strategies, criteria for advancement, and special considerations for the third phase of postoperative therapy.

EXPECTED OUTCOME

By 12 to 16 weeks post-surgery the patient should demonstrate improved motor control and be able to move the upper extremity independent of synergy patterns. At this time, improvements in hygiene, resting position of the arm, and functional independence are expected. The patient should be able to use his or her hand as an active assist in bimanual ADL during self-care, work, school, and leisure tasks.

DISCHARGE CRITERIA

Discharge from therapy is determined once the patient achieves the following degrees of AROM: 0 to 10

Postoperative Phase III (Week 8 to 6 Months)

GOALS

- Reinforce HEP and scar management
- Initiate strengthening
- Resume full participation in ADL and functional tasks in school/work
- Use splint for nighttime only

PRECAUTIONS

- Begin strengthening, only per surgeon's orders
- Do not strengthen forearm pronation
- Needs surgeon's approval to participate in gym and recess without splint protection

TREATMENT STRATEGIES

- Motion: AROM against gravity progressing toward resistance of the following:
  - elbow extension, forearm supination, wrist extension/flexion, digital extension, thumb extension and abduction, grasp, and prehension
- Neuromuscular reeducation
  - Use NDT or PNF patterns with functional activities to encourage new movement patterns
- Functional activities
  - Grasping objects that encourage spherical or cylindrical patterns
  - Pinching light objects that promote tip-to-tip or 3-jaw chuck prehension
  - School, art, athletic, self-care activities of low demand on muscles
  - Examples: carrying textbook, molding clay, wall push-ups, donning socks and shoes
- HEP
  - Modify program so that all exercises are performed against gravity
  - Continue scar management until week 12
  - Add grip-and-pinch strengthening as needed

CRITERIA FOR ADVANCEMENT

- Maintains good form as resistance increases
- Able to perform graded activities with minimal to no assistance
- Progress under guidance from surgeon

SPECIAL CONSIDERATIONS

- Integrate upper extremity into both unilateral and bilateral activities.
- Forearm procedure may result as a suspension in neutral rather than an active supinator; active supination may not evolve.
- Ulnar deviation preference may persist with active wrist extension; block this preference as patient strengthens wrist extension.

degrees of elbow extension, forearm supination to neutral (either actively or through passive positioning), wrist extension to neutral, MP extension to neutral, thumb radial abduction and palmar abduction to 45 degrees, and a +3/5 grade of strength of the involved muscles. Functional level of independence should reach or surpass the preoperative level. Therapy is discontinued once the patient resumes participation in all meaningful activities. Postoperative therapy can be followed with a school-based therapy program, which continues to focus on integration of the postoperative arm into functional activities. In addition to occupational and physical therapy, the patient is encouraged to engage in community-based physical activities that demand bilateral upper extremity use, such as karate, yoga, horseback riding, or kayaking.

REFERENCES

1. Bobath, K. *A Neurophysiological Basis for the Treatment of Cerebral Palsy*. Lippincott, Philadelphia, 1980.
2. Wong, D.L. *Whaley and Wongs Essentials of Pediatric Nursing*, 4th ed. Mosby, St. Louis, 1993.
3. Carlson, M.G. Cerebral Palsy. In Hotchkiss, R. (Ed). *Green's Operative Hand Surgery*. Elsevier, New York, 1999.
4. Samilson, R.L., Morris, J.M. *Surgical Improvement of the Cerebral-palsied Upper Limb: Electromyographic Studies and Results of 128 Operations*. J Bone Joint Surg 1964;46A:1203–1216.
5. Tachdjian, M.O., Minear, A.L. *Sensory Disturbances in the Hands of Children with Cerebral Palsy*. J Bone Joint Surg 1958;40A:85–90.
6. Renshaw, T.S. Cerebral Palsy. In Morrissy, R.T., Weinstein, S.L. (Eds). *Lovell and Winter's Pediatric Orthopedics*, 5th ed., vol. 1. Lippincott Williams & Wilkins, New York, 2001, pp. 563–599.
7. Stranger, M. Orthopedic Management. In Tecklin, J.S. (Ed). *Pediatric Physical Therapy*, 3rd ed. Lippincott Williams & Wilkins, New York, 1999, pp. 394–396.
8. Statistic from "How common is cerebral palsy?" Centers for Disease Control and Prevention (CDC). Available online at http://www.cdc.gov.
9. Gordon, K.Y., Schanzenbacher, K.E., Case-Smith, J., Carrasco, R.C. Diagnostic Problems in Pediatrics. In Case-Smith (Ed). *Occupational Therapy for Children*. Mosby, St. Louis, 1996.
10. Goldner, J.L. *Upper Extremity Tendon Transfers in Cerebral Palsy*. Orthop Clin North Am 1974;5(2):389–414.
11. Goldner, J.L. Surgical Reconstruction of the Upper Extremity in Cerebral Palsy. Hand Clin 1988;4(2):223–265.
12. Skoff, H., Woodbury, D.F. *Management of the Upper Extremity in Cerebral Palsy*. J Bone Joint Surg 1985;67A(3):500–503.
13. Van Heest, A.E., House, J.H., Cariello, C. *Upper Extremity Surgical Treatment of Cerebral Palsy*. J Hand Surg 1999;24A(2):323–330.
14. Cooper, W. *Surgery of Upper Extremity in Spastic Paralysis*. Q Rev Pediatr 1952;7:139–144.
15. Mital, M.A., Sakellarides, H.T. *Surgery of the Upper Extremity in the Retarded Individual with Spastic Cerebral Palsy*. Orthop Clin North Am 1981;12:127–141.
16. Waters, P.M., Zurakowski, D., Patterson, P., Bae, D.S., Nimec, D. *Interobserver and Intraobserver Reliability of Therapist-assisted Videotaped Evaluations of Upper-limb Hemiplegia*. J Hand Surg 2004;29A:328–334.
17. Leclercq, C. *General Assessment of the Upper Limb*. Hand Clin 2003;19:557–564.
18. Mowery, C.A., Gelberman, R.H., Rhoades, C.E. *Upper Extremity Tendon Transfers in Cerebral Palsy: Electromyographic and Functional Analysis*. J Pediatr Orthop 1985;5:69–72.
19. Chin, T.Y., Graham, H.K. *Botulinum Toxin A in the Management of Upper Limb Spasticity in Cerebral Palsy*. Hand Clin 2003;19(4):591–600.
20. Koman, L.A., Smith, B.P., Goodman, A. *Botulinum Toxin Type A in the Management of Cerebral Palsy*. Wake Forest University Press, Winston-Salem, NC, 2002.
21. Wall, S.A., Chait, L.A., Temlett, J.A., Perkins, B., Hillen, G., Becker, P. *Botulinum A Chemodenervation: A New Modality in Cerebral Palsied Hands*. Br J Plast Surg 1993;46:703–706.
22. Boyd, R.N., Morris, M.E., Graham, H.K. *Management of Upper Limb Dysfunction in Children with Cerebral Palsy: A Systematic View*. Eur J Neurol 2001;8(Suppl 5):150–166.
23. Autti-Ramo, I., Larsen, A., Taimo, A., von Wendt, L. *Management of the Upper Limb with Botulinum Toxin Type A in Children with Spastic Type Cerebral Palsy and Acquired Brain Injury: Clinical Implications*. Eur J Neurol 2001;8(Suppl 5):136–144.
24. Smith, K.L. Wound Healing. In Stanley, B.G., Tribuzi, S.M. (Eds). *Concepts in Hand Rehabilitation*. FA Davis, Philadelphia, 1992.
25. Scheker, L.R., Ozer, K. *Electrical Stimulation in the Management of Spastic Deformity*. Hand Clin 2003;19:601–606.
26. Wright, P.A., Granat, M.H. *Therapeutic Effects of Functional Electrical Stimulation of the Upper Limb of Eight Children with Cerebral Palsy*. Dev Med Child Neurol 2000;42:724–727.
27. Carmick, J. *Clinical Use of Neuromuscular Electrical Stimulation for Children with Cerebral Palsy, Part II: Upper Extremity*. Phys Ther 1993;73(8):514–522.

18

Ulnar Nerve Transposition

AMY BARENHOLTZ-MARSHALL, OTR, CHT

At the elbow, the ulnar nerve passes posterior to the medial epicondyle through a narrow space known as the cubital tunnel. Because of the anatomical configuration and the superficial course of the nerve, this is a common entrapment site and is referred to as *cubital tunnel syndrome*.[1,2] At this level the nerve is responsible for motor activity of the fourth and fifth flexor digitorum profundus (FDP) tendons, flexor carpi ulnaris (FCU) muscle, intrinsic hand muscles, and sensation of the fifth and ulnar one-half of fourth fingers. Injury to the nerve can be caused by a blunt trauma to the elbow (such as a fracture or fracture dislocation), compression, traction, friction, or subluxation.[1] Compression to the nerve can originate from external or internal sources. Externally sustained, prolonged pressure on the medial side of the elbow, or repetitive motion, results in compression of the nerve. Internal sources of compression include tight fascial bands, arthritic spurs, rheumatoid synovitis, and soft tissue tumors.[1,3] Other conditions that contribute to compression by lowering the nerve threshold include diabetes, chronic alcoholism, and renal disease.[1] Ulnar nerve compression symptoms can mimic other conditions. A differential diagnoses must be made to exclude thoracic outlet syndrome (TOS), cervical disc lesion with nerve root compression, and ulnar nerve entrapment at Guyon's canal.

Early symptoms of ulnar nerve compression include sharp or aching pain on the medial side of the proximal forearm, that radiates proximally or distally.[1] This is accompanied by intermittent paresthesias in the fourth and fifth fingers. Symptoms are aggravated by elbow flexion and frequently awaken the patient at night. Later symptoms include muscle atrophy of the intrinsics, slight clawing of the fourth and fifth digits accompanied by sensory changes (Figure 18-1, *A*), hand weakness, and impaired dexterity. The last changes to appear are FDP and FCU weakness.

Nerve compression that is detected early, with the compression attributed to external sources, is treated conservatively by anti-inflammatory medication, nighttime splinting (to avoid prolonged elbow flexion), postural education, and activity modification. If a 4- to 6-week trial of conservative treatment fails, surgery is considered.[4] Electromyography (EMG) testing before surgery confirms compression of the nerve.

Surgical procedures to decompress the nerve range from a simple ligament release (in situ decompression) to an anterior transposition of the nerve to a medial epicondylectomy. Functional results vary depending on the severity and duration of nerve compression, clinical symptoms, and surgical procedure. Symptoms that have been present for less than 6 months and limited to paresthesias can expect complete recovery.[4]

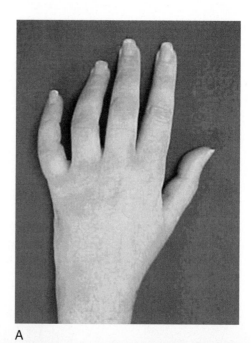

A

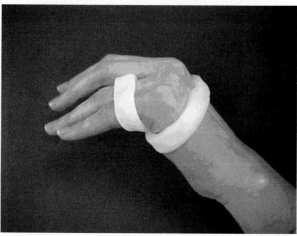

B

FIGURE **18-1** *A.* Claw hand deformity. The position of metacarpophalangeal (MP) joint hyperextension with interphalangeal (IP) joint flexion of ring and little fingers is the result of weakness or paralysis of the FDP and lumbricals to those fingers. *B.* Figure-eight splint. The MP joints are held in flexion, substituting for the lack of lumbrical motor function. This position redistributes the extensor force, which allows the patient to actively extend the interphalangeal joints.

ANATOMICAL OVERVIEW

The ulnar nerve arises from the medial cord of the brachial plexus. As the ulnar nerve courses medially toward the elbow, it pierces the medial intermuscular septum through the arcade of Struthers.[5] This is a fascial band that lies 8 cm proximally to the medial epicondyle and traverses the medial head of the triceps to the medial intramuscular septum.[4] The nerve descends subfascially on the medial aspect of the triceps muscle and changes to a more posterior course (Figure 18-2).

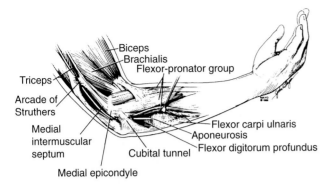

FIGURE **18-2** The ulnar nerve as it courses down the arm. (*From Mackin, E.J., Callahan, A.D., Skirven, T.M., Schneider, L.H., Hunter, J.M. [Eds].* Rehabilitation of the Hand and Upper Extremity, *5th ed. Mosby, St. Louis, 2002, p. 680, with permission.*)

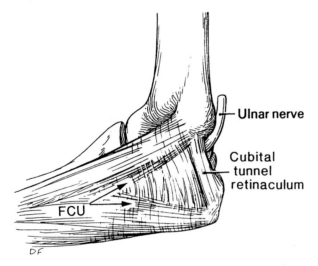

FIGURE **18-3** Anatomy of the cubital tunnel. The ulnar nerve lies posteriorly to the medial epicondyle and courses through the two heads of the FCU muscle. The triangular arcuate ligament forms the roof of the tunnel. (*From Green, D.P., Hotchkiss, R.N., Pederson, W.C.* Green's Operative Hand Surgery, *4th ed. Churchill Livingstone, New York, 1998, p. 1424, with permission.*)

Before the nerve enters the forearm, it passes posteriorly to the medial epicondyle through the cubital tunnel. The tunnel begins at the condylar groove between the medial epicondyle of the humerus and the olecranon of the ulna. The floor of the tunnel is composed of the medial collateral ligament of the elbow joint, and the two heads of the FCU form the sides. The roof is formed by the triangular arcuate ligament, which bridges the medial epicondyle of the humerus and the medial tip of the olecranon (Figure 18-3). The nerve then passes into the forearm between the ulnar and humeral heads of the FCU muscle. The capacity of the cubital tunnel is greatest when the elbow is extended, because this puts the arcuate ligament on slack.[1,3] Compression at the elbow can occur at various sites along the course of the nerve, including the arcade of Struthers, the medial intermuscular septum, the medial epicondyle,

the cubital tunnel, or between the two heads of the FCU origin.

SURGICAL OVERVIEW

The purpose of surgical intervention is to decompress the nerve while retaining adequate blood supply. If in situ decompression cannot adequately relieve compression, the nerve is removed from the tunnel and transposed anteriorly either subcutaneously or submuscularly. The nerve is moved to lie anteriorly to the elbow flexion/extension axis of motion to avoid compression and traction with elbow flexion. The approach is a posteromedial longitudinal incision approximately 8 to 10 cm long, with proximal exposure of the medial intermuscular septum and the arcade of Struthers and distal exposure of the nerve between the two heads of the FCU. The arcade of Struthers is released, and the intermuscular septum is removed. The nerve is then identified and freed in the proximal forearm at the level deep to the FCU origin. It is elevated from its bed and placed anteriorly to the medial epicondyle. At this point the nerve is placed in an intermuscular, subfascial, subcutaneous, or submuscular position.[5]

SUBCUTANEOUS TRANSPOSITION

The ulnar nerve and its neurovascular bundle are transposed anteriorly beneath the elevated skin flap. A loose fasciodermal sling, created from the flexor muscle mass or the intermuscular septum, is created to support the nerve in the new position. This approach is appropriate for mild cases of compression. Clinical symptoms are present, but EMG tests are normal[3,5] (Figure 18-4).

SUBMUSCULAR TRANSPOSITION (LEARMONTH PROCEDURE)

This procedure places the nerve in a protected position[4] and is indicated in moderate to severe neuropathies, thin-skinned individuals, or high demand elbows, such as throwing athletes.[3] It is also performed as a second procedure in people who had a failed anterior subcutaneous transposition. The muscles of the flexor-pronator group are detached 1 cm distally to the medial epicondyle. The ulnar nerve is moved beneath the flexor muscle group and aligned adjacently to the median nerve. The flexor-pronator origin is repaired and reattached to the epicondyle, with the forearm positioned in pronation[3] (Figure 18-5).

REHABILITATION OVERVIEW

Rehabilitation goals are to reduce pain, reduce paresthesias, optimize nerve glide, increase elbow range of motion (ROM), prevent deformity, increase muscle strength, restore full functional hand use, and educate the patient in sensory precautions, if necessary.

Protected ROM begins early to prevent nerve adhesions and joint stiffness. Full active elbow motion is

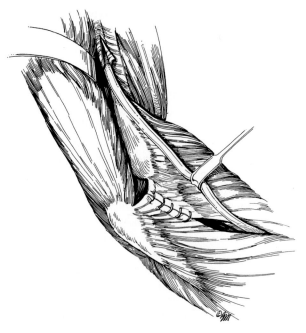

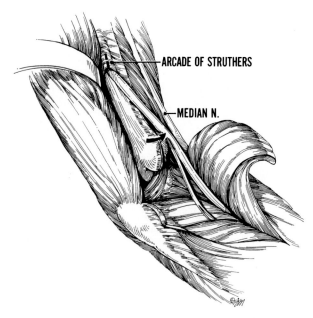

F I G U R E **18-4** *A.* Subcutaneous transposition. Exposure begins proximally at the medial intermuscular septum and the arcade of Struthers. The arcade is then released and the septum is removed. The nerve is then moved anteriorly to the elbow axis. *B.* A fascial sling is created from the fascia overlying the flexor-pronator mass. (*From Green, D.P., Hotchkiss, R.N., Pederson, W.C.* Green's Operative Hand Surgery, *4th ed. Churchill Livingstone, New York, 1998, p. 1426, with permission.*)

F I G U R E **18-5** Submuscular transposition. The flexor-pronator group is elevated off the medial epicondyle, and the nerve is brought forward to lie adjacently to the median nerve. The flexor-pronator group is then reattached. (*From Green, D.P., Hotchkiss, R.N., Pederson, W.C.* Green's Operative Hand Surgery, *4th ed. Churchill Livingstone, New York, 1998, p. 1427, with permission.*)

expected by 3 weeks post-surgery. Resistive exercises are initiated in accordance with the stages of soft tissue healing and are aimed at restoring normal upper extremity function to perform all relevant activities of daily living (ADL), vocational, and leisure activities.

POSTOPERATIVE PHASE I: INFLAMMATION (WEEKS 0 TO 2)

Immediately following surgery the elbow is immobilized in a bulky postoperative dressing and a posterior elbow splint. At the first postoperative visit, 7 to 10 days later, the patient is referred for therapy. The initial therapy visit includes wound care, instruction in ROM, edema reduction, instruction in a home program, and splint fabrication. Sensory precautions are reviewed if sensory loss is present. Usually, the elbow is supported in a sling, and a splint is not required. If the flexor-pronator group were reattached, a thermoplastic posterior elbow shell is fabricated with the elbow in 90-degree flexion and the forearm and wrist in neutral. This is worn full time and removed three to four times per day to perform exercises and wound care. In patients who have motor involvement in the hand, resulting in muscle imbalance, a corrective anti-claw splint is fabricated (see Figure 18-1, *B*). Restrictive dressings are avoided and light, nonbulky dressings are pre-

ferred to allow for full motion and adequate splint conformity. Instructions for daily wound care are provided, and isolated elbow and forearm exercises are emphasized. Exercises are performed while standing against a wall with the arm adducted and a towel roll behind the humerus to maintain correct alignment and prevent compensatory motions (see photos in Chapter 10). Active elbow flexion/extension is performed, and assistance is provided as needed. Elbow extension is limited to 90 degrees. For limited elbow flexion, gentle passive motion is performed. If the pronator-flexor origin is reattached, the patient performs elbow exercises with the forearm pronated and wrist flexed. Active forearm pronation, wrist flexion, and hand gripping are delayed. Active range of motion (AROM) for all uninvolved joints is reviewed. All exercises are performed four times a day. Edema control follows the standard procedure, as discussed previously.

Troubleshooting

Care is taken to avoid vigorous ROM, which leads to inflammation and pain. If this occurs, ROM exercises are avoided for 1 to 2 days, and measures are taken to decrease the pain and edema. Elbow motion is monitored carefully for early signs of flexion contracture, and treatment is adjusted accordingly. Any unusual situations, such as signs of infection or excessive pain indicating possible rupture, are reported to the physician for evaluation.

Postoperative Phase I: Inflammation (Weeks 0 to 2)

GOALS

- Edema and pain control
- Maximum elbow and forearm AROM within safe parameters
- Promote wound healing
- Awareness of precautions
- Full ROM of uninvolved joints
- Independence in HEP

PRECAUTIONS

- Avoid exacerbation of pain and inflammation
- Avoid neurovascular compromise
- No elbow extension beyond 90 degrees
- If the flexor-pronator group is reattached, no active wrist flexion or extension or forearm pronation
- Sensory precautions

TREATMENT STRATEGIES

Splinting
- Elbow positioned either in sling or splint (posterior elbow shell: elbow at 90 degrees with forearm and wrist in neutral) full-time, remove three to four times a day for Therex
- Splinting to prevent deformity
- Figure-eight splint for motor weakness and muscle imbalance (clawing of digits IV and V)

Wound care
- Wound care: maintain sterile protective dressing as thin as possible as not to impede motion

Edema control
- Elevated positioning at all times
- Compression wraps: coban or Ace wrapping
- Cryotherapy

Therapeutic exercises
- AROM elbow flexion and graded extension to pain tolerance
- AROM forearm pronation and supination to pain tolerance
- Gentle PROM elbow flexion
- AROM to uninvolved joints: shoulder, wrist and hand, tendon gliding exercises
  - If there is motor involvement in hand; intrinsic muscle exercises
- HEP

CRITERIA FOR ADVANCEMENT

- Evidence of wound healing
- Reduction in edema
- Minimal inflammatory responsiveness

POSTOPERATIVE PHASE II: FIBROPLASIA (WEEKS 3 TO 7)

Gradual weaning of the splint or sling begins during the day. The sling continues to be used for protection and sleep. Edema reduction techniques are continued as needed. Scar management commences when the sutures are removed and the incision is fully closed. The patient is instructed in scar massage and the use of silicone sheets. Compression should be added if hypertrophy is evident. All AROM exercises can be progressed to gentle passive exercises. The active arc of elbow flexion/extension is gradually increased. For flexor-pronator attachments, active forearm rotation and wrist flexion/extension is gradually introduced. Heat modalities are used before exercise, as long as no inflammation is present. Ulnar nerve gliding exercises are performed to prevent nerve and scar adhesions.[6] At 4 weeks postoperatively, midrange isometric exercises are initiated followed by grip-and-pinch strengthening with the use of putty or bands. This is delayed another 2 weeks if the flexor mass is reattached. The home program is continued and upgraded to include passive stretching. Repetitive elbow flexion/extension activities are avoided.

Troubleshooting

Occasionally, a flexion contracture may develop. If full active elbow ROM is not achieved by 6 weeks, corrective splinting is considered. Careful assessment must be made to differentiate possible causes, such as persistent edema, joint contracture, or heterotopic ossification[7] (see Chapter 9 on elbow contracture release). Pain symptoms and patterns are monitored closely. Persistent pain and localized point tenderness along the incision may be a sign of a neuroma. Pain and paresthesias with elbow flexion may indicate nerve subluxation or nerve adhesions. Any unusual symptoms must be communicated to the surgeon for further evaluation.

Postoperative Phase II: Fibroplasia (Weeks 3 to 7)

GOALS

- Scar management
- Promote scar mobility and minimize adhesions
- Promote nerve glide
- Reduce edema
- Maximize AROM/PROM
- Task modification
- Encourage functional hand use in light ADL

PRECAUTIONS

- Same as phase I
- Monitor soft tissue responses to treatment and upgrade techniques accordingly
- Watch for signs of nerve adhesions
- Sensory precautions
- Avoid provocative positioning
- Avoid repetitive elbow flexion/extension tasks

TREATMENT STRATEGIES

Splinting
- Wean splint/sling during day; use only for protection and sleep
- Splinting to prevent deformity

Edema reduction
- Elevation
- Retrograde massage
- Compression wrapping

Scar management (initiate after sutures are removed and incision is fully closed)
- Scar massage
- Silicone sheets
- Compression wraps during day and at night if tolerated

Therapeutic exercises
- Heat modalities pretreatment
- Elbow/forearm AROM and progress to PROM
- Graded progression of active elbow extension
- Upgrade forearm ROM
- Light soft tissue stretching
- Ulnar nerve gliding exercises
- Pain relief via appropriate modalities
- Hand strengthening with putty or bands
  ◦ Lumbricals
  ◦ Thumb adductor
  ◦ Dorsal/volar interossei
- Pinch strengthening
  ◦ Lateral pinch
  ◦ Three- and two-point pinch
- Isometric elbow exercises in midrange at 4 weeks
- Weeks 6 to 8: PREs to wrist begin at week 4 for subcutaneous transposition

Function
- Functional activities
- Sensibility retraining/ reeducation if necessary

CRITERIA FOR ADVANCEMENT

- Evidence of soft tissue healing without an inflammatory response
- Achieve full elbow AROM/PROM

Postoperative Phase III: Scar Maturation (Weeks 8 to 12)

GOALS
- Maximize AROM/PROM
- Improve upper extremity endurance
- Increase elbow/forearm strength
- Increase grip/pincher strength
- Return to full functional activity

PRECAUTIONS
- Grade introduction of PREs

TREATMENT STRATEGIES

Scar management
- ◦ Scar mobilization techniques

Therapeutic exercises
- Ulnar nerve gliding exercises
- Passive stretching
- Joint mobilizations if joint stiffness is present
- Continue with grip-and-pinch strengthening
- PREs to elbow
- Forearm and wrist strengthening
  - ◦ Free weights
  - ◦ Thera-Band
  - ◦ Putty
  - ◦ UBE
  - ◦ BTE

Function
- Functional activities
- Dexterity exercises

CRITERIA FOR DISCHARGE
- Minimal to no pain
- AROM/PROM has plateaued for 4 weeks
- Patient has resumed full use of extremity in all ADL, vocational, and recreational tasks.

POSTOPERATIVE PHASE III: SCAR MATURATION (WEEKS 8 TO 12)

Treatment is continued from the previous phases. The primary focus in phase III is strengthening and preparing the extremity for full return to all functional and recreational activities. Progressive exercises are provided for the shoulder, elbow, forearm, and wrist.

Troubleshooting

Signs of nerve irritation and tendonitis are monitored, and treatment is adjusted accordingly. Medial epicondylitis is an infrequent complication reported in the literature.[7]

REFERENCES

1. Omer, G. Diagnosis and Management of Cubital Tunnel Syndrome. In Mackin, E.J., Callahan, A.D., Skirven, T.M., Schneider, L.H., Hunter, J.M. (Eds). *Rehabilitation of the Hand,* 5th ed. Mosby, St. Louis, 2002, pp. 672–677.

2. Aeillo, B. Ulnar Nerve Compression. In Clark, G.L., Wilgis, E.F., Aiello, B., Eckhaus, D., Eddington, L.V. (Eds). *Hand Rehab, A Practical Guide,* 2nd ed. Churchill Livingstone, New York, 1998, pp. 213–220.

3. Szabo, R.M. Entrapment and Compression Neuropathies. In Green, D.P., Hotchkiss, R.N., Pederson, W.C. (Eds). *Green's Operative Hand Surgery,* 4th ed. Churchill Livingstone, New York, 1999, pp. 1422–1429.

4. Osterman, A.L., Davies, C.A. Subcutaneous Transposition of the Ulnar Nerve for Treatment of Cubital Tunnel Syndrome. In Plancher, K.D. (Ed). *Hand Clinics* 1996;12(2):421–433. WB Saunders, Philadelphia, 1996.

5. Spinner, R.J., Spinner, M. Nerve Entrapment Syndromes. In Morrey, B.F. (Ed). *The Elbow and Its Disorders,* 3rd ed. WB Saunders, Philadelphia, 2000, pp. 847–859.

6. Butler, D.S. *Mobilisation of the Nervous System.* Churchill Livingstone, Melbourne, Australia, 1991.

7. Jackson, L.C., Hotchkiss, R.N. Cubital Tunnel Surgery. In Plancher, K.D. (Ed). *Hand Clinics* 1996;12(2):449–455. WB Saunders, Philadelphia, 1996.

19

Thumb Carpometacarpal Joint Arthroplasty

CAROL PAGE, PT, DPT, CHT

Osteoarthritis, the most common type of arthritis, frequently affects the hands. The thumb carpometacarpal (CMC) joint is the second most frequently affected joint of the hand, following the distal interphalangeal (IP) joint. Thumb CMC joint osteoarthritis is more common in women than in men and is associated with aging.[1,2] Thumb CMC joint osteoarthritis may be degenerative or posttraumatic in origin. The chief complaint is thumb pain, with joint stiffness being a later finding. The severity of symptoms may not correspond radiographically to the degree of change in the joint. Initial treatment consists of nonoperative measures, such as splinting, education in joint protection principles, oral anti-inflammatory medications, and corticosteroid injections. Surgery is indicated when pain is no longer controlled by these nonoperative measures and when pain impairs sleep and functional use of the hand.[3]

ANATOMICAL AND SURGICAL OVERVIEW

The thumb CMC joint comprises the articulation of the trapezium and the first metacarpal. The scaphotrapezial joint may demonstrate degenerative changes as well. The most commonly performed surgery for thumb CMC osteoarthritis is resection arthroplasty of a portion of or the entire trapezium, with ligament reconstruction and use of filler for the excised bone.[3]

At the Hospital for Special Surgery (HSS), the two most commonly performed basal joint arthroplasties are ligament reconstruction tendon interposition (LRTI) arthroplasty and hematoma and distraction arthroplasty (HDA). LRTI arthroplasty involves excision of the distal portion of the trapezium, if the scaphotrapezial joint is in satisfactory condition. If not, the entire trapezium is excised. The base of the thumb metacarpal is excised and a hole is made in the radial base. Half of the flexor carpi radialis tendon is harvested, passed through the trapezial fossa into the medullary canal of the thumb metacarpal, and advanced through the hole in the metacarpal radial base. The tendon slip is pulled tightly and sutured to the periosteum of the metacarpal, resurfacing the metacarpal base. The remainder of the tendon slip is folded into the trapezial space to act as a spacer. Some surgeons use one or more longitudinal Kirschner's wires to stabilize the metacarpal in an abducted, distracted position[2] (Figure 19-1). LRTI arthroplasty has been shown to provide pain relief and thumb stability and restore grip-and-pinch strength for as long as 11 years after surgery.[4,5]

HDA involves excision of the entire trapezium without ligament reconstruction or tendon interposition. A Kirschner's wire is passed through the first metacarpal base into the trapezoid or second metacarpal with the thumb in palmar abduction, slight opposition,

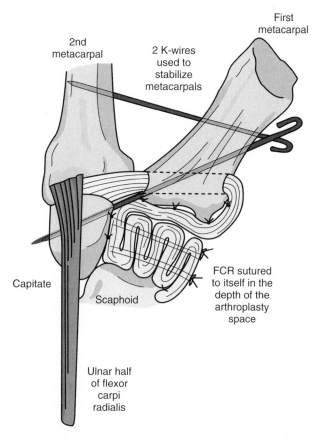

FIGURE **19-1** Ligament reconstruction tendon interposition arthroplasty. (*From Berger, R.A., Weiss, A.P. [Eds]. Hand Surgery. Lippincott Williams & Wilkins, Philadelphia, 2003, p. 1284, with permission; as reprinted in Young, S.D., Mikola, E.A. Thumb Carpometacarpal Arthritis. J Am Soc Surg Hand 2004;4(2):73.*)

and distraction. The Kirschner's wire is left in place for approximately 5 weeks. The hematoma filling the trapezial void becomes fibrotic, thus supporting the base of the second metacarpal.[6]

REHABILITATION OVERVIEW

The treatment guidelines that follow are designed for postoperative management of LRTI arthroplasty. However, they can be easily modified, as will be specified, for use following HDA. The goals of therapy after thumb CMC arthroplasty are to provide correct protective splinting; manage edema, pain, and the postoperative wound and resulting scar; and, ultimately, facilitate restoration of stable thumb and wrist motion and strength adequate to the functional demands of the individual. Individuals who underwent postoperative therapy following thumb CMC arthroplasty should be well versed in joint protection principles and able to consistently apply them during their daily activities. Overaggressive motion and strengthening exercises, as well as too rapid a return to full hand use, may increase pain and inflammation, delaying recovery.

POSTOPERATIVE PHASE I: INFLAMMATION/PROTECTION (WEEKS 0 TO 3)

A referral to therapy usually occurs at 7 to 10 days postoperatively, after the surgeon removes the bulky postoperative splint and sutures. A custom-molded thermoplastic splint is fabricated, with the thumb IP joint free (Figure 19-2). The thumb metacarpophalangeal (MP) and CMC joints are functionally positioned so that the thumb tip can oppose the index fingertip. The splint may rest on the volar or radial surface of the forearm,

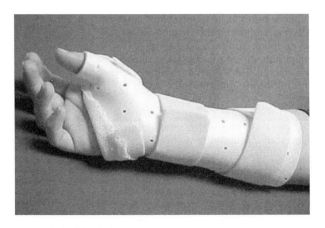

FIGURE **19-2** Volar-based thumb spica splint.

depending on the preferences of the surgeon and therapist. The volar splint is preferred because it is tolerated more easily by sensitive and painful joints. The wrist is included in a position of approximately 15- to 20-degree extension. Education in joint protection principles is started immediately and reinforced throughout the course of therapy. The splinted hand can be used for light activities to the tolerance of the patient (see section on troubleshooting phase I). Edema and pain are managed through consistent elevation of the upper extremity above the heart through positioning (rather than a sling) when possible. Intermittent use of cold packs during the day and light retrograde massage to the dorsum of the hand, avoiding the surgical site, are helpful. Active finger motion with the upper extremity elevated prevents finger stiffness and reduces edema. Patients are instructed to actively move the uninvolved joints of the upper extremity, specifically the fingers, thumb IP joint, forearm, elbow, and shoulder. If there are limitations, specific home exercises are prescribed.

Troubleshooting

Excessive pain in this phase may be the result of overuse of the thumb for functional activities. Although light activities may be performed with the thumb spica splint in place, forceful pinch is avoided as well as any activities that increase pain. For writing, a large grip, gel ink pen is recommended to reduce the force generated across the CMC joint.

Postoperative Phase I: Inflammation/Protection (Weeks 0 to 3)

GOALS
- Protect the arthroplasty through splinting and activity modification/joint protection
- Reduce edema and pain
- Maintain full AROM of uninvolved joints

PRECAUTIONS
- No ROM of thumb MP or CMC joints
- No ROM of wrist unless specifically prescribed by MD
- No strong pinching or other resistive activities

TREATMENT STRATEGIES
- Splinting: thumb spica splint when postoperative splint is discharged by MD
- Joint protection: avoid strong pinch and any aggravating activities; use hand for light ADL to tolerance only
- Edema and pain reduction: elevation, cold modalities, retrograde massage (avoiding surgical incision until fully closed)
- ROM exercises for uninvolved joints: fingers, thumb IP joint, elbow, forearm, and shoulder

CRITERIA FOR ADVANCEMENT
- Edema and pain controlled (minimal)
- Patient cleared by MD for thumb and wrist AROM, typically at 3 to 4 weeks postoperatively, depending on MD preference; some MDs may allow wrist AROM earlier.
- Note: If a Kirschner's wire is used, phase II does not begin until its removal, at 4 weeks following LRTI arthroplasty and at 5 weeks following HDA.

POSTOPERATIVE PHASE II: FIBROPLASIA (WEEKS 4 TO 8)

In phase II, the thumb spica splint is removed for hygiene and exercises and continues to be worn at all other times. Edema control techniques from phase I are continued as needed. When the surgical incision has healed, contrast baths are added. Light compression is used, as long as it is not overly constrictive. Scar management techniques are added when the surgical incision has closed. The patient performs scar massage for several minutes daily, and a silicone pad is worn on the scar at night.

Active motion exercises of the thumb MP and CMC joints (both isolated and composite) and wrist are begun in this phase and added to the home program. Assisted motion is indicated if motion is limited. Gentle passive motion is permitted with caution, only when range of motion (ROM) is significantly limited (see section on troubleshooting phase II). Resistive exercises are contraindicated in phase II. Although light, functional use of the hand should be encouraged, forceful pinch and resistive activities are avoided. Joint protection principles are reinforced as the patient gradually resumes functional hand use.

Troubleshooting

Gentle passive range of motion (PROM) is added as needed to restore functional mobility. Thumb stability is never sacrificed to gain motion. Because it is not unusual for mild pain to persist in phase II, care is taken to limit exercise and activity to individual tolerance. Overaggressive exercise and activity increase pain and inflammation and delay the recovery process.

POSTOPERATIVE PHASE III: SCAR MATURATION (WEEKS 8 TO 12)

The goals of therapy in phase III are to restore adequate thumb and wrist motion and strength for the pain-free performance of daily activities. Joint protection principles should be well understood and used consistently. For example, the palms are used whenever possible for lifting heavy objects rather than grasping with the thumbs.

As pain resolves, use of the splint is gradually discontinued. Some individuals continue to use the splint during this phase for protection while traveling on public transportation and sleeping at night. The motion exercises of phase II are continued with the emphasis on

---

Postoperative Phase II: Fibroplasia (Weeks 4 to 8)

GOALS

- Protect arthroplasty through continued splinting and activity modification
- Reduce residual edema and pain
- Minimize scarring
- Restore stable AROM of thumb CMC and MP joints and wrist within tolerance
- Restore independence in light ADL while maintaining joint protection

PRECAUTIONS

- No resistive activities or exercises

TREATMENT STRATEGIES

- Splinting: thumb spica splint is removed for therapeutic exercises and hygiene, until discharged by surgeon
- Phase I edema treatments continue; contrast baths and light compression wrapping, avoiding overly tight application
- Scar management when incision has healed: scar massage, silicone pad
- A/AAROM of thumb MP and CMC joints and wrist; PROM to regain functional motion (see section on troubleshooting phase II)
- Light, functional activities to encourage use of hand to tolerance, avoiding forceful pinch and any aggravating activities

CRITERIA FOR ADVANCEMENT

- Minimal pain with light activities and motion exercises
- Patient cleared by MD for strengthening exercises and discharge of splint

Postoperative Phase III: Scar Maturation (Weeks 8 to 12)

GOALS

- Restore functional, pain-free ROM in thumb and wrist
- Achieve functional strength for pinch, grip, and wrist
- Restore independent activities of daily living (ADL) while maintaining joint protection

PRECAUTIONS

- Avoid pain-provoking activities and overaggressive, resistive exercises

TREATMENT STRATEGIES

- Gradual weaning from splint
- Scar management until scar is pale and flat
- Thumb and wrist ROM exercises continue, with emphasis on functional motion vs extreme end range motion.
- Light resistance for wrist and grip strengthening for return to independent ADL
- Light resistance for pinch strength for return to independent ADL

CRITERIA FOR DISCHARGE

- Independence in home program
- Understanding and use of joint protection principles
- Functional thumb and wrist ROM
- Functional hand and wrist strength
- Independence in ADL with minimal discomfort

maximizing thumb and wrist motion, without causing undue pain or stress on the thumb and wrist joints. Hand strength begins to improve as functional activities are gradually resumed. Resistance exercises for the wrist and grip are added in therapy and to the home program, as necessary, to regain a functional level of strength. Thumb strengthening exercises are added, only if necessary, for resumption of daily functional activities. It is not unusual for therapy to continue for 12 weeks or more after surgery. Recovery varies in patients. For some, occasional therapy visits for progression of the home program are all that is required. Discharge from therapy is indicated when functional motion, strength, and pain-free independent hand function have been achieved.

Troubleshooting

Returning too quickly to full use of the hand may provoke pain and delay progress. A gradual return to function, respecting pain and avoiding stress to the thumb, is advisable.

REFERENCES

1. Chaisson, C.E., Zhang, Y., McAlindon, T.E., Hannan, M.T., Aliabadi, P., Naimark, A., Levy, D., Felson, D.T. *Radiographic Hand Osteoarthritis: Incidence, Patterns, and Influence of Pre-existing Disease in a Population Based Sample.* J Rheumatol 1997;24: 1337–1343.
2. Burton, R.I., Pellegrini, V.D. *Surgical Management of Basal Joint Arthritis of the Thumb. Part II: Ligament Reconstruction with Tendon Interposition Arthroplasty.* J Hand Surg 1986;11A: 324–332.
3. Berger, R.A., Beckenbaugh, R.D., Linscheid, R.L. Arthroplasty in the Hand and Wrist. In Green, D.P., Hotchkiss, R.N., Pederson, W.C. (Eds) *Green's Operative Hand Surgery,* 4th ed. Churchill Livingstone, New York, 1999, pp. 166–168.
4. Tomaino, M.M. *Ligament Reconstruction Tendon Interposition Arthroplasty for Basal Joint Arthritis.* Hand Clin 2001;17(2): 207–221.
5. Tomaino, M.M., Pellegrini, V.D., Burton, R.I. *Arthroplasty of the Basal Joint of the Thumb.* J Bone Joint Surg 1995;77A(3):346–355.
6. Kuhns, C.A., Emerson, E.T., Meals, R.A. *Hematoma and Distraction Arthroplasty for Thumb Basal Joint Osteoarthritis: A Prospective, Single-Surgeon Study Including Outcome Measures.* J Hand Surg 2003;28A:381–389.

20

Ulnar Collateral Ligament Repair

COLEEN T. GATELY, PT, DPT, MS

The ulnar collateral ligament (UCL) is the primary valgus stabilizer of the thumb metacarpophalangeal (MP) joint. The UCL is more frequently injured than the radial collateral ligament. A 10 to 1 ratio of injury is reported in the literature.[1,2] Historically, UCL laxity was observed in gamekeepers as a result of repetitive valgus stress placed on the thumb while pinning game between the thumb and index finger, and was subsequently referred to as "gamekeeper's thumb."[3] Acute injury to the UCL results from a fall on an extended thumb forced into hyperabduction. This is a common skiing injury and is frequently referred to as "skier's thumb" (Figure 20-1). The UCL can be ruptured or avulsed at the origin, with or without a bony fragment of the proximal phalanx. Symptoms following a UCL tear include pain, swelling, and instability of the MP during pinch activities.[4-6] Many patients do not seek immediate medical attention. If left untreated, this injury can lead to long-term weakness, joint deformity (subluxation), and arthritis.[4-7]

ANATOMICAL (SURGICAL) OVERVIEW

UCL ruptures may be treated conservatively with immobilization splinting for 6 to 8 weeks in a hand-based thumb immobilization splint with the interphalangeal (IP) joint free (Figure 20-2). Surgical indications for a UCL injury include failure of conservative management, clinical joint instability, fracture or displacement, and a Stener lesion.[8-11] A Stener lesion prevents the UCL from healing without surgery because of interposition of the adductor aponeurosis between the ligament's torn edges.[11] Several surgical techniques are used to repair a UCL tear.[4,12-18] They include a simple ligament repair and tendon reconstruction. Suture anchors are used for the repair, and a Kirschner's wire is used to stabilize larger avulsion fractures. In certain cases, a temporary transarticular pin is used to control stress across the repair site. The surgical technique is based on the extent of joint involvement and the time elapsed since injury. An acute injury is often treated with a simple repair, whereas a chronic injury may require a complex procedure.

REHABILITATION OVERVIEW

The amount of surgical stability achieved will determine the rate of progression of therapeutic techniques in each

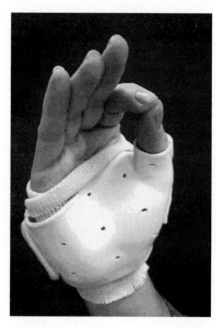

FIGURE 20-2 Short opponens splint with the IP joint free.

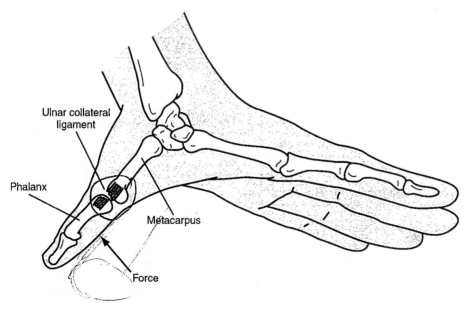

FIGURE 20-1 Acute injury to the UCL results from a fall on an extended thumb forced into hyperabduction.

phase of healing. Direct communication with the doctor is essential to determine the stability of the joint for appropriate therapeutic progression.

POSTOPERATIVE PHASE I: PROTECTION (WEEKS 0 TO 4)

While providing protective immobilization, the goals of phase I include protection of repair, wound care, minimizing edema and pain, and maintaining full range of motion (ROM) of the uninvolved joints and restoring involved thumb MP joint ROM. When the postoperative dressing is removed as early as 1 week, a custom thermoplastic hand-based thumb immobilization splint is molded with the thumb in functional opposition and the IP joint free. The thumb is positioned in a lateral pinch during the molding of the splint. This places less stress on the UCL while allowing function. The splint is modified to accommodate for protruding Kirschner's wires or transarticular pins as needed. The splint is remolded

and adjusted, as needed, to accommodate changes in edema and swelling. Standard wound care procedures are followed. Pin care varies from physician to physician. In most cases, the pins are cleaned twice daily with a solution of hydrogen peroxide and water or saline.[19] Edema control follows standard procedures and is described elsewhere in this book. Active range of motion (AROM) to the uninvolved joints—fingers, elbow, forearm and shoulder—begins immediately postoperatively. Participation in light, functional activities within the confines of the splint is encouraged. No motion is performed at the thumb MCP joint for the first 4 weeks following surgery.

Troubleshooting

During phase I, the thumb is immobilized in a hand-based thumb immobilization splint. Emphasis is placed on isolated IP ROM to prevent extensor hood and flexor pollicis longus (FPL) adhesions.[20]

Postoperative Phase I: Protection (Weeks 0 to 4)

GOALS
- Correct protective immobilization
- Edema and pain control
- Full ROM of uninvolved joints

PRECAUTIONS
- No thumb MP motion
- Valgus forces

PIN AND WOUND CARE
- Pin care regimens vary: commonly, 50% peroxide and sterile water two times per day
- Standard wound care procedures followed for ORIF

TREATMENT STRATEGIES
Protection options
- Hand-based thumb immobilization splint, IP free
  - Accommodate any pins
  - Remold to accommodate changes in edema

EDEMA/PAIN MANAGEMENT
- Elevation, rest, ice/cold
- Light, compressive garment or wrap (i.e., Coban™, compression sleeve, stockinette)

UNINVOLVED JOINTS ROM
- Tendon gliding exercises
- Thumb IP motion
- Shoulder, elbow, wrist, and forearm motion

LIGHT, FUNCTIONAL ACTIVITIES
- Restoration of normal movement patterns and light, functional activities with splint on

CRITERIA FOR ADVANCEMENT
- Determination by MD of ability of repair site to withstand stress and motion

POSTOPERATIVE PHASE II: STABILITY (WEEKS 4 TO 8)

By the fourth week the repair is strong enough to withstand stress, and motion at the MP joint begins. Goals from the previous phase continue to be addressed. The splint is weaned during the day and continued for protection during sleep and travel. Silicone gel sheeting, as described previously, can be used for scar management.[21-27]

Troubleshooting

MP joint stiffness is common with these injuries. Prolonged stretching via static progressive splinting is used to improve passive range of motion (PROM) of the MP and IP joints.[28,29] Care must continue to be taken to avoid excessive valgus stress to the thumb MP joint with splinting and other activities.

POSTOPERATIVE PHASE III: REPAIR CONSOLIDATION (WEEKS 8 TO 12)

The ability of the repair to withstand the stress of strengthening usually marks the beginning of phase III. Strengthening begins with lateral or key pinch and is gradually progressed to tip pinch.[20] The patient is cleared by the physician to return to work and/or a sport-specific activity. Although splints do not prevent re-injury, they provide protection during heavy labor and high impact sports. A "step down" transitional protective thumb MP splint is provided for use in sports (Figure 20-3). This is particularly important in athletes returning to play tennis or golf, because the racket and club place a slight stress on the repaired ligament.

Troubleshooting

A stiff thumb MP joint is common following UCL repairs. It is important to keep in mind that stiffness

---

Postoperative Phase II: Stability (Weeks 4 to 8)

GOALS
- Maximize ROM of the thumb MP and IP joints
- Restore functional use of the involved extremity
- Continue phase I goals as needed

PRECAUTIONS
- Avoid excessive PROM/stretching

TREATMENT STRATEGIES
Splinting
- Splint is weaned during the day and continued for sleep and travel.

SCAR MANAGEMENT
- Scar massage and silicone gel sheeting are initiated once the wound is fully healed (to avoid infection).

EDEMA/PAIN MANAGEMENT
- Cold pack
- Retrograde massage

TREATMENT STRATEGIES
MP joint ROM
- Thumb MP motion: flexion, abduction, and opposition
PROM and splinting
- PROM, stretching
- Serial static and static progressive splints to achieve end range potential
  ○ Examples: serial static thumb web spacer
Functional activities
- Restoration of normal movement patterns/activities of daily living (ADL)
- May require hand-based thumb immobilization splint, IP free for heavy activity

CRITERIA FOR ADVANCEMENT
- Determination by MD of ability of injury site to withstand stress

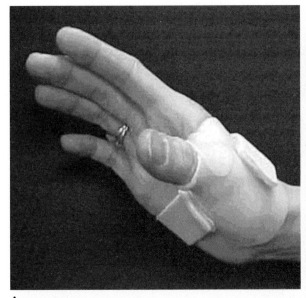

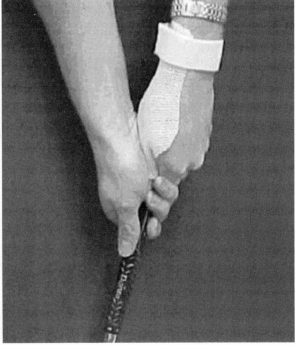

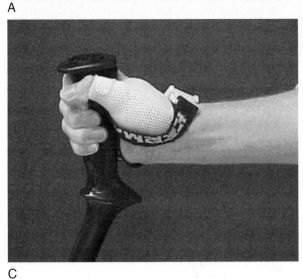

FIGURE **20-3** *A–C.* Examples of transitional protective thumb spica splints.

Postoperative Phase III: Repair Consolidation (Weeks 8 to 12)

GOALS

- Restore strength for return to functional activities and work
- Continue phase II goals as needed

PRECAUTIONS

- Progress strengthening exercises gradually, avoiding pain and compensations

STRENGTHENING

- Isometric and dynamic grip-and-pinch strengthening: putty, hand-helper, BTE PRIMUS (Baltimore Therapeutic Equipment Co., Hanover, MD), and Upper Limb Exerciser (ULE) (Biometrics LTD., UK)
- Wrist and forearm progressive resistive exercises (PREs): dumbbells, weight well, Thera-Band
- Work and sport conditioning: activity-specific activities

CRITERIA FOR DISCHARGE

- Restoration of functional AROM and strength, and return to prior ADL and work
- Independence in home exercise program

cannot be addressed at the risk of compromising stability.[30] Studies determine functional thumb ROM to be 21 degrees at the MP joint and 18 degrees at the IP joint.[31]

REFERENCES

1. Moutet, F. *Les entarse de la metacarpo-phalangienne due pouce a une experience de plus de 1000 cas.* Ann Chir Main Memb Super 1989;8:99.

2. Posner, M.A. *Metacarpophalangeal Joint Injuries of the Thumb.* Hand Clin 1992;8:713.

3. Campbell, C.S. *Gamekeeper's Thumb.* J Bone Joint Surg 1955; 37A:148.

4. Moberg, E., Stener, B. *Injuries to the Ligaments of the Thumb and Fingers.* Acta Chir Scand 1953;106:166–186.

5. Moberg, E. *Fractures and Ligamentous Injuries of the Thumb and Fingers.* Surg Clin North Am 1960;40:297–309.

6. Smith, R.J. *Post-traumatic Instability of the Metacarpophalangeal Joint of the Thumb.* J Bone Joint Surg 1977;59A:14–21.

7. Frykman, G., Johansson, O. *Surgical Repair of Rupture of the Ulnar Collateral Ligament of the Metacarpophalangeal Joint of the Thumb.* Acta Chir Scand 1956;112:58–64.

8. Bowers, W.H., Hurst, L.C. *Gamekeeper's Thumb. Evaluations by Arthrography and Stress Roentgenography.* J Bone Joint Surg 1977;59A(4):519–524.

9. Louis, D.S., Huebner, J.J., Hankin, F.M. *Rupture and Displacement of the Ulnar Collateral Ligament of the Metacarpophalangeal Joint of the Thumb. Preoperative Diagnosis.* J Bone Joint Surg 1986;6A(9):1320–1325.

10. Heyman, P., Gelberman, R.H., Duncan, K., Hipp, J.A. *Injuries of the Ulnar Collateral Ligament of the Thumb Metacarpophalangeal Joint.* Clin Orthop Relat Res 1993;292:165–171.

11. Stener, B. *Displacement of the Ruptured Ulnar Collateral Ligament of the Metacarpophalangeal Joint of the Thumb. A Clinical and Anatomical Study.* J Bone Joint Surg 1962;44B:869–879.

12. Strandell, G. *Total Rupture of the Ulnar Collateral Ligament of the Metacarpophalangeal Joint of the Thumb. Results of Surgery in 35 Cases.* Acta Chir Scand 1959;118:72–80.

13. Osterman, A.L., Hayken, G.D., Bora, W.M. *A Quantitative Evaluation of the Thumb Function after Ulnar Collateral Repair and Reconstruction.* J Trauma 1981;21:854–860.

14. Alldred, A.J. *Rupture of the Collateral Ligament of the Metacarpo-phalangeal Joint of the Thumb.* J Bone Joint Surg 1955;37B:443–445.

15. Frank, W.E., Dobyns, J.H. *Surgical Pathology of Collateral Ligamentous Injury of the Thumb.* Clin Orthop 1972;83:102–114.

16. Green, D. *Dislocations and Ligamentous Injuries of the Hand.* Churchill Livingstone, New York, 1990, pp. 385–448.

17. Kaplan, E.B. *The Pathology and Treatment of Radial Subluxation of the Thumb with Ulnar Displacement of the Head of the First Metacarpal.* J Bone Joint Surg 1961;43A:541–546.

18. Sennwald, G., Segmuller, G., Egli, A. *The Late Reconstruction of the Ligament of the Metacarpophalangeal Joint of the Thumb.* Ann Chir Main 1987;6:15–24.

19. Leibovic, S.J. *Bone and Joint Injury in the Hand: Surgeon's Perspective.* J Hand Ther 1999;12(2):111–120.

20. Campell, P.J., Wilson, R.L. Management of Joint Injuries and Intraarticular Fractures. In Mackin, E.J., Callahan, A.D., Skirven, T.M., Schneider, L.H., Osterman, A.L. (Eds). *Rehabilitation of the Hand and Upper Extremity,* 5th ed., vol. 1. Mosby, St. Louis, 2002, pp. 396–411.

21. Ahn, S.T., Monafo, W.W., Mustoe, T.A. *Topical Silicone Gel for the Prevention and Treatment of Hypertrophic Scars.* Arch Surg 1991;126:499–504.

22. Ahn, S.T., Monafo, W.W., Mustoe, T.A. *Topical Silicone Gel: A New Treatment for Hypertrophic Scars.* Surgery 1989;106: 781–787.

23. Quinn, K.J. *Silicone Gel in Scar Treatment.* Burns 1987;13: S33–S40.

24. Gibbons, M., Zuker, R., Brown, M., Candlish, S., Snider, L., Zimmer, P. *Experience with Silastic Gel Sheeting in Pediatric Scarring.* J Burn Care Rehabil 1994;15(1):69–73.

25. Carney, S.A., Cason, C.G., Gowar, J.P., Stevenson, J.H., McNee, J., Groves, A.R., Thomas, S.S., Hart, N.B., Auclair, P. *Cica-Care Gel Sheeting in the Management of Hypertrophic Scarring.* Burns 1994;20(2):163–167.

26. Sherris, D.A., Larrabee, W.F. Jr., Murakami, C.S. *Management of Scar Contractures, Hypertrophic Scars, and Keloid.* Otolaryngol Clin North Am 1995;28(5):1057–1068.

27. Tilkorn, H., Ernst, K., Osterhaus, A., Schubert, A., Schwipper, V. *The Protruding Scars: Keloids and Hypertrophic. Diagnosis and Treatment with Silicon-gel-sheeting.* Polym Med 1994; 24(1–2):31–44.

28. Lucas, S. Splinting the Stiff Wrist. In Skirven, T., Raphael, J. (Eds). *Contractures and Splinting.* WB Saunders, Philadelphia; Atlas Hand Clin 2001;6(1):77–106.

29. Schindeler-Grasse, P., Paynter, P. Splinting for Thumb Contractures. In Skirven, T., Raphael, J. (Eds). *Contractures and Splinting.* WB Saunders, Philadelphia; Atlas Hand Clin 2001;6(1):165–188.

30. Noyes, F.R., Torvik, P.J., Hyde, W.B. *Mechanics of Ligament Failure: An Analysis of Immobilization, Exercise and Reconditioning Effects in Primates.* J Bone Joint Surg 1974;56A: 1406.

31. Hume, M.C., Gellman, H., McKellop, H., Brumfield, R.H. Jr. *Functional Range of Motion of the Joints of the Hand.* J Hand Surg 1990;15A:240–243.

21

Volar Plate Arthroplasty

AVIVA WOLFF, OTR/L, CHT

Dislocations of the proximal interphalangeal (PIP) joint may be dorsal, lateral, or volar, depending on the position of the middle phalanx at the moment of joint deformation. The mechanism of injury in dorsal dislocations is usually hyperextension with longitudinal compression. In a more severe injury, rupture of the volar plate occurs proximally[1] (Figure 21-1).

ANATOMICAL OVERVIEW

Volar plate arthroplasty is a surgical technique used to treat unstable dorsal fracture dislocations of the PIP with disruption of the volar plate complex, the collateral ligaments, and greater than 40% of the volar articular surface of the middle phalanx. Because this is a complex injury that requires postoperative protection, it is often difficult to achieve adequate PIP range of motion (ROM). It is essential that postoperative management by the hand therapist begins in the early phases of wound healing. To avoid complications, such as contraction of the scarred volar plate and flexor tendons, protected motion must be initiated as early as possible.[2] The PIP joint is particularly prone to adhesions and contractures because multiple structures cross the joint. The structures include collateral ligaments, volar plate, central slip, lateral bands, transverse retinacular ligaments, oblique retinacular ligament, and flexor tendons. Even loose adhesions have been found to significantly limit motion.[3] Complications of volar plate arthroplasty include redisplacement, angulation, flexion contracture, distal interphalangeal (DIP) joint stiffness, oblique retinacular ligament (ORL) tightness, and flexor and extensor tendon adherence.

SURGICAL OVERVIEW

Surgical exposure is through a volar incision on the PIP joint surface. The flexor sheath is excised between the A2 and A4 pulleys and the tendons are retracted. The PIP joint is hyperextended, and the collateral ligaments are excised. Large fragments are reduced by K-wires, and loose bone fragments are debrided. The volar plate is mobilized to advance 4 to 6mm into the middle phalanx defect.

The plate is advanced by means of a pullout wire along the lateral margins of the volar plate and then exits the dorsal middle phalanx through the triangular ligament of the extensor mechanism. The pullout suture is then tied over a button. The lateral margins of the volar plate are sutured to the adjacent collateral ligament remnants. A longitudinal K-wire (Figure 21-2) or PIP compass hinge may be used to maintain the reduced joint in 30-degree flexion in severely unstable fractures (see chapter on PIP compass hinge).[1]

REHABILITATION OVERVIEW

POSTOPERATIVE PHASE I: INFLAMMATION/PROTECTION (WEEKS 0 TO 3)

The first priority of treatment is to decrease edema. In 1992, Agee[4] described edema as the number one culprit in causing adhesions. The patient is instructed to ice and elevate the hand repeatedly during the first postoperative week and referred for a dorsal protective splint 3 to 10 days post-surgery. The metacarpophalangeal (MP) is left free, and the PIP is blocked in 10- to 40-degree flexion, as determined by the surgeon (Figure 21-3). The DIP is splinted at 0 degrees. If indicated, a hand-based splint for extra stability is fabricated with the MP splinted in full flexion (Figure 21-4). Active DIP flexion exercises are begun immediately in the splint to encourage lateral band and flexor digitorum profundus (FDP) gliding. Active MP flexion and ROM of all uninvolved joints are encouraged to avoid stiffness. In most cases, a K-wire is used to maintain the reduced joint in 30- to 40-degree flexion. The K-wire is generally removed at 3 weeks, and PIP joint flexion exercises commence.

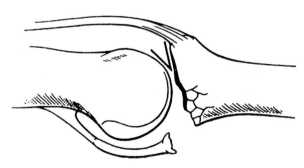

FIGURE 21-1 Dorsal dislocation with volar plate avulsion. *(From Kang, R., Stern, P. Fracture Dislocations of the Proximal Interphalangeal Joint. J Am Soc Surg Hand 2002;2[2].)*

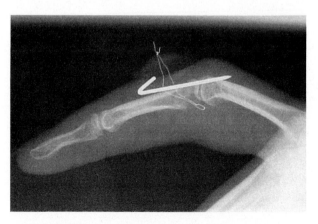

FIGURE 21-2 VPA: joint reduced in 30-degree flexion.

Postoperative Phase I: Inflammation/Protection (Weeks 0 to 3)

GOALS

- Provide correct splinting to maintain stability and protect repaired structures
- Control inflammation and reduce edema
- Maintain stability and protect repaired structures
- Maintain ROM in uninvolved joints
- Begin gentle protective active motion within the confines of the splint

PRECAUTIONS

- No active or passive PIP extension beyond prescribed position

TREATMENT STRATEGIES

Protective Immobilization

- Dorsal block splint in 35- to 40-degree PIP flexion

Edema Control

- Standard principles of edema control
- Gentle compressive wraps, such as Coban
- Avoid compression garments (such as Isotoner gloves) that place the digit in too much extension during donning

Protect Repaired Structures

- PIP joint not to be extended beyond prescribed limit
- Splint is not to be removed at home.

ROM Exercises of Uninvolved Joints

- Active DIP flexion exercises
- Active MP flexion and ROM of all uninvolved joints

Early Protective Mobilization

- Active PIP flexion when the K-wire is removed (3 weeks), or at 1 week (no K-wire)
- Gentle active composite flexion
- Active extension to the limit of the splint
- Active FDP and FDS glides

CRITERIA FOR ADVANCEMENT

- Removal of K-wire
- Joint stability determined by surgeon

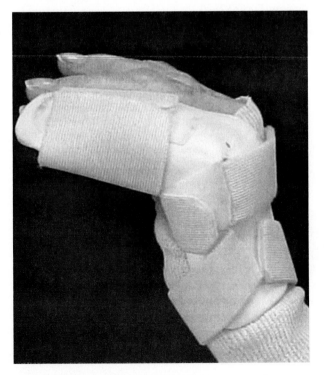

FIGURE **21-3** Dorsal block splint; PIP joint at 30 degrees.

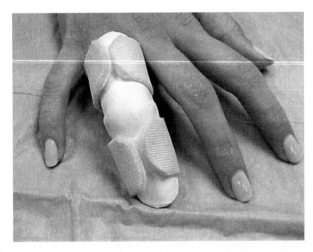

FIGURE **21-4** Hand-based protective splint.

Troubleshooting

Care must be taken to properly secure the proximal phalanx in the dorsal block splint to avoid loss of PIP extension[5] (Figure 21-5). Even for the experienced therapist, it is a challenge to obtain the proper joint position of the dorsal block splint. To obtain the desired position of flexion when molding the dorsal block splint it is best to position the joint in greater flexion (10 to 15 degrees) than desired.

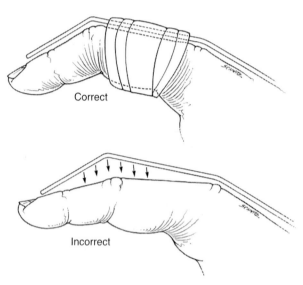

FIGURE **21-5** Care must be taken to properly secure the proximal phalanx in the dorsal block splint to avoid loss of PIP extension. *(From Kang, R., Stern, P. Fracture Dislocations of the Proximal Interphalangeal Joint. J Am Soc Surg Hand 2002;2[2].)*

POSTOPERATIVE PHASE II: FIBROPLASIA/EARLY REMODELING (WEEKS 3 TO 6)

Once the K-wire is removed (usually at 3 weeks), active and passive PIP flexion may commence. There are no limitations to joint flexion once the K-wire is removed. The importance of achieving maximum flexion as soon as possible cannot be overemphasized. Immobilization of 3 weeks or more has been found to cause permanent joint stiffness in the PIP joint.[6] Both active and passive flexion exercises are performed within the confines of the dorsal block splint four to five times daily. Isolated flexor digitorum superficialis (FDS) and FDP glides are added to the home program to prevent adhesion formation. The dorsal block splint is remolded to gradually increase PIP extension at the rate of 5 degrees per week under guidance of the surgeon. The dorsal button is usually removed at 5 or 6 weeks postoperatively. At this point, full PIP extension is permitted, and active PIP extension exercises begin. The MP is blocked in flexion to isolate PIP extension (Figure 21-6). Extensor digitorum communis (EDC) gliding exercises are performed to prevent adhesions of the extrinsic extensors. Treatment strategies are further listed in the following box.

Troubleshooting

Both flexor and extensor adhesions are common with PIP joint injuries. To encourage tendon glide, blocking exercises are performed. If gains in motion remain minimal, blocking splints are fabricated to encourage motion. An MP extension block splint described by Oyama,[7] in 1999, is effective in preventing MP hyperextension (Figure 21-7).

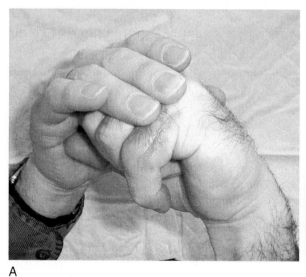

A

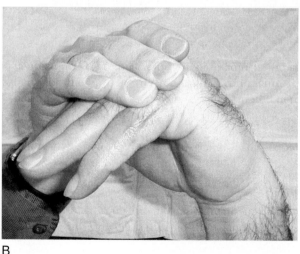

B

FIGURE **21-6** Isolated PIP extension. *A.* PIP is flexed. *B.* PIP is flexed with MP extended.

Postoperative Phase II: Fibroplasia/Early Remodeling (Weeks 3 to 6)

GOALS

- Achieve maximum PIP flexion
- Begin to progress PIP extension
- Encourage scar remodeling
- Encourage functional and protected use of hand

PRECAUTIONS

- No active or passive PIP extension beyond prescribed limits

TREATMENT STRATEGIES

PIP Flexion Exercises

- Gentle passive stretch into flexion at 3 to 4 weeks post-surgery
- Gentle hook and composite fisting

PIP Extension

- Progression of dorsal block splint into extension
- Active PIP extension following button removal
- The dorsal splint is worn between exercises and at night up to 6 weeks.

Scar Remodeling

- Begin gentle scar massage
- Use Otoform mold or silicone gel with Coban for night use
- Massage over the dorsal hood and lateral bands at 3 weeks

CRITERIA FOR ADVANCEMENT

- Removal of dorsal button
- Clinical union at fracture site
- Joint stability determined by surgeon

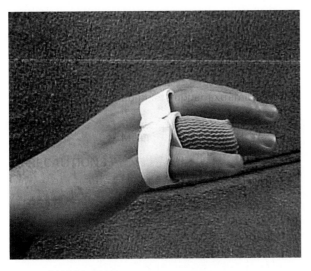

FIGURE **21-7** MP extension blocking splint.

POSTOPERATIVE PHASE III: SCAR MATURATION (WEEKS 6 TO 12)

By 6 weeks the joint is stable enough to withstand stronger motion. Depending on the stiffness of the joint, the therapist may use various techniques to gain motion.

Troubleshooting

If motion is not improving through passive stretching and joint mobilization, static progressive or serial static splinting is considered. Static progressive PIP flexion splinting is applied for a minimum of 15- to 20-minute intervals five to seven times daily. For an extension contracture of less than 30 degrees, a serial static finger gutter splint is applied at night; in addition, a dynamic extension splint (such as LMB) is used intermittently during the day. For a contracture of greater than 30 degrees, a static progressive extension splint or serial casting is the treatment of choice. The choice for serial casting must be carefully considered so as not to compromise PIP flexion.

Postoperative Phase III: Scar Maturation (Weeks 6 to 12)

GOALS
- To achieve full ROM (active and passive) at the PIP and DIP joints
- To prevent a PIP extension lag
- To prevent a PIP flexion contracture

TREATMENT PLAN
Achieve Maximum Range of Motion
- Splint to be discharged (6 to 8 weeks)
- Intensive ROM and blocking exercises initiated
- Blocking splints
- Joint mobilization in both directions with MD authorization
- Static progressive flexion splinting for end range flexion (6 to 8 weeks)
- NMES to encourage flexor tendon pull-through

Prevent PIP Extension Lag
- Finger gutter extension splint for night to prevent joint contracture
- Intrinsic exercises and progressive strengthening to the extensor mechanism
- Resistive exercises to decrease extensor mechanism adherence and cross adhesions of the FDS/FDP at Camper's chiasm

Prevent and Treat PIP Flexion Contractures
- Ultrasound to the PIP joint, followed by vigorous massage, exercise, and splinting
- Extension splinting/serial casting to the PIP

CRITERIA FOR DISCHARGE
- Maximum PIP flexion and extension
- Functional grip strength
- Return to premorbid level of function

REFERENCES

1. Glickel, S.Z., Baron, O.A., Eaton, R. Dislocations and Injuries in the Digits. In Green, D.P. (Ed). *Operative Hand Surgery*, 4th ed., vol. 1. Churchill Livingstone, Philadelphia, 1999, pp. 772–800.
2. Kiefhaber, T.R., Stern, P. *Fracture Dislocations of the Proximal Interphalangeal Joint.* J Hand Surg 1998;23A:368–380.
3. Lanz, U., H.P. Tendon Adhesions. In G.A. Bruser, P. (Eds). *Finger, Bone and Joint Injuries.* Dunitz, UK, 1999.
4. Agee, J. *Treatment Principles for Proximal and Middle Phalanx Fractures.* Orthop Clin North Am 1992;23(1):35–40.
5. Kang, R., Stern, P. *Fracture Dislocations of the Proximal Interphalangeal Joint.* J Am Soc Surg Hand 2002;2(2):.
6. Phair, I.C., Quinton, D.N., Allen, M.J. *The Conservative Management of Volar Avulsion Fractures of the PIP Joint.* J Hand Surg 1989;14B:168–170.
7. Oyama, M., Kino, Y., Machida, M., Onishi, M., Yamamoto, S. *Postoperative Management of the Dorsal Fracture-Dislocation of the Proximal Interphalangeal Joint.* Tech Hand Up Extrem Surg 1999;3(1):66–73.

22

Proximal Interphalangeal (PIP) Joint Replacement

EMILY ALTMAN, PT, CHT

The proximal interphalangeal (PIP) joint can be affected by posttraumatic arthritis and osteoarthritis.[1] Impairments typically include pain, weakness, joint stiffness, and deformity.[1] Even though patients often present with only one affected digit, the impact on the function of the entire hand is significantly impacted secondary to the quadriga effect. Because the four tendons of the flexor digitorum profundus (FDP) share a common muscle belly, a surgical procedure results in limited proximal tendon excursion (in this case, because of limited PIP flexion range of motion [ROM]).[1] When the ulnar digits are involved, grip is impaired. When the index is involved, pinch strength and dexterity are affected.[2] Surgical options for this condition include joint fusion, joint replacement (arthroplasty), and amputation.[1-3] Joint replacement is the only option that preserves joint motion. To date, options for joint replacement include fibrous interposition, volar plate advancement, metallic or metalloplastic hinges, or one-piece polymeric plastic hinge devices.[1] Surgical placement of early prostheses requires extensive resection of the joint, including the collateral ligaments.[1] This compromises the postoperative stability of the PIP joint. At the Hospital for Special Surgery (HSS), the Avanta PIP finger prosthesis (Avanta Orthopaedics, San Diego) is the option most often used. It is a *semiconstrained* prosthesis that more closely mimics the anatomy and kinematics of the PIP joint than other, earlier prostheses. The proximal phalanx component is a metallic cobalt chromium (CoCr) alloy, and the middle phalanx component is titanium with an ultra high molecular weight polyethylene surface.[1] Minimal bony excision is required for placement of the Avanta prosthesis, permitting preservation of the collateral ligaments and enhanced joint stability.

ANATOMICAL (SURGICAL) OVERVIEW

The Avanta prosthesis replaces the articular surfaces of the head of the proximal phalanx and the base of the middle phalanx. The surgery can be done via a dorsal, lateral, or volar approach.[1] The dorsal approach is preferred because there is better exposure of the joint and easier placement of the prosthesis.[1] Flexor tendon adherence can be a complication of the volar approach. With the dorsal approach, the author recommends that the central slip *not* be dissected from its insertion on the middle phalanx. Instead, the central slip is isolated proximal to the dorsal rim of the middle phalanx for 1 to 2 cm (via parallel incisions on either side of the central slip) then cut transversely and reflected distally, exposing the PIP joint.[1] This technique permits a larger (and therefore stronger) area of repair of the central slip/extensor apparatus once the prosthesis has been placed. The distal end of the proximal phalanx and the proximal end of the middle phalanx are excised, and the implant is fitted and placed. The extensor apparatus is repaired with multiple fine sutures, the skin is closed, and the finger is immobilized in full extension.

If a volar approach is used, the flexor tendons are released and retracted, and the volar plate is released to obtain access to the volar aspect of the PIP joint.[1] The distal end of the proximal phalanx and the proximal end of the middle phalanx are excised, and the implant is fitted and placed. The volar plate and the tendon sheath complex (annular pulleys) are repaired.[1] Immediately postoperatively the finger is immobilized in 15- to 20-degree PIP flexion for 1 to 3 days to protect the repaired volar plate.

REHABILITATION OVERVIEW

The goal of rehabilitation following PIP joint arthroplasty is to regain a pain-free functional arc of PIP joint motion. With both dorsal and volar approaches, certain structures must be protected following surgery. Appropriate postoperative splinting is essential. Once the protection phase is over, gradually regaining ROM of the joint is the goal of therapy. Strengthening is not a priority.

POSTOPERATIVE PHASE I (DAYS 1 TO 14)

The initial phase of postoperative rehabilitation focuses on patient education, protective splinting, wound care, edema control, and instruction in a home exercise program. The first therapy visit is generally around postoperative days 4 to 7, when the postoperative dressing is removed.

Patient Education

The patient is instructed in standard wound care, and the splinting regimen is explained.

Splinting

Two splints are fabricated at the first follow-up visit, when the postoperative dressing is removed. A forearm-based, dynamic PIP extension outrigger splint is used during the day (Figures 22-1 and 22-2). For a dorsal surgical approach, the splint extends far enough over the PIP joint to prevent hyperextension of the prosthesis. If a volar approach is used, the splint is designed to block PIP extension at 20-degree flexion. Blocks (small beads of thermoplastic) are placed on the lines of the outrigger to limit active range of motion (AROM) into PIP flexion to 30 degrees for the dorsal approach and 40 degrees for the volar approach (Figure 22-3).

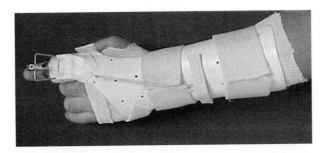

FIGURE **22-1** Dorsal view of a postoperative dynamic PIP extension splint.

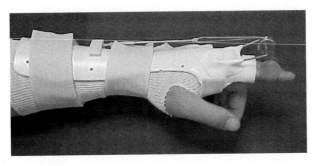

FIGURE **22-2** Lateral view of a postoperative dynamic PIP extension splint.

The dynamic component is used as an extensor assist, not for an aggressive, passive stretch. A finger gutter splint is fabricated for use at night. For a dorsal approach, the PIP joint is splinted in full extension; for a volar approach, the PIP joint is splinted in 20-degree flexion.

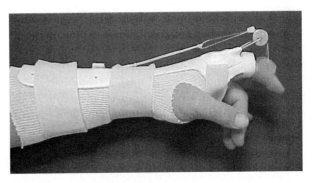

FIGURE **22-3** Thermoplastic bead on outrigger line used to limit AROM of PIP joint flexion.

Edema Control

Standard edema control techniques are used, including elevation, light Coban wrapping, and cryotherapy.

Therapeutic Exercise

AROM is initiated at the first therapy visit. Early controlled motion facilitates collagen remodeling during the encapsulation process, which results in a stable joint.[4] The exercise program includes (1) AROM of the uninvolved joints; (2) AROM of the distal interphalangeal (DIP) of the involved digit (DIP blocking), which promotes distal glide of the dorsal apparatus and lateral band excursion[3]; and (3) AROM of the involved PIP joint (PIP blocking). The PIP joint AROM is performed in the dynamic outrigger splint. The uninvolved hand is used

---

Postoperative Phase I (Days 1 to 14)

GOALS
- Edema reduction
- Patient education
  - Wound care
  - Signs of infection
- Independence in home exercise program
- Independence in splint regimen

PRECAUTIONS
- No hyperextension force at the PIP joint
- Passive range of motion (PROM) of the PIP joint is contraindicated
- No strengthening

TREATMENT STRATEGIES
- Splint fabrication-static and dynamic splints
- Instruction in specific home exercise program
- Instruction in precautions
- Instruction in edema reduction techniques

CRITERIA FOR ADVANCEMENT
- Wound closure
- PIP joint stability (determined by surgeon)

to hold the metacarpophalangeal (MP) joints of II–V at 0-degree flexion. For a dorsal approach, flexion is limited to 30 degrees; for a volar approach, flexion is limited to 40 degrees. The flexion blocks on the lines of the dynamic outrigger will prevent motion beyond these limits. Flexion is limited to protect the dorsal apparatus. *Returning to full extension (or 20 degrees for volar approach) between each repetition is important.* The amount of flexion should be gradually increased over the first 6 weeks postoperatively to a target of 70 to 80 degrees, and three sets of 10 repetitions are performed four to six times per day.

If an extension lag is noted and appears to increase after the dynamic splinting regimen is initiated, use of the dynamic splint is temporarily discontinued, and static splinting in full extension is resumed for an additional 2 to 4 weeks.[1] This helps the central slip heal at the correct length and recover its function.[1] The static splint is removed four to six times per day for performance of exercises, as described previously. A dynamic splint (or manual assist) is used to assist PIP joint extension.

Wound Care

Standard surgical wound care and dressing techniques are used.

Troubleshooting

Poor progression of PIP joint AROM can be an issue in phase I as a result of persistent edema, which must be addressed. Pain also inhibits the progression of AROM.

Cryotherapy, more frequent exercise sessions with fewer repetitions, and the use of a volar template splint to serve as a goal for flexion exercises are possible strategies for these problems. The inability to maintain full active PIP extension must be addressed with a period of static PIP extension splinting. Extensor lags at the PIP joint are unacceptable.

POSTOPERATIVE PHASE II (WEEKS 2 TO 6)

Phase II of postoperative rehabilitation includes the continuation of dynamic extension splinting until postoperative weeks 3 to 4,[3] the gradual progression of the PIP joint's arc of AROM, the continuation of night extension splinting, and the initiation of scar management.

Scar Management

Mechanical massage (small circular movements) to the incision line is started when the incision is fully closed. Use of the preferred form of silicone gel sheeting is initiated as well. Many over-the-counter products are now available.

Splinting

Use of a dynamic PIP extension splint is continued until postoperative weeks 3 to 4, and use of the night static PIP extension splint is continued until postoperative week 6. The 20-degree extension block required for the volar approach can be discontinued at postoperative weeks 2 to 3, with the surgeon's approval.

Postoperative Phase II (Weeks 2 to 6)

GOALS
- Independence in scar management
- AROM PIP joint 0 to 70 degrees

PRECAUTIONS
- No PROM of PIP joint
- No strengthening
- Careful monitoring for PIP joint extension lag
- Prevent scar adherence to dorsal apparatus

TREATMENT STRATEGIES
- Precise progression of PIP AROM
- Template exercise splinting for PIP AROM
- Scar mobilization

CRITERIA FOR ADVANCEMENT
- Acceptable arc of motion at PIP joint

Therapeutic Exercise

The exercise program continues to focus on regaining AROM of the involved PIP joint and maintaining AROM of the uninvolved joints. Beginning treatments with moist heat can be very effective. The splint is removed for exercises. Over the course of phase II, the manual assist for extension of the involved PIP joint during exercises is gradually reduced. The involved PIP joint flexion arc of AROM is gradually progressed to a target of 70 to 80 degrees by postoperative week 6. Extension exercises for the involved PIP joint are critical for regaining effective central slip function and preventing adhesions. Other AROM exercises include PIP and DIP blocking exercises, tendon gliding exercises, and extensor digitorum communis (EDC) gliding exercises.

Troubleshooting

Close monitoring for PIP extension lag continues to be a priority in this phase. Using static extension splints and emphasizing PIP extension exercises, including repeated PIP extension with the MP joints held in flexion, are effective in treating extension lags. The occurrence of extensor adhesions (dorsal approach) is reduced by the early initiation of AROM exercises.[2] Flexor tendon adhesions (volar approach) can occur. Proper scar management and mobilization, and differential tendon gliding exercises, will prevent adherence of the scar to the tendon sheath below as well as adhesions between the repaired tendon sheath and structures below.

POSTOPERATIVE PHASE III (WEEKS 6 TO 14)

Postoperative phase III focuses on regaining functional use of the involved hand and upper extremity. The daily performance of digit ROM should be gradually replaced with increased use of the hand for activities of daily living (ADL).

Scar Management

Scar management techniques initiated in phase II are continued. Scar mobilization and AROM exercises prevent scar adherence to the dorsal apparatus.

Splinting

All splinting is discontinued by postoperative week 6, unless specific extension deficit issues need to be addressed.

Therapeutic Exercises

The AROM exercise program of phase II is continued. Strengthening is not recommended following PIP joint replacement. The increased use of the hand for ADL is encouraged.

Troubleshooting

Severely limited PIP joint ROM can occur. Even though PROM of the joint is not recommended, if cleared by the surgeon, very gentle, low-load static progressive splinting can be used at postoperative weeks 8 to 10. A flexion glove is a good option. Care must be taken to avoid gaining PIP joint flexion at the expense of losing extension.

Postoperative Phase III (Weeks 6 to 14)

GOALS
- To regain full functional use of hand for grasping, holding, lifting, and manipulating objects
- Greater than 1/10 pain

PRECAUTIONS
- No strengthening
- No aggressive PROM of PIP joint

TREATMENT STRATEGIES
- Replace tendon gliding and AROM exercises with functional activities

CRITERIA FOR DISCHARGE
- Able to perform ADL without assistance

REFERENCES

1. *Proximal Interphalangeal (PIP) Finger Prosthesis—Surgical Technique.* Available online at http://www.avanta.org.
2. Kobayashi. K.Y., Terrono, A. *Proximal Interphalangeal Joint Arthroplasty of the Hand.* J Am Soc Surg Hand 2003;3(4):219–226.
3. Sauerbier, M., Cooney, W.P., Linscheid, R.L. *Operative Technique of Surface Replacement Arthroplasty of the Proximal Interphalangeal Joint.* Tech Hand Up Extrem Surg 2001;5(3):141–147.
4. Kirkpatrick, W.H., Kozin, S.H., Uhl, R. *Early Motion after Arthroplasty.* Hand Clin 1996;12(1):73–86.
5. Berger, R.A., Beckenbaugh, R.D., Linscheid, R.L. Arthroplasty in the Hand and Wrist. In Green, D.P., Hotchkiss, R.N., Pederson, W.C. (Eds). *Green's Operative Hand Surgery,* 4th ed. Churchill Livingstone, New York, 1999, pp. 147–191.
6. Uchiyama, S., Cooney, W.P., Linscheid, R.L., Neibur, G. *Kinematics of the Proximal Interphalangeal Joint of the Finger after Surface Replacement.* J Hand Surg 2000;25A:305–312.

23

Dynamic External Fixation of the Proximal Interphalangeal (PIP) Joint

EMILY ALTMAN, PT, CHT

Injury to the proximal interphalangeal (PIP) joint is frequently the result of a fall or participation in sports.[1] Many injuries are managed with closed reduction, open reduction and internal fixation (ORIF), or splinting. However, complex, unstable fracture dislocations are very difficult to successfully treat. Poor results include severely limited joint range of motion (ROM), chronic joint pain, posttraumatic arthritis, and chronic joint instability. ROM impairments affect the patient's ability to grasp objects. Severe PIP joint flexion contractures make it very difficult to open the hand enough to get around objects, don a glove, slip a hand in a garment pocket, or shake another person's hand. Use of the Compass PIP joint hinge (Smith & Nephew, Orthopedic Division, Memphis, TN) can be an effective way to treat complex PIP joint injuries. The Compass PIP joint hinge (hereafter referred to as "hinge") is an external fixation device composed of a unilateral external hinge that attaches with skeletal fixation to either side of the joint[1] (Figures 23-1 and 23-2). The design permits controlled passive motion of the joint when the gear is engaged and protected active motion when the gear is not engaged. Indications for use of the hinge include acute fracture dislocations with comminution, volar plate arthroplasty, contracture release of the PIP joint, and chronic boutonniere reconstruction.[1]

ANATOMICAL (SURGICAL) OVERVIEW

The PIP joint is a ginglymus, or hinge joint, whose instant center of rotation moves only slightly as the joint moves through its arc of motion.[1] This kinematic fact permits the use of this hinged external fixator whose axis of rotation is fixed. For the hinge to work effectively, its axis of rotation must be aligned *perfectly* with the joint's axis of rotation.

The hinge is attached to the skeleton by two pins in the proximal phalanx and two pins in the middle phalanx. Exactly four pins are necessary to handle the mechanical requirements of maintaining joint stability (two pins), applying distraction, if needed (one pin), and controlling joint rotation (one pin). Distraction creates tension in the ligaments and capsule, which maintains reduction (the principle of ligamentotaxis).[2]

The hinge is often used in conjunction with other surgical procedures, such as volar plate arthroplasty, internal fracture fixation, extensor tendon reconstruction, or tenolysis. The hinge is usually removed after 5 to 6 weeks.[3] It can be removed as early as 3 weeks, depending on the specifics of the injury and surgery.

REHABILITATION OVERVIEW

Because the hinge can be used in the surgical management of several different diagnoses (e.g., fracture dislocations, volar plate arthroplasties, contracture releases), postoperative rehabilitation guidelines will vary widely. Variables include the duration of immediate postoperative immobilization, the preferred resting position for the hinge, the rate of progression of ROM, the initiation of active range of motion (AROM), and specific precautions. The therapist *must* communicate with the surgeon and obtain the details of the original injury and the operative procedure and confirm an appropriate plan of care.

POSTOPERATIVE PHASE I (DAYS 1 TO 14)

The initial phase of postoperative rehabilitation focuses on patient education, protective splinting, wound and pin care, edema control, initiation of passive range of motion (PROM) program for the PIP joint (using the hinge's worm gear), and AROM/PROM for the uninvolved joints of the hand, paying particular attention to the distal interphalangeal (DIP) and metacarpophalangeal (MP) of the involved digit. The first therapy visit is on postoperative days 5 to 7, when the postoperative dressing is removed. Starting movement after the initial

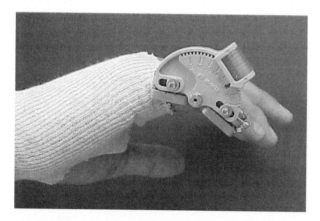

FIGURE 23-1 Compass PIP joint hinge on fifth digit. Note pen mark used as visual cue for ROM limit.

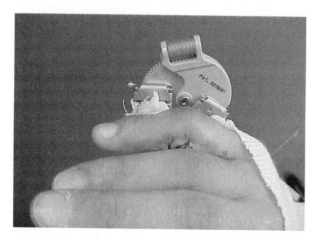

FIGURE 23-2 Compass PIP joint hinge on fifth digit. Note worm gear mechanism.

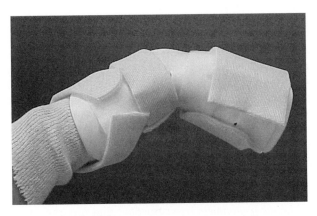

FIGURE **23-3** Protective thermoplastic splint.

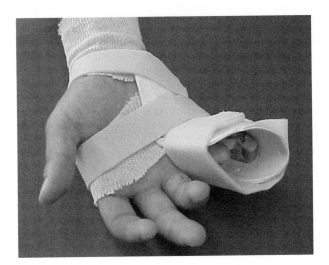

FIGURE **23-4** Protective thermoplastic splint.

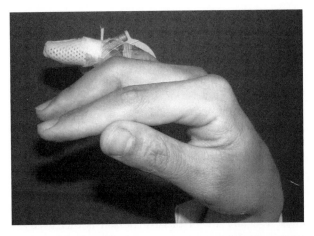

FIGURE **23-5** Mallet-type splint for PIP joint.

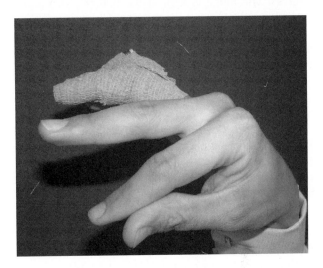

FIGURE **23-6** Coban wrap for edema management.

stage of the acute inflammation reduces the incidence of infection.[2]

Splinting

A hand-based protective splint that positions the involved digit in the intrinsic plus position is fabricated (Figures 23-3 and 23-4). This position prevents the MP joint from posturing in MP hyperextension and protects the hinge. The splint is worn outside the home and at night. If necessary, a simple static DIP extension splint (mallet-type splint) is fabricated (Figure 23-5). It is used to prevent prolonged posturing in DIP flexion and isolate flexor digitorum superficialis (FDS) function during PIP blocking exercises.

Standard edema control protocols are followed. Coban wrapping (3M Health Care, St. Paul, MN) is performed carefully to accommodate the pins (Figure 23-6).

AROM Uninvolved Joints

Both the flexor and extensor mechanisms lie very close to the PIP joint and are at risk for developing adhesions.[4] Active MP flexion/extension ("duck fist") and DIP

blocking exercises for the involved digit are started on the first therapy visit. These exercises help glide the lateral bands, minimizing scarring and adherence.[4] Gentle PROM of the MP and DIP joints is permitted if indicated. Active abduction/adduction of the MP joints of II–V helps glide the intrinsic muscles.

Wound and Pin Care

The surgeon's preference varies somewhat, but pins are commonly cleaned once per day, using a cotton swab and a solution of 50% hydrogen peroxide and 50% sterile water or saline solution. The incision is dressed as with any other surgical wound.

Hinge Protocol

Fracture Dislocation. For the first 2 to 3 weeks postoperatively, only PROM is performed, using the hinge's gear system. Salter[5] demonstrated that cartilage heals better with passive motion than immobilization. Cartilage needs nutrition and motion for repair. Four times daily, the hinge is passively cranked to 30-degree flexion and then returned to maximum extension, which is usually either 0 degrees (no protection necessary) or 15 degrees (protection necessary to preserve stability). The surgeon sets the range limitations. This is repeated 10 times. The hinge is again passively cranked to 30 degrees, and this position is maintained for 15 to 30 minutes, providing a sustained, end range stretch. During this time, the patient gently, isometrically flexes the PIP joint, holding for a count of 10. The contraction is repeated 10 times. The hinge is returned to the patient's maximum extension. In this position, the patient gently, isometrically extends the PIP joint, holding for a count of 10. The contraction is repeated 10 times. The amount of passive flexion is increased by about 5 to 10 degrees per week from the initial 30 degrees. The hinge is kept at the patient's maximum extension when not exercising.

Volar Plate Arthroplasty. The PROM program is performed as described previously (for fracture dislocation), but full extension is contraindicated for 4 weeks[2] to protect the volar plate arthroplasty (see chapter on volar plate arthroplasty). The extension block is set at 15 to 20 degrees.[2]

Flexion Contracture Release. *Capsular release:* The PROM program is performed as described previously (for fracture dislocation). However, because acute fractures and surgical repairs of bone and soft tissue are not involved, the weekly increase in flexion ROM is greater (10 degrees per week), and PIP AROM (unlocking hinge gear) is initiated at the first therapy visit. Details of AROM program are described later in phase II. If the preoperative PIP flexion contracture were long-standing, the neurovascular bundle may not be able to tolerate extended periods of time in full extension between exercise sessions.[6] The patient should be taught to monitor the digit for ischemia and sensory changes.

Tenolysis: The program used for capsular release is also used for tenolysis. However, details of tendon tissue quality should be obtained from the surgeon. PROM and AROM may need to be adjusted to protect the extensor or flexor tendons.

Chronic boutonniere reconstruction: The program used for capsular release is also used for chronic boutonniere reconstruction. Keeping the hinge at 0-degree extension between exercises is important. If weekly gains in flexion are difficult to achieve, more frequent sustained, end range flexion stretches are recommended. The patient passively locks the hinge at end range flexion and maintains that position for 30 minutes.

Troubleshooting

Difficulty meeting the goals of weekly increases in PIP flexion PROM is common. Addressing edema is critical for maximizing ROM. More frequent bouts of sustained, passive end range positioning may be helpful. Some cases respond well to increasing the frequency of the passive home program from 4 to 8 times a day and reducing the repetitions from 10 to 5.

Postoperative Phase I (Days 1 to 14)

GOALS
- Effective edema reduction
- Thorough patient education
  - Hinge use
  - Signs of infection
  - Pin and wound care
- Independence in HEP targeting uninvolved joints
- Independence in appropriate hinge program for PROM of PIP joint

PRECAUTIONS
- Close monitoring for pin tract infection
- Close monitoring for pin loosening

TREATMENT STRATEGIES
- Instruction in very specific HEP
- Cryotherapy instruction
- Instruction in edema reduction techniques
- Marks on hinge itself (with permanent ink marker) to monitor progress and/or delineate boundaries of "safe" PIP ROM

CRITERIA FOR ADVANCEMENT
- Wound closure
- Suture removal
- Independence in hinge management, independence in HEP
- Bone and soft tissue able to tolerate initiation of PIP AROM

POSTOPERATIVE PHASE II (WEEKS 2 TO 6)

Phase II of postoperative rehabilitation includes the continuation of the PIP joint PROM program, continuation of the splinting program, continuation of the AROM/PROM program for uninvolved joints, initiation of scar management, and initiation of the PIP joint AROM program (unlocking the hinge).

Scar Management

Mechanical massage (small circular movements) to the incision line is started when the incision is fully closed. Use of a preferred form of silicone gel sheeting is initiated as well. Many over-the-counter products are now available.

Hinge Protocol

Fracture Dislocation. At postoperative weeks 2 to 3, AROM of the PIP joint is initiated.[3] The worm gear is disengaged by pulling the cylindrical barrel outward. An audible click is heard when the gear fully disengages. The following AROM exercises are performed 4 times per day, 10 repetitions each[7]:

1. The patient flexes and extends the PIP joint while holding the MP joint in flexion. This position of the MP joint tensions the dorsal apparatus via the extensor digitorum communis (EDC) tendon, thus assisting PIP extension.
2. The patient flexes and extends the PIP joint while holding the MP joint in full extension (*not* hyperextension). This position of the MP joint emphasizes the contribution of the intrinsics to PIP joint extension via their insertion on the lateral bands on the dorsal apparatus.

3. The patient flexes digits II–V into a composite fist, paying particular attention to emphasizing the normal cascade of digit flexion: MP extension is maintained as the DIP joints initiate digit flexion and digits II–V move into a hook fist. MP flexion is then permitted and the digits are rolled into a composite fist. From the composite fist position, the digits return to the hook fist and then to full digit extension.

Volar Plate Arthroplasty. The previously described AROM program is initiated. The extension block is continued until postoperative week 4.

Flexion Contracture Release. Capsular release, tenolysis, and chronic boutonniere reconstruction: The previously described AROM program is initiated at the first therapy visit.

Troubleshooting

Difficulty meeting the goals of weekly increases in PIP flexion PROM/AROM continues to be an issue in phase II. Recommendations made in "Troubleshooting Phase I" can still be effective.

Posturing in MP hyperextension to compensate for loss of PIP extension is common. Hyperextension at the MP joint decreases the mechanical advantage of the EDC by putting it on slack and thereby limiting its ability to tension of the dorsal apparatus. This can contribute to the development of an extension lag at the PIP joint. Cues to avoid MP joint hyperextension during the performance of exercises are given to the patient.

Loss of extension at the PIP (extensor lag, flexion contracture) following PIP joint fractures is more common and more difficult to treat than loss of flexion.[8] Keeping the hinge at maximum extension between exercise

---

Postoperative Phase II (Weeks 2 to 6)

GOALS

- Independence in scar management
- Independence in progressed HEP
- AROM PIP joint 15 to 70 degrees

PRECAUTIONS

- Persistent edema
- Poor progression of ROM
- Pin site infection
- Pin loosening
- Strengthening is contraindicated.

TREATMENT STRATEGIES

- Precise instruction in AROM program to normalize digit flexion
- Instruction in scar management

CRITERIA FOR ADVANCEMENT

- Joint is ready for hinge removal = fracture has healed sufficiently and joint is stable.
- Maximum PROM/AROM of involved PIP joint has been achieved.

sessions and at night, and maximizing glide of the dorsal apparatus, cannot be overemphasized.

With fracture dislocations of the PIP joint, disruption of the collateral ligaments and the volar plate can be assumed. These damaged ligaments will tend to become fibrotic and thickened, and the volar plate will tend to shorten.[4] The benefits of PROM on the prevention of fibrosis have been well demonstrated.[5]

POSTOPERATIVE PHASE III: HINGE REMOVAL (WEEKS 6 TO 14)

Postoperative phase III focuses on regaining functional use of the involved hand and digit. The fracture and joint are now stable enough to withstand more aggressive therapeutic interventions. This phase usually begins at 6 weeks but may begin as early as 3 weeks, depending on when the surgeon removes the hinge.

Scar Management

Scar massage and the use of preferred silicone sheeting are continued.

AROM/PROM

The patient continues to actively flex and extend the PIP joints with the MP joints held in flexion and extension (as described previously). The patient continues to perform EDC gliding and tendon gliding exercises, including composite fist, hook fist, and duck fist. The patient performs isolated DIP and PIP blocking exercises. PROM of all joints is performed by the therapist and patient.

Splinting

The splinting program mimics the function of the hinge and addresses any mechanical deficits. If ordered by the surgeon, a static progressive PIP joint flexion splint is fabricated and worn intermittently during the day for periods of 15 to 45 minutes. A static digit extension splint (finger gutter) is worn at night to increase or maintain PIP joint extension. The use of an MP joint blocking splint (MP joints at full extension) during AROM exercises will help isolate and improve the patient's active hook fist and address lumbrical and/or interosseous tightness. A PIP joint blocking splint is used to isolate and promote active DIP flexion to promote flexor digitorum profundus (FDP) excursion and distal glide of dorsal apparatus. Dynamic PIP joint extension splints are used for PIP joint flexion contractures of 30 to 50 degrees. The MP joints are splinted in flexion, and the dynamic outrigger is mounted over the dorsum of the proximal phalanx to maximize the passive tension of the dorsal apparatus over the PIP joint.

Therapeutic Exercises

Resistive exercises using therapeutic putty are initiated. Putty stamping is used to increase grip strength. The patient is encouraged to maximize the use of the hand in the performance of all activities of daily living (ADL).

Troubleshooting

Persistent PIP joint extension lags can develop. Resistive extension, using putty or a Velcro board, and extension splinting are emphasized.

Especially after chronic boutonniere reconstructions, PIP joint flexion contractures can reoccur. Serial casting is an option. However, serial casting to increase extension at the expense of decreased flexion is a poor choice. A slight (15 to 20 degrees) PIP flexion contracture is preferred over the inability to make an acceptable fist.

Postoperative Phase III: Hinge Removal (Weeks 6 to 14)

GOALS
- Increased use of hand and digit in performance of ADL
- Continued increase in PIP AROM/PROM

PRECAUTIONS
- Inability to maintain PIP extension that was obtained in surgery (return to flexion contracture)
- Poor progression of ROM

TREATMENT STRATEGIES
- Therapeutic putty activities/exercises
- Exercise splints (MP blocking splint, PIP blocking splint)
- Dynamic PIP extension splinting

CRITERIA FOR DISCHARGE
- Functional composite fist
- Acceptable PIP active extension (25 degrees)
- Independent in advanced HEP
- Full use of hand in performance of ADL

References

1. Hotchkiss, R. *Surgical Technique: Compass Proximal Interphalangeal (PIP) Joint Hinge.* Available online at http://www.ortho.smith-nephew.com.
2. Bain, G.I., Mehta, J.A., Heptinstall, R.J., Bria, M. *Dynamic External Fixation for Injuries of the Proximal Interphalangeal Joint.* J Bone Joint Surg Br 1998;80B:1014–1019.
3. Meals, R.A., Foulkes, G.D. *Hinged Device for Fractures Involving the Proximal Interphalangeal Joint.* Clin Orthop 1996;327:29–37.
4. Hastings, H., Ernst, M.J. *Dynamic External Fixation for Fractures of the Proximal Interphalangeal Joint.* Hand Clin 1993;9(12):659–674.
5. Salter, R.B. *The Physiologic Basis of Continuous Passive Motion for Articular Cartilage Healing and Regeneration.* Hand Clin 1994;10:211–219.
6. Innis, P.C. Surgical Management of the Stiff Hand. In Hunter, J.M., Mackin, E.J., Callahan, A.D. (Eds). *Rehabilitation of the Hand and Upper Extremity,* 5th ed. Mosby, St. Louis, 2002, pp. 1057, 1058.
7. Feldscher, S.B., Blank, J.E. *Management of a Proximal Interphalangeal Joint Fracture Dislocation with Compass Proximal Interphalangeal Joint Hinge and Therapy: A Case Report.* J Hand Ther 2002;15:266–273.
8. Hastings, H., Carroll, C. *Treatment of Closed Articular Fractures of the Metacarpophalangeal and Proximal Interphalangeal Joints.* Hand Clin 1988;4(3):503–527.

24

Dupuytren's Fasciectomy

CAROL PAGE, PT, DPT, CHT

Dupuytren's disease is a condition of increased fibrous tissue growth in the hand, characterized by nodule and cord formation.[1] The changes in the palmar and digital fascia result in flexion contractures of the proximal interphalangeal (PIP) and metacarpophalangeal (MP) joints. The distal interphalangeal (DIP) joints may also become contracted. Although any of the digits can be involved, the fourth and fifth fingers are most commonly affected.[2] As the flexion contractures progress, hand function becomes increasingly impaired.

Although Dupuytren's disease is considered to be idiopathic,[1] there is evidence of a genetic component. The disorder occurs more commonly in Northern European populations, particularly in men and with advancing age. Additional links have been made with diabetes, epilepsy, alcohol use, and cigarette smoking.[3]

ANATOMICAL AND SURGICAL OVERVIEW

Dupuytren's disease typically presents with a nodule in the palm of the hand. The disease progresses more quickly in some individuals than others. The normal fibrous tissue changes into fibrous cords that form longitudinally along the lines of tension placed on the tissue with hand motion and use. Formation of the cords causes joint contractures of the MP and PIP joints.[1]

Indications for surgical intervention include impairment of hand function as a result of digital flexion contractures and demonstrated disease progression. Impairment of digital extension may interfere with the ability to perform various functions, such as reaching into pockets, purses, and briefcases, and opening the hand for face washing and hand shaking.[1]

The purpose of surgery is to restore the ability to straighten the digits to promote hand function. The surgical approach to treating contractures resulting from Dupuytren's disease ranges from the less frequently performed simple fasciotomy, the division of contracted tissue, to various types of fasciectomy. In a limited fasciectomy, the diseased tissue in the digits is excised. In a radical fasciectomy, the diseased palmar fascia is excised in addition. A dermofasciectomy, in which the skin as well as the diseased fascia are excised, may be performed in the attempt to minimize the rate of recurrence. Closure of surgical incisions is handled in several ways. The incisions made on the digits are usually primarily closed, and the surgical wounds on the palm are either left open to heal by secondary intention or primarily closed, with or without skin grafting.[1]

REHABILITATION OVERVIEW

Preoperative rehabilitation for Dupuytren's contracture has not been demonstrated to be effective and is therefore not indicated.[4] However, rehabilitation is widely recognized to be a critical component in a successful postoperative outcome.[5-8]

The purpose of postoperative therapy is to use interventions, such as scar and edema management techniques, splinting, and therapeutic exercise, to promote motion, strength, and function. Scar management is particularly important to prevent loss of digit extension gained in surgery and flexor tendon adherence. Extension splinting, which is used throughout the course of therapy, continues at night until scar tissue is mature to prevent recurrence of flexion contractures resulting from scar contraction. Although passive motion is helpful for regaining motion, it should never substitute for the active gliding of the tendons that can adhere in the scarred region, causing impairment of hand function.

Continuous passive motion machines have not been found to be useful for this diagnosis and are therefore not recommended.[9]

Therapists treating patients following Dupuytren's fasciectomy need to be on the alert for the onset of complications and communicate with the referring surgeon if signs are present. The most common complications are hematoma, skin loss, loss of digital flexion, and complex regional pain syndrome (formerly known as *reflex sympathetic dystrophy*).[10] Additional complications include infection, excessive edema, and persistent or recurrent proximal phalangeal joint flexion contractures.[7,8,10-12] Complications are best caught and addressed early. They will be discussed in further detail in the following sections.

POSTOPERATIVE PHASE I: INFLAMMATION/PROTECTION (WEEKS 0 TO 2)

Therapy is initiated when the initial postoperative edema begins to diminish, ideally between 3 and 7 days after surgery. If skin grafting has been used, initiation of therapy is delayed until the graft is well vascularized, as early as 7 to 10 days postoperatively. The graft must then be protected from shearing forces for an additional 10 days and compressive wraps avoided until after the graft is well vascularized.[13]

The first session begins with an examination and evaluation. The surgical wounds are inspected for signs of infection or hematoma, and the digits are inspected for signs of impaired circulation, such as coolness and pallor. The amount, type, and location of edema are noted. Patient reports of sensory changes are documented, and a formal sensibility evaluation is performed in a future session if indicated. Range of motion (ROM) measurements are taken of the involved digits, and the other upper extremity joints are screened to check for impairment of motion.

The patient is fitted with a custom-molded thermoplastic static extension splint (Figure 24-1). The MP and

Postoperative Phase I: Inflammation/Protection (Weeks 0 to 2)

GOALS

- Provide correct positioning in splint for reduction of inflammation and maintenance of tissue length
- Facilitate wound healing
- Reduce edema and pain
- Prevent tendon adherence and joint stiffness in involved joints
- Maintain full AROM of uninvolved joints

PRECAUTIONS

- Positioning in excessive digit extension can compromise circulation and prolong the inflammatory phase.
- In cases of skin grafting, delay ROM exercises until graft is well vascularized and protect from shearing forces.
- Alert physician to signs of hematoma or infection.

TREATMENT STRATEGIES

- Splinting: volar-based extension splint for involved digits and wrist
- Wound care: dressing changes and patient education, monitoring of wound status
- Edema and pain reduction: elevation, cold modalities, retrograde massage on dorsum of hand and wrist (avoid surgical wounds)
- ROM exercises for uninvolved joints: uninvolved digits, wrist, elbow, forearm, shoulder
- AROM/AAROM/PROM to involved digits when acute postoperative edema has diminished (and skin graft, if present, is well vascularized): tendon gliding, blocking, and extension exercises

CRITERIA FOR ADVANCEMENT

- Sutures removed and well-vascularized skin graft, if present
- Controlled (minimal) edema and pain

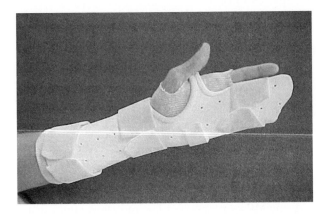

FIGURE 24-1 Custom-molded thermoplastic static extension splint.

interphalangeal (IP) joints of the involved digits are positioned in a comfortably extended position, taking care to avoid excessive extension that may compromise circulation and increase the risk of complications.[14] The wrist is usually included in the splint in approximately 15-degree extension. Occasionally, the wrist is left free if the surgery was of a limited nature. A volar-based splint is the preference at the Hospital for Special Surgery (HSS) because it can be used in later treatment phases for scar compression with a silicone insert. The splint is

initially worn at all times, except for dressing changes and exercises. Following removal of the sutures, the splint is worn at night only, unless it is needed on an intermittent basis during the day to improve digit extension.

At the first therapy visit, the patient is instructed in dressing the surgical wounds. The bulky postoperative splint is removed, and a nonadherent dressing is placed on wounds with the presence of exudates. All wounds are covered with sterile gauze dressings. The patient and therapist continue to monitor wound and circulation status on a regular basis.

Edema is addressed in phase I by elevation of the upper extremity above the heart as often as possible. Cold packs are used intermittently during the day. Light retrograde massage over the dorsum of the hand and wrist, avoiding contact with the surgical wounds, is helpful.

Active exercises of both the uninvolved upper extremity joints (uninvolved digits, wrist, forearm, elbow, and shoulder) and the involved digits begin in phase I at 3 to 7 days postoperatively. The presence of open wounds with minimal exudate is not a contraindication to beginning motion exercises of the involved digits. Open wounds remain covered with nonrestrictive dressings during exercise to prevent contamination. Active tendon gliding exercises (hook, straight, and composite fisting) and isolated DIP and PIP exercises differentially glide the tendons of flexor digitorum profundus (FDP) and flexor digitorum superficialis (FDS) in the digits and palm.[15] Active finger extension exercises are performed, including composite finger extension and IP extension with MP flexion. Patients are instructed to perform 10 repetitions of each exercise 4 times daily and provided with written instructions and photographs of the exercises. Assisted and gentle passive motion is indicated in phase I for individuals who have limited active motion. Overaggressive passive motion increases pain and edema, prolonging the inflammatory phase.

Troubleshooting

Signs of infection, such as excessive pain, edema, exudate, or heat, are reported immediately to the referring surgeon. Hematoma formation, a commonly reported wound complication, is less likely to occur in open palm surgical techniques.[11] If signs of a hematoma are present, such as localized swelling and discoloration at a surgical site, the physician should be contacted for possible drainage. Excessive edema without infection or hematoma may result from other causes. Overaggressive passive digital motion exercises increase edema, whereas active digit motion with the upper extremity elevated helps to decrease edema. Care is taken to ensure that dressings and splint straps are not too tight, thus compromising circulation. Strict upper extremity elevation is encouraged through positioning on pillows, rather than constant use of a sling, which may contribute to cervical and shoulder pain and stiffness.

POSTOPERATIVE PHASE II: FIBROPLASIA (WEEKS 2 TO 6)

Sutures are removed 10 to 14 days after surgery. The extension splint is remolded in maximum tolerated extension during the fibroplastic (scar formation) phase and worn at night only while sleeping, unless digit extension becomes progressively worse during the day. The splint can be worn intermittently during the day to maintain digit extension, but active motion and light, functional use of the hand is encouraged.

The surgical wounds can take as long as 6 weeks to fully heal. Portions of the wounds may heal more quickly than others. Incisions on the digits treated with primary closure will heal more quickly than an open wound in the palm. Wound inspection and wound care continue until all wounds have fully closed. Scar management techniques begin on the portions of the wounds that have healed. Scar massage with oil or thick lotion, avoiding contamination of any open areas, is performed for several minutes daily to minimize scar

adherence. When all areas of the wounds have healed, a silicone pad or mold worn on the scars at night will facilitate scar remodeling. It may be necessary to remold the splint to accommodate the silicone insert. The volar-based splint is useful in holding the insert in place and providing light compression to the scar.

Edema control measures continue as needed. Contrast baths are added once the wounds have fully closed. Light compression wraps are helpful, but if they are too constrictive, they contribute to the problem they are meant to address.

Active and passive motion exercises are continued. Emphasis is placed on balancing flexion and extension exercises, which are individualized according to findings on reevaluation. The home exercise program is progressed with added stretching exercises to improve passive range. Caution is required because overaggressive stretching may increase pain and inflammation. Passive exercises cannot substitute for active motion exercises. Active gliding of the tendons through the scarred region is critical for the prevention of tendon adherence. Heat modalities, such as moist hot packs, paraffin, and ultrasound, are helpful in preparing the soft tissues for motion and scar massage, if edema is not excessive and the wounds have healed.

Use of the hand for light, functional activities is encouraged and will speed recovery. If spontaneous use of the hand is not observed, activities are included in the therapy sessions.

Troubleshooting

Passive flexion of the involved digits that exceeds active flexion indicates poor flexor tendon gliding with possible scar adherence. Loss of flexion in the uninvolved fingers, known as quadrigia, can occur if scar adherence limits the glide of FDP. Active motion exercises and scar management techniques (e.g., scar massage, silicone inserts, and compression) decrease adhesion formation. Neuromuscular electrical stimulation to the FDP may be added to facilitate active recruitment of this muscle. An exercise splint that maintains the MP joints in extension and allows full PIP and DIP joint motion, while active hook fisting is performed, also facilitates FDP glide.

Excessive edema, persistent pain, vasomotor changes, and impaired hand function may be indicative of complex regional pain syndrome. The referring physician should be contacted for possible treatment with medications or stellate ganglion blocks. McFarlane and McGrouther[10] report that over 4% of patients developed reflex sympathetic dystrophy (now known as complex regional pain syndrome) after surgery for Dupuytren's contracture. In this situation, techniques that increase pain, such as stretching, are avoided, and active use of the hand and upper extremity is encouraged.

Postoperative Phase II: Fibroplasia (Weeks 2 to 6)

GOALS

- Reduce residual edema and pain.
- Minimize scar adherence.
- Maximize AROM and PROM of involved digits.
- Restore independence in light activities of daily living (ADL).

PRECAUTIONS

- Overzealous stretching and resistive exercises may increase inflammation.
- Compression wraps that are too tight may increase rather than decrease edema.

TREATMENT STRATEGIES

- Splinting: remold extension splint if needed to maximize MP and IP joint extension or to accommodate silicone insert; splint worn at night only
- Edema control: continue treatments from phase I, adding (if needed) light compression, contrast baths (when wounds are fully healed)
- Scar management when wounds have healed: scar massage, silicone scar pad or mold
- Heat modalities to prepare soft tissues for ROM
- AROM, AAROM to promote tendon gliding, balancing focus on flexors and extensors
- PROM, gentle stretching
- Light, functional activities to encourage use of hand to tolerance

CRITERIA FOR ADVANCEMENT

- Complete wound closure
- Minimal edema and pain with light activities and motion exercises

POSTOPERATIVE PHASE III: SCAR MATURATION (WEEKS 6 TO 12)

Night extension splinting and scar management techniques begun in phase II continue until the scar tissue is mature, 6 months to a year postoperatively, to prevent recurrence of flexion contractures secondary to scar contraction. Edema measures continue until the edema has resolved.

Active and passive motion exercises continue with an emphasis on achieving maximum end range motion in both directions. Heat modalities are useful in preconditioning the tissues. If passive digit extension remains more limited than the motion achieved intraoperatively, additional splinting or serial casting to increase extension is considered (see "Troubleshooting Phase III").

Light resistive flexion and extension exercises are added to the treatment sessions and home exercise program during phase III. Examples of resistive exercises include lumbrical and composite grasping of therapy putty, pressing of a gripped wooden dowel into putty, digit extension against the resistance of looped putty, and resistive dowel rolling. Resistive exercise promotes tendon gliding as well as improving hand strength. To prevent loss of extension, flexion exercises are balanced with extension exercises. If edema persists in phase III, resistive exercise is delayed or minimized. Patients are cautioned against overzealous performance of repetitive, resistive flexion, because this may cause

an overuse of inflammatory response in the flexor tendons.

Gradual return to all functional activities by the end of phase III is encouraged. The patient who is independent in splinting, scar management, and a home exercise program, who has maximized digit motion, and who has sufficient hand strength to perform ADL, is ready for discharge from therapy. It is not unusual for therapy to continue 12 or more weeks postoperatively for achievement of these goals.

Troubleshooting

PIP joint extensor lag (decreased active PIP extension) may result from attenuation of the extensor mechanism as a result of prolonged preoperative flexion positioning. For treatment of this complication, active and resistive extension exercises are emphasized.

If passive PIP extension remains limited or worsens, recurrence of PIP joint flexion contracture may be secondary to scar contraction or joint stiffness. If consistent use of night extension splinting, exercise, and scar management techniques do not resolve the contracture, intermittent use of a serial static digit extension splint during the day is indicated. The splint is periodically remolded by the therapist into greater PIP extension as improvement is made. PIP joint contractures that are resistant to improvement with splinting and other therapy techniques respond to remodeling through

Postoperative Phase III: Scar Maturation (Weeks 6 to 12)

GOALS

- Achieve flat, nonadherent scars.
- Achieve maximum AROM/PROM in involved digits, without flexion contractures.
- Achieve functional strength.
- Restore independence in ADL.

PRECAUTIONS

- Night extension splinting with silicone insert should continue until scar maturity (up to a year postoperatively) to avoid digital flexion contractures.

TREATMENT STRATEGIES

- Continue night extension splinting and scar management until scar is mature.
- Heat modalities, including ultrasound, as needed, to prepare soft tissues for ROM and scar techniques
- Edema control measures as needed
- AROM, PROM, and stretching with emphasis on end range flexion and extension
- Resistance exercises to promote tendon gliding and strengthening of digits (flexors and extensors) and wrist
- Functional activities to promote restoration of independent ADL

CRITERIA FOR DISCHARGE

- Independence in home program of night splinting, scar management, and therapeutic exercise
- Full or maximum digit AROM with freely gliding tendons
- Functional hand strength
- Independence in ADL

the use of full-time serial casting.[16] The digit extension cast is changed several times weekly as PIP extension increases. When the cast is removed in therapy, exercises for flexion and extension are performed. The patient is closely monitored to ensure that digit flexion does not become impaired during the period that extension casting is being used.

REFERENCES

1. McGrouther, D.A. Dupuytren's Contracture. In Green, D.P., Hotchkiss, R.N., Pederson, W.C. (Eds). *Green's Operative Hand Surgery*, 4th ed. Churchill Livingstone, New York, 1999, pp. 563–591.
2. McFarlane, R.M., MacDermid, J.C. Dupuytren's Disease. In Hunter, J.M., Mackin, E.J., Callahan, A.D. (Eds). *Rehabilitation of the Hand: Surgery and Therapy*, 5th ed. Mosby, St. Louis, 2002, pp. 971–988.
3. Ross, D.C. *Epidemiology of Dupuytren's Disease.* Hand Clin 1999;15(1):53–62.
4. Abbott, K., Denney, J., Burke, F.D., McGrouther, D.A. *A Review of Attitudes to Splintage in Dupuytren's Contracture.* J Hand Surg Br 1987;12:326–328.
5. Fietti, V.G. Jr., Mackin, E.J. Open-palm Technique in Dupuytren's Disease. In Hunter, J.M., Mackin, E.J., Callahan, A.D. (Eds). *Rehabilitation of the Hand: Surgery and Therapy*, 4th ed. Mosby, St. Louis, 1995, pp. 995–1006.
6. Gosset, J. Dupuytren's Disease and the Anatomy of the Palmodigital Aponeuroses. In Hueston, J., Tubiana, R. (Eds). *Dupuytren's Disease*, 2nd ed. Churchill Livingstone, London, 1985, pp. 13–26.
7. Mullins, P.A. *Postsurgical Rehabilitation of Dupuytren's Disease.* Hand Clin 1999;15(1):167–174.
8. Prosser, R., Conolly, W.B. *Complications Following Surgical Treatment for Dupuytren's Contracture.* J Hand Ther 1996;9: 344–348.
9. Sampson, S.P., Badalamente, M.A., Hurst, L.C., Dowd, A., Sewell, C.S., Lehmann-Torres, J., Ferraro, M., Semon, B. *The Use of a Passive Motion Machine in the Postoperative Rehabilitation of Dupuytren's Disease.* J Hand Surg Am 1992;17:333–338.
10. McFarlane, R.M., McGrouther, D.A. Complications and Their Management. In McFarlane, R.M., McGrouther, D.A., Flint, M.H. (Eds). *Dupuytren's Disease: Biology and Treatment.* Churchill Livingstone, Edinburgh, Scotland, 1990, pp. 377–382.
11. Boyer, M.I., Gelberman, R.H. *Complications of the Operative Treatment of Dupuytren's Disease.* Hand Clin 1999;15:161–166.
12. Watson, H.K., Fong, D. *Dystrophy, Recurrence, and Salvage Procedures in Dupuytren's Contracture.* Hand Clin 1991;7:745–755.
13. Singer, D.I., Moore, J.H. Jr., Bryon, P.M. Management of Skin Grafts and Flaps. In Hunter, J.M., Mackin, E.J., Callahan, A.D. (Eds). *Rehabilitation of the Hand: Surgery and Therapy*, 4th ed. Mosby, St. Louis, 1995, pp. 277–290.
14. Evans, R.B., Dell, P.C., Fiolkowski, P. *A Clinical Report of the Effect of Mechanical Stress on Functional Results after Fasciectomy for Dupuytren's Contracture.* J Hand Ther 2002;15: 331–339.
15. Wehbe, M.A., Hunter, J.M. *Flexor Tendon Gliding in the Hand. Part II: Differential Gliding.* J Hand Surg 1985;10A:575–579.
16. Bell-Krotoski, J.A. Plaster Cylinder Casting for Contractures of the Interphalangeal Joints. In Hunter, J.M., Mackin, E.J., Callahan, A.D. (Eds). *Rehabilitation of the Hand: Surgery and Therapy*, 5th ed. Mosby, St. Louis, 2002, pp. 1839–1845.

III

PEDIATRIC
REHABILITATION

DEBORAH CORRADI-SCALISE, PT, DPT

C H A P T E R

25

Lower Extremity Surgical Intervention in Patients with Cerebral Palsy: Bone and Musculotendinous Procedures

DEBORAH CORRADI-SCALISE, PT, DPT

CATHI WAGNER, PT, MBA

AMANDA R. SPARROW, PT

CEREBRAL PALSY AND SURGICAL CONSIDERATIONS

Cerebral palsy (CP) is defined as a condition characterized by a chronic, nonprogressive disorder of movement or posture of early onset.[1] It presents as abnormal control of motor function/coordination as a result of damage to one or more specific areas of the brain.[2] The damage to the brain can occur during the prenatal, perinatal, postnatal, as well as the infancy period.[2] The primary lesion is static; however, the manifestations can change, especially in the musculoskeletal system, because of muscle imbalances, growth, development, and the effects of gravity.[3,4] CP occurs in approximately 1 to 7 per 1000 children worldwide, and diagnosis in the United States is reported to be 5.2 per 1000 children.[4,5] There are many causes of CP; however, in most cases, only risk factors can be identified and not the specific cause of the condition. Some risk factors include prematurity, low birth weight, infection, hypoxia, anoxia, trauma, placental complications, genetic abnormalities, teratologic agents, and maternal risk factors (i.e., toxemia, drug/alcohol abuse) that affect the developing fetus.[2,4]

CP can be classified by both anatomical and neuromotor involvement.[4] The most common type of motor dysfunction in CP is spasticity. Spasticity is characterized by an increase in muscle tone and the presence of hyperactive stretch reflexes. Weakness; loss of active muscle control; problems with coordination, balance, dexterity; and poverty of movement are often seen with spasticity. Simultaneous contraction of antagonistic muscles and joint contractures is often noted in this type of CP.[4] Orthopedic surgery is frequently performed in this population with overall positive results. Orthopedic surgery is less predictable in other neuromotor classifications of CP, such as athetoid CP (characterized by writhing movements), ataxic CP (characterized by uncoordinated movements, tremors, balance problems), and mixed CP (characterized by a combination of spasticity, athetosis, or ataxia).[4] The main anatomical classifications of CP are quadriplegia (total body involvement with equal involvement of all four extremities), diplegia (total body involvement with the lower extremities more involved than the upper extremities), hemiplegia (involvement of one side of the body; typically, the upper extremity is more involved than the lower extremity),[4,5] and monoplegia (involvement of one extremity). The anatomical and neuromotor classifications are typically combined to further describe CP (Figures 25-1 through 25-3). Although anatomical and neuromotor classifications exist, CP is a complex condition, and extensive variability exists regarding presentation, severity, and abilities among patients.

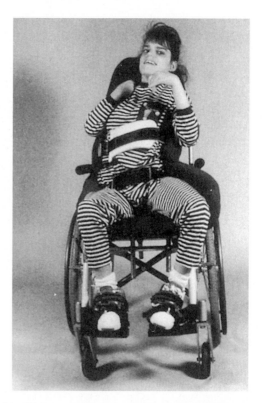

FIGURE **25-1** A 15-year-old girl with spastic quadriplegia. *(From Herring, J.A. Tachdjian's Pediatric Orthopaedics, 3rd ed. WB Saunders, Philadelphia, 2002, p. 1125, with permission.)*

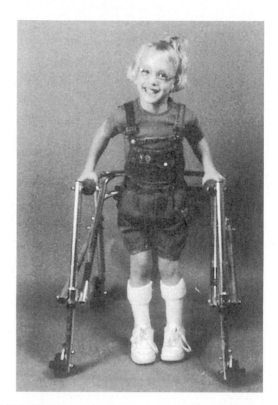

FIGURE **25-2** A 5-year-old girl with spastic diplegia. *(From Herring, J.A. Tachdjian's Pediatric Orthopaedics, 3rd ed. WB Saunders, Philadelphia, 2002, p. 1125, with permission.)*

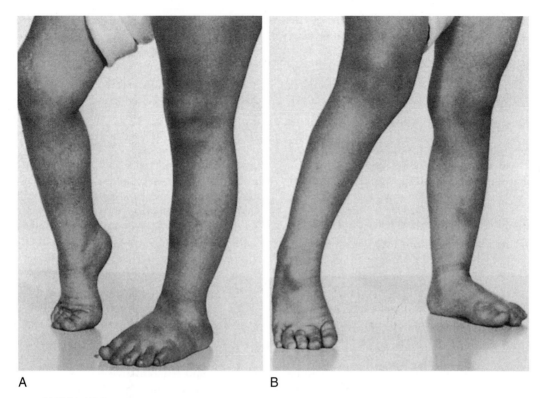

A   B

FIGURE 25-3 A child with right spastic hemiplegia. *(From Herring, J.A.* Tachdjian's Pediatric Orthopaedics, *3rd ed. WB Saunders, Philadelphia, 2002, p. 1125, with permission.)*

REHABILITATION OVERVIEW

Preoperative Considerations

Orthopedic management of a child with CP is best accomplished via a team approach. It is essential that the surgeon and medical/rehabilitation team consider the "total" child when evaluating a patient with CP for surgical intervention. An understanding of atypical development and movement compensations is imperative to determine how surgery will likely impact the child's future function.[6] Muscular tightness and joint limitations at any one joint impact the alignment and function of adjacent muscles and joints. Surgically treating one problem, without consideration of the rest of the body in CP, may have a poor outcome.[3] Additionally, one must also remember that lengthening a muscle also weakens it.[4] This is very important to remember when considering any surgical procedure in the ambulatory patient. The current trend in orthopedic surgery is to develop a strategy and prepare an operative plan that addresses all of the patient's impairments at one time.[7]

Additionally, a differentiation must be made between primary impairments and secondary compensations to adequately address CP. Often the basic ability to activate a muscle for isolated or coordinated joint movement is absent in CP. The patient subsequently develops secondary compensations in an effort to move and obtain maximum function with the least amount of energy expenditure. If the primary problem is surgically addressed first, the need for the secondary compensation may be eliminated. If, however, the secondary problem is addressed first, or in lieu of the primary problem, the presentation of the condition may actually get worse.[3] The result of a careful and thorough team evaluation frequently leads to a single-stage, multiple-level surgical treatment, simultaneously correcting bone and soft tissue problems.[3] This avoids additional hospitalizations for subsequent operations, when all of the patient's impairments are considered at one time.[7]

Typically, there is no specific preoperative therapeutic protocol for children with CP because they are usually actively involved in some form of a physical therapy program that addresses their individual impairments and functional disabilities. A comprehensive physical therapy examination for each presurgical candidate should be performed and the findings discussed with the team. Another tool that may be used in the preoperative evaluation process is quantitative gait analysis.[4,7] Gait analysis, using a three-dimensional (3-D) motion analysis laboratory, provides the clinician with important objective data. Kinematic, kinetic, and electromyographic (EMG) data collected in this fashion help identify, simultaneously, the presence of multiple abnormalities (bone and soft tissue) at multiple levels, in three anatomical planes. Gait analysis provides the team with data to assist in the differentiation of primary gait deviations and secondary coping strategies.[3] Consultation with the surgeon to discuss the orthopedic and physical therapy examination findings, observational videotaped gait analysis, and quantitative gait analysis is key in presurgical planning and decision making (Figure 25-4). Team collaboration and open communication between the surgeon, physical therapist, patient, and family will assist the surgeon in formulating an operative plan and developing postoperative therapy goals.

POSTOPERATIVE CONSIDERATIONS

Immediate postoperative concerns for any surgical procedure in the patient with CP include pain and spasm management and decreasing the anxiety level of both the child and caregiver/family.[4] It is important to overcome the early weakness, stiffness, and discomfort postoperatively. Rapid mobilization following surgery is essential in overcoming early postoperative stiffness and weakness; however, traumatized muscles should be given enough time to recover, and the child should be as comfortable as possible when beginning therapy.[8] Analgesic medication and muscle relaxants (to control or lessen the muscle spasms) are used immediately postoperatively. A compassionate and supportive staff is also essential to help the patient and family during the postoperative rehabilitation phase.[4]

Postoperative rehabilitation focuses on the restoration of range of motion (ROM), regaining preoperative muscle strength, and optimizing mobility/gait and functional ability.[4,9] All goals will be directly related to and dependent upon the overall functional ability of the patient. During the initial rehabilitative period, it may be beneficial to use splints for comfort and prevent joint

positioning that could contribute to recurrent contractures.[4] If only soft tissue procedures have been performed, ambulation typically begins on postoperative day one (POD 1). If bone procedures are performed, radiographic evidence of bone healing and physician clearance are necessary before initiating weight-bearing activities.[4,10] When multiple surgical procedures are performed on the lower extremity, it may take a long time for the patient to regain preoperative level of strength and function.[4]

During the rehabilitation period of POD 1 and beyond, the physical therapist must take great care in assessing the patient's neuromuscular capability as well as the ability of the patient to progress. The treatment and goals must be individually based, and progressing the patient is always based on a thorough physical therapy examination. Modifications to therapeutic programs must continually be addressed to remediate or safely progress the therapeutic exercise program and the patient's functional ability. At the Hospital for Special Surgery (HSS), home exercise programs (HEPs) are emphasized. A HEP will greatly assist the patient in the recovery and rehabilitative process. The patient's HEP is continually updated based on evaluative findings. Compliance to the HEP is very important and should be reinforced with the patient and family. In the rehabilitation process of a patient with a primary neurological impairment, it is important to incorporate principles of motor learning into the treatment program. Direct hands-on therapeutic input, in addition to providing the patient with feedback through all of the sensory systems, is important. Repetition is necessary for learning a movement skill, and a focus on functional tasks will provide meaning to the activity for the patient.

The goal of orthopedic management is to help each individual patient reach his or her optimal functional

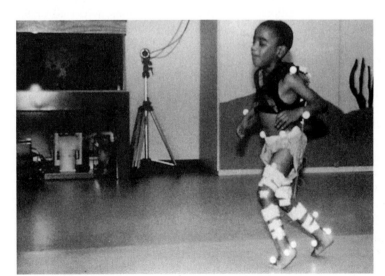

FIGURE **25-4** A young boy with spastic diplegia undergoing preoperative gait analysis. *(From Herring, J.A. Tachdjian's Pediatric Orthopaedics, 3rd ed. WB Saunders, Philadelphia, 2002, p. 1126, with permission.)*

ability, prevent deformity and structural changes, which may become disabling later in life, and decrease pain and/or discomfort.[5] For ambulatory patients the goal of surgery might be to improve the ability, quality, efficiency, and cosmesis of gait. In the nonambulatory patient the goal of surgery may be to maintain the ability to sit, facilitate transfer activities and activities of daily living (ADL), and/or decrease deforming forces that will impact postural alignment. It is interesting to note that the functional priorities of a person with CP, who has severe involvement, are (in order of importance) communication, ADL, mobility in the environment, and, last, the ability to walk.[4,6] It is very important that the medical team identify and address the patient/family goals when making decisions regarding surgical interventions. Typically, there is an increase in frequency of physical therapy intervention postoperatively for a period of time to address the immediate weakness and functional limitations/disability associated with surgical lengthening, bone procedures, and immobilization. Once the acute and subacute phase of rehabilitation is complete, the patient typically returns to his or her preexisting, preoperative therapeutic program.

The following pages set forth postoperative guidelines following bone and soft tissue surgical procedures commonly performed at HSS for the treatment and rehabilitation of CP. For the sake of clarity, only one anatomical deformity/surgery is presented at a time. The reader must realize that, characteristically, many of the deformities coexist in patients with CP and therefore multiple surgical procedures are typically performed simultaneously. The total rehabilitation course must reflect this and be coordinated/modified according to the surgical procedures performed on each individual patient. As always, the physical therapist should maintain open communication with the treating surgeon on how to progress each individual patient.

At HSS, the Pediatric Physical Therapy Department is an integral part of the presurgical evaluation process, including gait analysis and collaboration with the physicians regarding surgical decision making for patients with CP.

VARUS ROTATIONAL OSTEOTOMY

Children with CP commonly present with coxa valga and excessive femoral anteversion, as reported on radiograph.[6,11] Both of these findings can contribute to hip subluxation and dislocation.[3,11–13] Coxa valga is described as an increase in the neck shaft angle of the femur[6] (Figures 25-5 and 25-6). At birth the neck shaft angle is typically 150 to 160 degrees.[14] This angle decreases to 120 to 135 degrees in adulthood.[14] As reported by Bobroff et al.,[13] children with CP displayed a significant increase in neck shaft angles as compared to the neck shaft angles of normal children. Femoral anteversion is the degree of forward projection of the femoral neck as measured by the angular difference between the axis of the femoral neck and the transcondylar axis of the knee[14,15] (Figure 25-7). In the normal population, femoral anteversion is greatest at birth, ranging from 30 to 40 degrees and decreases with age.[12,13] By adulthood, the average amount of femoral anteversion is 8 degrees in men and 14 degrees in women.[16] Bobroff et al.[13] report that the angles of femoral anteversion are similar at early ages between children with typical development and children with CP. As the age of both groups of children increased, however, those with CP showed little change in anteversion angles, whereas the typical children had progressively decreasing angles of femoral anteversion as they approached adulthood. Other authors report that femoral anteversion often remains excessive in individuals with CP.[11,17] According to Novacheck, the degree of femoral anteversion in CP is frequently between 50 to 65 degrees.[3] Children with CP appear to have a decreased ability to resolve/reduce congenital anteversion. This may, in part, be a result of the persistence of

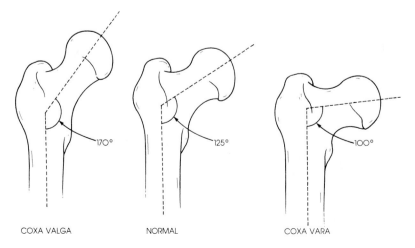

FIGURE **25-5** Neck shaft angles in adults: normal and coxa valga. *(Modified from Magee, D.J. Orthopedic Physical Assessment, 3rd ed. WB Saunders, Philadelphia, 1997, p. 481, with permission.)*

COXA VALGA   NORMAL   COXA VARA

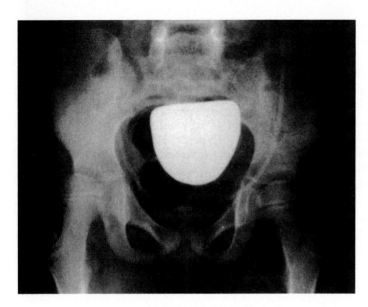

FIGURE **25-6** AP pelvic radiograph of a 5-year-old girl with spastic quadriplegia. The right hip is subluxed, and coxa valga is apparent. *(From Herring, J.A.* Tachdjian's Pediatric Orthopaedics, *3rd ed. WB Saunders, Philadelphia, 2002, p. 1188, with permission.)*

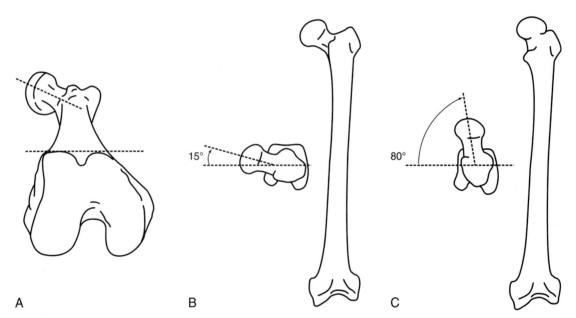

A   B   C

FIGURE **25-7** *A.* Femoral anteversion of the hip. *B.* Normal angle. *C.* Excessive angle. *(From Magee, D.J.* Orthopedic Physical Assessment, *3rd ed. WB Saunders, Philadelphia, 1997, pp. 474 and 475, respectively; Hoppenfeld, S.* Physical Examination of the Spine and Extremities. *Appleton-Century-Crofts, New York, 1976, p. 158, with permission.)*

abnormal patterns of posture and movement, delayed lower extremity weight-bearing, and muscle imbalances resulting from spasticity[6,10,13] (Figure 25-8).

Functionally, increased femoral anteversion presents as an in-toeing gait pattern (Figure 25-9). Excessive hip internal rotation during gait carries with it an associated cosmetic and functional disability.[18] Increased femoral anteversion can result in hip flexion and adduction contractures with shortening of the psoas muscles.[3] This can lead to hip instability and subsequent hip subluxation or dislocation.[3,11,12]

Clinically, femoral anteversion is evaluated by palpating the greater trochanter and assessing passive internal and external rotation of the hips in the prone position with the pelvis stabilized[14,19] (Figure 25-10). Excessive hip internal rotation and limited hip external rotation is clinically indicative of femoral anteversion.[10,16] Radiographs, CAT scans (computed axial tomography), and fluoroscopy are valuable to the surgeon in measuring femoral anteversion and neck-shaft angles.[3]

Quantitative gait analysis, using a 3-D gait system, is useful in confirming the presentation and the location

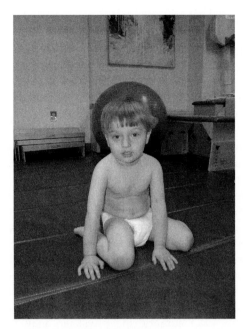

FIGURE **25-8** W-sitting, which perpetuates the patterns of hip flexion, adduction, and internal rotation.

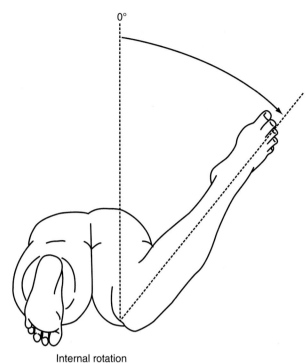

Internal rotation

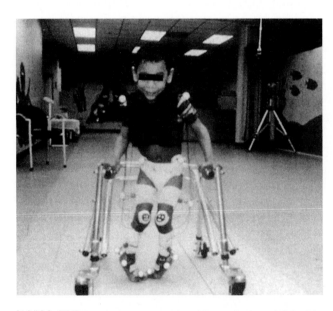

FIGURE **25-9** Excessive anteversion bilaterally in a child with cerebral palsy. Tape outlines the patellas. He has difficulty clearing his foot forward in swing phase owing to in-toeing from the anteversion and exacerbated by hip adduction. *(From Herring, J.A. Tachdjian's Pediatric Orthopaedics, 3rd ed. WB Saunders, Philadelphia, 2002, p. 1178, with permission.)*

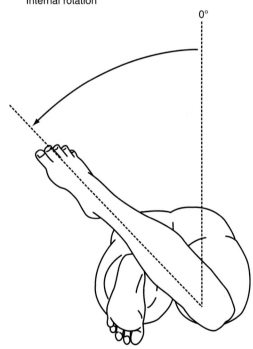

External rotation

FIGURE **25-10** Assessment of hip rotation in the prone position. *(From Bleck, E.E. Orthopaedic Management in Cerebral Palsy. JB Lippincott, Philadelphia, 1987, p. 51; Herring, J.A. Tachdjian's Pediatric Orthopaedics, 3rd ed. WB Saunders, Philadelphia, 2002, p. 66; Magee, D.J. Orthopedic Physical Assessment, 3rd ed. WB Saunders, Philadelphia, 1997, p. 464, with permission.)*

of rotation abnormalities. An in-toeing gait pattern can be a result of rotational deformities of the femur, tibia, and/or foot. Three-dimensional gait analysis assists the surgeon in identifying the primary site of the rotational deformity[18] (Figure 25-11).

The varus rotational osteotomy (VRO) is a surgical intervention performed to correct femoral anteversion, coxa valga, and hip subluxation.[11] The goal of this procedure in individuals with CP is to improve cosmetic and functional gait parameters as well as stabilize the hip joint.[16,18] In individuals with CP, VRO outcomes have reportedly included an increase in hip external rotation and extension, a decrease in anterior pelvic tilt, and an increase in knee extension strength.[16,18]

Surgical indications are based on clinical examination, gait analysis, and radiographic findings. Indications for a VRO are

- In-toeing gait with excessive femoral anteversion greater than 40 to 45 degrees[3,4,10]
- Clinically, passive internal rotation greater than 45 degrees with less than 30 degrees of external rotation on physical exam[10]
- Hip subluxation[3]

SURGICAL OVERVIEW

The VRO procedure is performed prone, as described by Dr. Leon Root.[10,16] An osteotomy is performed at the upper level of the lesser trochanter in the inter-trochanteric aspect of the femur. The osteotomy is positioned to prevent extension or flexion. The blade portion is inserted through the greater trochanter into the neck of the femur. The distal femur is then clamped to a plate. The distal femur is rotated externally, and the head and neck are placed in decreased valgus. The femoral head is centered into the acetabulum, and the femoral anteversion is corrected.[16] The proximal screw is inserted, and the ROM is evaluated.[10,20] The goal is to have an approximate 2 : 1 ratio (60 to 30 degrees) of hip external to internal rotation.[20,21] If the desired rotation is achieved, then the remaining screws are inserted. If not, the proximal screw is removed, and the degree of rotation is modified[10,16,20,21] (Figures 25-12 and 25-13). In addition to the bone VRO surgery, the physician may need to perform concurrent soft tissue procedures, such as hip flexor and/or adductor muscle lengthening to address either the presence of muscle contractures or spasticity that may impact passive and active hip motion.[4,6,9]

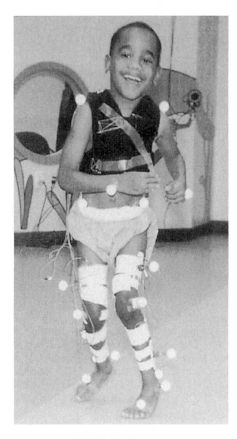 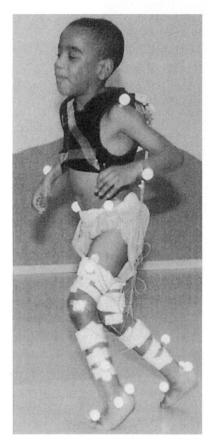 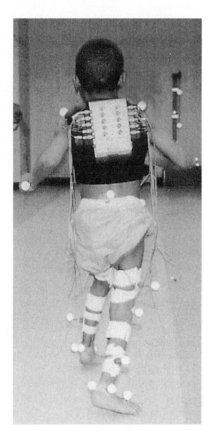

FIGURE **25-11** A 6-year-old boy with cerebral palsy spastic diplegia undergoing gait analysis. Markers are used to collect kinematic data; electromyographic data is being gathered simultaneously. (*From Herring, J.A. Tachdjian's Pediatric Orthopaedics, 3rd ed. WB Saunders, Philadelphia, 2002, p. 81, with permission.*)

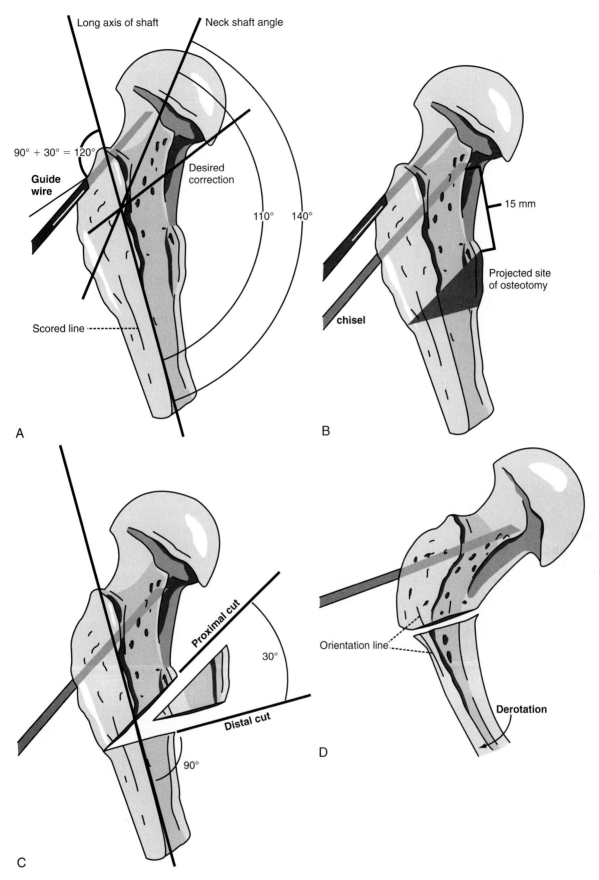

Long axis of shaft   Neck shaft angle

90° + 30° = 120°

Guide wire

Desired correction

110°   140°

Scored line

A

15 mm

Projected site of osteotomy

chisel

B

Proximal cut

30°

Distal cut

90°

C

Orientation line

Derotation

D

FIGURE **25-12** Varus rotational osteotomy surgical procedure. *A.* A reference point is made for the correction of anteversion. *B.* The projected site for the osteotomy is identified. *C.* The wedge is removed. *D.* The distal femur is externally rotated to a predetermined position.

Continued

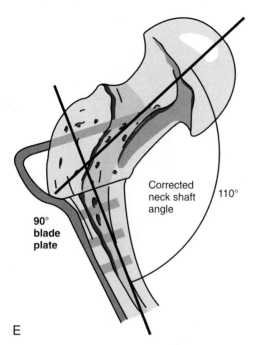

E

FIGURE **25-12, cont'd** *E.* The neck shaft angle is corrected, and the blade plate is secured to the distal section of the femur. *(Courtesy of Dr. Leon Root, New York.)*

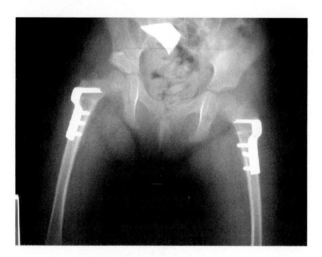

FIGURE **25-13** Radiograph of a 4-year-old child with cerebral palsy who underwent bilateral varus rotation osteotomies. *(Courtesy of Dr. Leon Root, New York.)*

REHABILITATION OVERVIEW

The rehabilitation following a VRO is designed to progressively increase range of joint motion, muscle strength, and the patient's ability to resume lower extremity weight-bearing activities. Communication between the physical therapist and the surgeon is imperative. The surgeon will assess bone healing via radiograph and advise the therapist when the healing is sufficient to begin weight-bearing activities in therapy. Each individual with CP is unique, and the time frame of his or her rehabilitation progression will vary because

of the level of function before surgical intervention and the ability of the body to heal. The patient and the caregiver must be involved in the rehabilitation process to ensure a successful outcome.

PREOPERATIVE CONSIDERATIONS

There is no specific preoperative therapeutic protocol before a VRO procedure. Before a VRO the patient with CP may undergo a gait analysis to have objective data from motion analysis confirm clinical and radiographic findings of increased hip internal rotation and femoral anteversion.

POSTOPERATIVE REHABILITATION OF VRO: PHASE I (DAYS 2 TO 4)

The patient is typically on bed rest at POD 1. Rehabilitation begins on POD 2. Two different postoperative courses may be encountered following a VRO. The direction that the postoperative course will follow is determined by the surgeon. The patient with CP may be immobilized in a spica cast (Figure 25-14), or immobilization may be accomplished via the use of removable long leg splints only (Jordan splints) (Figure 25-15). Factors that contribute to this decision include the age of the patient, the degree of involvement/severity of CP, the size of the patient, and/or the type of plate that is used intraoperatively. Children under age 8, and those patients who present with severe physical or cognitive involvement, are typically placed in a spica cast. This will ensure immobilization to provide a safe environment for the surgical correction to heal. Hip precautions are in place post-VRO and consist of no hip adduction or internal rotation past midline and no hip flexion past 90 degrees. Early motion/mobilization within established movement precautions is the benefit of using Jordan splints rather than a spica cast during the

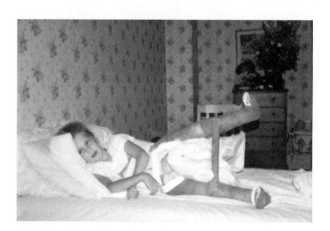

FIGURE **25-14** A 7-year-old girl with cerebral palsy who underwent bilateral VROs. She was placed in a spica cast postoperatively. Note positioning of patient is side-lying with spica cast.

Postoperative Rehabilitation of VRO: Phase I (Days 2 to 4) with Spica Cast

GOALS

- Control of postoperative pain/spasm
- Frequent changes of position: side-lying/prone and sitting in a reclining wheelchair (typically days 2 to 3)
- Ensure that the cast fits appropriately and does not impede circulation or cause irritation
- Maintain patient non–weight-bearing status
- Caregiver independent in patient transfers

PRECAUTIONS

- Avoid prolonged periods of lying in supine
- Monitor skin for irritation/breakdown from cast and positioning
- Monitor distal extremities for signs of edema

TREATMENT STRATEGIES

- Caregiver instructed to monitor the cast for fit and skin irritation
- Caregiver education in importance of position changes
    Prone (Figure 25-16, *A*)
    Side-lying (Figure 25-14)
    Supine (Figure 25-16, *B*)
    Sitting (Figure 25-16, *C*)
- Caregiver instructed in proper body mechanics for transfers

CRITERIA FOR ADVANCEMENT

- Dependent upon bone healing seen on radiograph; determined by the surgeon

Postoperative Rehabilitation of VRO: Phase I (Days 2 to 4) with Jordan Splints; No Casting

GOALS

- Control of postoperative pain/spasm
- Educate patient/caregivers regarding hip precautions
- Frequent changes of position (maintaining hip precautions) to prevent decubiti and decrease fear of movement
- Develop ability to sit in a reclining wheelchair (Figure 25-17)
- Develop/maintain passive range of motion (PROM) of lower extremities maintaining hip precautions
- Educate caregivers on transfers and importance of maintaining non–weight-bearing status

PRECAUTIONS

- Avoid prolonged periods of lying in supine
- Maintain hip precautions of no adduction or internal rotation past neutral; no flexion past 90 degrees
- Hip external rotation; extension and abduction as tolerated
- The patient is typically non–weight-bearing for at least 3 weeks, but this is dependent on bone healing and clearance by the surgeon

THERAPEUTIC STRATEGIES

- Frequent change of position
  - From supine to side-lying with pillows to maintain hip abduction and neutral rotation
  - Reclining wheelchair with knees flexed if tolerated (typically PODs 2 to 3)
- Gentle PROM of the hips, within precautions of hip flexion to 90 degrees, hip internal rotation to neutral, hip adduction to neutral; hip external rotation, extension, and abduction as tolerated
- Gentle PROM of the knees and ankles may begin POD 2
- Active ankle pumps
- Training patient/caregiver regarding hip precautions and the importance of position change

CRITERIA FOR ADVANCEMENT

- Dependent upon bone healing seen on radiograph; determined by the surgeon

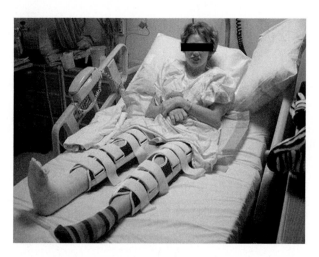

FIGURE **25-15** Patient is an adolescent female with CP who underwent multiple lower extremity procedures, including bilateral VROs. Patient is using bilateral Jordan splints.

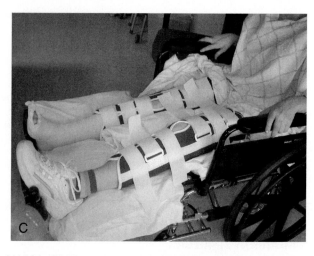

FIGURE **25-17** Patient is an adolescent female with CP who underwent multiple lower extremity procedures, including bilateral VROs. Patient is using bilateral Jordan splints.

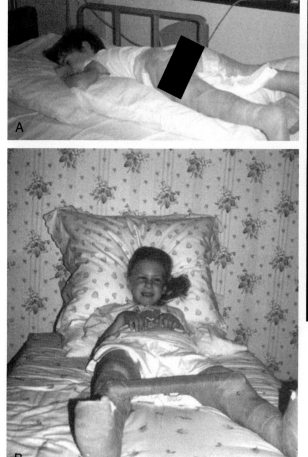

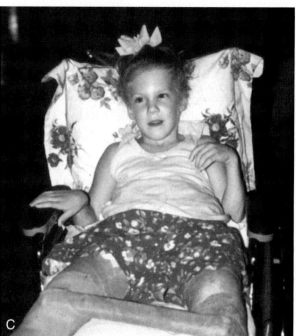

FIGURE **25-16** Patients with CP who underwent bilateral VROs and were placed in a spica cast postoperatively: *A.* Prone positioning with pillows. *B.* Supine positioning. *C.* Positioning in a reclining wheelchair.

postoperative period. For clarity sake, as needed, the postoperative rehabilitative care has been separated into two courses: rehabilitation of the patient immobilized in a spica cast and rehabilitation of the patient immobilized in Jordan splints.

Troubleshooting

Postoperative planning for home accommodations is imperative for all patients, regardless of the type of postoperative immobilization. A reclining wheelchair is necessary because the patient must avoid hip flexion beyond 90 degrees and hip adduction or internal rotation past midline. The patient immobilized in a spica cast may not fit into his or her current wheelchair because of the increased girth of the spica cast. A reclining wheelchair with elevating leg rests is the best way to accommodate a patient with a spica cast. Patients in Jordan splints may also initially require a reclining wheelchair and elevating leg rests on a short-term basis. The use of Jordan splints allows progression to the upright sitting position, with appropriate knee flexion, typically during the second postoperative week. For patients who were ambulatory before the surgery, caregiver education in performing non–weight-bearing transfers must be taught and emphasized. Transfer training and education are very important during the postoperative non–weight-bearing phase. Education stressing proper body mechanics will help the entire family during recovery.

POSTOPERATIVE REHABILITATION OF VRO: PHASE II (DAYS 5 TO 21)

Rehabilitative phase II for the patient in a spica cast remains the same as in phase I. Occasionally, the surgeon will allow the patient to be placed in standing position in the spica cast with supervision and support at home (Figure 25-18).

The patient immobilized in Jordan splints is afforded more mobility during this phase of rehabilitation. The caregiver is instructed to begin weaning the patient out of the Jordan splints during the day for early mobility

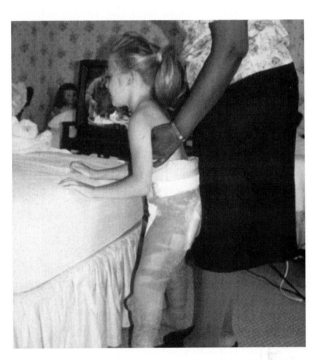

FIGURE 25-18 A 7-year-old patient who underwent bilateral VROs. Patient was placed in a spica cast. Note positioning in standing with assistance.

Postoperative Rehabilitation of VRO: Phase II (Days 5 to 21) with Spica Cast

GOALS
- Controlling postoperative pain/spasm
- Ensure that cast fits appropriately and does not impede circulation or cause irritation.
- Frequent changes of position to side-lying, prone, and up to reclining wheelchair
- Patient maintains non–weight-bearing until clearance from surgeon.

PRECAUTIONS
- Avoid prolonged periods of lying in supine.
- If patient is allowed to stand in the spica cast at home, supervision and support must be given at all times.

TREATMENT STRATEGIES
- Caregiver/patient education and importance of position changes
- Caregiver instructed in transfers
- The surgeon may allow the patient to stand in the spica cast at home.

CRITERIA FOR ADVANCEMENT
- Dependent upon the bone healing seen on radiograph; determined by the surgeon

Postoperative Rehabilitation of VRO: Phase II (Days 5 to 21) with Jordan Splints

GOALS

- Control of pain/spasm
- Decrease fear of movement
- Sitting in a wheelchair for longer periods of time
- Active and active-assisted motion of the lower extremities

PRECAUTIONS

- Avoid prolonged periods of lying in supine.
- Maintain hip precautions of no adduction or internal rotation past neutral; no hip flexion past 90 degrees
- Hip external rotation; extension and abduction as tolerated
- The patient is typically non–weight-bearing for at least 3 weeks, but this is dependent upon the bone healing and clearance by the surgeon.

TREATMENT STRATEGIES

- Control of postoperative pain and swelling
- Frequent change of position
  - To side-lying with pillows between legs to maintain hip abduction and neutral rotation
  - Reclining wheelchair, moving the trunk toward an upright position with knees flexed
- Passive, active-assisted, or active range of motion (AROM) of the hips, knees, and ankles as tolerated, to include heel slides, hip abduction with neutral hip rotation, quad sets, ankle pumps
- Review with caregiver/patient the importance of position changes and sitting in wheelchair with the knees flexed

CRITERIA FOR ADVANCEMENT

- Dependent upon the bone healing seen on radiograph; determined by the surgeon

and motion of the lower extremities. The patient must be encouraged to change positions frequently to prevent decubiti and actively perform the therapeutic exercises as instructed. The Jordan splints continue to be used at night throughout the postoperative period to maintain overall hip and knee extension during sleep. Following these recommendations will afford the patient improved range of passive joint motion. The patient begins active assistive and active exercises in phase II. Active movements will help the patient regain postoperatively his or her lower extremity muscle control and strength and prepare the patient for weight-bearing in phase III of rehabilitation.

Troubleshooting

Some patients/caregivers are reluctant to perform the HEP of active-assisted range of motion (AAROM) to the hips and knees in fear of disrupting the surgical procedure and/or causing pain to the child. Children are also fearful to move because of pain and weakness. It is very important that early mobilization be emphasized to prevent stiffness and occurrence of contractures, as well as ease the transition from a non–weight-bearing to a weight-bearing status. Postoperative movement pre-

cautions must continue to be emphasized during positioning and transfers.

POSTOPERATIVE REHABILITATION OF VRO: PHASE III (POSTOPERATIVE WEEKS 3 TO 6)

Initiation of weight-bearing activities typically begins in this phase, dependent upon bone healing on radiograph and physician clearance. The physical therapist must consider that postoperative immobility typically results in muscle weakness and atrophy, especially for the patient who is just coming out of the spica cast. A thorough physical therapy examination is necessary to determine both the appropriate therapeutic intervention and the plan for progression of the therapeutic program. Weight-bearing should be progressive, with appropriate therapeutic strategies and the use of assistive devices. Initially, the patient will be weak and fearful of standing. Weight-bearing can be progressed from sitting to standing gradually. The emphasis is on decreasing the amount of upper extremity support given by the physical therapist/assistive device for the patient to gradually take more weight through the lower extremities. Additionally, moving from prone on a therapy ball to

Postoperative Rehabilitation of VRO: Phase III (Weeks 3 to 6) with Spica Cast— Cast Removal

If there is adequate bone healing on radiograph at 3 weeks, the orthopedist may choose to remove the cast. Following cast removal, physical therapy will begin when prescribed by the physician.

GOALS

- Control pain and spasm.
- Decrease fear of movement.
- Upright sitting in wheelchair
- Increase ROM of hips/knees/ankles, maintaining hip precautions.
- Initiate weight-bearing.
- Begin lower extremity active movement and strengthening

PRECAUTIONS

- Continue to avoid periods of prolonged static positioning.
- Maintain hip precautions.
- Weight-bearing to patient's tolerance, with appropriate therapist support and assistive device

TREATMENT STRATEGIES

- Frequent changes of position: prone/supine/sitting/side-lying with pillows between legs to maintain neutral hip abduction and rotation
- Passive, progressing to AAROM and AROM of hips, knees, and ankles as tolerated, maintaining hip precautions
- Gluteal sets
- Quadriceps sets
- AROM/AAROM of the hips, knees, and ankles
  - Supine hip abduction, adduction to neutral
  - Heel slides for hip and knee flexion
  - Ankle dorsiflexion and plantar flexion
- Gentle stretching/elongation of the hip flexors, hamstrings, quadriceps, and gastrocsoleus as tolerated
- Initiation of weight-bearing can be achieved using the therapy ball to move from prone to standing with support. Increasing the amount of time and decreasing the amount of support as the patient progresses
- Weight-bearing with appropriate assistive device to begin as prescribed by surgeon
- Weight-shifting facilitated in sitting/standing to assist body to readjust to new lower extremity orientation
- HEP—warm water bath may aid in relaxation for performance of gentle ROM exercises

CRITERIA FOR ADVANCEMENT

- Dependent upon strength and ROM in the lower extremities as well as patient tolerance

supported standing with therapist assistance is also a good way to gradually increase tolerance to weight-bearing on the lower extremities. The physical therapist will offer adequate support until the patient has enough strength to maintain erect standing with an assistive device, such as a walker. Strengthening the lower extremities and decreasing fear to achieve standing and ambulation are the focus of this phase.

Troubleshooting

At times, the surgeon may not remove the spica cast because of inadequate bone healing. In this case, the patient would continue with the guidelines as detailed in postoperative phase II until the surgeon modifies the therapeutic program. Once the spica cast is removed the patient may experience stiffness and discomfort because of the immobilization.

Patients in this phase of rehabilitation innately recognize the weakness in their lower extremities and tend to be fearful and resistant to initiate weight-bearing activities. When adequate strength is achieved, the physical therapist should encourage progressive weight-bearing and begin gait training with the appropriate assistive device. It is important to address ROM limitations and continue to emphasize hip precautions to safely progress the patient.

Postoperative Rehabilitation of VRO: Phase III (Weeks 3 to 6) with Jordan Splints

If there is adequate healing on radiograph at 3 weeks, the orthopedist may allow the patient to begin weight-bearing.

GOALS

- Control pain and spasm.
- Decrease fear of movement.
- Initiate weight-bearing.
- Improve ROM of the lower extremities.

PRECAUTIONS

- Maintain hip precautions of no adduction or internal rotation past neutral; no hip flexion past 90 degrees
- Weight-bearing to patient's tolerance

TREATMENT STRATEGIES

- Frequent position changes as previously described
- Passive, progressing to AAROM to AROM of the hips, knees, and ankles as tolerated; heel slides for hip and knee flexion, supine hip abduction with neutral rotation, adduction to midline
- Begin lower extremity active-assistive/active movements against gravity if able.
- Ankle pumps
- Gluteal sets
- Quadriceps sets
- Ankle dorsiflexion and plantar flexion
- Gentle stretching/elongation of the hip flexors, hamstrings, quadriceps, and gastrocsoleus as tolerated
- Facilitate weight-shifting in sitting forward over feet to assist body to readjust to new lower extremity orientation and begin to accept weight through lower extremities
- Progressive weight-bearing with appropriate assistive device as prescribed by orthopedist

CRITERIA FOR ADVANCEMENT

- Dependent upon strength and ROM in the lower extremities

POSTOPERATIVE REHABILITATION OF VRO: PHASE IV (WEEK 6 TO MONTH 9 OR FULL RECOVERY)

In the beginning of this phase, the patient uses an assistive device for ambulation. The goal of phase IV is to decrease the amount of external support that is needed for ambulation as well as improve the parameters of gait. In this phase, normalizing the patient's gait pattern and developing core muscle strength should be emphasized to promote improved balance and stability.

Troubleshooting

The ability to progress the patient through phase IV is largely dependent upon the patient's level of functional ability and his or her neuromuscular capability. Physical therapy should emphasize lower extremity strengthening and gait training as well as functional skill ability. Specifically, the physical therapy should promote foot clearance during swing and coactivation of typical force couples during stance for control. Now that the lower extremities are in neutral rotation, the therapist should work on developing a heel-toe gait pattern with improved hip extension and graded knee control at mid-stance. Functional activities, such as stair and obstacle negotiation, should also be emphasized. It is important to note that overall lower extremity alignment has been changed by this surgery and, therefore, therapeutic intervention should provide a proprioceptive "cue" to assist the patient into his or her new lower extremity alignment/position. Stasikelis et al.[22] found that an average of 9 months of rehabilitation was needed following a femoral osteotomy in children with CP for the patient to return to, or surpass, the level of function before surgery. The protocol at HSS is that at 1 year post-surgery, the patient will return to the hospital to undergo removal of the hip plates. This typically requires a 1-night stay in the hospital and physical therapy intervention to assist the patient out of bed before discharge home.

Postoperative Rehabilitation of VRO: Phase IV (Week 6 to Month 9 or Full Recovery)

GOALS

- Develop/increase lower extremity ROM
- Strengthen lower extremities
- Improve quality of ambulation and progress ability and endurance ambulation with or without assistive device
- Return to or surpass the patient's functional level before surgery

PRECAUTIONS

- Avoid pain with therapeutic exercise and functional activities
- Avoid jumping/ballistic or high impact activities

TREATMENT STRATEGIES

- Core muscle strengthening exercises
- Sit to stand with facilitation; grade assistance as needed
- Qualitative gait training; work toward normalized gait pattern
- Endurance gait training
- Total gym activities (progressive weight-bearing and strengthening)
- Stationary bicycle
- Treadmill walking—forward, sideways, and retroambulation
- Stair negotiation
- Hip abduction in standing
- Single leg stance activities
- Side stepping with neutral rotation
- Return to typical physical therapy routine/program

HIP FLEXORS RELEASE

Excessive hip flexion is a common deformity in CP (Figure 25-19). Most hip flexor deformities are caused by a tight iliopsoas unit. A physical exam may reveal hip flexor spasticity or a hip flexion contracture.[3,4] Impairments associated with excessive hip flexion are restricted stride length during gait, excessive anterior pelvic tilt, excessive lordosis, hip dysplasia, subluxation, and dislocation.[23] A hip flexion contracture of more than 20 degrees is clinically significant because it may contribute to hip instability.[21] Hip flexor contractures can be assessed using the Thomas test (Figure 25-20) and/or the Staheli test (Figure 25-21).[3,19] Radiographic assessment of a hip flexion deformity is made by measuring the sacrofemoral angle.[9] The sacrofemoral angle is the angle formed between the top of the sacrum and the axis of the extended femoral shaft (Figure 25-22). The normal sacrofemoral angle is reported to range between 40 and 60 degrees. The sacrofemoral angle decreases with a hip flexion deformity.[9]

The goal of a hip flexor release is to decrease static contractures, rebalance the muscles around the hip joint to aid in hip stability, allow for functional hip extension during gait in ambulatory children, and preserve the ability of the psoas to function appropriately in a concentric fashion.[6] It is well reported in the literature that release of the iliopsoas tendon via tenotomy at the lesser trochanter may excessively weaken the hip flexors. The

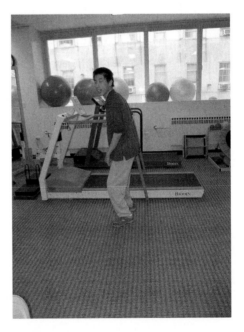

FIGURE **25-19** Patient with cerebral palsy who displays a crouched gait pattern with hip, knee, and ankle flexion deformity.

aforementioned procedure may cause such a significant decrease in hip flexor strength that the patient's ability to lift the limb to climb stairs or negotiate curbs becomes impaired.[4,6,23,25] Therefore, ambulatory children should

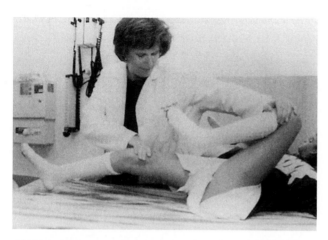

FIGURE **25-20** The Thomas test revealing a 20-degree hip flexion contracture. The opposite hip is fully flexed to flatten lumbar lordosis. *(From Herring, J.A. Tachdjian's Pediatric Orthopaedics, 3rd ed. WB Saunders, Philadelphia, 2002, p. 1178, with permission.)*

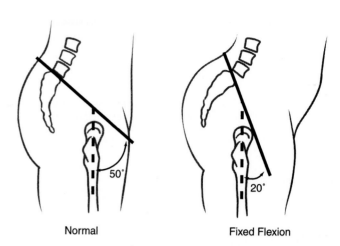

FIGURE **25-22** The sacrofemoral angle is formed between a line drawn along the superior aspect of the sacrum, and the femoral shaft decreases with flexion of the hip. With increasing hip flexion contracture, the pelvis tips forward and the sacrum becomes more vertical. *(From Herring, J.A. Tachdjian's Pediatric Orthopaedics, 3rd ed. WB Saunders, Philadelphia, 2002, p. 1179, with permission.)*

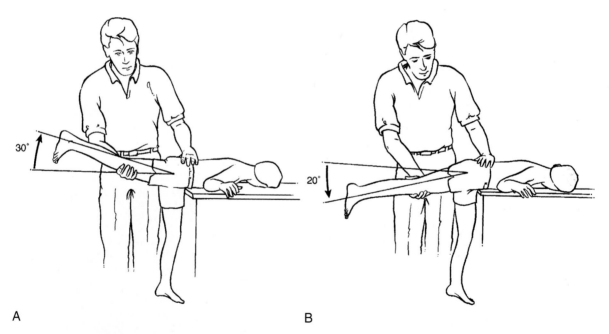

A   B

FIGURE **25-21** The Staheli test, used to determine hip flexion deformity with the patient prone. The pelvis is stabilized, the patient's thigh is raised toward the ceiling, and the tested hip is extended. The degree by which the hip fails to reach neutral position is the degree of deformity. A. Normal hip extension. B. Hip flexion contracture of 20 degrees. *(From Herring, J.A. Tachdjian's Pediatric Orthopaedics, 3rd ed. WB Saunders, Philadelphia, 2002, p. 1179, with permission.)*

have tenotomy of the psoas tendon alone (not the iliacus fibers) performed over the brim of the pelvis.[4,23] The most common procedure performed to address hip flexor contracture/spasticity at HSS is the release of psoas tendon over the pelvic brim.[10] As reported by Sutherland et al.,[23] this anterior approach psoas tenotomy at the pelvic brim increases hip extension in stance, increases stride length, and yet maintains hip flexion strength. This procedure preserves all of the muscle fibers of the iliacus and lengthens the psoas muscles—the portion of the muscle complex most directly related to the lordotic posture and pelvic alignment.[23]

Indications for a hip flexor release are

• Hip flexion contracture greater than 15 to 20 degrees[4,6,10,21]

- Radiographic measurement of the sacrofemoral angle is less than normal (40 to 60 degrees).[9]
- Hip flexor contracture associated with hip instability (subluxation)[10]

SURGICAL OVERVIEW

The major muscles responsible for flexion of the hip are the psoas major and the iliacus. The iliopsoas is considered the primary and most powerful flexor of the hip. It is composed of the iliacus muscle (which originates from the medial wall of the ilium) and the psoas muscles, which arise from the transverse processes and the sides of the bodies of all the lumbar vertebrae and the intervertebral disc annular ligaments from T12–L5 interspaces. The psoas major muscle terminates below the pelvic brim as a broad tendon that inserts into the lesser trochanter of the femur and the fibers of the iliacus muscle unite to form the tendon[6,26,27] (Figure 25-23).

The surgical procedure for release of the psoas muscles is performed with the patient supine. An oblique incision is made 2 cm below the anterior superior iliac spine to visualize the sartorius, tensor fascia lata (TFL), and the lateral femoral cutaneous nerve. The TFL is reflected to visualize the anterior inferior iliac spine and rectus femoris. The iliacus is retracted to reveal the tendon of the psoas, where it lies under the iliacus muscle. The psoas is then transected. In selected cases, when applicable, the TFL can be lengthened by incising the aponeurosis through the same incision[10,23] (Figure 25-24).

REHABILITATION OVERVIEW

Rehabilitation for a hip flexor release focuses on early ROM, positioning the patient to maintain the new muscle length, mobility out of bed to include ambulation (as functional level permits), and the return of the patient to his or her preexisting therapeutic program as soon as possible. No casting or splinting is used postoperatively post hip flexor release. Patient/caregiver education is important to address positioning and ROM exercises. In the ambulatory patient, ambulation with an appropriate assistive device should be initiated on POD 1. There is no specific preoperative therapeutic protocol prior to a hip flexor release.

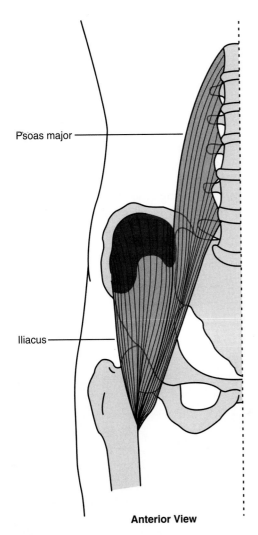

Anterior View

FIGURE **25-23** Anatomy of the psoas major and the iliacus muscles. *(From Daniels, L., Worthingham, C. Muscle Testing: Techniques of Manual Examination, 4th ed. WB Saunders, Philadelphia, 1980, p. 169, with permission.)*

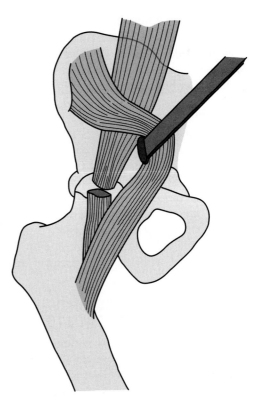

FIGURE **25-24** Surgical procedure depicting release of the psoas muscles over the brim of the pelvis. *(Courtesy of Dr. Leon Root, New York.)*

Postoperative Rehabilitation of Hip Flexor Release: Phase I (Days 1 to 2)

GOALS

- Control postoperative pain/swelling/spasms
- Full passive hip extension
- Caregiver able to perform gentle passive hip extension in prone
- Early weight-bearing—standing and ambulation as tolerated with appropriate assistive device
- Independence in HEP

PRECAUTIONS

- Avoid prolonged periods of hip flexion (sitting)

TREATMENT STRATEGIES

- Educate patient/caregiver in positioning to promote hip extension, prone-lying positioning
- Teach caregiver gentle passive and active assistive hip extension in prone
- Gait training with assistive device as appropriate. Educate patient/caregiver in importance of good posture; trunk/hip extension in standing/ambulation

CRITERIA FOR ADVANCEMENT

- Discharge from hospital PODs 1 to 2
- Dependent upon level of functioning before surgery

POSTOPERATIVE REHABILITATION OF HIP FLEXOR RELEASE: PHASE I (DAYS 1 TO 2)

Rehabilitation begins immediately on POD 1. The patient/caregiver is educated in the importance of prone-lying three to five times per day to maintain the new length of the hip flexors. If the patient did not have any bone procedures performed concurrently, weight bearing as tolerated (WBAT) is initiated at POD 1. Painful muscle spasms are particularly common in the first few days after hip surgery.[4]

Troubleshooting

A common finding in this phase is the tendency for pediatric patients to avoid movement because of pain/discomfort or muscle spasms. Caregivers may be unwilling to progress their children because of pain. The physical therapist needs to be supportive, yet firm, and encourage the patient/caregiver to strive for the attainment of full, gentle, passive hip extension. If pain and spasm are an issue, modalities to control pain/spasm should be discussed with both the caregiver and the physician.

POSTOPERATIVE REHABILITATION OF HIP FLEXOR RELEASE: PHASE II (DAY 3 TO WEEK 6)

During this phase of rehabilitation, standing and ambulation are emphasized to encourage active hip extension and strengthening of the gluteal muscles within their new and improved length-tension relationship. An HEP consisting of passive, active, and active assistive hip extension in prone or side-lying and prone positioning to tolerance three to five times per day is recommended.

Troubleshooting

During rehabilitation status post hip flexor release, the physical therapist will want to pay specific attention to the patient's ability to perform active isolated hip flexion. The patient may attempt to compensate for hip flexor weakness by substituting hip external or internal rotation for hip flexion or hike the pelvis to lift the limb. Additionally, developing the typical force couple between the abdominal muscles and the hip extensor muscles should be emphasized through core muscle activation exercises and strengthening activities. Qualitative gait training emphasizing trunk and hip extension is important for ambulatory patients.

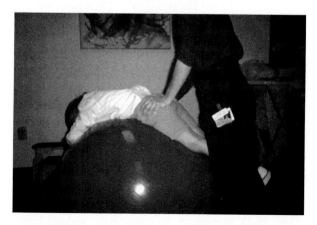

FIGURE **25-25** A 7-year-old girl status post (s/p) hip flexor release over therapy ball to passively extend the hip in prone.

Postoperative Rehabilitation of Hip Flexor Release: Phase II (Day 3 to Week 6)

GOALS
- Promote/maintain full passive and active hip extension in prone and side-lying
- Strengthening gluteals in new end range
- Improve hip extension in stance phase of gait
- Independence in HEP

PRECAUTIONS
- Avoid increased pain with therapeutic exercise and functional activities
- Avoid prolonged periods of hip flexion (sitting)

TREATMENT STRATEGIES
- Gluteal sets
- Passive/active/active-assistive hip extension in prone and side-lying (Figure 25-25)
- Bridging exercises
- Sit to stand with facilitation (Figure 25-26)
- Standing activities that promote gluteal and abdominal co-contraction
- Core muscle activation/exercises
- Stair climbing/step-up activities
- Treadmill walking when able (forward and retroambulation)
- HEP

CRITERIA FOR ADVANCEMENT
- Dependent upon level of functioning before surgery
- Resume preoperative physical therapy program

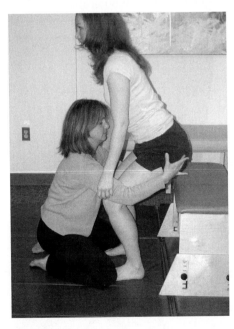

FIGURE 25-26 Moving from sit to stand with facilitation to activate the hip extensors.

HIP ADDUCTOR TENOTOMY

Hip adductor spasticity is common in many patients with CP, regardless of their ambulatory status. A physical exam may reveal the presence of a true hip adductor contracture.[3,9] Impairments associated with hip adductor spasticity or contractures are a scissoring type gait pattern demonstrating a decreased stride length and a decreased base of support (Figure 25-27), a predisposition to hip dysplasia or subluxation, and the inability of the caregiver to perform adequate perineal care in the more severely involved patient.[6,9,10] It is considered clinically significant if passive hip abduction is limited to 30 degrees or less.[10] Hip adductor contractures can be assessed in supine with the patient's knees and hips flexed or extended[4,6] (Figure 25-28). Radiographic assessment of the hip will determine the presence of hip instability, such as hip dysplasia or subluxation.[4,6] Improving the overall integrity and stability of the hip is one primary goal of hip adductor tenotomy in both the ambulatory and nonambulatory patient with CP. More specifically, in the ambulatory patient, the goal of surgery is to obtain a base of support during gait, which is similar to that of a normal gait pattern: 5 to 10 cm from heel to heel.[6] In the nonambulatory patient the goal of surgery may be to balance the muscles about the hip joint to improve or preserve the integrity and stability of the hip and pelvis, aid in an improved sitting posture with a leveled pelvis and neutral lower extremity alignment, and assist the caregiver in performing perineal care.[6,10]

Indications for a hip adductor tenotomy are

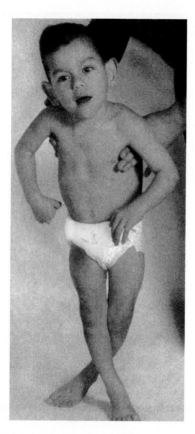

FIGURE **25-27** A 3-year-old boy with CP and scissoring of the lower extremities. *(From Herring, J.A. Tachdjian's Pediatric Orthopaedics, 3rd ed. WB Saunders, Philadelphia, 2002, p. 1179, with permission.)*

- Passive hip abduction is 30 degrees or less, with hips and knees flexed[10] or extended[4,6]
- Presence of scissoring gait, which interferes with functional ambulation[9]
- Radiographic evidence of hip subluxation (or potential)[9]
- The need to facilitate perineal care in patients with total body involvement[6,9]

Typically, an adductor release or lengthening is performed bilaterally in patients with diplegia and quadriplegia, unless the patient presents with a windswept deformity. A windswept deformity presents as persistent hip adduction, internal rotation of one lower extremity, and hip abduction, external rotation of the other lower extremity.[6] During assessment, if one hip is found to be less adducted than the other, both hips should typically be released, because there is a tendency for the nonoperated hip to subsequently become unstable if a unilateral release is performed.[28]

SURGICAL OVERVIEW

The major muscles responsible for adduction of the hip are the adductor magnus, adductor brevis, adductor longus, pectineus, and gracilis.[27] The hip adductor release most often performed in children with spastic diplegia is an adductor longus tenotomy.[6] The adductor longus originates from the outer margin of the inferior surface of the ischial tuberosity, the inferior ramus of the ischium, and the anterior surface of the inferior

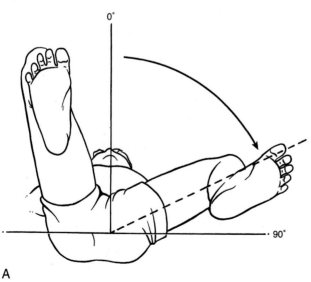

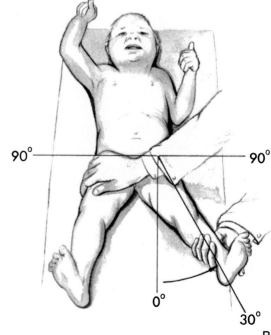

FIGURE **25-28** *A.* Hip abduction assessed with the patient's knees and hips in 90-degree flexion. *B.* Hip abduction assessed in supine with the hips and knees extended; the pelvis is steadied by the examiner's hand. *(From Herring, J.A. Tachdjian's Pediatric Orthopaedics, 3rd ed. WB Saunders, Philadelphia, 2002, p. 40, with permission.)*

ramus of the pubis. It inserts by a broad aponeurosis into the linea aspera via a tendon into the adductor tubercle on the medial condyle of the femur[27] (Figure 25-29).

Adductor tenotomy is performed with the patient supine. A transverse incision is made over the adductor longus tendon. The adductor longus and brevis, as well as the gracilis, are identified with blunt dissection. The adductor longus is transected. Simple percutaneous adductor longus tenotomy may be sufficient to achieve a release in ambulatory patients.[10] PROM of hip abduction is then assessed. The goal of this procedure is to obtain at least 50 to 60 degrees of passive hip abduction on each side, with the hips and knees flexed to 90 degrees[10] or at least 45 degrees of passive abduction, with the hips and knees extended.[4] Excessive lengthening beyond that leads to pelvic instability.[10] If passive abduction remains limited after the initial adductor longus tenotomy, the adductor brevis and gracilis may also be released[4,10,19] (Figure 25-30).

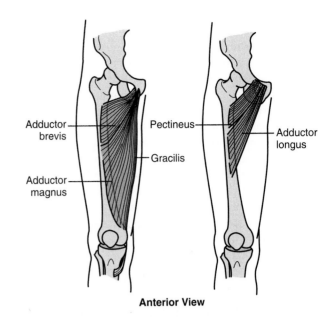

Anterior View

FIGURE **25-29** Anatomy of the hip adductor muscles. *(From Daniels, L., Worthingham, C. Muscle Testing: Techniques of Manual Examination, 4th ed. WB Saunders, Philadelphia, 1980, p. 190, with permission.)*

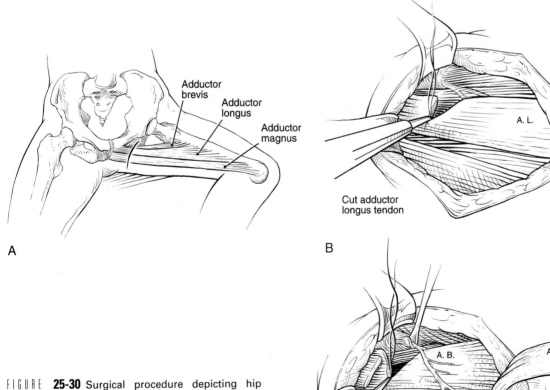

A

B

Cut adductor longus tendon

• Cut adductor brevis
• Keep obturator branches intact

C

FIGURE **25-30** Surgical procedure depicting hip adductor tenotomy. *A.* A transverse incision is made in the groin crease and centered over the adductor longus tendon, which is easily palpated. *B.* The adductor longus tendon is identified, isolated from the deeper adductor brevis, and divided. *C.* The adductor brevis is then divided, if necessary. *(From Herring, J.A. Tachdjian's Pediatric Orthopaedics, 3rd ed. WB Saunders, Philadelphia, 2002, p. 1181, with permission.)*

REHABILITATION OVERVIEW

Rehabilitation for a hip adductor tenotomy is similar to that for the hip flexor release focusing on early mobilization and out-of-bed mobility, including gait training, ROM/positioning to maintain the new muscle length, and return to the preexisting therapeutic program as soon as possible. If hip adductor release is the sole procedure performed, there is no postoperative casting or splinting. If other procedures are performed in conjunction with a hip adductor tenotomy, then the postoperative rehabilitation must be reflective of that. Patient/caregiver education to address positioning and ROM exercises is important. In the ambulatory patient, ambulation with an appropriate assistive device should be initiated on POD 1. There is no specific preoperative therapeutic protocol before an adductor tenotomy.

POSTOPERATIVE REHABILITATION OF HIP ADDUCTOR TENOTOMY: PHASE I (DAYS 1 TO 2)

Rehabilitation begins immediately while the patient is in the hospital on POD 1. The patient/caregiver is educated in the importance of positioning the patient with a pillow in between the lower extremities to maintain hip abduction in supine (Figure 25-31). If the patient did not have any bone procedures performed concurrently, then WBAT is started on POD 1. Discharge from the hospital is typically on POD 1 to 2.

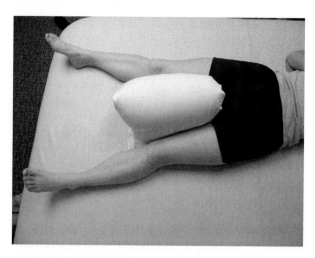

FIGURE **25-31** A pillow is placed between the lower extremities to maintain hip abduction in supine.

Troubleshooting

Muscle spasms and pain are common postoperatively and should be addressed as previously mentioned in this chapter. The physical therapist should instruct the patient/caregiver in an HEP that strives for the attainment of full, gentle, passive hip abduction ROM in supine. During passive hip abduction the therapist should instruct the caregiver to stabilize the pelvis with one hand while simultaneously abducting the opposite hip with the other hand. Compliance with the HEP and

---

Postoperative Rehabilitation of Hip Adductor Tenotomy: Phase I (Days 1 to 2)

GOALS

- Control postoperative pain/swelling/spasms
- Full passive hip abduction in supine
- Caregiver to perform gentle passive and active-assistive hip abduction in supine
- Early weight-bearing—standing and ambulation as tolerated with appropriate assistive device
- Independence in HEP

PRECAUTIONS

- Avoid increased pain with therapeutic exercise and functional activities
- Avoid prolonged periods of hip adduction (side-lying) to maintain lengthened muscle position

TREATMENT STRATEGIES SPECIFIC TO INCREASING HIP ABDUCTION

- Educate patient/caregiver in positioning to promote hip abduction
- Supine/sitting/side-lying positioning; pillow placement between legs to maintain hip abduction
- Teach caregiver gentle passive and active-assistive hip abduction in supine (Figure 25-32)
- Gait training with assistive device as appropriate. Educate patient/caregiver in the importance of proper foot placement and adequate base of support in standing

CRITERIA FOR ADVANCEMENT

- Discharge from the hospital postoperative days 1 to 2
- Dependent upon level of functioning before surgery

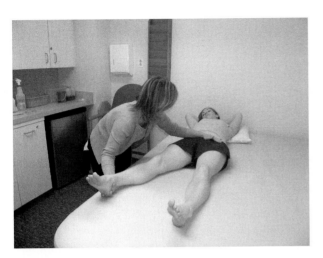

FIGURE **25-32** Passive hip abduction in supine with the pelvis stabilized.

early weight-bearing/ambulation as tolerated should be emphasized.

POSTOPERATIVE REHABILITATION OF HIP ADDUCTOR TENOTOMY: PHASE II (DAY 3 TO WEEK 6)

During this phase, standing and ambulation are emphasized to encourage hip abductor activity, with the patient being able to demonstrate a leveled pelvis in static standing and an adequate base of support during ambulation. The abductors are inherently weak in patients with CP, and excessive weakening of the adductors may create greater side-to-side swaying of the trunk and pelvis during walking.[21] Therefore, it is important to focus on developing a balance of muscle strength between the hip abductor and adductor muscles for improved pelvic stability and functional control during ambulation. The therapist should watch for the use of compensations for inefficient muscle recruitment and strength. The therapeutic goal of this phase of rehabilitation is to improve overall function and quality of movement. The HEP is progressed based on evaluative findings.

Troubleshooting

Children with CP often have difficulty isolating specific muscles, leading to compensatory movement patterns and synergy patterns during exercises and functional activities. During rehabilitation post-adductor tenotomy, the physical therapist should pay specific attention to the patient's ability to maintain neutral alignment of the hip and pelvis during hip abduction exercises, because compensatory hip flexion or pelvic hiking is common during this activity. Gait training should emphasize the ability to maintain a neutral

---

Postoperative Rehabilitation of Hip Adductor Tenotomy: Phase II (Day 3 to Week 6)

GOALS
- Promote/maintain full passive and active hip abduction in supine
- Strengthening hip abductors in new end range
- Develop a balance between hip adductor/abductor musculature
- Improve hip abductor control in standing/stance phase of gait/unilateral stance
- Independence in home exercise program (HEP)

PRECAUTIONS
- Avoid pain with therapeutic exercise and functional activities
- Avoid prolonged periods of hip adduction (side-lying, sitting)

TREATMENT STRATEGIES SPECIFIC TO INCREASING HIP ABDUCTION
- Supine active hip abduction
- Side-lying A/AA hip abduction
- Clamshell exercises (25-33, *A* and *B*)
- Sit to stand while straddling a bolster
- Facilitate single leg stance
- Standing active hip abduction (Figure 25-34)
- Side-stepping/cruising with facilitation
- Treadmill walking sideways, if able
- Step up and down to the side off a step

CRITERIA FOR ADVANCEMENT
- Dependent upon level of functioning before surgery
- Resume preoperative physical therapy program

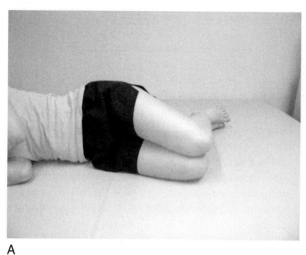
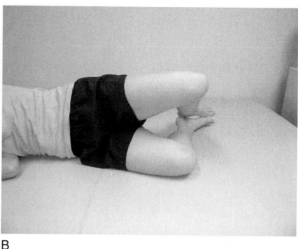

A   B

FIGURE **25-33** *A, B.* Clam shell exercises.

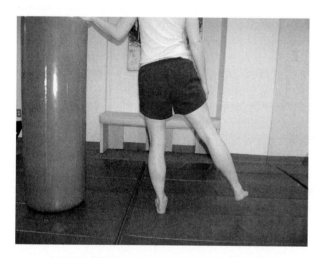

FIGURE **25-34** Standing active hip abduction.

pelvis in the frontal plane in double support and single limb stance. The hip adductors function to stabilize the hip against excessive abduction during gait, allowing for more effective hip flexor and extensor activity.[4] It is therefore important to work on control of both the hip adductors and abductors to improve overall quality of gait and movement.

RECTUS FEMORIS TRANSFER

In children with CP, spasticity of the quadriceps muscle leading to continuous rectus femoris activity throughout the swing phase (and sometimes throughout the entire gait cycle) severely limits knee flexion in swing and subsequent foot clearance to take steps.[29–31] Functionally, the child displays a stiff knee gait pattern (Figure 25-35) with decreased ability to step up to negotiate a curb-step or stairs and may frequently trip and drag his or her toes on the floor. Observation of the

child's footwear typically reveals scuff marks on the toe box. Distal rectus femoris transfer is a commonly performed operation in children with CP who present with a stiff knee gait. Transferring the distal rectus femoris posterior to the axis of the knee into either the gracilis or semitendinosus enhances knee flexion in the swing phase.[4,29]

Additionally, in children with CP, there may be cospasticity of the rectus femoris muscle and hamstring muscles, limiting overall knee ROM to less than 80% of normal.[4] Therefore, distal rectus femoris transfers are frequently combined with hamstring lengthenings.[30,32,33] In a child with CP who presents with a crouched knee gait, if only hamstring lengthenings are performed to gain more knee extension, yet the rectus femoris muscle is spastic (active during swing), then the result may be a stiff knee gait pattern.[30,31,33] A preoperative gait analysis is extremely important to assess the firing pattern of the rectus femoris to determine the amount of peak knee flexion during the swing phase of gait. Normally, the rectus femoris muscle begins to fire at terminal swing along with the other quadriceps muscles to prepare the limb for acceptance of weight.[30,31] Clinically, rectus femoris tightness or contracture can be assessed using the Duncan Ely test[14] (Figure 25-36).

Indications for a rectus femoris muscle transfer are

- Stiff knee gait pattern (decreased knee flexion in swing) and positive Duncan Ely test[3,32]
- Poor foot clearance and rectus femoris activity in the swing phase of gait confirmed by 3-D motion analysis with EMG[32]

SURGICAL OVERVIEW

The rectus femoris is part of the quadriceps muscle group and acts as a primary knee extensor. It originates

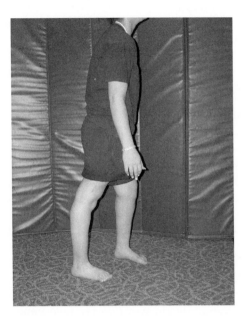

FIGURE **25-35** A 13-year-old girl with a stiff knee gait pattern.

by two tendons: the straight head from the anterior inferior iliac spine and the reflected head from a groove just above the brim of the acetabulum.[26] The muscle fibers attach into the base of the patella via the tendon of the quadriceps femoris into the tibial tuberosity[27] (Figure 25-37). The rectus femoris thus acts on both the knee and hip joints because it is a two-joint muscle. The rectus femoris is more effective as a hip flexor if the knee flexes simultaneously because this permits the muscle to contract within a favorable range. Conversely, the rectus is more efficient as a knee extensor if the hip extends simultaneously with the knee.[26]

Rectus femoris transfer is performed with the patient supine. A longitudinal incision is performed at the mid to distal anterior thigh, and the incision is extended distally. The quadriceps tendon is identified, and the rectus femoris tendon is isolated from the tendinous portion of the vastus medialis and lateralis. The rectus femoris is further separated from the intermedialis. Next, the rectus femoris tendon is released from its distal insertion at the patella, ensuring that the knee joint is not disturbed. The tendon, which is flat, is then surgically "tubed" to have the shape of a typical tendon. The tendon is brought from the anterior thigh through a sub-

FIGURE **25-36** Duncan Ely test. *A.* The Duncan Ely test is performed with the patient in prone. *B.* The knee is passively flexed. *C.* A positive result occurs when the ipsilateral buttock rises, which may indicate rectus femoris spasticity. *(From Herring, J.A. Tachdjian's Pediatric Orthopaedics, 3rd ed. WB Saunders, Philadelphia, 2002, p. 1172, with permission.)*

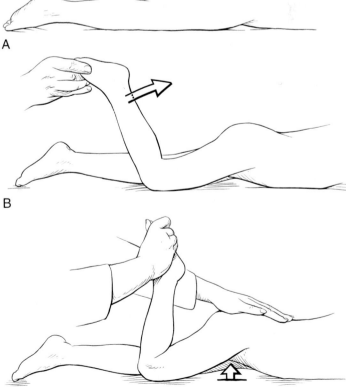

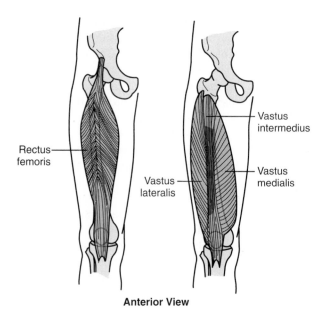

Anterior View

FIGURE **25-37** The anatomy of the quadriceps muscle. *(From Daniels, L., Worthingham, C. Muscle Testing: Techniques of Manual Examination, 4th ed. WB Saunders, Philadelphia, 1980, p. 207, with permission.)*

cutaneous tunnel and is sewn into either the semitendinosus or gracilis, thus making the rectus femoris muscle act as a knee flexor by changing its insertion.[10,19,34] The tendon transfer should be fixed with the knee in about 15 to 20 degrees of flexion[10] (Figure 25-38).

REHABILITATION OVERVIEW

The rehabilitation program following rectus femoris transfer is designed to facilitate increased knee ROM passively and actively immediately after surgery. In the immediate postoperative phase, the patient may have significant spasms in the quadriceps muscle. Jordan splints (Figure 25-39) are used during ambulation because of quadriceps weakness and decreased ability to maintain knee extension during the stance phase of gait. The physical therapist will begin to remove the Jordan splints during ambulation, based upon the patient's ability to extend his or her knee during gait. The physical therapist should focus on the neuromuscular re-education of the transferred muscle and using its new function to facilitate increased knee flexion during ambulation on level surfaces and during stair negotiation.

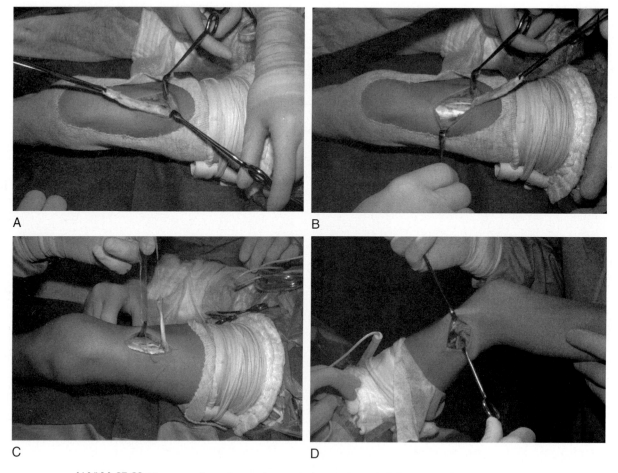

FIGURE **25-38** The rectus femoris transfer surgical procedure. *A, B.* The rectus femoris is released from the distal insertion at the patella and isolated from the other quadriceps muscle. *C.* The tendon is "tubed" and ready to be transferred. *D.* The tendon is brought through the subcutaneous tunnel and sewn into the semitendinosus or gracilis. *(Courtesy of Dr. Leon Root, New York.)*

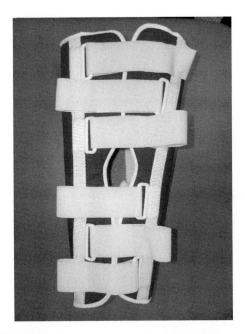

FIGURE **25-39** Jordan splints are worn around leg between the hip and the ankle to maintain the knee in extension.

Traditional therapeutic and neurodevelopmental techniques should be incorporated to improve ROM and strength. Strengthening activities should be progressed and incorporated during functional activities. The patient and his or her family must play an active role in the recovery from rectus femoris transfer surgery to optimize the knee motion gained by the surgery.

PREOPERATIVE CONSIDERATIONS

The preoperative phase is critical in determining the need for a rectus femoris transfer. The surgeon should be provided with complete information inclusive of a thorough physical therapy examination that presents objective measurements and clinical observation of the patient's ability to flex his or her knee(s) during gait as well as when negotiating stairs and curbs. The patient should also be referred for a 3-D gait analysis with muscle EMG to determine the knee ROM and the firing pattern of the rectus femoris during the swing phase of gait. The clinical assessment and the results of the gait analysis are invaluable in assisting the surgeon in making the decision as to whether to perform a rectus femoris transfer. There is no specific preoperative therapeutic protocol before rectus femoris transfer surgery.

POSTOPERATIVE REHABILITATION

Physical therapy is initiated on POD 2 because the patient is typically on bed rest on POD 1. Postoperative spasms are very common with rectus femoris transfers. The patient and caregiver should be aware of this postoperative finding, and the physician will typically prescribe pain and antispasmodic medication for the

patient as appropriate. It is important to stress early knee ROM, into both knee flexion and extension. As previously mentioned, it is not uncommon that a rectus femoris transfer be performed concurrently with a hamstring lengthening. The patient will use Jordan splints to maintain knee extension during ambulation, as a result of the initial presentation of knee flexion in stance postoperatively. The patient is encouraged to remove the splints in sitting to allow for the knee to flex.

POSTOPERATIVE REHABILITATION OF RECTUS FEMORIS TRANSFER: PHASE I (DAYS 2 TO 3)

During phase I, the patient and caregiver are instructed in active-assisted knee flexion and passive knee extension. It is imperative that the patient perform active-assisted ROM of the knee to begin to use the rectus femoris in its new role as a knee flexor (Figure 25-40). If the patient did not have any bone procedures performed concurrently, ambulation WBAT is initiated on POD 2, with an appropriate assistive device and Jordan splints.

Troubleshooting

In phase I, following rectus femoris transfers, the physical therapist should be attentive to the postoperative

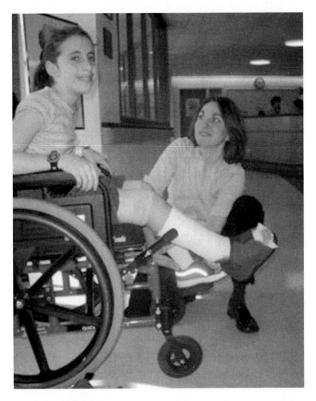

FIGURE **25-40** Patient is a 12-year-old girl with CP who underwent multiple soft tissue procedures in the lower extremities, including bilateral rectus femoris transfers. The therapist and patient are working on knee ROM.

Postoperative Rehabilitation of Rectus Femoris Transfer: Phase I (Days 2 to 3)

GOALS

- Control of postoperative spasm, which is common with rectus femoris transfers
- Control of postoperative pain and swelling
- Improve PROM knee extension and active-assistive knee flexion
- Sitting with knees in a flexed position, working toward 45 degrees of knee flexion
- Early weight-bearing for standing and ambulation with the use of Jordan splints and appropriate assistive device
- Educate/train caregiver for independence in HEP
  - Knee ROM exercises in sitting (passive knee extension and AA knee flexion)
  - Gentle passive SLR
  - Positioning—no prolonged periods of knee flexion or extension
  - Ankle pumps
  - Ambulation, as tolerated, with appropriate assistive device and Jordan splints

PRECAUTIONS

- Avoid prolonged periods of knee flexion (sitting) or knee extension
- Avoid increased pain with therapeutic exercise and functional activities
- Monitor use/tolerance of Jordan splints application/fit/tolerance/irritation
- Monitor surgical scar for color changes/swelling/discharge/drainage
- Jordan splints must be on at night for sleeping for 6 weeks

TREATMENT STRATEGIES

- Positioning, as noted above
- Training patient in ambulation with improved knee extension in stance phase
- Passive knee extension in supine/sitting
- AAROM knee flexion in sitting at edge of bed; goal is to obtain 45 degrees knee flexion
- Ankle pumps
- Progress ambulation with Jordan splints and appropriate assistive device, as tolerated, with specific focus on quality of gait pattern to gain better control of knee flexion during swing and extension during stance

CRITERIA FOR ADVANCEMENT

- Discharge from the hospital is typically on POD 3, depending on patient comfort level as a result of postoperative pain and spasm.
- Active-assistive knee flexion to 45 degrees
- Ability to passively extend the knee in supine
- Dependent upon level of functioning before surgery

spasms that patients often experience following this surgical procedure, especially with movement into knee flexion. The therapist and caregiver should take care with knee ROM to ensure pain- and spasm-free movement. Ice packs may provide comfort to the patient. PROM should be performed gently and slowly. Deep breathing exercises may be useful to assist the patient in relaxation. Sitting is the optimal position to slowly progress knee flexion ROM. If the patient is in a wheelchair, an alternate manner to progress knee flexion is to gradually lower the elevating leg rests to allow for a comfortable increase in knee flexion ROM. It is imperative to mobilize the knee early via active-assistive knee flexion to gain optimal results.

POSTOPERATIVE REHABILITATION OF RECTUS FEMORIS TRANSFER: PHASE II (DAYS 4 TO 14)

Typically, the patient will present with a postoperative knee flexion lag in standing and ambulation. The Jordan splints will be used until the patient can maintain adequate knee extension during stance and gait. Rehabilitation emphasizes active-assistive knee flexion and passive knee extension ROM exercises, the ability to extend the knee in standing and walking, as well as to obtain co-activation of the quadriceps and the hamstrings around the knee joint for stability. Core muscle control and trunk/abdominal strengthening should also be emphasized throughout the next phases of rehabilitation.

Postoperative Rehabilitation of Rectus Femoris Transfer: Phase II (Days 4 to 14)

GOALS

- Control of postoperative spasm, which is common with rectus femoris transfer
- Control of postoperative pain and swelling
- Postoperative weeks 1 to 2 removal of Jordan splints during waking hours
- Emphasis on both passive extension and active-assistive flexion of the knee
- Sitting with knees in a flexed position with a goal of 90 degrees
- Progress ambulation with appropriate assistive device and begin to wean patient out of Jordan splints
- Advance out of Jordan splints if able to actively extend knee during ambulation
- Independence in the HEP
  - Positioning so as not to be in prolonged periods of knee flexion or extension
  - Knee ROM exercises—AA flexion, passive extension
  - Gentle passive SLR
  - Quadriceps sets
  - Assisted heel slides in supine
  - Ambulation as tolerated with appropriate assistive device

PRECAUTIONS

- Avoid prolonged periods of knee flexion (sitting) or knee extension.
- Avoid pain with therapeutic exercise and functional activities.
- Monitor use/tolerance of Jordan splints application/fit/tolerance/irritation.
- Monitor surgical scar for color changes/swelling/discharge/drainage.
- Jordan splints must be on at night for sleeping for 6 weeks.

TREATMENT STRATEGIES

- Gait training: improved knee extension in stance phase, improved knee flexion in swing, and ability to co-activate hamstrings and quadriceps for knee stability
- AAROM knee flexion—working toward obtaining active knee flexion
- Passive extension in sitting
- Ankle pumps, quadriceps sets, passive SLR
- Progress ambulation with Jordan splints and appropriate assistive device as tolerated with specific focus on endurance

CRITERIA FOR ADVANCEMENT

- Ability to actively flex the knee to 90 degrees
- The ability to actively extend the knee in standing is very important. Jordan splints may be discontinued when the patient is able to display full knee extension in stance. If there is any lag into knee flexion, the splints should continue to be used.
- Dependent upon level of functioning before surgery

Troubleshooting

A common finding following rectus femoris transfers is the lack of full and fluid knee motion during gait. Because patients with CP may have a tendency to get "stuck" in a mid-range position, it is important to monitor and promote the full arc of knee flexion and extension during the appropriate phases of gait. The treatment and goals of this phase must be individually based and continually updated, according to the patient's progress and functional level.

POSTOPERATIVE REHABILITATION OF RECTUS FEMORIS TRANSFER: PHASE III (WEEKS 2 TO 6)

Overall knee ROM must continue to be addressed during this phase of rehabilitation. At the end of phase III the patient should display full passive ROM of knee flexion and extension, and the therapist should be working toward the attainment of full arc of active motion of the knee joint in isolation and during gait. Strengthening of the lower extremities for functional activities must also be emphasized through open and closed chain exercises and activities. It is very important to work toward developing the appropriate timing of knee flexion during swing as well as knee extension during stance to obtain a more normalized gait pattern.

Troubleshooting

A common finding following rectus femoris transfer is a decreased ability to fully extend the knee during stance and/or decreased knee flexion during the swing phase of gait. In the first instance, emphasis should be on strengthening the quadriceps. For patients who have

Postoperative Rehabilitation of Rectus Femoris Transfer: Phase III (Weeks 2 to 6)

GOALS
- Discontinue use of Jordan splints during waking hours at 2 weeks postoperatively
- Discontinue use of Jordan splints at night 6 weeks postoperatively
- Increase knee flexion passively and actively
- Promote/maintain knee extension passively and actively
- Strengthening lower extremities
- Improved foot clearance during swing phase of gait
- Return to stair/curb negotiation as functional level permits

PRECAUTIONS
- Avoid pain with therapeutic exercise and functional activities
- Monitor use/tolerance of Jordan splints application/fit/tolerance/irritation
- Monitor surgical scar for color changes/swelling/discharge/drainage
- Jordan splints must be on at night for sleeping for 6 weeks to maintain knee extension

TREATMENT STRATEGIES
- Active knee flexion in sitting
- Active/active-assisted knee flexion in prone
- Standing activities with facilitation for co-activation of quadriceps and hamstrings
- Activities to promote knee flexion in standing (i.e., low step up, stepping over small obstacles)
- Activities to promote concentric and isometric quadriceps strengthening
- Transitions from sit to and from stand with therapeutic assistance as needed
- Total gym squats, progressing to wall squats
- Ascending stairs emphasizing graded control and progress to descending stairs with control
- Treadmill/gait training
- Weight-shifting in stance progressing toward single limb stance activities—emphasizing knee control
- Continue with HEP: evaluation-based

CRITERIA FOR ADVANCEMENT
- Dependent on the level of functioning before surgery
- Ability to extend knee in stance phase of gait
- Ability to flex knee in swing phase of gait
- Discontinue use of Jordan splints at night 6 weeks postoperatively.

difficulty with decreased knee flexion in swing, special attention during rehabilitation should focus on the strength and timing of the knee flexion to be able to lift the leg to step forward or over obstacles (Figure 25-41).

POSTOPERATIVE REHABILITATION OF RECTUS FEMORIS TRANSFER: PHASE IV (WEEKS 6 TO 14)

This phase of rehabilitation is evaluation-based, and the patient is progressed accordingly.

It is the therapist's role to ascertain which patients can be progressed to this level. Given the variability of functional levels in CP, some patients may never progress to this phase of rehabilitation.

Troubleshooting

Emphasis should be placed on improving the quality of gait. A full observational gait analysis should be performed at this time to assess postoperative functional gains. The therapist should assess both the available

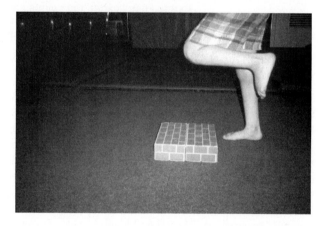

FIGURE **25-41** A child with CP who underwent bilateral rectus femoris transfers. The patient is working on stepping over blocks to increase knee flexion.

Postoperative Rehabilitation of Rectus Femoris Transfer: Phase IV (Weeks 6 to 14)

GOALS

- Enhance co-activation of quadriceps and hamstrings in single limb stance.
- Improve eccentric hamstring activation for deceleration during swing.
- Improve eccentric quadriceps control for functional activities (stair descension, stand to sit).
- Increase functional muscle strength.
- Continue to improve quality of ambulation.
- Return to or surpass functional level before surgery.

PRECAUTIONS

- Avoid pain with therapeutic exercise and functional activities

TREATMENT STRATEGIES

- Stair-stretch for increased knee flexion; single-leg stance activities to promote co-activation
- Swing phase activities
- Stand to sit, emphasizing eccentric control of quadriceps
- Total gym progressive
- Wall squats
- Step-ups/step over
- Stair negotiation, emphasizing eccentric control
- Treadmill walking
- Stationary bicycle
- Gait training
- HEP: evaluation-based

CRITERIA FOR ADVANCEMENT

- Dependent on the level of functioning before surgery
- Ability to flex knee in swing phase of gait and allow for heel strike at initial contact
- Resume existing preoperative physical therapy program

range of knee joint motion and the timing of muscle activation during the specific phases of the gait cycle, and the therapeutic program should proceed based on the findings.

HAMSTRING LENGTHENING

Many patients with CP exhibit excessive knee flexion because of spastic or tight hamstring musculature. A knee flexion deformity may be the result of a fixed capsular contracture, but, typically, it is caused by simply spastic and tight hamstring muscles.[4] In normal gait, the hamstring muscles are active eccentrically as they decelerate the forward flexing limb during the latter part of the swing phase of gait.[35] In ambulatory patients with CP, the hamstrings tend to be active throughout the entire stance phase, thus leading to persistent knee flexion during the stance phase of gait, as well as a shortened stride length during swing phase.[35] Additionally, with a knee flexion deformity, there is often an associated hip flexion contracture, and a crouched gait pattern is observed[4] (see Figure 25-19). If the child with CP displays knee flexion at mid-stance, significant work

must be performed by the quadriceps to prevent the knee from collapsing. Patients who exhibit this type of a crouch gait pattern present with decreased walking endurance as well as increased energy consumption.[35] Walking in a crouched gait pattern also produces increased stresses at the knee, which can lead to pain and degenerative changes later in life. In most children with spastic diplegia, once a knee flexion pattern in gait develops, the deformity will typically increase over time, eventually limiting ambulation ability.[35]

Clinically, hamstring tightness can be assessed by performing a straight leg raise (SLR) (Figure 25-42) or measuring the popliteal angle (Figure 25-43). The normal ROM of an SLR is 90 degrees, and a normal popliteal angle is considered full knee extension to 180 degrees, with the hip flexed to 90 degrees.[14,21] A preoperative gait analysis may support surgical decision making because it is helpful in assessing the firing pattern of the hamstring musculature as it corresponds to the various phases of gait. It also provides objective data of the ROM at the knee joint during gait.

Indications for a hamstring lengthening are

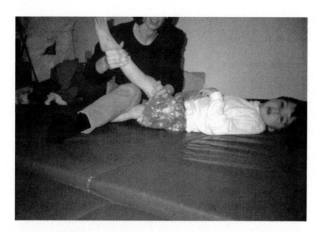

FIGURE **25-42** Performance of an SLR to assess hamstring tightness.

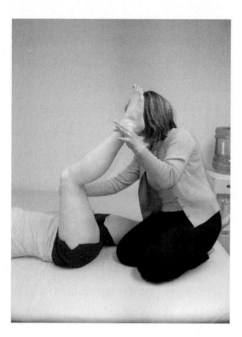

FIGURE **25-43** Assessing the popliteal angle to evaluate hamstring tightness.

- Knee flexion of 15 degrees or more during the stance phase of ambulation[6,21]
- Decreased stride length[10]
- Straight leg raise less than 70 degrees or popliteal angle less than 135 degrees[4]
- Knee pain during transfers in nonambulatory patients or patients with limited ambulation ability[9]
- Increased posterior pelvic tilt, which impacts postural alignment and/or ability to sit upright[6,10]

SURGICAL OVERVIEW

The primary muscles responsible for knee flexion are the hamstring muscles. The hamstrings are comprised of the biceps femoris, semitendinosus, and semimembranosus. The accessory muscles that act to flex the knee are the popliteus, sartorius, gracilis, and gastrocnemius.[27] The long head of the biceps femoris originates from the distal and medial aspect of the ischial tuberosity and the inferior part of the sacrotuberous ligament. The short head of the biceps femoris originates at the lateral lip of the linea aspera and lateral condyle of the femur. Both tendons insert into the head of the fibula and lateral tibial condyle.[27] The semitendinosus originates at the ischial tuberosity and inserts into the proximal part of the anteromedial surface of the tibia. The semimembranosus originates at the ischial tuberosity and inserts into the horizontal groove on the posteromedial aspect of the medial tibial condyle and into the posterior aspect of the lateral femoral condyle[27] (Figure 25-44).

The medial hamstrings are usually the tighter muscle group and are typically surgically addressed first.[4] Lengthening of the hamstrings can be performed in supine or prone.[10] Lengthening the medial hamstrings is performed by incising the fascial aponeurosis of the semimembranosus muscle at one or two levels and step-cut lengthening or tenotomizing the semitendinosus and gracilis tendons. If adequate ROM is not obtained after these procedures, the lateral hamstrings are

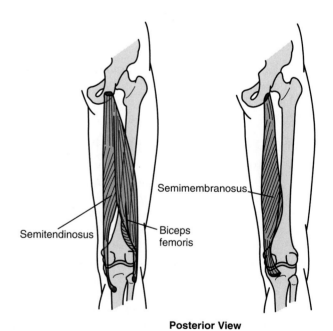

Semimembranosus

Semitendinosus

Biceps femoris

Posterior View

FIGURE **25-44** Anatomy of the hamstring muscles. *(From Daniels, L., Worthingham, C. Muscle Testing: Techniques of Manual Examination, 4th ed. WB Saunders, Philadelphia, 1980, p. 202, with permission.)*

addressed and the biceps femoris may then also require aponeurotic lengthening[4,10,19] (Figure 25-45).

At times, a proximal lengthening of the hamstrings is performed. Results have shown, however, that after this procedure lumbar lordosis may increase because of overactivity of the hip flexors, and the distal hamstrings may still remain tight.[4]

REHABILITATION OVERVIEW

Rehabilitation following hamstring lengthening is designed to both maintain and actively use the newly obtained length of the hamstrings in all positions. In the initial postoperative phase, the patient will use Jordan splints for ambulation and during sleeping hours to maintain knee extension. Rehabilitation will focus on decreasing the use of the Jordan splints during ambulation based on the patient's ability to extend the knees during the stance phase of gait. Additionally, rehabilitation will focus on functionally integrating the newfound hamstring length by facilitation of an upright pelvis in sitting or a greater step length during ambulation. Knee ROM and ambulation with an assistive device is begun early, and all activities should be progressed as strength improves.

PREOPERATIVE CONSIDERATIONS

To determine the most appropriate treatment for the patient with CP one must first determine the primary impairments and the cause of the impairment. As with many issues in CP, this analysis is difficult because the deformity is usually the result of not just a single problem but a combination of problems, all of which must be identified and addressed appropriately to improve this dynamic deformity.[35] The knee is a pivotal joint in lower extremity biomechanics. In a patient who is being considered for hamstring lengthenings, the hip and ankle joints should be carefully evaluated to ascertain their role in the presentation of a crouched gait. Specific ROM measurements should include popliteal angle, SLR, and the Thomas test. Other aspects of the physical therapy examination should include a functional and qualitative movement assessment and observational gait analysis, with possibly a 3-D gait analysis with EMG data collection. Identification of the primary impairments vs the secondary compensations will help ensure a positive and more predictable surgical outcome.

There is no specific preoperative therapeutic protocol before a hamstring lengthening procedure.

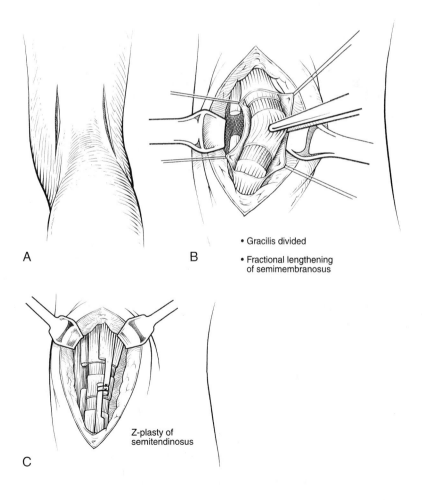

FIGURE **25-45** Surgical procedure depicting hamstring lengthening. *A.* The hamstrings are approached through two longitudinal incisions. *B.* The gracilis tendon is divided, and the aponeurosis of the semimembranosus is cut. *C.* The semitendinosus is either simply transected or Z-lengthened. *(From Herring, J.A. Tachdjian's Pediatric Orthopaedics, 3rd ed. WB Saunders, Philadelphia, 2002, p. 1171, with permission.)*

A

B

• Gracilis divided

• Fractional lengthening of semimembranosus

Z-plasty of semitendinosus

C

POSTOPERATIVE REHABILITATION OF HAMSTRING LENGTHENING: PHASE I (DAYS 1 TO 2)

Physical therapy is initiated on POD 1. The patient and caregiver are educated in the importance of positioning to maintain the elongated position of the hamstrings. Typically, patients use Jordan splints to maintain knee extension. Postoperatively, Jordan splints are worn 1 to 2 weeks during waking hours. The Jordan splints are removed for gentle PROM of the knee and hip, as well as for short periods during the day for sitting. If the patient did not have any bone procedures performed concurrently, WBAT is initiated on POD 1 while wearing the Jordan splints and using an appropriate assistive device. Splints are used for ambulation until there is adequate ability to maintain knee extension during the stance phase of gait (Figure 25-46).

Patients are typically discharged from the hospital on POD 1 or 2. The patient is instructed to wear the Jordan splints at night postoperatively for 1 to 6 weeks, dependent upon the individual surgeon's recommendations.

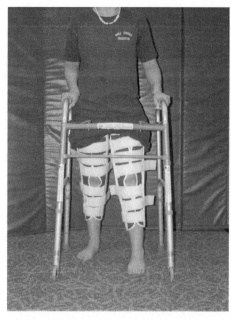

FIGURE 25-46 A patient status post hamstring lengthenings using Jordan splints to maintain the knees in extension during ambulation with assistive device.

Postoperative Rehabilitation of Hamstring Lengthening: Phase I (Days 1 to 2)

GOALS
- Control postoperative pain/swelling/spasms
- Emphasis on positioning to increase knee extension when in supine
- Optimize knee extension ROM, emphasizing hip flexion with knee extension
- Maintain knee flexion ROM for function (sitting and gait)
- Early weight-bearing—standing and ambulation WBAT with Jordan splints and appropriate assistive device
- Independence in HEP
  - Positioning to maintain hamstring muscle length
  - ROM exercises of hip and knee
  - Gentle passive SLR
  - Gait training

PRECAUTIONS
- Avoid prolonged periods of knee flexion (sitting) or knee extension.
- Avoid increased pain with therapeutic exercise and functional activities.
- Avoid overstretching lengthened muscle in any position.
- Monitor use/tolerance of Jordan splints application/fit/tolerance/irritation.
- Monitor surgical scar for color changes/swelling/discharge/drainage.
- Jordan splints must be on at night for sleeping up to 6 weeks.

TREATMENT STRATEGIES
- Training patient/caregiver in positioning to maintain new hamstring muscle length
- PROM knee extension in supine/sitting
- PROM knee flexion in supine/sitting
- Ankle pumps
- In supine, towel roll may be placed under heel to allow for passive stretch of the knee in supine.
- Training patient in ambulation with improved knee extension in stance phase (if ambulatory)

CRITERIA FOR ADVANCEMENT
- Discharge from the hospital is typically on PODs 1 to 2.
- Dependent on the level of functioning before surgery
- At discharge from the hospital, patient may resume preoperative therapeutic physical therapy program of upper extremity and proximal core musculature strengthening.

Troubleshooting

In phase I the physical therapist must pay careful attention to the patient's pelvic position in sitting. Because Jordan splints are worn for 1 to 2 weeks postoperatively during waking hours, the importance of an upright pelvis in sitting needs to be emphasized to the patient and caregiver. Because the hamstrings are a two-joint muscle, the patient may attempt to create a shortened range of the hamstring muscles by posteriorly tilting the pelvis. A neutral pelvic position with the knee extended in the Jordan splints will promote the elongation of the hamstrings at both joints. Jordan splints are used during ambulation until there is adequate ability to maintain knee extension during the stance phase of gait.

POSTOPERATIVE REHABILITATION OF HAMSTRING LENGTHENING: PHASE II (DAY 2 TO WEEK 2)

During this phase of rehabilitation, physical therapy should focus on improving hip and knee joint ROM, improving soft tissue flexibility and lengthening of the hamstring muscles, maximizing muscle strength, and optimizing gait and functional ability. The patient may discontinue the use of the Jordan splints at this phase of rehabilitation during waking hours. The splints will continue to be worn during gait training and at night.

Troubleshooting

Complications and/or compensatory mechanisms can occur if the patient is allowed to resume old habits, that is, crouched gait. The physical therapist should be sure to check for tightness of the hip flexors and stretch those muscles, if indicated, to help prevent the recurrence of a crouched gait pattern. Postoperatively, genu recurvatum may also occur because of weakness of the hamstring muscles. Phase II is an opportune time to promote strength in a newly lengthened muscle.

Postoperative Rehabilitation of Hamstring Lengthening: Phase II (Day 2 to Week 2)

GOALS
- Control postoperative pain/swelling/spasms
- Optimize knee extension ROM emphasizing hip flexion with knee extension
- Optimize/maintain hip extension; stretching of hip flexors may be indicated
- Emphasis on positioning to increase knee extension when in supine
- Maintain knee flexion ROM for function (sitting and gait)
- Strengthen quadriceps for knee extension during stance to allow for removal of Jordan splints
- Progress standing and ambulation WBAT with Jordan splints and appropriate assistive device
- Independence in HEP
  - As noted in Phase I, add heel slides in supine

PRECAUTIONS
- As noted in Phase I

TREATMENT STRATEGIES
- Training patient and caregiver in positioning optimizing knee extension
- Towel roll may be placed under heel to allow for passive stretch of the knee in supine
- Training patient in ambulation with improved knee extension in stance phase (if ambulatory)
- Gentle SLR
- P/AAROM knee extension in supine/sitting
- PROM knee flexion in supine/sitting
- AAROM hip and knee flexion in supine-heel slides
- Begin AAROM knee flexion in prone if patient can tolerate
- PROM hip extension and stretching of hip flexors if appropriate
- Quad sets
- Ankle pumps
- Resume preoperative therapeutic physical therapy program of upper extremity and proximal/core muscle strengthening
- Progress ambulation with Jordan splints and appropriate assistive device as tolerated. Specific focus should be on the quality of the gait pattern to gain better control of knee extension during stance.

CRITERIA FOR ADVANCEMENT
- Depends on the level of functioning prior to surgery
- Ability to extend knee in stance phase of gait will dictate discontinuation of Jordan splints during ambulation

Postoperative Rehabilitation of Hamstring Lengthening: Phase III (Weeks 2 to 6)

GOALS

- Promote/maintain knee extension passively and actively
- Promote/maintain hip extension passively and actively
- Discontinue use of Jordan splints during waking hours
- Wean patient out of Jordan splints for ambulation: based on ability to extend knee in stance
- Strengthen quadriceps in new end range
- Strengthen hamstrings throughout range of motion
- Return to preoperative ambulatory status
- Return to stair/curb negotiation as functional level permits

PRECAUTIONS

- As noted in Phase I

TREATMENT STRATEGIES

- ROM knee flexion/extension and SLR
- Quad sets
- Prone hamstring curls (Figure 25-47)
- Standing activities with facilitation for co-activation of quadriceps and hamstrings
- Activities to promote concentric and isometric quadriceps strengthening at end range
- Activities to promote concentric and isometric hamstring strengthening throughout ROM
- Emphasize core muscle strength and control
- Sit to stand
- Step-ups and stair negotiation
- Continue with HEP: evaluation-based

CRITERIA FOR ADVANCEMENT

- Depends on the level of functioning prior to surgery
- Ability to extend knee in stance phase of gait
- Discontinue use of Jordan splints at night 6 weeks postoperatively

POSTOPERATIVE REHABILITATION OF HAMSTRING LENGTHENING: PHASE III (WEEKS 2 TO 6)

This phase of rehabilitation is evaluation-based, and the patient is progressed accordingly.

Troubleshooting

A common finding during this phase of rehabilitation is for the patient to experience difficulty actively extending the knee during the stance phase of gait. The Jordan splints should continue to be used during ambulation until the patient can actively extend the knee during the stance phase, if therapeutically possible.

POSTOPERATIVE REHABILITATION OF HAMSTRING LENGTHENING: PHASE IV (WEEKS 6 TO 8)

Typically, after week 6, the nonambulatory patient will not progress to rehabilitative phase IV but will resume his or her preoperative therapeutic program, whereas the ambulatory patient will continue to progress to rehabilitative phase IV. This phase of rehabilitation is evaluation-based, and the patient is progressed accordingly.

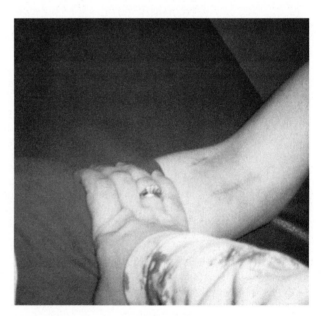

FIGURE **25-47** A patient status post hamstring lengthenings performing prone hamstring curls.

Postoperative Rehabilitation of Hamstring Lengthening: Phase IV (Weeks 6 to 8)

GOALS FOR THE AMBULATORY PATIENT
- Enhance co-activation of quadriceps and hamstrings
- Develop concentric and eccentric hamstring and quadriceps strengthening
- Maintain or increase passive and active knee extension range of motion
- Maintain passive knee flexion range of motion
- Increase lower extremity functional muscle strength
- Continue to improve quality of ambulation
- Resume full preoperative physical therapy program
- Discontinue use of Jordan splints completely

PRECAUTIONS
- Avoid pain with therapeutic exercise and functional activities

TREATMENT STRATEGIES
- ROM knee flexion/extension and SLR
- Single leg stance activities to promote co-activation
- Swing phase activities to develop improved stride length
- Sit to stand exercises
- Emphasize core muscle strength and control
- Total Gym Progressive Exercises for strengthening of the LEs (Figure 25-48, *A* and *B*)
- Step-ups
- Stair negotiation (Figure 25-49, *A* and *B*)
- Treadmill walking (Figure 25-50)
- Stationary bicycle
- HEP: evaluation-based

CRITERIA FOR ADVANCEMENT
- Depends on the level of functioning prior to surgery
- Ability to extend knee in stance phase of gait

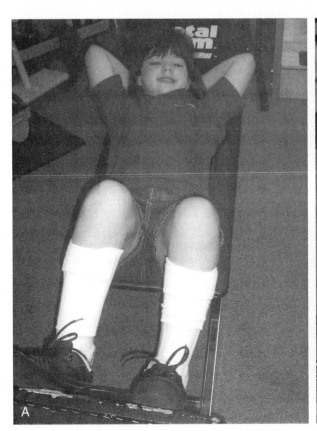 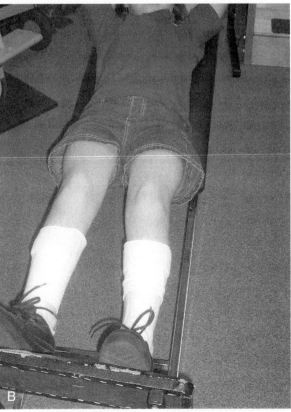

FIGURE **25-48** Using the total gym to increase lower extremity strength. *A.* Moving from knee flexion to knee extension to increase quadriceps strength. *B.* Moving from knee extension to a flexed position to develop eccentric quadriceps control.

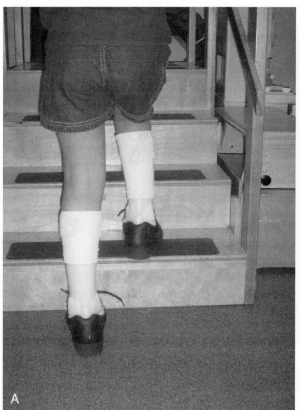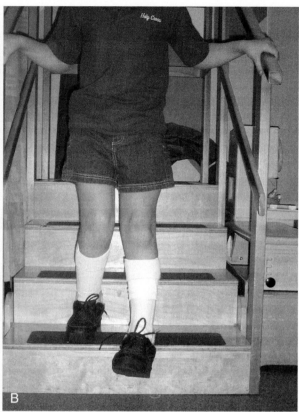

FIGURE **25-49** Stair negotiation. *A.* Patient ascending stairs to develop lower extremity muscle strength. *B.* Patient descending stairs to develop eccentric control of the lower extremity.

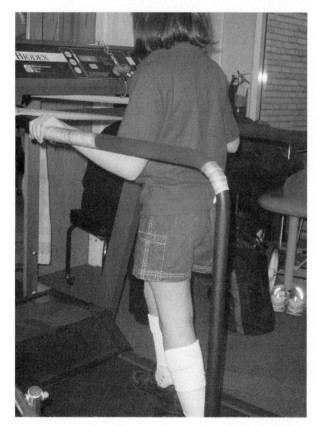

FIGURE **25-50** The treadmill is a useful piece of equipment to facilitate gait. The therapist can address the timing and sequencing of the lower extremity musculature during the specific phases of gait.

Troubleshooting

Complications of hamstring lengthening may include genu recurvatum because of weak hamstring muscles, or, if the gastrocnemius muscle is tight, the patient may attempt to get the heel flat in mid-stance via knee hyperextension. A careful and thorough physical therapy examination is the key to determining the root of the problem and thereby the most appropriate course of treatment. If genu recurvatum is observed, functional exercises that emphasize the use of the hamstrings in a shortened range (i.e., during swing phase of gait or hamstring curls) may be helpful. An increased lordosis may occur with a proximal lengthening, if inadequate abdominal muscle strength is present, or if the hip flexors are tight. The physical therapist also needs to continue to monitor for the possible recurrence of a crouch gait pattern.

TENDO ACHILLES LENGTHENING

Children with CP typically present with spasticity of the ankle plantar flexor muscles, resulting in shortening of the gastrocsoleus musculature and an equinus gait pattern[36] (Figure 25-51). Abnormal frequent contraction of the calf muscles may result in the inability to dorsiflex the foot during functional activities, such as ambulation. The inability to obtain heel strike during gait does not allow for the ankle plantar flexors to obtain periodic elongation in the stance phase.[6] This combination of failure to passively elongate the ankle plantar flexors during gait, with diminished ability to functionally activate the ankle dorsiflexors, inhibits the normal elasticity of the calf muscles. Additionally, rapid skeletal growth in children may impact the muscle's ability to keep up with bone length, thus contributing to the occurrence of muscle contracture in children with CP.[6] Children with spastic ankle plantar flexors typically toe-walk or display a toe-heel gait pattern.

Though equinus deformity of the ankle is the most common cause for toe-walking or a toe-heel gait pattern, increased knee flexion can also cause this foot contact pattern.[35] Treatment of an equinus gait with gastrocsoleus lengthening, when the true problem is knee flexion spasticity or contracture, will universally result in profound weakness and calcaneus gait[35] (Figure 25-52, A and B). It is well reported in the literature that a calcaneus deformity is much more functionally debilitating than a moderate degree of equinus.[6,9,35]

The major muscle of the lower extremity responsible for ankle plantar flexion is the gastrocnemius. It is the primary action muscle, and through physical examination it is oftentimes found to be the tighter muscle of the group.[4] To determine whether the muscle tightness is originating from the gastrocnemius muscle or the soleus muscle, the Silverskiold test is performed. Ankle joint ROM is assessed with the knee flexed and extended. A positive Silverskiold test indicates that there is more equinus with the knee extended, thereby targeting the gastrocnemius as the primary tight muscle[1,9] (Figure

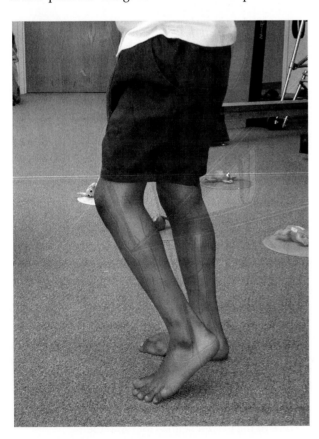

FIGURE 25-51 A patient with an equinus gait pattern.

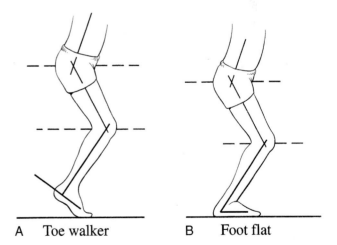

A   Toe walker   B   Foot flat

Post-Op Calcaneal Gait

FIGURE 25-52 A. Child with a crouched knee and toe-toe gait. The ankle is actually in a neutral position, but the child walks on the toes to compensate for the flexed knee. B. Following inappropriate Achilles tendon lengthening, flexion at the knee remains unchanged, and the ankle is now excessively dorsiflexed, resulting in calcaneus gait. (From Herring, J.A. Tachdjian's Pediatric Orthopaedics, 3rd ed. WB Saunders, Philadelphia, 2002, p. 1142, with permission.)

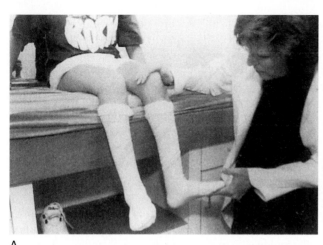
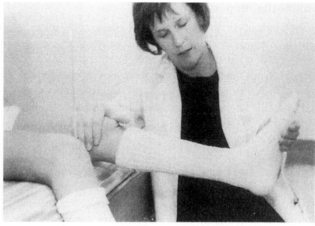

A   B

FIGURE **25-53** Silverskiold test. *A.* With the knee in flexion, the gastrocnemius muscle is relaxed and plantar flexion is caused by tightness of the soleus muscle. *B.* With the knee in extension, the tightness of the gastrocnemius is assessed. (From Herring, J.A. *Tachdjian's Pediatric Orthopaedics,* 3rd ed. WB Saunders, Philadelphia, 2002, p. 1135, with permission.)

25-53). In an equinus gait pattern, the soleus muscle is usually not the major problem.[4]

Indications for a tendo Achilles lengthening (TAL) are

- Passive ankle dorsiflexion less than zero degrees[6,10]
- A fixed equinus deformity is present such that the ankle cannot be dorsiflexed to neutral with the hind-foot locked in varus in an ambulatory patient.[6]

SURGICAL OVERVIEW

The major muscles of the lower leg that are responsible for ankle plantar flexion are the gastrocnemius and soleus. The gastrocnemius originates from two heads—the medial head originates from the medial femoral condyle and popliteal surface, and the lateral head originates from the lateral femoral condyle. The gastrocnemius muscle inserts via the tendo calcaneus (Achilles tendon) into the calcaneus.[27,37] The soleus originates from the upper portion of the fibula and tibia and inserts via Achilles tendon into the calcaneus. The muscle fibers of the two heads of the gastrocnemius unite into a broad tendon-aponeurosis that blend with aponeurosis of the soleus muscle to form the Achilles tendon[37] (Figure 25-54). The combined soleus and gastrocnemius muscles make up the triceps surae.[37]

The goal of a TAL is to correct an equinus deformity and relieve the contracture without excessively weakening the muscle. Excessive lengthening of the gastrocnemius can result in a crouch gait and an actual decrease in functional ambulation over time because of the inability to push-off during the stance phase of gait.[6,35] Although several surgical procedures may be used to lengthen the ankle plantar flexors, only two procedures will be presented: the Vulpius and the Hoke procedures.[6,9,10] The Silverskiold tests assist the surgeon in determining which procedure to use because it differentiates between

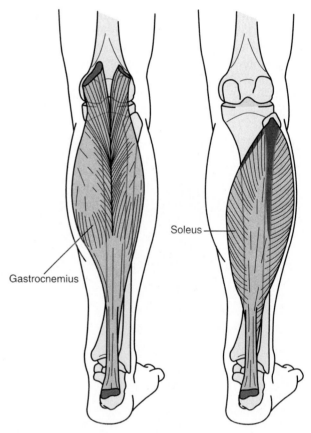

Gastrocnemius   Soleus

Posterior View

FIGURE **25-54** Anatomy of the gastrocnemius and soleus muscles. *(From Daniels, L., Worthingham, C. Muscle Testing: Techniques of Manual Examination, 4th ed. WB Saunders, Philadelphia, 1980, p. 211, with permission.)*

contracture of the gastrocnemius alone or combined contracture of the gastrocnemius and the soleus.[6,19]

The Vulpius procedure lengthens the gastrocnemius and spares the soleus muscle.[6] It consists of making an inverted V incision in the gastrocnemius tendinous aponeurosis and passively dorsiflexing the ankle with the knee in extension. The aponeurosis separates and thus lengthens the gastrocnemius[6,10] (Figure 25-55). This method is advantageous because it preserves the soleus muscle, which can be used as a muscle for push-off.[4]

The Hoke procedure is performed by making three incisions, each one half way through the tendon. Two incisions are made on the medial aspect of the Achilles tendon, one proximal and one distal, and a single lateral incision is performed halfway between the previous two. The surgeon then dorsiflexes the ankle to neutral, causing a sliding lengthening of the tendon. No sutures are necessary with the Hoke procedure[9,10] (Figure 25-56). This procedure weakens both the soleus and the gastrocnemius musculature.

Regardless of the procedure used by the surgeon to lengthen the Achilles tendon, the patient is placed in a short leg cast for 3 to 6 weeks postoperatively.[10] Duration of cast use is based on the individual surgeon's protocol.

REHABILITATION OVERVIEW

The patient is permitted to ambulate immediately postoperatively in the short leg cast, with cast boots and appropriate assistive device. While in the short leg cast, it is important to position and maintain the knee in extension. Once the cast is removed the physical therapist will need to address the ROM limitations of the ankle as well as strengthening the muscles about the ankle foot complex for functional mobility and control. The goal post-TAL is for the patient to display a heel-toe gait pattern.

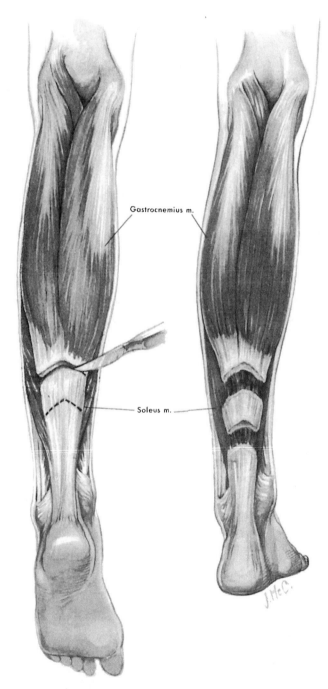

Gastrocnemius m.

Soleus m.

FIGURE **25-55** Lengthening of the gastrocnemius via the Vulpius procedure. *(From Herring, J.A. Tachdjian's Pediatric Orthopaedics, 3rd ed. WB Saunders, Philadelphia, 2002, p. 1137, with permission.)*

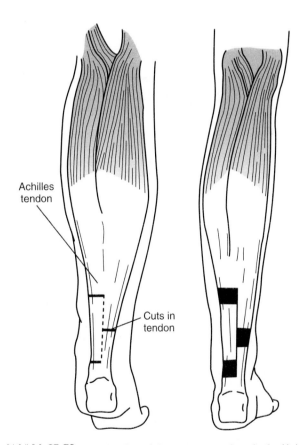

Achilles tendon

Cuts in tendon

FIGURE **25-56** Lengthening of the gastrocnemius via the Hoke procedure. *(From Rinsky, L.A. Surgery for Cerebral Palsy. In Chapman's Orthopaedic Surgery, 3rd ed. Lippincott Williams & Wilkins, Philadelphia, 2001, p. 487; Bleck, E.E. Orthopaedic Management in Cerebral Palsy. JB Lippincott, Philadelphia, 1987, p. 249; and courtesy of Amanda Sparrow, PT, With permission.)*

PREOPERATIVE PHASE

The physical therapist will perform a comprehensive examination, inclusive of ROM, functional ability, quality of movement, and observational gait analysis. These findings will be presented to the surgeon, and a decision will be made as to the course of treatment. There is no specific preoperative therapeutic protocol prior to a TAL.

POSTOPERATIVE REHABILITATION OF TENDO ACHILLES LENGTHENING: PHASE I (DAYS 1 TO 2)

Rehabilitation begins immediately on POD 1. The lower leg will typically be placed in a short leg cast postoperatively for 3 to 6 weeks. As reported in the literature, the shortest duration of immobilization is ideal to allow for a quick return to normal function.[38] Because the gastrocnemius is a two-joint muscle, caregivers must be educated in the importance of encouraging knee extension during positioning to maintain the elongated position of the gastrocnemius at both the knee and ankle joints. Additionally, the family should be educated on the anatomy of the hamstring musculature and its impact on knee position. It is important to perform passive, gentle SLR exercises while the ankle is positioned in dorsiflexion to ensure adequate ROM at the hip, knee, and ankle joint for future function. Standing and ambulation begin on POD 1, with cast boots, WBAT with an appropriate assistive device. Patients are encouraged to obtain full knee extension during ambulation. During this phase of rehabilitation, passive and active knee extension exercises may be performed if tolerated by the patient.

Troubleshooting

The child may initially stand with increased knee, hip, and trunk flexion because of pain/spasms and/or in an attempt to maintain a shortened position of the gastrocnemius muscle. In this instance, it is important to educate the caregivers on the need to emphasize good posture to obtain active elongation of the gastrocnemius muscle in standing.

The HEP should emphasize positioning of the knee in extension when in supine and avoiding sitting for long periods of time (as a result of time spent with the knee flexed), active and passive knee ROM, stretching of the hamstrings, postural alignment in standing and walking, and progression of ambulation distance as tolerated.

Postoperative Rehabilitation of Tendo Achilles Lengthening: Phase I (Days 1 to 2)

GOALS

- Control postoperative pain/swelling/spasms
- Emphasis on positioning to increase knee extension when in supine
- Maintain overall knee range of motion
- Encourage active toe movements
- Early weight-bearing: standing and ambulation WBAT with appropriate assistive device
- Independence in HEP

PRECAUTIONS

- Avoid prolonged periods of knee flexion (i.e., sitting)
- Monitor skin for signs of irritation or constriction from cast
- Monitor exposed foot/toes for signs of edema

TREATMENT STRATEGIES

- Educate and train patient/caregivers in positioning. Towel roll may be placed under the ankle to allow for passive stretching of the knee in supine. Initially, operated extremity is elevated to control postop edema
- Encourage toe wiggling
- Teach patient/caregivers PROM of knee extension
- Gentle SLR to elongate the hamstrings
- Quad sets may be performed if tolerated
- Gait training emphasizing good posture and knee extension in stance phase (for ambulators)

CRITERIA FOR ADVANCEMENT

- Patient is typically discharged PODs 1 and 2
- Assistance will be necessary for distance mobility (stroller, wheelchair)
- Depends upon level of functioning prior to surgery

Postoperative Rehabilitation of Tendo Achilles Lengthening: Phase II (Day 3 to Cast Removal)

GOALS

- Control postoperative pain/swelling/spasms
- Emphasis on positioning to increase knee extension when in supine
- Maintain overall passive and active knee range of motion
- Encourage active toe movements
- Increase standing and ambulation distance WBAT with appropriate assistive
- Independence in HEP
- Resume preoperative physical therapy program to tolerance

PRECAUTIONS

- Same as in Phase I

TREATMENT STRATEGIES

- Continue with treatment strategies from Phase I
- Active knee extension exercises may be performed
- Resume preoperative physical therapy program to tolerance
- Gentle passive SLR (Figure 25-57)
- Quad sets
- Gait training emphasizing good posture and knee extension in stance phase (for ambulators)

CRITERIA FOR ADVANCEMENT

- Assistance will be necessary for distance mobility (stroller, wheelchair)
- Depends upon level of functioning prior to surgery

POSTOPERATIVE REHABILITATION OF TENDO ACHILLES LENGTHENING: PHASE II (DAY 3 TO CAST REMOVAL)

Phase II of rehabilitation is similar to phase I. The patient is typically able to resume his or her preoperative physical therapy program to tolerance.

Troubleshooting

Patients may have a tendency to externally rotate the casted extremity (or extremities) to avoid full weight-bearing and transitioning forward over their foot. Physical therapy should focus on neutral rotation of lower extremities during standing and walking.

POSTOPERATIVE REHABILITATION OF TENDO ACHILLES LENGTHENING: PHASE III (DAY OF CAST REMOVAL TO 3 WEEKS POST CAST REMOVAL)

This phase of rehabilitation focuses on the initiation and/or return of active ankle movement and progression of independent ambulation. Emphasis is placed on active ROM of ankle dorsiflexion and plantar flexion and strengthening of both muscle groups about the ankle. Therapeutic sequence should first initiate activation and strengthening of the ankle dorsiflexors followed by activation and strengthening of the ankle plantar flexors in their newly elongated range (dorsiflexion with knee extension). Ankle foot orthoses are recommended during this phase of rehabilitation to prevent the recurrence of ankle plantar flexion during walking and/or

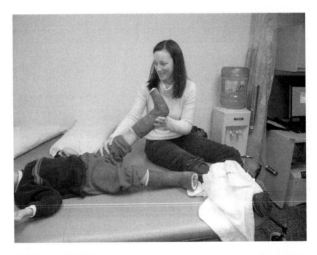

FIGURE **25-57** Therapist performing passive SLR to the patient's tolerance.

overlengthening of the triceps surae muscle group during weight-bearing. The specific type of orthoses is determined via a thorough physical therapy examination in conjunction with physician consultation. Initially, the patient may be placed in a custom-made solid ankle foot orthosis (SAFO) to allow him or her to accommodate to the new muscle length (Figure 25-58). Other types of orthoses may also be used initially, such as a hinged ankle foot orthosis (AFO) with a check strap, which allows the therapist to control the amount of dorsiflexion available to the patient (Figure 25-59).

Postoperative Rehabilitation of Tendo Achilles Lengthening: Phase III (Day of Cast Removal to 3 Weeks Post Cast Removal)

GOALS

- Promote/maintain ankle dorsiflexion with knee extension passively and actively
- Strengthening dorsiflexors
- Strengthening plantarflexors in elongated range of motion (with dorsiflexion and knee extension)
- Patient/caregiver education regarding the importance of utilizing AFOs during the day to maintain ankle joint range of motion
- Progress ambulation endurance and independence as appropriate

PRECAUTIONS

- Avoid pain with therapeutic exercise and functional activities
- Avoid overstretching into dorsiflexion
- Monitor incision/scar for irritation and continued adequate healing

TREATMENT STRATEGIES

- Gentle stretching into dorsiflexion with subtalar neutral, not to exceed normal ROM
- Myofascial release of the plantar fascia if indicated
- Passive great toe extension for push-off
- Ankle pumps (emphasis on dorsiflexion)
- Standing activities to promote isometric contraction of ankle plantar flexion in an elongated position
- Sit to stand activities with emphasis on tibial translation forward over foot with neutral STJ
- Work in step stance-ability to control transition of tibia over foot (Figure 25-60)
- Begin to work on push-off during gait
- Continue with HEP: evaluation-based

CRITERIA FOR ADVANCEMENT

- Assistance may be necessary for distance mobility (stroller, wheelchair)
- Depends upon level of functioning prior to surgery

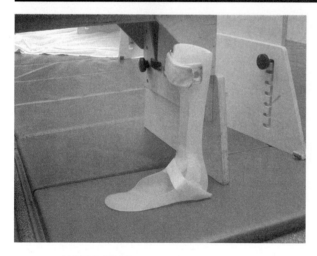

FIGURE 25-58 A solid ankle foot orthotic.

Troubleshooting

A potential complication during this phase of rehabilitation is an overstretching of the lengthened musculature, which may result from failure to comply with AFO wear or from aggressive plantar flexor stretching. Patient/caregiver education is essential to prevent this problem. Additionally, the fit of the AFO should be closely monitored for areas of increased pressure, especially around the scar. A hinged AFO with posterior check strap is a nice adjunct to postoperative therapy.

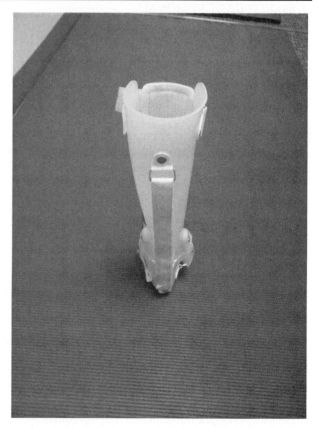

FIGURE 25-59 A hinged ankle foot orthotic with a check strap to control the amount of ankle dorsiflexion.

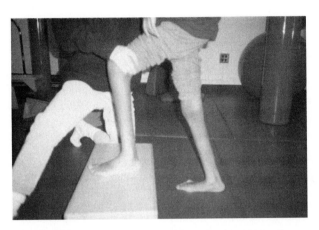

FIGURE **25-60** Therapeutic exercise in step stance position to control forward tibial translation over the foot.

This type of orthosis allows the therapist to work with the patient in varied ranges of ankle dorsiflexion to develop control of both active dorsiflexion and eccentric plantar flexion during functional activities. The check strap can be set and secured to maintain the ankle at 90 degrees, essentially presenting as an SAFO if needed. The therapist should focus on the ability of the patient to activate the ankle dorsiflexors and plantar flexors throughout the available ROM. In some cases, the therapeutic need will be to stress active ankle dorsiflexion, and, in other cases, the need will be to emphasize activation of the ankle plantar flexors. Isolated active movement of both muscle groups as well as co-activation of both muscle groups are needed for optimal ankle function and stability.

POSTOPERATIVE REHABILITATION OF TENDO ACHILLES LENGTHENING: PHASE IV (WEEKS 3 TO 6 POST CAST REMOVAL)

As the patient progresses in this phase, the need for orthotic needs should be continually assessed and appropriately addressed.

Troubleshooting

It may be difficult during this phase of rehabilitation to obtain functional dorsiflexion during gait, even if the patient can actively isolate dorsiflexion of the ankle. Spasticity and synergistic muscle activity may impact timing and sequencing of movement, thus impairing the patient's ability to obtain heel strike upon initial contact. Additionally, dynamic foot reactions as well as ankle/foot proprioception should be evaluated because deficits in these areas will impact functional ankle control and stability. When working with children with CP, attention to subtle compensations is necessary throughout the phases of rehabilitation to promote appropriate muscle activation. An orthotic may be necessary to maintain the correction. Night splinting is reserved for those patients who show early signs of recurrent tightness.[4]

In summary, this chapter presents postoperative rehabilitation considerations and guidelines for children with CP who have undergone bone and musculotendinous surgical procedures. CP is a complex and multifaceted condition. There is extensive variability regarding presentation, severity, functional ability, and neuromuscular capability in the patient with CP. The concept of treating the total child in orthopedics via a

---

Postoperative Rehabilitation of Tendo Achilles Lengthening: Phase IV (Weeks 3 to 6 Post Cast Removal)

GOALS

- Enhance co-activation of postural plantarflexors, and dorsiflexors
- Promote appropriate ankle kinematics during gait
- Progress ambulation endurance and independence to level at or greater than presurgery

PRECAUTIONS

- Same as Phase III

TREATMENT STRATEGIES

- Continue with treatment strategies from Phase II
- Single leg stance activities to promote co-activation
- Strengthening of anterior tibialis, and dorsiflexors to improve heel strike during gait (heel walking)
- Eccentric plantar flexion activities (retro ambulation, step-ups, squat to stand . . .)
- Dynamic foot reactions
- Walking balance beam, tandem walking
- HEP: evaluation-based

CRITERIA FOR ADVANCEMENT

- Assistance may be necessary for distance mobility (stroller, wheelchair)
- Depends upon level of functioning prior to surgery
- Progress ambulation endurance/distance as tolerated

team approach is essential in both preoperative decision making and postoperative rehabilitation. Treatment and goals must be individually based, and each patient is progressed at his or her own pace and capability. Direct, open communication with the patient/family and surgeon is of paramount importance for an optimal surgical outcome. Scientific-based knowledge must be combined with the art of caring throughout the entire therapeutic healing process. Once the acute and subacute phases of rehabilitation are completed, the child typically returns to his or her preexisting, preoperative therapeutic program.

REFERENCES

1. Nelson, K. *What Proportion of Cerebral Palsy is Related to Birth Asphyxia?* J Pediatr 1988;113:572–574.
2. Press Room/Facts and Figures, January 2005. Available online at http://www.ucp.org.
3. Novacheck, T.F. Surgical Intervention in Ambulatory Cerebral Palsy. In Harris, G.F., Smith, P.A. (Eds). *Human Motion Analysis.* IEEE Press, Piscataway, NJ, 1996, pp. 231–254.
4. Renshaw, T.S. Cerebral Palsy. In Morrissy, R.T., Weinstein, S.L. (Eds). *Lovell and Winter's Pediatric Orthopaedics,* 5th ed., vol. 1. Lippincott Williams & Wilkins, New York, 2001, pp. 563–599.
5. Stanger, M. Orthopedic Management. In Tecklin, J.S. (Ed). *Pediatric Physical Therapy,* 3rd ed. Lippincott Williams & Wilkins, New York, 1999, pp. 394–396.
6. Bleck, E.E. *Orthopaedic Management in Cerebral Palsy.* JB Lippincott, Philadelphia, 1987.
7. Sutherland, D.H., Kaufman, K.R. Human Motion Analysis and Pediatric Orthopaedics. In Harris, G.F., Smith, P.A. (Eds). *Human Motion Analysis.* IEEE Press, Piscataway, NJ, 1996, pp. 219–230.
8. Sussman, M.D., Aiona, M.D. Treatment of Spastic Diplegia in Patients with Cerebral Palsy. J Pediatr Orthop B 2004;13(2): S1–S128.
9. Rinsky, L.A. Surgery for Cerebral Palsy. In *Chapman's Orthopaedic Surgery,* 3rd ed. Lippincott Williams & Wilkins, New York, 2001, pp. 4485–4506.
10. Personal communication, Dr. Leon Root, Medical Director of Rehabilitation, Hospital for Special Surgery, November 2004; May 2005.
11. Laplaza, F.J., Root, L. *Femoral Anteversion and Neck-shaft Angles in Hip Instability in Cerebral Palsy.* J Pediatr Orthop 1994;14:719–723.
12. Staheli, L.T. *Medial Femoral Torsion.* Orthop Clin North Am 1980;11:39–50.
13. Bobroff, E.D., Chambers, H.G., Sartoris, D.J., Wyatt, M.P., Sutherland, D.H. *Femoral Anteversion and Neck-shaft Angle in Children with Cerebral Palsy [Section II: Original Articles: Knee].* Clin Orthop Relat Res 1999;1(364):194–204.
14. Magee, D.J. *Orthopedic Physical Assessment,* 3rd ed. WB Saunders, Philadelphia, 1997.
15. Wheeless' Textbook of Orthopaedics. Available online at http://www.wheelessonline.com.
16. Murray-Weir, M., Root, L., Peterson, M., Lenhoff, M., Daly, L., Wagner, C., Marcus, P. *Proximal Femoral Varus Rotation Osteotomy in Cerebral Palsy: A Prospective Gait Study.* J Pediatr Orthop 2003;23(3):321–329.
17. Fabry, G., MacEwen, G.D., Shands, J.R. *Torsion of the Femur.* J Bone Joint Surg Am 1973;55:1726–1738.
18. Ounpuu, S.M., DeLuca, P., Davis, R., Romness, M. *Long-term Effects of Femoral Derotation Osteotomies: An Evaluation Using Three-dimensional Gait Analysis.* J Pediatr Orthop 2002;22(2): 139–145.
19. Herring, J.A. *Tachdjian's Pediatric Orthopaedics,* 3rd ed. WB Saunders, Philadelphia, 2002.
20. Root, L., Siegal, T. *Osteotomy of the Hip in Children: Posterior Approach.* J Bone Joint Surg Am 1980;62:571–575.
21. Renshaw, T., Green, N.E., Griffin, P.P., Root, L. *Cerebral Palsy: Orthopaedic Management—Instructional Course Lectures.* J Bone Joint Surg Am 1995;77A(10):1590–1606.
22. Stasikelis, P.J., Davids, J.R., Johnson, B.H., Jacobs, J.M. *Rehabilitation after Femoral Osteotomy in Cerebral Palsy.* J Pediatr Orthop B 2003;12:311–314.
23. Sutherland, D.H., Zilberfarb, J.L., Kaufman, K.R., Wyatt, M.P., Chambers, H.G. *Psoas Release at the Pelvic Brim in Ambulatory Patients with Cerebral Palsy: Operative Technique and Functional Outcome.* J Pediatr Orthop 1997;17(5):563–570.
24. Novacheck, T.F., Trost, J.P., Schwartz, M.H. *Intramuscular Psoas Lengthening Improves Dynamic Hip Function in Children with Cerebral Palsy.* J Pediatr Orthop 2002;22(2):158–164.
25. Matsuo, T., Hara, H., Tada, S. *Selective Lengthening of the Psoas and Rectus Femoris and Preservation of the Iliacus for Flexion Deformity of the Hip in Cerebral Palsy Patients.* J Pediatr Orthop 1987;7:690–698.
26. Brunnstrom, S. *Clinical Kinesiology,* 3rd ed. FA Davis, Philadelphia, 1972.
27. Daniels, L., Worthingham, C. *Muscle Testing: Techniques of Manual Examination,* 4th ed. WB Saunders, Philadelphia, 1980.
28. Carr, C., Gage, G.R. *The Fate of the Nonoperated Hip in Cerebral Palsy.* J Pediatr Orthop 1987;7:262.
29. Perry, J. *Distal Rectus Femoris Transfer.* Dev Med Child Neurol 1987;29:153–158.
30. Ounpuu, M.S., Davis, R.B., Gage, J.R., DeLuca, P.A. *Rectus Femoris Surgery in Children with Cerebral Palsy. Part I: The Effect of the Rectus Femoris Transfer Location on Knee Motion.* J Pediatr Orthop 1993;13:325–330.
31. Sutherland, D.H., Santi, M.D., Abel, M.F. *Treatment of Stiff Knee Gait in Cerebral Palsy: A Comparison by Gait Analysis of Distal Rectus Femoris Transfer vs Proximal Rectus Release.* J Pediatr Orthop 1990;10:433–441.
32. Delp, S.L. *Computer Modeling and Analysis of Movement Disabilities and Their Surgical Corrections.* In Harris, G.F., Smith, P.A. (Eds). *Human Motion Analysis.* IEEE Press, Piscataway, NJ, 1996, pp. 114–132.
33. Yngve, D.A., Scarborough, N., Goode, B., Haynes, R. *Rectus and Hamstring Surgery in Cerebral Palsy: A Gait Analysis Study of Results by Functional Ambulation Level.* J Pediatr Orthop 2002;22:672–676.
34. Morrissy, R.T., Weinstein, S.L. *Atlas of Pediatric Orthopedic Surgery,* 3rd ed. Lippincott Williams & Wilkins, Philadelphia, 2001.
35. Aiona, M.D., Sussman, M.D. *Treatment of Spastic Diplegia in Patients with Cerebral Palsy: Part II.* J Pediatr Orthop 2004; 13(3):S13–S38.
36. Grant, A.D., Feldman, R., Lehman, W.B. *Equinus Deformity in Cerebral Palsy: A Retrospective Analysis of Treatment and Function in 39 Cases.* J Pediatr Orthop 1985;5(6):678–681.
37. Kendall, F.P., McCreary, E.K., Provance, P.G. *Muscles Testing and Function,* 4th ed. Lippincott Williams & Wilkins, New York, 1993.
38. Rattey, T.E., Leahey, L., Hyndman, J., Brown, D.C., Gross, M. *Recurrence after Achilles Tendon Lengthening in Cerebral Palsy.* J Pediatr Orthop 1993;13(2):184–187.

CHAPTER

26

Spinal Fusion in Adolescent Idiopathic Scoliosis

LORETTA AMOROSO, DPT

KELLY SINDLE, PT

The Scoliosis Research Society defines idiopathic scoliosis as a lateral curvature of the spine of unknown etiology that is greater than or equal to a 10-degree Cobb angle with rotation.[1] Adolescent idiopathic scoliosis (AIS) appears before the onset of puberty and before skeletal maturity.[1] AIS occurs in roughly 2% to 3% of the pediatric population, with 10% of those children requiring some type of medical intervention—conservative or surgical.[2,3] The incidence of occurrence varies depending on the severity of the curve. In curves less than or equal to 30 degrees, the incidence is equal in women and men.[3-5] In curves greater than 30 degrees, the incidence in women increases significantly to a 4:1 female to male ratio, as reported by Weinstein[3] and as great as 8:1, as reported by Lovell and Winter.[4] Research suggests that there is a genetic component to adolescent idiopathic scoliosis. In a study done by Risenborough and Wynne-Davies,[6] an 11.1% incidence was found among first-degree relatives. Studies of twins also support this finding, reporting a 73% incidence of AIS in monozygotic twins and a 36% incidence in dizygotic twins.[6]

The diagnosis of AIS and the subsequent course of treatment of AIS are determined by the size of the curve and the skeletal maturity of the patient. Once AIS is diagnosed, the physician determines the risk of curve progression. Two major considerations are taken into account: curve factors and growth factors. Curve factors describe the curve magnitude and its pattern. Curve magnitude describes the size of the curve and is determined by measuring the Cobb angle. The Cobb angle, or the degree of curvature, is formed by the intersection of perpendicular lines drawn to the end plates of the most tilted vertebrae[7] (Figure 26-1). The Cobb angle must be greater than 10 degrees for a diagnosis of AIS to be made.[1] In a typical spine, the angle measures 0 degrees. In general, the larger the curve, the greater the incidence of progression (Figure 26-2). Curve patterns can describe where and how many curves are present and are named by the terms *single*, *double*, *minor*, and *major*. Major curves tend to be structural and more deforming, whereas minor curves are most often compensatory curves (Figure 26-3). The larger the curve at the time of diagnosis and/or the presence of a double curve, the greater the risk of progression.

Growth factors describe the skeletal maturity of the patient and his or her remaining growth at the time of diagnosis. The degree of skeletal maturity at the time of curve identification is noted radiographically, using Risser's sign. Risser's sign is the amount of ossification across the top of the iliac crest which is graded on a scale of 0 to 5 (Figure 26-4). The skeletally immature patient (i.e., Risser's grade of 0 to 2) has a much higher risk of progression than the skeletally mature patient (i.e.,

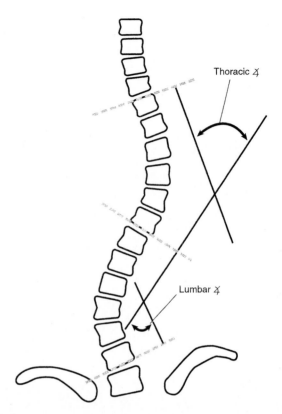

FIGURE **26-1** The Cobb measurement. The vertebras with the greatest amount of tilt are selected as the end vertebra. Lines are drawn perpendicularly to the end plates of the vertebras. The angle formed at the intersection of these lines is the Cobb angle. If a second curve is present below the primary curve, the original curve's lower vertebra becomes the top vertebra for measuring the second curve, and the same line along its surface is used. *(From Herring, J.A. Tachdjian's Pediatric Orthopaedics, 3rd ed., vol. 1. WB Saunders, New York, 2002, p. 225; fig. 11-17, with permission.)*

Risser's grade of 5).[3] Research reveals that the progression of curves in AIS occurs most rapidly between the time of detection and skeletal maturity.[1,9] The younger the patient and the lower the Risser's grade at the time of initial detection, the greater the risk for curve progression.[3,4,10-14]

The degree of curvature and risk of progression will dictate whether treatment will be managed conservatively or surgically. Conservative management of AIS consists of observation and/or bracing. Curves that are 20 degrees or less before the time of skeletal maturity are considered mild and are usually observed every 6 months for progression.[15] Bracing is indicated for individuals with curves of 25 to 45 degrees who have not reached skeletal maturity and/or those curves that progress 5 to 10 degrees in 6 months.[15]

Research has proven bracing to be the most effective conservative treatment in maintaining or correcting a scoliotic curve.[15,16] According to a study by

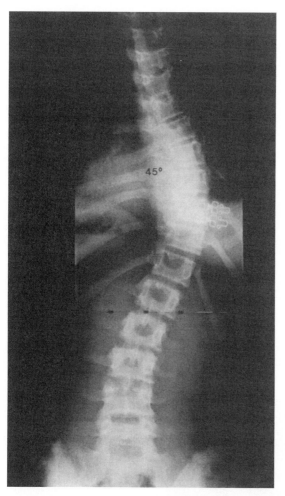

FIGURE **26-2** PA radiograph of the thoracolumbar spine of a 13-year-old girl showing a 45-degree right thoracic scoliosis. *(From Herring, J.A. Tachdjian's Pediatric Orthopaedics, 3rd ed., vol. 1. WB Saunders, New York, 2002, p. 214; fig. 11-1, with permission.)*

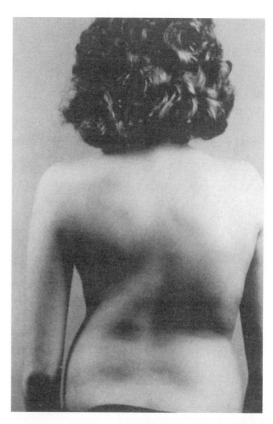

FIGURE **26-3** Clinical appearance of a 13-year-old girl with a right thoracic and left lumbar scoliosis. *(From Herring, J.A. Tachdjian's Pediatric Orthopaedics, 3rd ed., vol. 1. WB Saunders, New York, 2002, p. 222; fig. 11-11, with permission.)*

Nachemson and Peterson,[16] bracing has a 74% success rate for curve maintenance or correction of the curve. It is hypothesized that scoliosis correction through bracing provides constant corrective molding of the trunk and spine during growth.[4] Therefore, there must be some skeletal growth remaining for bracing to positively affect the curve. The type of brace used will vary depending on the type of curve, degree of curvature, and the individual surgeon. At the Hospital for Special Surgery (HSS), a custom molded TLSO or CTLSO (Milwaukee brace) is used most often with a bracing protocol of 23 hours a day[4,24] (Figures 26-5 and 26-6). This protocol is based on research that demonstrates that bracing for 23 hours a day had a 93% success rate vs bracing for only 8 or 16 hours a day, which had success rates of 60% and 62%, respectively.[15] This protocol must be strictly followed for bracing to be effective (Figure 26-7).

In recent years at HSS, there has been increased use of a tension-based scoliosis bracing system for treatment of AIS. Correction of the scoliotic curve is achieved by a series of elastic straps that apply dynamic corrective forces to the spine, altering posture and derotating the spinal column. Indications for using this bracing system at HSS are curves less than 35 degrees and a Risser's grade of 2 or less. The tension-based brace is worn for 20 hours a day, with 2 hours off in the morning and 2 hours off in the afternoon. Patients report a higher compliance rate secondary to increased flexibility and better cosmesis in the tension system compared to the rigid brace. Studies done in Europe with the Spine Cor brace (a tension-based system) have successful results equal to those of a rigid brace.[25] Currently, no other treatments, including physical therapy[1-3,15,20] and electrical stimulation,[21-23] have proven to be effective in managing a patient's curve.

Surgical intervention may be indicated depending on the degree of curvature, the risk for progression, the secondary effects of the scoliosis, and the failure or success of conservative treatment. Surgery is indicated for curves greater than 50 degrees in the skeletally immature patient and 60 degrees in the skeletally mature

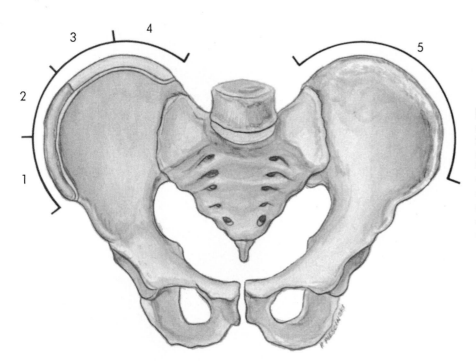

FIGURE **26-4** The Risser's sign proceeds from grade 0 (no ossification) to grade 4 (all four quadrants show ossification of the iliac apophysis). When the ossified apophysis has fused completely to the ilium (Risser's grade 5), the patient is skeletally mature. *(From Herring, J.A. Tachdjian's Pediatric Orthopaedics, 3rd ed., vol. 1. WB Saunders, New York, 2002, p. 215; fig. 11-2, with permission.)*

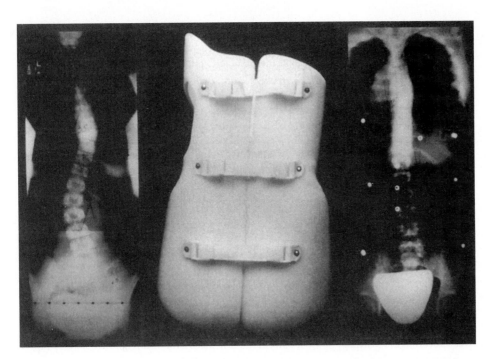

FIGURE **26-5** Custom-molded TLSO. *(From Herring, J.A. Tachdjian's Pediatric Orthopaedics, 3rd ed., vol. 1. WB Saunders, New York, 2002, p. 231; fig. 11-23, with permission.)*

patient. Surgery may be indicated for those who have failed conservative treatment, that is, bracing, secondary to a severe scoliosis and/or decreased patient compliance with the bracing protocol.[15] If a progressing curve is left untreated, it can lead to deformity, pain, decreased pulmonary function, and/or negative psychological effects[3,17–19] (Figure 26-8).

SURGICAL OVERVIEW

When surgical management is optimal for correction of the curve, the surgeon must consider (1) what curves to fuse, (2) how many and what spinal levels to fuse, (3) the type of instrumentation to use, and (4) the surgical approach.[3] The curve fused and levels of fusion are

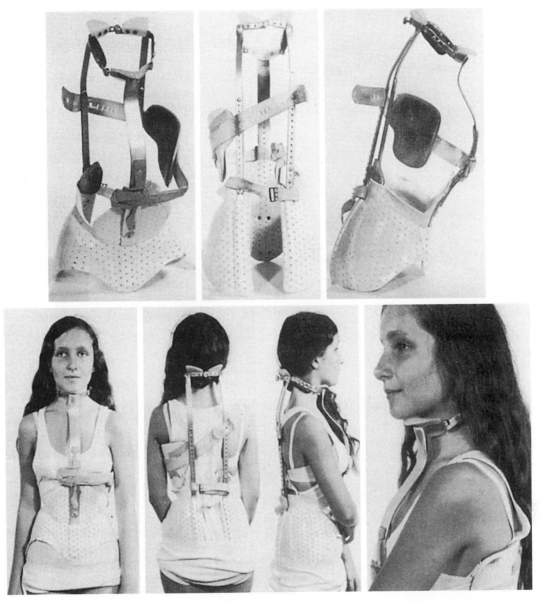

FIGURE **26-6** Milwaukee brace (CTLSO). *(From Herring, J.A. Tachdjian's Pediatric Orthopaedics, 3rd ed., vol. 1. WB Saunders, New York, 2002, p. 230; fig. 11-22, with permission.)*

determined by the identification of the primary and secondary curves as well as the severity of the curve. The first and the last vertebra of the major curve(s) are identified and all included vertebras are fused. To achieve a neutrally rotated spine, the fusion must often extend one level above the scoliotic curve. The fusion is extended one level below the curve to achieve a stable base.[24]

The possible surgical approaches for correction of scoliosis include a posterior spinal fusion (PSF), an anterior spinal fusion (ASF), or a combination of both. The most common surgical procedure performed for correction of AIS is a posterior spinal fusion in conjunction with posterior instrumentation. In a PSF, a subperiosteal exposure

is made followed by facet excision, and fusion is achieved with bone obtained from the iliac crest or ribs[24] (Figure 26-9). Instrumentation is added to the fusion to achieve and maintain correction (Figure 26-10). An anterior approach is often chosen when there is a single lumbar curve or for a thoracolumbar curve (Figures 26-11 and 26-12). For this surgical approach, the segments included in the fusion are those central to the structural central area of the curve. In an ASF, exposure is made on the convex side of the curve with complete disc excision. The disc space is packed with autologous rib bone graft, then stabilized with compression instrumentation on the convex side.[24] A combined anterior/posterior spinal

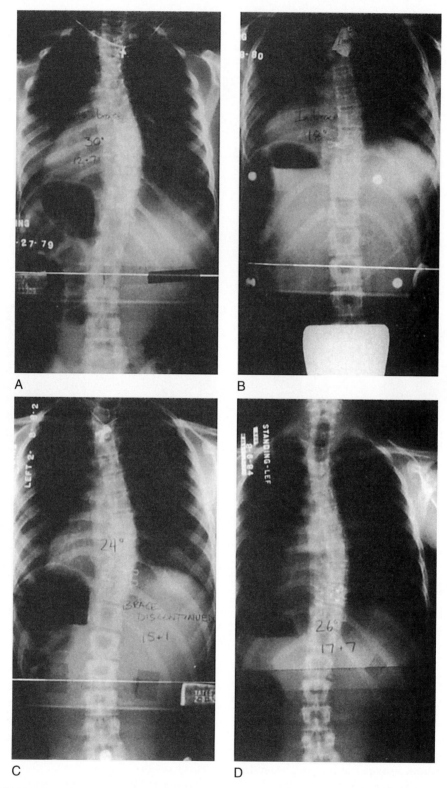

A

B

C

D

FIGURE **26-7** Radiographic findings with brace wear in a premenarchal girl age 12 years, 7 months. *A.* Initially, she had a 30-degree thoracic curve with a Risser's grade of 0. *B.* Treatment in a TLSO was begun, with in-brace correction to 18 degrees. *C.* Brace wear was continued until the patient was 2 years postmenarchal and had a Risser's grade of 4. *D.* Two and a half years later curve remained stable at 26 degrees. *(From Herring, J.A. Tachdjian's Pediatric Orthopaedics, 3rd ed., vol. 1. WB Saunders, New York, 2002, p. 233; fig. 11-25, with permission.)*

Treatment	Cobb Angle (degrees)	Skeletal Maturity (Risser's sign)
Observation	0–20	0–1
	0–30	2–3
Brace	20–40	0–1
	30–40	2–3
	40–50	0–3
Surgery	40–50	0–3
	>50	0–4

Adapted from information in *Scoliosis Research Society* Web site http://www.SRS.org.

FIGURE **26-8** Indications for treatment.

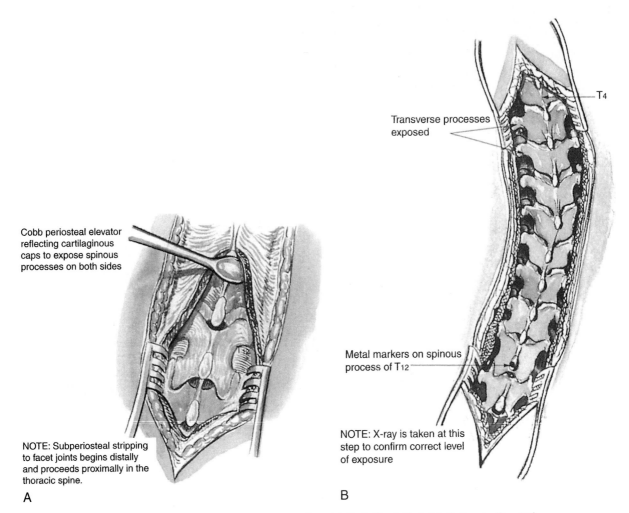

Cobb periosteal elevator reflecting cartilaginous caps to expose spinous processes on both sides

NOTE: Subperiosteal stripping to facet joints begins distally and proceeds proximally in the thoracic spine.

A

T4

Transverse processes exposed

Metal markers on spinous process of T12

NOTE: X-ray is taken at this step to confirm correct level of exposure

B

FIGURE **26-9** Posterior spinal fusion. *(From Herring, J.A. Tachdjian's Pediatric Orthopaedics, 3rd ed., vol. 1. WB Saunders, New York, 2002, p. 251; plate 11–2, figs. I and K, with permission.)*

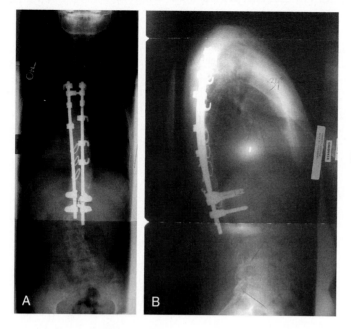

FIGURE **26-10** Radiograph of a 15-year-old boy status post PSF depicting third generation spine instrumentation.

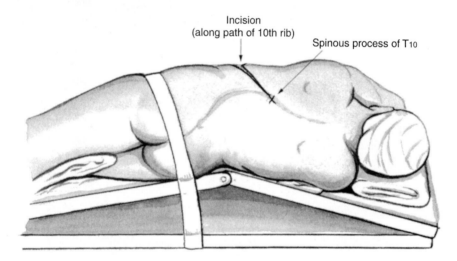

Incision
(along path of 10th rib)

Spinous process of T10

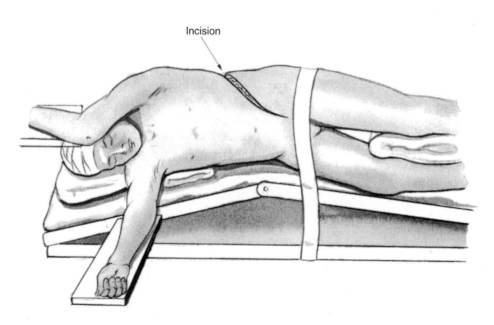

Incision

FIGURE **26-11** Anterior spinal fusion. *(From Herring, J.A. Tach-djian's Pediatric Orthopaedics, 3rd ed., vol. 1. WB Saunders, New York, 2002, p. 263; plate 11–3, fig. A, with permission.)*

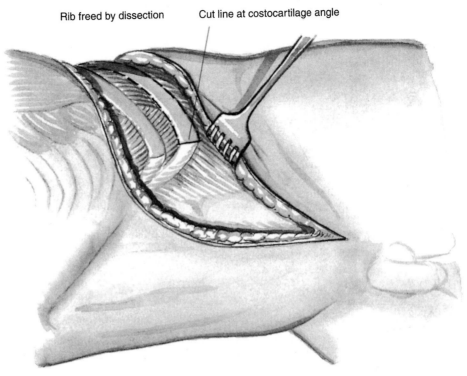

Rib freed by dissection   Cut line at costocartilage angle

FIGURE **26-12** Anterior spinal fusion. *(From Herring, J.A. Tach-djian's Pediatric Orthopaedics, 3rd ed., vol. 1. WB Saunders, New York, 2002, p. 265; plate 11–3, fig. B, with permission.)*

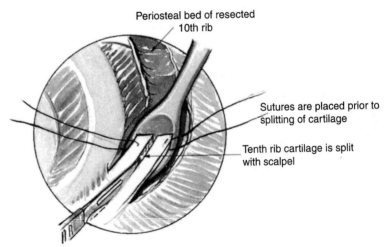

Periosteal bed of resected 10th rib

Sutures are placed prior to splitting of cartilage

Tenth rib cartilage is split with scalpel

fusion for AIS is indicated for large, stiff curves and/or a progressing curve that demonstrates a rotational deformity, especially in a skeletally immature patient.[24]

Instrumentation combined with a spinal fusion assists in correcting spinal deformity, improves spinal stability, and allows for early mobilization resulting in a lower pseudoarthrosis rate as the fusion heals.[24] The original instrumentation was introduced by Harrington[24] and consisted of two rods, a distraction rod on the concave side of the curve, and a compression rod on the convex side of the curve. Modifications have been made to the original Harrington system, which currently affords the surgeon to have many options for instrumentation. At HSS, surgeons prefer to use third generation systems or modern spine systems. Such systems are comprised of two interlinked rods made of titanium and/or stainless steel, with hooks, wires, and screws that allow for segmental fusion.[24] Spinal fusion combined with instrumentation takes between 6 and 12 months to be completely healed.[3] Most patients do not require removal of hardware from this surgery.

REHABILITATION OVERVIEW

At HSS, physical therapy plays a primary role in the post-surgical rehabilitation of AIS. The rehabilitation program following ASF and/or PSF surgery is designed to pro-

Preoperative Rehabilitation

GOALS

- Patient/caregiver education
- Maximize trunk extensor strength
- Maximize core abdominal strength
- Demonstrate independence in log rolling
- Demonstrate understanding of all spine precautions

TREATMENT STRATEGIES

- Patient/parent education in spine precautions, body mechanics, and proper postural alignment
- Breathing exercises: incentive spirometry
- Log rolling
- Hamstring/hip flexor stretching
- Trunk extension strengthening
- Core abdominal strength: neutral spine stabilization exercises, Physio ball Therex
- LE strengthening: quadriceps sets, bridges, wall squats, total gym
- Endurance training/general conditioning: stationary bike, treadmill, elliptical

gressively return patients to their prior level of function. The focus of physical therapy is to restore trunk and core abdominal strength, upper and lower extremity flexibility and strength, as well as educate the patient in proper posture and body mechanics. Both the anatomy and biomechanics of the spine pre- and post-surgery must be considered throughout the course of treatment. The biomechanics of the fused levels are altered post-surgically as well as those levels just above and below the fusion. Continuous communication between the surgeon, therapist, and patient is key for a successful outcome. Throughout the rehabilitation course, the patient should play an active role in his or her recovery by setting and working toward functional goals. The patient must be compliant with all spine precautions to protect the healing fusion and be diligent in performing his or her home exercise program (HEP) to ensure carryover and success in the rehabilitative process.

PREOPERATIVE REHABILITATION

When a child is referred for preoperative physical therapy, the goals are to improve overall endurance, general conditioning, flexibility, trunk strength, and abdominal and lower extremity strength in preparation for surgery. Special focus is given to hamstring and hip flexor flexibility, trunk extensor strength and core lower abdominal strength, and proper breathing techniques.

In addition, the preoperative program emphasizes patient education. All patients and their caregivers are instructed in postoperative spine precautions as well as proper posture and body mechanics during functional activities. Postoperative spine precautions/movement contraindications are in place for at least 6 months and include the following: no flexion of the lumbar or thoracic spine, no rotation of the lumbar or thoracic spine,

and no lifting of heavy objects (<8 to 10 pounds). The 6-month time frame in which these precautions are maintained is fairly consistent but may vary slightly depending on the individual patient and physician. To abide by these precautions, patients are taught proper transfers in and out of bed via log rolling, transfers from sit to stand and vice versa, emphasizing the lower extremities, and proper body mechanics during all movements and activities of daily living (ADL).

POSTOPERATIVE REHABILITATION ACUTE/INPATIENT PHASE I (WEEK 1)

Postoperative rehabilitation begins on postoperative day 1 in the hospital. Following a spinal fusion, patients are seen twice a day for physical therapy, with an emphasis on functional activities. On postoperative day 1, all patients are evaluated by a physical therapist and both the patient and the caregivers are instructed in all spine precautions and proper body mechanics. Patients are given quadriceps sets for lower extremity strength and ankle pumps to aid in the reduction of swelling, prevention of blood clots, and increase circulation. The goal for postoperative day 1 is for the patient to dangle at bedside for as long as tolerated (usually 1 to 2 minutes). The patient is instructed in supine to sit transfers via log rolling and is assisted to sit at the edge of the bed (dangle) for as long as tolerated (Figure 26-13). On postoperative day 1, most patients require maximum assistance for this task. While dangling, patients are asked to perform incentive spirometry and deep breathing exercises. During the treatment session, patients should be monitored for increased pain and signs that would indicate orthostatic hypotension, such as nausea and increased dizziness. On postoperative day 2, log rolling is reinforced and instruction is

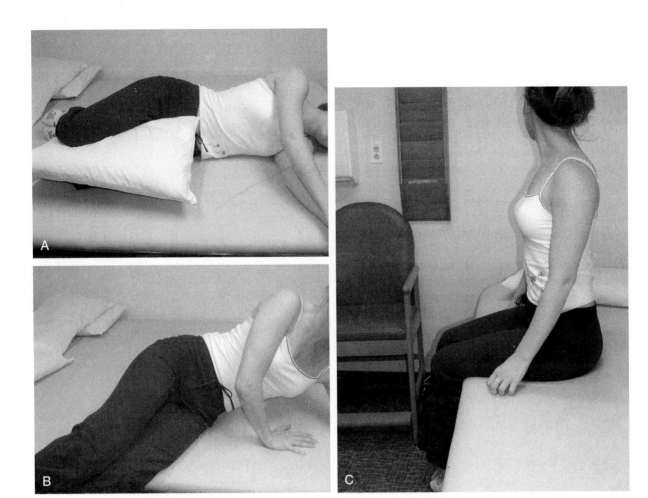

FIGURE 26-13 Patient is taught log rolling and how to maintain the spine in a neutral position during the transition. During log rolling, spine precautions are maintained to protect the healing fusion. *A.* Patient has rolled from supine to left side-lying with spine in neutral. *B.* Patient transitions from side-lying to sit, maintaining spine in neutral position. *C.* Patient dangling at edge of bed.

given on sit-to-stand transfers. If tolerated, the patient progresses to standing and ambulation. Ambulation is performed with a rolling walker and assistance from the physical therapist. On postoperative days 3 and 4, the focus of rehabilitation is on reinforcing precautions, progressing toward independent transfers in and out of bed via log rolling, progressing ambulation with a rolling walker, and building endurance through ambulation. At this time, patients are encouraged to spend part of their day sitting in a chair to further build up their endurance and improve tolerance for out-of-bed activities. On days 5 and 6, patients progress to ambulating with hand-held assistance and begin stair climbing. Before a patient is discharged, he or she is required to be independent with all spine precautions, required minimal to no assistance during log rolling/transferring in and out of bed, required to ambulate independently without an assistive device, and climb stairs using one rail. Upon discharge, which

is typically day 6 or 7, patients continue to follow all spine precautions until otherwise directed by their surgeon and are encouraged to gradually progress ambulation distance to improve overall endurance. The previously described protocol is an average approximation based on the authors' typical postoperative patient. Patients are not discharged until they have met their individual discharge goals.

Troubleshooting

Most of the issues encountered that delay progress in post-surgery physical therapy are medically related. Following major surgery, patients often experience nausea, vomiting, dizziness, orthostatic hypotension, and pain. In some patients, these symptoms can last for a few days, thus delaying their progress in physical therapy and achievement of functional goals. For a patient suffering from severe nausea and vomiting, medications can be administered or changed by the

Postoperative Rehabilitation Acute/Inpatient Phase I (Week 1)

GOALS

- Independent with all spine precautions
- Independent or minimally assisted transfers
- Independent ambulation
- Independent stair climbing with one railing
- Independent with proper posture and body mechanics
- Independent with donning/doffing brace, if applicable

PRECAUTIONS

- No lumbar or thoracic flexion
- No lumbar or thoracic rotation
- No lifting of heavy objects (<8 to 10 pounds)

TREATMENT STRATEGIES

Day 1

- Patient education regarding spine precautions to protect the healing fusion
- Incentive spirometry
- Assisted log rolling for transfers in and out of bed
- Assisted dangle at bedside
- Ankle pumps and quadriceps sets 10 times per hour

Day 2

- Review spine precautions
- Incentive spirometry
- Log rolling for transfers in and out of bed
- Stand and ambulate at bedside with rolling walker and assistance
- Ankle pumps and quadriceps sets 10 times per hour

Days 3 and 4

- Review spine precautions
- Incentive spirometry
- Log rolling for transfers in and out of bed
- Progress ambulation with rolling walker, with emphasis on decreasing use of upper extremities—assess ability to ambulate with hand-held assistance
- Patient comfortable sitting in chair for 20 minutes
- Ankle pumps and quadriceps sets 10 times per hour

Days 5 and 6

- Review spine precautions
- Deep breathing exercises
- Log rolling for transfers in and out of bed
- Ambulation with hand-held assistance to supervised ambulation
- Stairs with supervision and one rail

Day 7—Discharge

- Review all spine precautions and discharge instructions
- Independent with donning/doffing brace, if applicable (caregiver can assist if needed)
- Independent/minimal assistance for log rolling for transfers in and out of bed
- Independent ambulation
- Independent stairs with one rail
- Patient comfortable sitting in chair for all meals
- Independent with HEP (quadriceps sets, ankle pumps, endurance training with walking program)

physician, depending on individual medical needs. Patients may also require the change in the amount and/or type of pain medication administered. For a patient suffering from orthostatic hypotension, slow but more frequent mobilization throughout the day may be beneficial to help these symptoms resolve at a faster rate. It is often necessary to have other members of the health care team, such as nursing and rehabilitation aids, involved in this mobilization process.

For patients who are suffering from increased dizziness, increased pain, muscle spasms, and atelectasis, deep breathing can be a key component to their recovery. Deep breathing exercises should be emphasized during all positions, that is, supine through standing, and given to the patient to practice with family members supervising throughout the day. Deep breathing can aid in not only alleviating complications postoperatively, but also in preventing their occurrence.

Another issue that may delay progress in physical therapy is a patient's need for the external support of a custom-made brace to dangle and/or ambulate. If this is the case, physical therapy will be postponed until the brace is available.

POSTOPERATIVE REHABILITATION OUTPATIENT PHASE I (WEEKS 1 TO 6)

Postoperative outpatient physical therapy at HSS typically begins 1 to 6 months post-surgery, depending on

the surgeon. When beginning the rehabilitation course with a patient who recently underwent a spinal fusion, all spine fusion precautions must remain in place until the surgeon discontinues or modifies the precautions. The precautions should be continually reinforced to provide a safe environment for healing of the fusion. Before beginning treatment, the level of fusion should be known to protect the surrounding thoracic and lumbar segments because the levels just below and above the fusion are at increased risk for becoming hypermobile. The following rehabilitation protocol uses the core stabilization program of Shirley Sahrmann. The Sahrmann core program is devised for patients to learn to contract the abdominal muscles to prevent motions of the spine during movements of the lower extremities (Figures 26-14, 26-15, 26-16).[26]

Postoperative Rehabilitation Outpatient Phase I (Weeks 1 to 6)**

GOALS
- Patient can verbalize and demonstrate spine precautions, proper body mechanics, positioning, and posture.
- Maximize core strengthening
- Maximize postural strength
- Maximize flexibility of upper and lower extremities
- Maximize strength of upper and lower extremities
- Maximize endurance
- Independent with HEP

PRECAUTIONS
- No lumbar or thoracic flexion
- No lumbar or thoracic rotation
- No lifting of heavy objects (8 to 10 pounds)
- Sports/gym activities, as per surgeon
- No weights or resistance training
- Hamstring stretching, as per surgeon (reinforce use of abdominal stabilization as to stretch only hamstrings and reduce pull on lumbar spine)

TREATMENT STRATEGIES
- Review log rolling, bed mobility, resting/sleep positioning
- Review and facilitate proper posture in sitting and standing
- Core stabilization (Sahrmann) at appropriate level: neutral spine stabilization exercises with emphasis on abdominal contraction
- Lower extremity flexibility, as per surgeon (*gentle stretching only*)
- *Active* shoulder girdle mobilization—shoulder shrugs, forward/backward shoulder rolls, scapular retraction
- Postural strengthening—scapular retraction (progressive), shoulder forward flexion in scapular plane on bench, sitting posture with visual cueing, chin tucks, prone scapular retraction with upper and middle trapezius, shoulder extension, scapular stabilization
- Soft tissue/myofascial to trunk and shoulder girdle
- Endurance/general conditioning: treadmill, stationary bike

ADVANCEMENT CRITERIA
- Patient exhibits symmetrical shoulders and pelvis 50% of the time
- Ambulation with reciprocal arm swing
- Improved core strength, Sahrmann level II
- Independent in log rolling, bed mobility

**Postoperative rehabilitation begins 1 to 6 months after surgery.*

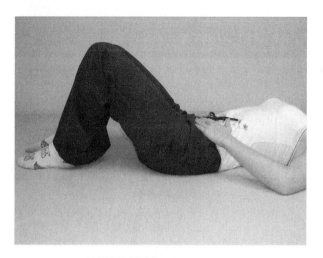

FIGURE **26-14** Abdominal set.

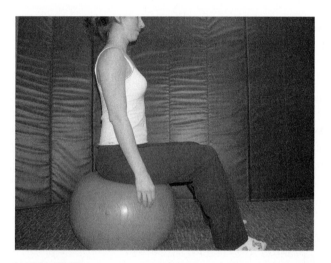

FIGURE **26-15** Postural reeducation on physio ball, emphasizing chin tuck and abdominal activation. A mirror can be used for visual cueing of straight spine and symmetrical shoulders.

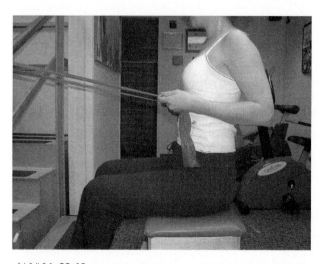

FIGURE **26-16** Seated scapular retraction with Thera-Band.

Troubleshooting

During phase I of the postoperative outpatient rehabilitation of the child who has undergone a spinal fusion, emphasizing spine precautions continues to be critical. In most cases, by this time, pain levels are decreasing, discomfort is subsiding, and patients begin to have minimal to no limitations during ADL. However, once a patient's level of pain is decreased, he or she tends to disregard the spine precautions that are still in place to protect the surgery. It is therefore necessary to reinforce spine precautions for all functional activities, from bed mobility to self-care, and especially when returning to recreational activities.

Persistent asymmetry of the shoulders and pelvis may be observed postoperatively in some individuals (Figure 26-17). This may be as a result of habitual posturing, postural holding, muscle imbalance, tightness/restriction of the trunk fascia, or, in severe scoliotic curves, a residual asymmetry that was not able to be surgically corrected. It is important to assess the etiology of all trunk asymmetries and implement appropriate treatment before new postural habits are formed. Useful therapeutic techniques in the correction of

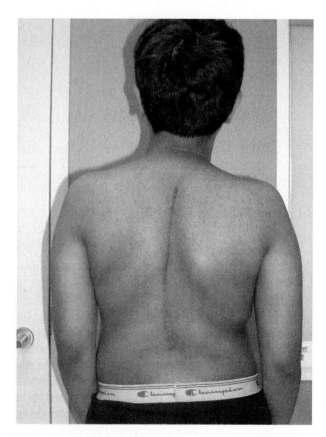

FIGURE **26-17** A 15-year-old boy 12 weeks postoperative PSF. Note the asymmetry of the shoulders and pelvis as well as increased scapular winging and shortening on the right side.

persistent asymmetry include elongation of shortened structures with myofascial release techniques and stretching, (active and passive) as well as muscle strengthening, with an emphasis on postural reeducation. Visual feedback with a mirror can be a useful tool, especially for carryover at home.

Particular weakness of scapular muscular may be noted with asymmetrical scapular winging. Strengthening of such musculature and stabilizing the scapula against thoracic wall are important for maintaining proper scapulohumeral rhythm and the prevention of pain and future shoulder problems.

At this stage of the outpatient rehabilitation process, a patient who complains of persistent and intense pain should be referred back to his or her surgeon for a follow-up. As previously stated, it is very important that the therapist and surgeon are in contact throughout the rehabilitation process. This will allow the therapist to have a solid basis for progression of each patient and constant information regarding the status of fusion healing. Continued reinforcement of spine precautions and a daily HEP is necessary throughout the rehabilitation course.

POSTOPERATIVE REHABILITATION OUTPATIENT PHASE II (WEEKS 6 TO 12)

The primary focus of this phase of rehabilitation is to improve posture and develop overall muscle strength. Emphasis is placed on core stabilization and lower extremity strength because patients will be given physician clearance to return to light recreational activities and noncontact sports in the next few months. It is important that they develop the strength, endurance, and good postural support to further protect their spinal fusion. As a patient is preparing to return to sports/recreational activities, the therapist should perform an activity-specific evaluation with special attention paid to strength deficits and biomechanical movement of the spine. Movements should be distributed throughout the mobile segments rather than just above and below fusion (Figures 26-18, 26-19, 26-20).

Troubleshooting

During phase II of the outpatient postoperative rehabilitation, patients may experience difficulties with many of the same issues as in phase I. Strong communication

---

Postoperative Rehabilitation Outpatient Phase II (Weeks 6 to 12)

GOALS
- Independent with proper posture and body mechanics during advanced functional activities
- Core strength Sahrmann level III
- Maximize postural strength
- Maximize postural endurance
- Maximize flexibility of upper and lower extremities
- Maximize lower extremity strength, proximal hip strength (5/5)
- Maximize endurance and general conditioning

PRECAUTIONS
- Same as phase I
- Hamstring stretching, as per surgeon (reinforce use of abdominal stabilization so as to stretch hamstrings only and reduce pull on lumbar spine)

TREATMENT STRATEGIES
- Body mechanics with regard to squatting to pick objects off floor; use hip flexion not lumbar motion
- Postural strengthening—emphasis on scapular stabilization, scapular retraction, shoulder forward flexion in prone
- Advanced core stabilization—therapeutic ball, quadruped with neutral spine
- Lower extremity flexibility—gentle stretching with abdominals activated
- *Continue active* shoulder girdle mobility
- Soft tissue/myofascial release
- Continue and progress endurance

CRITERIA FOR DISCHARGE
- Symmetrical shoulders and pelvis 100% of the time
- Proper posture and body mechanics 100% of the time
- Pre-surgical level of endurance
- Sahrmann level III

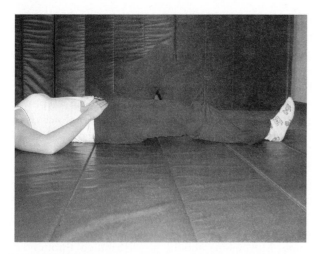

FIGURE **26-18** Abdominal set with heel slide and spine maintained in neutral alignment.

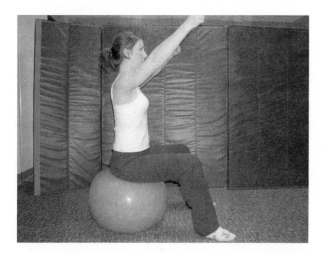

FIGURE **26-19** Forward shoulder flexion in the scapular plane done on physio ball to incorporate reeducation of postural muscles.

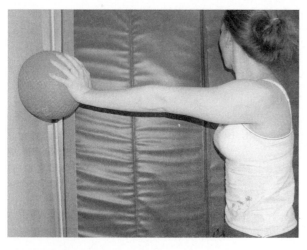

FIGURE **26-20** Scapular stabilization for scapular winging and strengthening of shoulder girdle.

with the surgeon will again help guide the rehabilitation course. The rehabilitation program continues to emphasize flexibility and strengthening. Pain should no longer be a primary and/or daily complaint. A patient who has unusual complaints at anytime throughout during the rehabilitation course should be immediately referred back to his or her surgeon. During phase II, it becomes even more necessary to emphasize the importance of spine precautions in higher level functional activities and recreational/sport activities. As patients have less pain and begin to resume normal activities, they tend to disregard spine precautions. It will be necessary to demonstrate and practice how to perform these activities while maintaining all spine precautions, so that carryover is ensured. Finally, emphasizing the importance of carryover with the HEP is necessary to achieve adequate strength and flexibility for return to sports and other functional activities. At HSS each patient with scoliosis is treated individually to achieve his or her maximum functional goals and potential.

REFERENCES

1. *SRS Terminology and Working Group on Spinal Classification* (Chair Larry Lenke, MD). Revised Glossary of Terms, 2000. Available online at http://www.SRS.org.
2. Tecklin, J. *Pediatric Physical Therapy,* 3rd ed. Lippincott Williams & Wilkins, New York, 1999.
3. Weinstein, S.L. *The Pediatric Spine, Principles and Practice,* 2nd ed. Lippincott Williams & Wilkins, Philadelphia, 2001.
4. Lovell, W.W., Winter, R.B. *Pediatric Orthopaedics,* 4th ed., vol. 2. Lippincott and Raven, New York, 1996.
5. Rogala, E.J., Drummond, D.S., Gurr, J. *Scoliosis Incidence and Natural History. A Prospective Epidemiological Study.* J Bone Joint Surg Am 1978;60(2):173–176.
6. Risenborough, E.J., Wynne-Davies, R. *A Genetic Survey of Idiopathic Scoliosis in Boston, Massachusetts.* J Bone Joint Surg Am 1973;55(5):974–982.
7. Benzel, E. *Spine Surgery: Techniques, Complication Avoidance, and Management,* vol. 1. Churchill Livingstone, New York, 1999.
8. Herring, J.A. *Tachdjian's Pediatric Orthopaedics,* 3rd ed., vol. 1. WB Saunders, New York, 2002, pp. 215, fig. 11-2.
9. Weinstein, S.L. Idiopathic scoliosis. *Natural History.* Spine 1986;11(8):780–783.
10. Lonstein, J., Carlson, J. *The Prediction of Curve Progression in Untreated Idiopathic Scoliosis During Growth.* J Bone Joint Surg 1984;66:1061–1071.
11. Peterson, L.E., Nachemson, A.L. *Prediction of Progression of the Curve in Girls Who Have Adolescent Idiopathic Scoliosis of Moderate Severity. Logistic Regression Analysis Based on Data from The Brace Study of the Scoliosis Research Society.* J Bone Joint Surg Am 1995;77(6):823–827.
12. Duval-Beaupere, G., Lamireau, T. *Scoliosis at Less than 30 Degrees. Properties of the Evolutivity (Risk of Progression).* Spine 1985;10(5):421–424.
13. Perdriolle, R., Vidal, J. *Thoracic Idiopathic Scoliosis Curve Evolution and Prognosis.* Spine 1985;10(9):785–791.
14. Weinstein, S.L., Ponseti, I.V. *Curve Progression in Idiopathic Scoliosis.* J Bone Joint Surg Am 1983;65(4):447–455.

15. Rowe, D.E., Bernstein, S.M., Riddick, M.F., Adler, F., Emans, J.B., Gardner-Bonneau, D. *A Meta-analysis of the Efficacy of Nonoperative Treatments for Idiopathic Scoliosis.* J Bone Joint Surg 1997;79:664–674.

16. Nachemson, A.L., Peterson, L.E. *Effectiveness of Treatment with a Brace in Girls Who Have Adolescent Idiopathic Scoliosis. A Prospective, Controlled Study Based on Data from The Brace Study of the Scoliosis Research Society.* J Bone Joint Surg Am 1995;77(6):815–822.

17. Clayson, D., Luz-Alterman, S., Cataletto, M.M., Levine, D.B. *Long-term Psychological Sequelae of Surgically Versus Nonsurgically Treated Scoliosis.* Spine 1987;12:983–986.

18. Payne, W., Ogilvie, J. *Does Scoliosis Have a Psychological Impact and Does Gender Make a Difference?* Spine 1997;22(12):1380–1394.

19. Winter, R.B., Lovell, W.W., Moe, J.H. *Excessive Thoracic Lordosis and Loss of Pulmonary Function I Patients with Idiopathic Scoliosis.* J Bone Joint Surg Am 1975;57(7):972–977.

20. Stone, B., Beekman, C., Hall, V., Guess, V., Brooks, L. *The Effect of an Exercise Program on Change in Curve in Adolescents with Minimal Idiopathic Scoliosis.* Phys Ther 1979;59:759–763.

21. Bertrand, S.L., Drvaric, D.M., Lange, N., Lucas, P.R., Deutsch, S.D., Herndon, J.H., Roberts, J.M. *Electrical Stimulation for Idiopathic Scoliosis.* Clin Orthop Relat Res 1992;276:176–181.

22. Durham, J.W., Moskowitz, A., Whitney, J. *Surface Electrical Stimulation Versus Brace Treatment of Idiopathic Scoliosis.* Spine 1990;15(9):888–892.

23. O'Donnell, C.S., Bunnell, W.P., Betz, R.R., Bowen, J.R., Tipping, C.R. *Electrical Stimulation in the Treatment of Idiopathic Scoliosis.* Clin Orthop Relat Res 1988;229:107–113.

24. Lonstein, J., Bradford, D., Winter, R., Ogilvie, J. *Moe's Textbook of Scoliosis and Other Spinal Deformities,* 3rd ed. WB Saunders, Philadelphia, 1995.

25. Coillard, C., Leroux, M., Zabjek, K., Rivard, C. *SpineCor—A Non-rigid Brace for the Treatment of Idiopathic Scoliosis: Post-treatment Results.* Eur Spine J 2003;12(2):141–148.

26. Sahrmann, S. *Diagnosis and Treatment of Movement Impairment Syndromes.* Mosby, Philadelphia, 2002.

27

Congenital Muscular Torticollis

DEBORAH CORRADI-SCALISE, PT, DPT

AMANDA R. SPARROW, PT

LORETTA AMOROSO, DPT

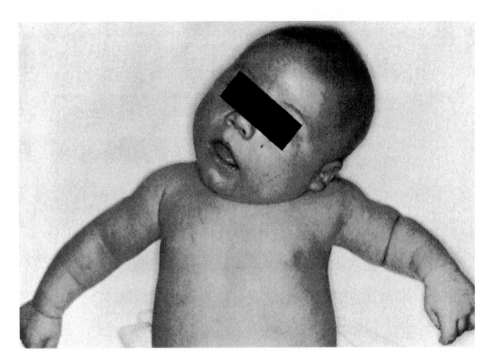

FIGURE **27-1** CMT due to a contracted left SCM. *(From Herring, J.A. Tachdjian's Pediatric Orthopaedics, 3rd ed. WB Saunders Co, Philadelphia, 2002, p. 173.)*

Congenital muscular torticollis (CMT) is defined as a unilateral shortening or contracture of the sternocleidomastoid (SCM) muscle, present at birth. It presents as a persistent tilt of the head toward the involved side with the chin rotated toward the opposite shoulder[1] (Figure 27-1). Torticollis (*tortus* ["twisted"], *collum* ["neck"]) is also referred to as "wry neck."[2] The reported incidence of occurrence ranges from 0.4% to 1.9% of births.[3] Diagnosis of CMT can be as early as ages 2 to 3 weeks.[4] Three of four diagnosed cases present with the lesion on the right side.[1] The coexistence of CMT with developmental hip dysplasia has been reported with variations of 0 to 20%.[5,6] Additionally, babies with CMT have a higher incidence of breech presentation, associated congenital musculoskeletal disorders, and foot deformities.[4] The exact etiology of CMT is unknown; however, many causative theories have been postulated, including intrauterine malposition, birth trauma, uterine compression/crowding, possible ischemic event causing a compartment syndrome of the SCM, faulty SCM cell differentiation, or possible entrapment of the spinal accessory nerve due to fibrosis.[1,4] An infant with right CMT presents with cervical lateral flexion to the right side and cervical rotation to the left shoulder (Figure 27-2). Facial asymmetry and plagiocephaly (flattening of the occiput on the contralateral side as the tilt) are also often associated with CMT (Figure 27-3). Occasionally, a palpable mass or pseudotumor is associated with CMT. This fibrotic mass is within the SCM muscle belly and will gradually resolve[4] (Figure 27-4).

Conservative management of CMT, which includes physical therapy and a home exercise program (HEP),

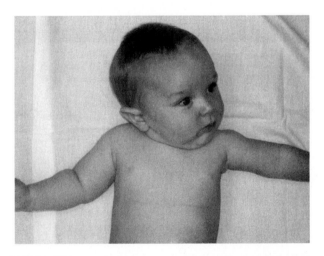

FIGURE **27-2** A 7-month-old infant with right CMT. Note cervical lateral flexion to the right and rotation to the left.

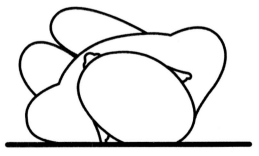

FIGURE **27-3** Flattening of the left occipital area and left ear deformation due to supine positioning of a child with right CMT. *(From Herring, J.A. Tachdjian's Pediatric Orthopaedics, 3rd ed. WB Saunders Co, Philadelphia, 2002, p. 173.)*

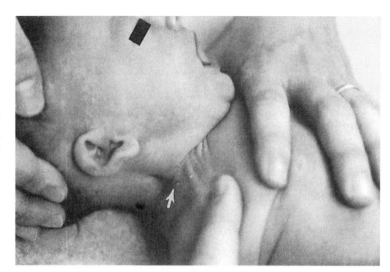

FIGURE 27-4 Palpable mass in right SCM (*arrow*) of a newborn. *(From Herring, J.A. Tachdjian's Pediatric Orthopaedics, 3rd ed. WB Saunders Co, Philadelphia, 2002, p. 173.)*

is recommended during the first year of life.[1,4] There is evidence in the literature that complete resolution of CMT occurs in greater than 90% of those babies treated by conservative means.[7-9] CMT cases that do not resolve with conservative management after age 1 may require surgical intervention for correction.[10] If left untreated, CMT can lead to increased facial and cranial asymmetries, positional deformity of the ear, cervical scoliosis with thoracic kyphosis, ocular and vestibular impairments, and functional asymmetry resembling hemiplegia, without neurological deficits.[4,11]

ANATOMICAL OVERVIEW

The SCM is composed of two muscles, one located on each side of the neck. The SCM is the most superficial of the anterior neck muscles.[12] It originates from two heads: the sternal head, originating from the ventral border of the manubrium sterni partly covering the sternoclavicular joint; and the clavicular head, originating from the superior border and anterior surface of the medial one-third of the clavicle. The SCM inserts by a thin aponeurosis into the lateral one-half of the superior nuchal line of the occipital bone (Figure 27-5). The SCM muscle is innervated by the spinal accessory nerve and ventral primary divisions of cranial nerves 2 and 3. The two SCM muscles working in synergy will flex the neck. Unilateral SCM muscle activation will produce lateral flexion to the same (ipsilateral) side and rotation to the opposite (contralateral) side, with slight cervical extension.[13]

Although the SCM muscle is the muscle primarily responsible for CMT, other musculature around the neck, shoulder girdle, chest, and trunk may display tightness and/or shortening. Performing a thorough

examination to identify the impairments to be addressed in treatment is important.

DIFFERENTIAL DIAGNOSIS

CMT is present at birth. As previously stated, it can be diagnosed as early as ages 2 to 3 weeks, but it may not be diagnosed until the infant is noted to be unable to hold his or her head in midline at ages 4 to 5 months. Medical differential diagnosis is important to rule out other causative factors of positional head/neck asymmetry. Other causative factors, such as viral infection, muscular strain, postnatal trauma (clavicular fracture), congenital anomalies of the base of the skull, congenital anomalies of the upper cervical spine, ocular pathology, imbalance of the extraocular muscles, rotary subluxation of the atlantoaxial joints (following URI), tumor of the posterior fossa, brain stem, or cervical spinal cord, all need to be ruled out as the cause of the presenting neck asymmetry.[1] Neurological evaluation may be required to rule out an underlying neurological cause, especially in the event of sudden onset torticollis in the infant.[1]

Additionally, syndromes that may present with associated torticollis should be considered in the differential diagnosis (Figure 27-6). Routine radiography of the cervical spine will frequently rule out congenital anomalies of the cervical spine and rotary subluxation of the atlantoaxial junction. Computed tomography (CT) scanning or magnetic resonance imaging (MRI) may be necessary for more precise evaluation and in ruling out the presence of tumors or growths.[1]

Evidence shows that a thorough clinical examination is necessary to assist in differential diagnosis as it relates to CMT. As previously stated, ocular pathologies, bony deformities of the spine, neurological impairments, syndromes, and congenital deformities can present with an

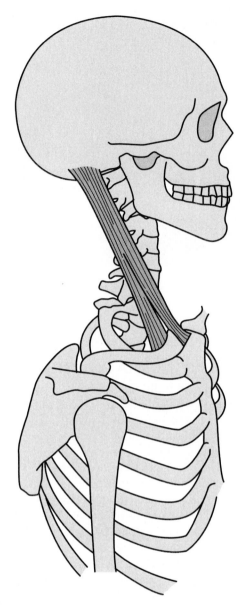

FIGURE **27-5** Anatomy of the SCM muscle. *(From Daniels, L., Worthingham, C. Muscle Testing: Techniques of Manual Examination, 4th ed. WB Saunders Co, Philadelphia, 1980, p. 16.)*

Syndrome	Typical Presentation
Klippel Feil Syndrome	Congenital fusion of the cervical vertebrae, triad of low posterior hairline, short neck, and limited range of neck motion[1]
Sandifer Syndrome	Gastroesophageal reflux, abnormal posturing of the neck and trunk typically as torticollis, may present with opisthostonus or neural tics that often mimic central nervous system disorders[1]
Paroxysmal Torticollis of Infancy	Rare episodic torticollis lasting for minutes or days, attacks occur in the morning, 1–4 episodes per month, trunk movements, eye movements alternating sides of the Torticollis[1]
Arnold Chairi Malformation	Caudal displacement of the hindbrain often associated with other congenital deformities of the brainstem and cerebellum. May present with torticollis, headaches and Paracervical muscle spasms[1]

FIGURE **27-6** Syndromes that should be considered in differential diagnosis of CMT because each may present with an associated torticollis. *(Adapted from Loder, R.T. The Cervical Spine. In Morrissy, R.T., Weinstein, S.L. [Eds]. Lovell and Winter's Pediatric Orthopaedics, 5th ed., vol. 2. Lippincott Williams & Wilkins, New York, 2001, pp. 811–815.)*

evaluation and treatment as needed. When examining an infant with a diagnosis of CMT, it is important for the pediatric physical therapist to perform a standard pediatric developmental, as well as an orthopedic, evaluation. Advanced evaluation skills are needed in infant assessment. Specific evaluation procedures are beyond the scope of this chapter. If CMT is diagnosed or suspected, specific focus should be placed on assessing neck ROM both passively and actively, using a universal goniometer. Neck measurements of lateral flexion and rotation are performed in supine (Figure 27-7, *A* and *B*). Additionally, at the Hospital for Special Surgery (HSS) all CMT infants referred for physical therapy by the Pediatric Orthopedic Department have been evaluated for developmental dysplasia of the hip.

REHABILITATION OVERVIEW
PRIMARY IMPAIRMENTS
- The baby postures with a lateral tilt toward the involved side and rotation away from the tight SCM.
- Limited passive range of motion (PROM) into lateral flexion toward the uninvolved side and decreased rotation toward the involved side.
- Decreased active head righting (i.e., muscle weakness with weight shift toward shortened SCM).
- Decreased active rotation toward the involved side in all developmental positions (Figure 27-8, *A* and *B*).

associated torticollis. In conditions such as cerebral palsy, an infant may present with a head tilt and asymmetrical neck muscle control. In infants with cerebral palsy, however, typically, assessment of passive neck range of motion (ROM) of lateral flexion and rotation is symmetrical, thus ruling out CMT. The influence of gravity and the presence of muscle weakness, coupled with poor head righting reactions, and the persistent influence of the asymmetrical tonic neck reflex may lead to an initial misdiagnosis of CMT. Based on clinical findings, the physical therapist may need to make referrals to other appropriate medical professionals for further

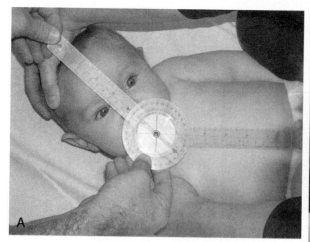

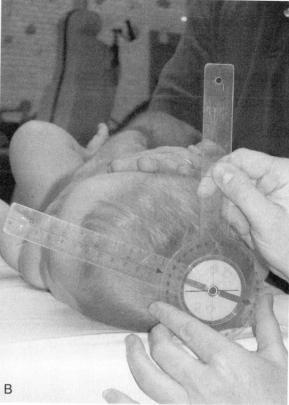

FIGURE **27-7** *A.* Measuring PROM of cervical lateral flexion in supine with a universal goniometer. *B.* Measuring PROM of cervical rotation in supine with a universal goniometer.

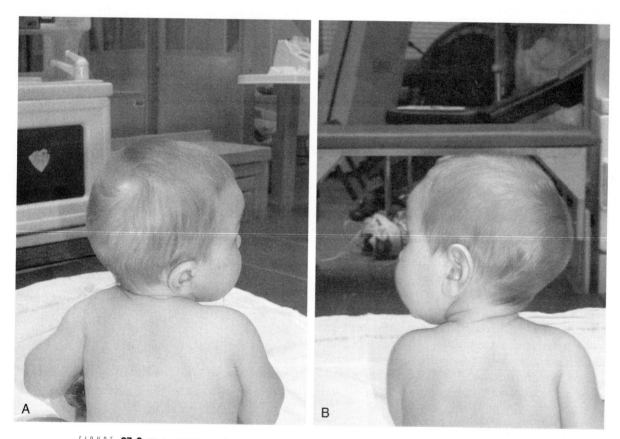

FIGURE **27-8** Right CMT—active neck ROM: *A.* Active cervical rotation to the right. *B.* Active cervical rotation to the left. Note decreased amount of active cervical rotation to the right side as compared to the left side. The infant is also enlisting trunk rotation to rotate to the right side; this is a means to compensate for decreased ability to rotate to the right through the cervical spine.

SECONDARY IMPAIRMENTS

- Plagiocephaly and facial deformity: Flattening on the posterior lateral portion of the skull on the uninvolved side due to the child's positioning in supine; associated facial deformities include posterior displacement of the ear on the same side of the involved SCM, posterior recession of the same side eyebrow and forehead, and the tip of the chin skewed toward the involved side. Less commonly noted is that the eye on the involved side is inferior to the opposite eye, and the nose may be deviated with the tip displaced toward the tight SCM.[14-16] Orthoplastic helmets may be used to treat plagiocephaly; however, at HSS they are not routinely used in standard treatment practices (Figure 27-9, A–C).

- Secondary muscle shortening: Tightness in secondary muscle(s) such as the platysma, scalene muscles, trapezius muscles, cervical extensors, pectoral muscles, as well as limitation of scapulohumeral ROM and trunk flexibility; shoulder elevation and protraction on the involved side may also be present.

- Developmental delays: As mentioned earlier, an infant diagnosed with CMT postures in a position that maintains a shortened position of the involved SCM. This habitual posturing leads to asymmetrical strength between sides, because the baby prefers to weight-bear over the unaffected side. A weakness in the ipsilateral trunk and scapular musculature due to the decreased active and controlled weight-bearing to and on that side (Figure 27-10) may also be present. Delays or asymmetrical movement patterns can develop, which include delayed rolling or rolling toward/over the unaffected side only, decreased weight-bearing and/or use of the arm on the involved side (prone prop and reaching), in sitting asymmetrical weight-bearing that fosters lateral flexion to the involved side, delayed creeping, pull to stand, and ambulation. Additionally, infants with CMT have a decreased awareness of midline orientation and may exhibit persistent expression of the asymmetrical tonic neck reflex to the uninvolved side (Figure 27-11). Therefore, delayed development of midline orientation and the following functional abilities of hands to midline, hands crossing midline, and bilateral upper extremity use, hands to knees and hands to feet may not be present.

REHABILITATION

The severity of the CMT upon initial diagnosis may affect the length of physical therapy treatment. The guidelines presented in the following section are based on the typical referral where initial diagnosis of CMT is made between ages 2 and 4 months.

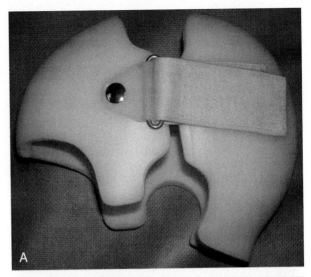

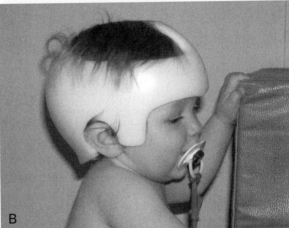

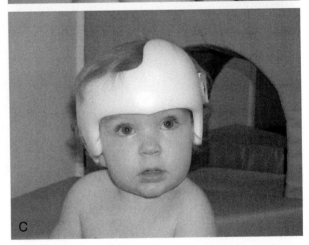

FIGURE 27-9 *A.* Orthoplastic helmet used to treat plagiocephaly—left side view. *B.* An infant, wearing an orthoplastic helmet, with right CMT and plagiocephaly—sagittal view. *C.* Frontal view.

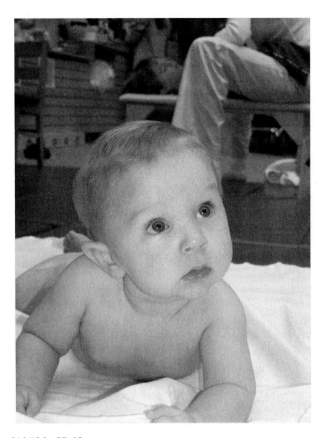

FIGURE **27-10** A 7-month-old infant with right CMT. Note decreased weight-bearing on the right shoulder and arm.

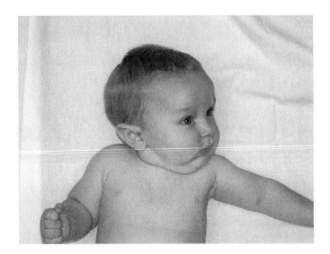

FIGURE **27-11** A 7-month-old infant with right CMT. Note influence of the asymmetrical tonic neck reflex (ATNR) to the uninvolved side.

TREATMENT GUIDELINES

When treating babies and children with CMT, early diagnosis and intervention as well as caregiver compliance with HEP is the key to a successful outcome. Complete recovery occurs in over 90% of all cases of CMT, if the diagnosis is made early and the infant receives physical

therapy, including HEP, before age 12 months.[8,9] After this age, conservative treatment through physical therapy and home stretching is less effective, with a greater percentage of the cases requiring surgical intervention.[14] At HSS, infants are seen for physical therapy intervention two to three times per week for 30 to 45 minute-sessions, depending on the severity of the CMT and the child's tolerance to therapeutic intervention. A HEP is recommended to be performed a minimum of four to five times per day or at every diaper change.

Physical therapy treatment for CMT consists of gentle passive and active stretching of the affected muscle, strengthening of the contralateral SCM muscle, positioning and facilitation of active midline head control, positioning of the child to promote lateral flexion to the uninvolved side, and rotation to the involved side. A specific HEP is given for the family/caregiver to perform. Some therapeutic techniques used in the management of CMT are traditional passive stretching methods of identified shortened muscles of the neck, shoulder, scapula, upper chest and trunk; myofascial release of the SCM, pectoralis, and upper trapezius muscles; disassociation of the scapulohumeral muscles on the involved side; active scapula adduction for shoulder girdle stability during weight-bearing activities; the use of postural adjustment reactions to promote head righting and antigravity neck strengthening (Figure 27-12); prone positioning to promote symmetrical cervical extension (Figure 27-13); functional activities

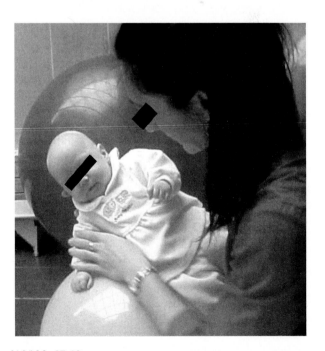

FIGURE **27-12** Active scapula adduction for shoulder girdle stability during weight-bearing activities; the use of postural adjustment reflexes to promote head righting and antigravity neck strengthening in an infant with right CMT.

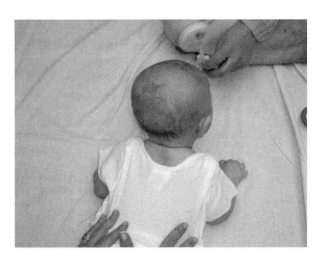

FIGURE **27-13** Prone positioning to promote symmetrical cervical extension.

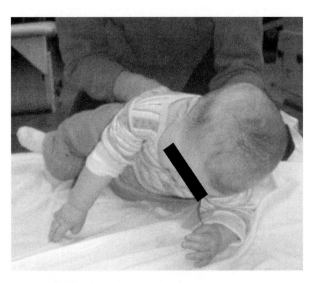

FIGURE **27-14** Transition from prone to left side-lying toward sitting to facilitate lateral head righting reactions and age-appropriate developmental skills.

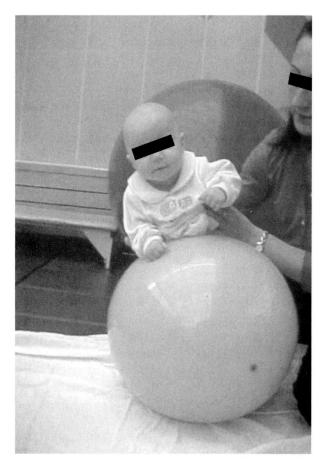

FIGURE **27-15** Facilitation of balance reactions on the therapy ball.

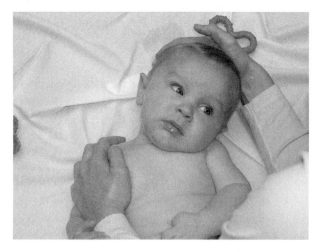

FIGURE **27-16** A 7-month-old infant with right CMT. Stretching exercise performed in physical therapy and taught to caregivers as part of the HEP; lateral cervical flexion toward the uninvolved side to stretch the tight right SCM muscle.

that promote strengthening of the contralateral SCM such as facilitation for rolling (Figure 27-14); and transitioning from supine to side-lying to sit from the involved side and facilitation of balance reactions on the therapeutic ball (Figures 27-15).

During the initial evaluation, the parent and/or caregiver should be instructed in a home stretching program of lateral flexion toward the uninvolved side (Figure 27-16) and rotation toward the involved side (Figure 27-17), to be performed at a minimum of four to five times per day. Each stretching exercise should be held for a minimum of 30 seconds if tolerated. The parents should be shown various positions in which to perform stretching activities and should be able to demonstrate all of the exercises independently in front of the therapist before beginning them at home. Positioning is also an

important adjunct to therapy, and family/caregivers should be educated in ways to position the infant (Figure 27-18), hold/carry the infant (Figure 27-19), and play/stimulate the infant in ways that encourage rota-

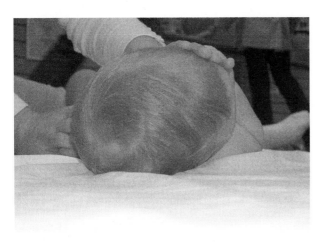

FIGURE **27-17** A 7-month-old infant with right CMT. Stretching exercise performed in physical therapy and taught to caregivers as part of the HEP; cervical rotation to the involved side.

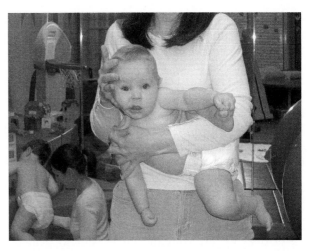

FIGURE **27-19** A 7-month-old infant with right CMT. Side-carrying position performed in physical therapy and taught to caregivers as part of the HEP as means of carrying the infant to stretch the tight SCM muscle on the right side.

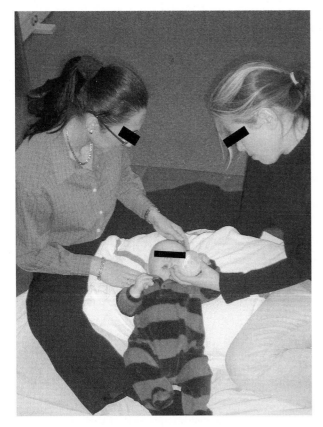

FIGURE **27-18** Positioning for midline orientation during feeding.

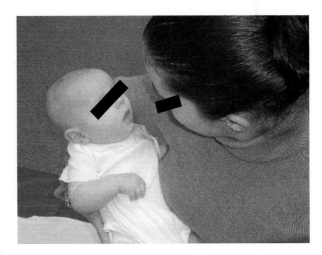

FIGURE **27-20** Visually engage/stimulate baby toward midline orientation.

position. This HEP remains in place 3 to 6 months after discharge with decreased frequency.

PRECAUTIONS

Before beginning any torticollis treatment or evaluation, it is important to remember that you are dealing with an infant's cervical spine. All patients should have had medical clearance before the physical therapy examination. Infants cry to express themselves; they will cry if they are experiencing negative symptoms associated with stretching, such as pain, numbness, or burning; they will also cry if they are afraid, tired, or hungry. The therapist should develop a sense of the infant's personality and his or her tolerance for stretching and exercise. Performing gentle stretching and constantly monitoring the baby for signs of discomfort or distress throughout the treatment session are extremely important. Signs of

tion toward the involved side and lateral flexion away from the involved side as well as midline orientation (Figure 27-20). Supervised time spent in prone is important for the development of symmetrical neck extension and upper extremity weight-bearing. Active neck ROM can also be encouraged through positioning of toys, positioning during feeding, and varying the carrying

discomfort can include clenching of teeth or grimacing, increase or decrease in tone, increased heart and/or respiratory rate, and/or inconsolable crying.[17]

While passively stretching the SCM into lateral flexion, the neck must be kept in a neutral position within both the sagittal and transverse planes. Functional strengthening exercises or positions that promote strengthening (antigravity control) should be age-appropriate and should not be included in the treatment until the infant begins to develop independent head control.

RECOMMENDATIONS

The best time to work with an infant is when he or she is well fed and rested. The therapist should take time to develop a rapport with the infant and to gain the infant's trust through interaction and play before initiating stretching. Stretching can typically be accomplished without eliciting crying if the therapist is gentle and can develop strategies to distract the infant, such

as using singing and/or sensory stimulating and age-appropriate toys during treatment.

REHABILITATION PHASE I (WEEKS 1 TO 8)

During phase I, physical therapy treatment should focus primarily on improving neck PROM and ensuring caregiver competency of HEP. Two-thirds of each treatment session should focus primarily on gentle manual stretching of the identified tight musculature around the neck, shoulders, scapula, and trunk, with specific focus on the identified tight SCM muscle. During the remaining one-third of the session, focus should be on muscle activation for active ROM. The therapist should facilitate active midline head control, visual tracking in all planes (with specific focus on horizontal tracking toward the involved side), attempts at eliciting graded antigravity head control and righting reactions, midline orientation, cervical lateral flexion toward the uninvolved side, and age-appropriate developmental skills.

Rehabilitation Phase I (Weeks 1 to 8)

GOALS

- Increase PROM of cervical lateral flexion to the uninvolved side by 10–15 degrees
- Increase PROM of cervical rotation to the involved side by 10–15 degrees
- Actively bring head into midline in supine and hold it there 50% of the time
- Actively rotate head from side to side in supine to visually track a toy in available ROM
- Actively begin to right head to midline against gravity in side-lying and supported sitting positions from the involved side
- Hold head in cervical extension for 10 seconds in the prone position (if infant has head control)
- Prone prop on forearms with good weight-bearing on the UE on the affected side
- Demonstrate head righting reactions 50% of the ROM during facilitated rolling
- Caregiver is independent and compliant with HEP.

PRECAUTIONS

- Keep the infant's neck in a neutral position; do not stretch in a flexed or hyperextended position.
- Keep the stretching gentle.
- Look for signs of discomfort or pain throughout the treatment session.

TREATMENT STRATEGIES

- Parent education of positioning, gentle manual stretching, and HEP
- Passive manual stretching of the SCM in cervical lateral flexion to the uninvolved side
- Passive manual stretching of the SCM in cervical rotation to the involved side
- Myofascial/soft tissue techniques to the SCM, upper chest, shoulder girdle, and scapulohumeral muscles. Maintain distance/mobility between neck and shoulders
- Positioning of musical or visually attractive toys to promote active rotation to the involved side
- If independent head control is beginning, begin strengthening of the uninvolved side to bring the head into midline through hands on facilitation and the use of the righting reactions if present
- Mild vestibular activities to encourage eyes horizontal in space
- Facilitation of all age-appropriate developmental skills, such as rolling, prone prop on forearms and extended elbows, reaching in prone, midline orientation in supine as appropriate

CRITERIA FOR ADVANCEMENT

- Increase in neck PROM of lateral flexion toward the uninvolved side and rotation toward the involved side
- Increase in neck active range of motion (AROM), with observation of midline head control

Troubleshooting

Caregivers/parents may be apprehensive to perform neck stretching exercises on their infant. Encouragement and support need to be given if the family is apprehensive. Frequent review of the HEP with the caregiver is necessary to ensure correct understanding and correct performance. The physical therapist must take the time to explain the precautions (as noted previously in this chapter) to the caregiver and to provide appropriate feedback regarding his or her ability to perform the exercises. Once the caregiver is competent in performing the exercises, providing reassurance to the caregiver may be necessary to decrease any fear or anxiety that may arise while performing these exercises. Carryover of the physical therapy treatment via the HEP is of utmost importance and needs to be stressed to the caregiver. The recommendation is that the HEP be performed four to five times per day.

REHABILITATION PHASE II (WEEKS 8 TO 16)

In addition to improving neck ROM, attention should be placed on the child's developmental skill level in

---

Rehabilitation Phase II (Weeks 8 to 16)

GOALS

- Full PROM of both cervical lateral flexion and cervical rotation (to equal the ROM of the uninvolved side)
- Midline head control in supine 100% of the time
- Midline head control in highest age-appropriate developmental position 50%–75% of the time
- Actively rotate head to both sides in full ROM in supine
- Actively hold head in midline against gravity for 10–15 seconds in side-lying and supported sitting positions on both sides
- Hold head in cervical extension in prone for an appropriate amount of time to play with a toy
- Prone prop on forearms or extended elbows with good weight-bearing on the UE on the affected side
- Bring head into midline in supported sitting and hold it there to play with a toy for 20 seconds
- Visually track an object 180 degrees in the horizontal plane in supine and if developmentally appropriate supported sitting
- Demonstrate head righting reactions during facilitated rolling over on either side
- Head in midline and chin tuck evident in pull to sit
- Demonstrate the ability to reach forward for a toy with two hands in supported sitting, without head tilt
- Caregiver is independent and compliant with HEP

PRECAUTIONS

- Same as noted in Phase I

TREATMENT STRATEGIES

- Passive manual stretching of the SCM muscle into cervical lateral flexion to the uninvolved side and rotation to the involved side
- Myofascial/soft tissue techniques to maintain mobility of the upper chest and shoulder girdle musculature
- Promote active cervical rotation toward the involved side in all-age appropriate developmental positions via toy placement and manual facilitation
- Manual facilitation and/or positioning of toys to promote head in midline in supine, supported/unsupported sitting.
- Vestibular input and manual facilitation to elicit appropriate head righting reactions in all planes
- Therapeutic ball activities to grade antigravity head control
- Facilitation of all age-appropriate developmental skills such as rolling, prone prop on forearms and extended elbows, reaching in prone, midline orientation in supine, hand to hand, hand to mouth, hands to feet, and feet to mouth focusing on active head control and midline orientation without compensations. Facilitation of sitting and creeping with midline head control if appropriate.

CRITERIA FOR ADVANCEMENT

- Increase in neck PROM of lateral flexion toward the uninvolved side and rotation toward the involved side
- Increase in neck AROM, with observation of midline head control

phase II. Approximately half of the treatment session focuses on neck PROM and the other half on muscle activation for active neck ROM and antigravity control in all age-appropriate developmental positions. The therapist should continue to review the HEP with the caregiver and update it, as necessary, to keep pace with the child's developmental progression.

Troubleshooting

The physical therapist should note a significant improvement in both passive and active neck range of motion and the attainment of age-appropriate gross motor skills. If not, lack of compliance to the HEP may be the culprit and reiterating the importance of the HEP with the caregiver is necessary. In addition to achieving full passive neck range of motion, attention should be placed on the child's developmental skill level. Discrepancy between full range of cervical ROM and inability to actively maintain head control can be an indication of a developmental problem or a different problem other than CMT. Additionally, if gains are not being made as expected, the child is recommended to return to the referring physician for a follow-up examination.

The therapist should pay close attention to compensatory movements that the child may exhibit to substitute for weak muscles or inadequate PROM. The HEP continues to be stressed as an important adjunct to therapy and continues to be performed four to five times per day. If compliance to the HEP program is inadequate, and child is not making gains in PROM, direct

physical therapy contact frequency may need to be increased.

REHABILITATION PHASE III: DISCHARGE (WEEKS 16 TO 24)

Typically, the baby is becoming more active. Slight asymmetry may be present initially but is resolved by the end of phase III. Full, symmetrical, passive, and active neck ROM needs to be present, as well as good neck strength, and the baby needs to display age-appropriate developmental skills to be discharged from therapy.

Troubleshooting

The infant typically has obtained full PROM, and focus is on maintaining neutral head alignment during dynamic functional activities. Occasionally, during stressful activities or during the acquisition of new developmental skills, a slight head tilt may be observed, but this is never persistent. If at this phase of rehabilitation, passive range of neck motion is still limited, the recommendation is to return for follow-up with the referring physician. As with all other phases, frequent review of the HEP with the caregiver is necessary to ensure correct performance. The HEP is kept in place after discharge from physical therapy and is performed three times per day for 3 to 6 months after discharge.

SURGICAL MANAGEMENT

Stretching and conservative intervention is effective in greater than 90% of CMT cases; however, conservative treatment is usually unsuccessful after age 12

Rehabilitation Phase III: Discharge (Weeks 16 to 24)

GOALS

- Full passive and active ROM of both cervical lateral flexion and rotation
- Head is in midline 95% of the time in all age-appropriate developmental positions
- Able to hold head in midline and play with a toy in all age-appropriate developmental positions
- Full active cervical rotation in highest developmental positions without compensations
- Demonstrates no preference when performing functional activities such as rolling, reaching, and UE weight-bearing
- Age-appropriate antigravity neck strength
- Parents are independent with and understand the importance of continuing the HEP

PRECAUTIONS

- Same as noted in Phase 1

TREATMENT STRATEGIES

- Same as noted in Phase II

CRITERIA FOR ADVANCEMENT

- Physical therapy discontinued if the child has met all phase III goals

months.[1,8,9] When conservative methods fail, surgery may be indicated. Indications for surgical intervention include facial deformity or cervical ROM limitations of 30 degrees or more.[1,10,16] Optimal surgical results are obtained when the surgery is performed on patients between ages 1 and 4.[1,10]

Typically, a unipolar release is performed at the distal or clavicular end of the SCM muscle. If this muscle remains tight, a bipolar release is performed with the second lengthening performed at the proximal or mastoid end[18] (Figure 27-21).

Depending on physician recommendation, physical therapy may begin immediately or within the first 2 weeks postoperatively.[18] The postoperative patient is typically placed in a soft cervical collar for comfort, which is removed for physical therapy treatment (Figure 27-22). The collar begins to be removed during the day as the patient develops sufficient neck strength and endurance to maintain midline head control. Consultation with the surgeon is necessary to safely and appropriately progress the patient throughout the postoperative treatment period.

Control of postoperative pain and early PROM are key to a successful rehabilitation outcome. Treatment techniques and goals for the initial postoperative period emphasize maintaining the surgical lengthening, gaining passive and active neck ROM, developing proprioceptive awareness and muscle balance for midline head orientation, and developing functional strength of the neck musculature (Figure 27-23, A–C). Postural training, using a mirror for feedback, may assist the patient in orienting his or her head to a midline position. Because of the patient's new head alignment in

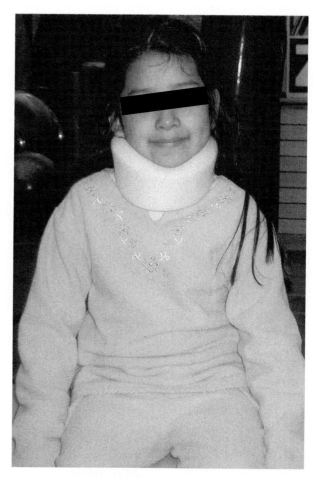

F I G U R E **27-22** Patient using a soft cervical collar status post right SCM surgical lengthening.

space, visual training may be indicated to assist in coordinating eye movements and visual functioning while maintaining a midline head position. Additionally, scar management must be taken into consideration after an SCM release. Once the incision is well healed, a silicon-based patch may be applied to aid in flattening and softening of the scar. Physical therapy should be provided until functional integration of midline head orientation and control are present and the patient displays symmetrical neck ROM and strength.

The HEP is kept in place after discharge from physical therapy and is performed once a day for 4 to 8 weeks after discharge.

Troubleshooting

Care should be taken with the postoperative patient, being mindful of the incision site and the healing process. Stretching should never be so aggressive that it irritates the incision site. The proprioceptive aspect of developing midline head control of the postoperative patient must not be overlooked. Vestibular and visual

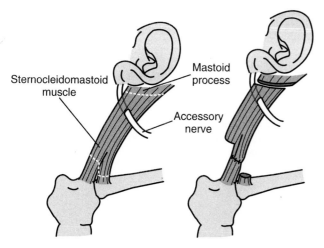

F I G U R E **27-21** Illustration of surgical lengthening of the SCM muscle. *(From Herring, J.A. Tachdjian's Pediatric Orthopaedics, 3rd ed. WB Saunders Co, Philadelphia, 2002, p. 173.)*

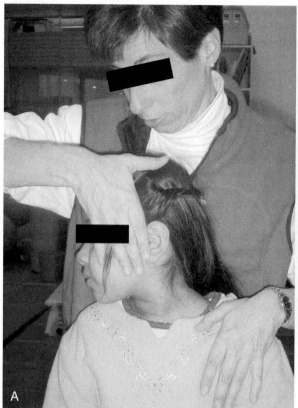

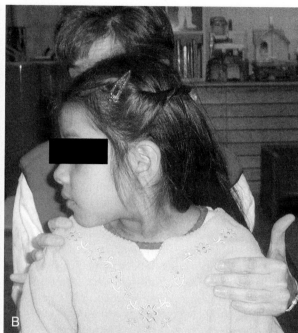

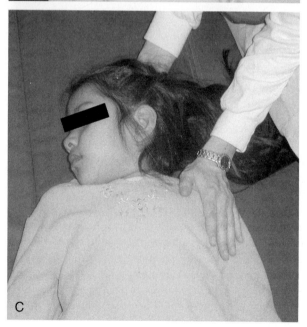

FIGURE **27-23** *A.* PROM cervical rotation to the involved side. *B.* Active ROM cervical rotation to the involved side. *C.* Active-assisted ROM cervical rotation to the involved side.

Postoperative Phase I (Weeks 1 to 8)

GOALS

- Patient and caregiver education
- Control of postoperative pain, as per physician recommendation
- Monitor healing of surgical incision
- Maintain/gain passive range of all cervical motions
- Develop head and neck midline postural awareness and control
- Develop active head righting reactions in all planes
- Maximize cervical muscle strength
- Scar management
- Patient/caregiver is independent with HEP

PRECAUTIONS

- Same as noted in Phase I, Conservative Treatment
- Keep the child's neck in a neutral position; do not stretch in a flexed or hyperextended position
- Keep the stretching gentle
- Look for signs of discomfort or pain throughout the treatment session
- Do not cause irritation to the incision

TREATMENT STRATEGIES

- Parent education of positioning and instruction of HEP for gentle manual stretching
- Caregiver and patient education in wear schedule for soft cervical collar
- Caregiver and patient education in monitoring incision site
- Upon physician approval, use of silicon-based patch to aid in flattening and softening of the scar
- Passive manual stretching of the SCM in cervical lateral flexion to the uninvolved side.
- Passive manual stretching of the SCM in cervical rotation to the involved side.
- Myofascial/soft tissue techniques to the SCM, upper chest, shoulder girdle, and scapulohumeral muscles. Maintain distance/mobility between neck and shoulders.
- Facilitate midline head orientation through visual and vestibular cues/feedback
- Develop head righting reactions in all planes, especially in antigravity positions
- Develop ability to chin tuck in pull to sit or sit up with head in midline, with emphasis on symmetrical muscle activation into flexion
- Develop ability to extend the cervical spine against gravity in midline, with emphasis on symmetrical muscle activation into extension
- Strengthening of the uninvolved side via active lateral cervical flexion against gravity in side-lying
- Therapeutic ball activities to grade antigravity head control, and develop functional head righting skills in all planes

DISCHARGE CRITERIA

- Functional integration of midline head orientation without soft cervical collar
- Symmetrical neck ROM
- Symmetrical neck muscle strength

stimulation should be incorporated in the physical therapy program to promote automatic midline head orientation.

TAKE HOME MESSAGE

- Physical therapy is the "Gold Standard" of care for the initial treatment of CMT.
- Differential diagnosis is extremely important in dictating type of treatment.
- Early diagnosis of CMT and initiation of physical therapy treatment are the key to the success of conservative management.

- HEP and caregiver compliance/participation is critical for the optimal results.
- Infants are unable to fully express themselves; *remember precautions at all times.*
- When conservative methods fail, surgical intervention may be indicated in children over age 1 year.

REFERENCES

1. Loder, R.T. The Cervical Spine. In Morrissy, R.T., Weinstein, S.L. (Eds). *Lovell and Winter's Pediatric Orthopaedics*, 5th ed., vol. 2. Lippincott Williams & Wilkins, New York, 2001, pp. 811–815.

2. Cailliet, R. *Neck and Arm Pain,* 2nd ed. FA Davis Co, Philadelphia, 1981, p. 46.

3. Cheng, J.C., Au, A.W. *Infantile Torticollis: A Review of 624 Cases.* J Pediatr Orthop 1994;14:802–808.

4. Stanger, M. Orthopedic Management. In Tecklin, J.S. (Ed). *Pediatric Physical Therapy,* 3rd ed. Lippincott Williams & Wilkins, New York, 1999, pp. 394–396.

5. Tein, Y.C., Su, J.Y. *Ultrasonographic Study of the Coexistence of Muscular Torticollis and Dysplasia of the Hip.* J Pediatr Orthop 2001;21(3):343–347.

6. Weiner, D.S. *Congenital Dislocations of the Hip Associated with Congenital Muscular Torticollis.* Clin Orthop 1976;121:163.

7. Cheng, J.C., Wong, M.W. *Clinical Determinants of the Outcome of Manual Stretching in the Treatment of Congenital Muscular Torticollis in Infants. A Prospective Study of 821 Cases.* J Bone Joint Surg 2001;83A(5):679–687.

8. Taylor, J.L., Stamos, N.E. *Developmental Muscular Torticollis: Outcomes in Young Children Treated by Physical Therapy.* Pediatr Phys Ther 1997;9:173–178.

9. Emery, C. *The Determinants of Treatment Duration for Congenital Muscular Torticollis.* Phys Ther 1994;74:921–929.

10. Cheng, J.C., Tang, S.P. *Outcome of Surgical Treatment of Congenital Muscular Torticollis.* Clin Orthop Relat Res 1999;1(362):190–200.

11. Binder, H., Eng, G.D., Gaiser, J.F., Koch, B. *Congenital Muscular Torticollis: Results of Conservative Management with Long-term Follow-up in 85 Cases.* Arch Phys Med Rehabil 1987;68:222–225.

12. Brunnstrom, S. *Clinical Kinesiology,* 2nd ed. FA Davis Co, Philadelphia, 1972, p. 269.

13. Daniels, L., Worthingham, C. *Muscle Testing: Techniques of Manual Examination,* 4th ed. WB Saunders Co, Philadelphia, 1980, p. 16.

14. Hollier, L., Kim, J.D. *Congenital Muscular Torticollis and the Associated Craniofacial Changes.* Plast Reconstr Surg 2000;105(3):827–835.

15. Gupinar, A., Kiristioglu, I. *Surgical Correction of Muscular Torticollis in Older Children with Peter G. Jones Technique.* J Pediatr Orthop 1998;18(5):598–601.

16. Yu, C., Wong, F.H., Lo, L.J., Chen, Y.R. *Craniofacial Deformity in Patients with Uncorrected Congenital Muscular Torticollis: An Assessment from Three-dimensional Computed Tomography Imaging.* Plast Reconstr Surg 2004;113(1):24–33.

17. Byers, J.F., Thornely, K. *Cueing into Infant Pain.* Am J Matern Child Nurs 2004;29(2):84–89.

18. Verbal Conversation with Dr. Daniel Green, Attending Pediatric Orthopedic Surgeon, Hospital for Special Surgery, May 2005.

IV

SPINE REHABILITATION

HOLLY RUDNICK, PT, Cert MDT

28

Lumbar Microdiscectomy

TODD GAGE, PT, CSCS

LUMBAR DISC HERNIATION

Lumbar disc herniation (LDH) is one of the most common injuries to the lumbar spine. LDH most commonly occurs between ages 30 and 50. Approximately 95% of LDH occur at the L4/L5 and L5/S1 levels. Disc herniations are broken into two classifications: contained and sequestered. Contained herniations include protruded/bulging discs, in which the nucleus has not perforated the annulus fibrosis, and prolapsed discs, in which the nucleus has perforated the annulus but is contained by the posterior longitudinal ligament (PLL). A sequestered disc is described as perforation of the PLL by the disc, with a fragment in the epidural space.

Flexion/rotation of the lumbar segments has been shown to lead to an increase in intradiscal pressure and LDH.[1] The greatest amount of lumbar flexion/extension range of motion (ROM) occurs at the L4/L5 and L5/S1 segments, which creates an increased risk for herniation at these levels. Because combined motions are a part of activities of daily living (ADL), there is the potential for breakdown of the annulus and migration of nuclear material beyond the confines of the disc and surrounding ligaments leading to mechanical or chemical irritation of the nerve roots or spinal cord.

Many herniations will spontaneously disappear or decrease in size over the course of several months.[2] Less than 2% of disc herniations require surgery and less than 15% of patients with disc herniations will have underlying nerve root compression.[3,4] Indications for microdiscectomy include evidence of cauda equina syndrome, significant motor weakness, or intractable pain. In addition, the patient will have failed conservative treatment, which includes nonsteroidal anti-inflammatory drugs (NSAIDs), physical therapy for 8 to 12 weeks, and epidural steroid injections.

SURGICAL OVERVIEW

A lumbar microdiscectomy (LMD) is performed in the reverse Trendelenburg's position (Figure 28-1). A small incision (ranging from 3 to 6 cm) is made along the midline, over the interspace of the affected level. The paraspinal musculature is stripped subperiosteally, and a retractor with a 5-pound weight is placed over the facet to open the interspace. The interspinous ligament is kept intact. The microscope is then introduced, part of the lateral aspect of the ligamentum flavum is resected, and a foraminotomy is performed (Figure 28-2). The nerve root is then retracted medially. The PLL and nucleus are cut laterally to the nerve root, and a nucleotomy is performed (Figure 28-3). Insult to the ligamentum flavum and paraspinal musculature is routinely not repaired; however, the lumbar fascia is closed with absorbable sutures.[5]

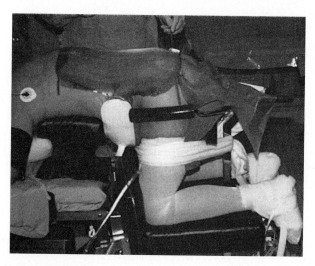

FIGURE 28-1 Reverse Trendelenburg's or kneeling position for lumbar disc excision.

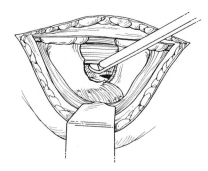

FIGURE 28-2 Resection of the ligamentum flavum.

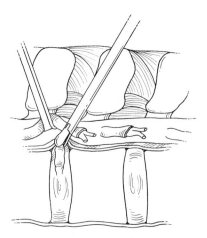

FIGURE 28-3 Nerve root is retracted medially, and a nucleotomy is performed.

REHABILITATION OVERVIEW

The rehabilitation program following an LMD begins on the day of surgery. Patients who undergo an LMD are hospitalized for approximately 1 to 2 days.

The treatment in the acute stage is primarily one of education. Patients must have a basic understanding of the mechanism of injury for disc herniations, to avoid the risk of reherniation following microdiscectomy. The recurrence rate following LMD is reported as being between 3% and 19%.[6-10] Morgan-Hough et al.[11] performed a retrospective analysis of 531 patients who underwent primary microdiscectomy over a 16-year period. They calculated a revision rate of 7.9% and reported that contained protrusions were almost three times more likely to require revision surgery compared to extruded or sequestered discs. Seventy-six percent of the recurrent herniations occurred between 3 and 48 months following primary LMD.[11]

The physical therapist must consider the work done by Nachemson[12] on intradiscal pressure and loads when educating the patient on body mechanics, posture, and exercise. At the Hospital for Special Surgery (HSS), all patients are instructed in log-roll transfers, when performing supine to sit, and a basic home exercise program consisting of abdominal setting, gluteal sets, and ankle pumps, before leaving the hospital.

Patients are discharged from the hospital on the first or second postoperative day. Criteria for discharge include patient demonstration of proper supine-sit transfers, a basic understanding of body mechanics during ADL to avoid lumbar flexion, independent ambulation, with or without an assistive device, and demonstration of independence with donning/doffing a lumbar orthosis. Patients are provided with an activity guide upon discharge from the hospital, to provide a basic framework for the progression of activity following LMD before initiating formal physical therapy.

During the first 4 weeks postoperatively, patients are encouraged to walk and continue with the basic exercise program described previously. Patients must continue to avoid lifting, bending, twisting, and prolonged sitting during this period in an attempt to allow healing and diminish postoperative pain.

Patients begin formal outpatient physical therapy between 4 and 6 weeks postoperatively and are seen two to three times per week for 8 to 14 weeks. The phases of tissue healing, along with symptom behavior, recovery of motor deficits, and the restoration of muscle imbalances, will dictate the progression in the rehabilitation program following LMD. Ahlgren et al.[13] looked at the effect of annular repair on the healing strength of the intervertebral disc in sheep spines following a partial discectomy. They determined that at 6 weeks following partial discectomy, disc strength ranged between 60% and 75% of the control values. As a result, patients must make every attempt to minimize intradiscal pressures during the first 6 weeks post-LMD.

A systematic review of randomized controlled trials was conducted by Ostelo et al.[14] to determine the effectiveness of active treatments following primary lumbar disc surgery. After looking at 13 studies that fulfilled the inclusion criteria, they determined that there is strong evidence that intensive exercise programs initiated 4 to 6 weeks postoperatively are more effective on functional status and faster return to work.

PREOPERATIVE PHASE: CONSERVATIVE MANAGEMENT

Before considering surgery, patients diagnosed with LDH should undergo various conservative interventions. They may include anti-inflammatory drugs, activity modification, epidural steroid injections, and physical therapy. Those patients who are referred for physical therapy should receive a thorough evaluation, which includes assessment of posture and body mechanics, ROM and movement (static and repeated), strength/motor control, sensation, and reflexes. The goal of the initial assessment is to identify the lesion behavior. Lesion behavior refers to the manner in which the signs and symptoms behave with movement and position. During the initial assessment, the therapist is looking to identify provocative movements and positions, as well as determine a directional preference to diminish and/or abolish symptoms. The therapist is also interested in such lesion behaviors as centralization and peripheralization of symptoms that are commonly associated with LDH. Centralization, in particular, has been shown to be a predictor of good to excellent outcome for conservative management, using the McKenzie method of assessment and treatment.[15,16] The therapist may also assess the patient for a directional susceptibility to movement (DSM), using Shirley Sahrmann's[17] evaluation to categorize and treat the patient according to the movement impairment syndromes. Regardless of the method of assessment and treatment used, avoiding positions that increase intradiscal pressure during the acute phase of an LDH is crucial to minimize symptoms and is repeatedly stressed during this phase.

The patient is considered to have failed physical therapy if all movements worsen or have no effect on symptoms, are unable to tolerate loaded positions, and have intractable pain, progressive neurological signs, or cauda equina syndrome. A patient has failed conservative treatment when all conservative interventions have been unsuccessful.

Preoperative Phase: Conservative Management

GOALS

- Education
  - Anatomy/biomechanics of lumbar disc
  - Patients are educated on proper body mechanics during transfers
  - Mechanism of injury
  - Proper sitting posture to avoid loss of lumbar lordosis
  - Instruct on pain-relieving positions
  - Educate patient on the principles of centralization
- Decrease pain/centralize/abolish symptoms
- Patient to demonstrate proper abdominal setting with activation of transversus abdominis during spinal stabilization exercise
- Independent with home exercise program

PRECAUTIONS

- Avoid prolonged sitting/driving (>20 min) or flexed postures
- Avoid lifting and carrying
- Avoid flying
- Avoid activities that involve repetitive loading of the spine (i.e., jogging)

TREATMENT STRATEGIES

- Relative rest
- Soft tissue mobilization/joint mobilization
- Modalities for pain control (US, TENS, Ice)
- Repeated movement of the lumbar spine (direction determined by evaluation) to decrease, abolish, or centralize symptoms
- Lumbar stabilization initiated in unloaded position progressing to loaded positions as tolerated
- Neural mobilization

CRITERIA FOR SURGERY

- Failed conservative management
- Intractable pain
- Neurological signs that have worsened or do not respond to conservative therapy
- Cauda equina syndrome

POSTOPERATIVE PHASE I: PROTECTED MOBILIZATION (WEEKS 4 TO 6)

The protected mobilization phase begins between 4 and 6 weeks after surgery. All patients undergo a thorough physical therapy evaluation, which includes active range of motion (AROM) of the lumbar spine as tolerated, neurological assessment, strength assessment, and lower extremity flexibility before beginning a formal physical therapy program.

The goals of this phase are to educate the patient on basic spinal anatomy, proper posture and body mechanics, and lay the groundwork for a lumbar stabilization program.

Nachemson[12] determined that intradiscal pressure can be decreased as much as 300%, with the use of a lumbar roll to maintain lordosis and by reclining the backrest of the chair. As a result, patients are instructed not to sit for greater than 20 minutes and are also encouraged to use a lumbar roll to diminish lumbar flexion, as well as sit semi-reclined (between 100 and 130 degrees) during the first 2 to 4 weeks following surgery.

Patients must understand the importance of using correct body mechanics to avoid repetitive lumbar flexion and rotation during ADL and transfers. They are also instructed to avoid lifting/carrying anything greater than 10 pounds.

Hodges and Richardson[18] have shown that a delayed postural contraction of the transversus abdominis exists in subjects with LBP. Yoshihara et al.[19] showed that atrophy of the multifidus muscle occurs in patients with nerve root involvement secondary to an L4/L5 LDH.[20] Therefore, abdominal setting and lumbar stabilization should be incorporated into the program to increase trunk stiffness and reduce motion at the injured segment during ADL and transfers. Abdominal and lumbar stabilization exercises should first begin with the spine fully supported in an unloaded position (i.e., supine/prone). Patients who complain of pain with walking are encouraged to perform abdominal setting during ambulation to improve control and diminish pain.

Modalities, such as ultrasound, TENS, ice, and/or moist heat, are also used during this phase to minimize pain, edema, and muscle spasm. These modalities are used as an adjunct to therapeutic exercise and education, not as a sole form of treatment. It is crucial that the patient understands the importance of avoiding positions and movements that exacerbate his or her symptoms, rather than relying on modalities and pain medication to provide temporary relief.

Neural mobilization is initiated during this stage in an attempt to decrease the risk of nerve root adhesions. It is important when beginning neural mobilization exercises to maintain the lumbar spine in a protected position and progressively apply force to the nerve root. Patient response is crucial. The decision to incorporate hamstring stretching should be considered carefully.

Subjects are progressed from the protected mobilization phase, when the patient demonstrates proper sitting posture, body mechanics during transfers, a basic understanding of LDH, and the ability to perform abdominal setting. These criteria will create a good healing environment, as well as the tools to progress to the next phase: neutral stabilization.

Troubleshooting

Pain and fear are the most limiting factors encountered during phase I. The degree and location of pain experienced postoperatively depends greatly upon the preoperative symptoms. Following an LMD, most patients experience less overall pain than preoperatively; however, there is a group of patients who either have no relief or complain of more pain. The postoperative pain is considered to be largely the result of inflammation from the soft tissue trauma caused by the surgical procedure. Radicular symptoms may be produced or

---

Postoperative Phase I: Protected Mobilization (Weeks 4 to 6)

GOALS

- Education
  - Anatomy/biomechanics of lumbar disc
  - Patients are educated on proper body mechanics during transfers
  - Mechanism of injury
  - Proper sitting posture to avoid loss of lumbar lordosis
  - Instruct on pain-relieving positions
  - Educate patient on the surgical procedure
- Decrease pain/centralize symptoms
- Patient to demonstrate proper abdominal setting with activation of transversus abdominis
- Improve neural mobility
- Independent with home exercise program

PRECAUTIONS

- Avoid prolonged sitting/driving (>20 min) or flexed postures
- Avoid lifting and carrying >10 pounds
- Avoid flying
- Avoid activities that involve repetitive loading (i.e., jogging) and/or repetitive flexion of the lumbar spine in a loaded position
- Avoid all sporting activities at this time

TREATMENT STRATEGIES

- Relative rest—walking, unloaded cycling
- Soft tissue mobilization/joint mobilization
- Education on sitting posture, avoiding prolonged lumbar flexion
- Modalities for pain control (US, TENS, Ice)
- Basic lumbar stabilization initiated in unloaded position (supine/prone) (Figures 28-4 and 28-5)
- Neural mobilization (sciatic and/or femoral nerve) (Figures 28-6 and 28-7)

CRITERIA FOR ADVANCEMENT

- Patient demonstrates understanding of proper sitting posture, body mechanics during transfers, and pain-relieving positions
- Patient to demonstrate understanding of LDH mechanism of injury
- Patient demonstrates basic principles of abdominal stabilization in an unloaded position

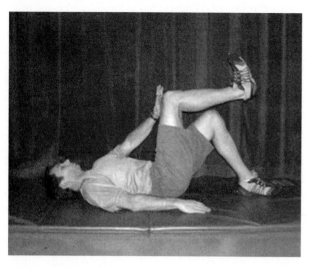

FIGURE 28-4 Supine isometric hip flexion with abdominal setting.

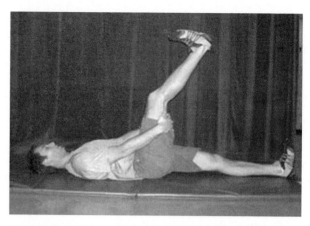

FIGURE 28-6 Supine knee extension with ankle dorsiflexion for sciatic nerve mobilization, with spine supported.

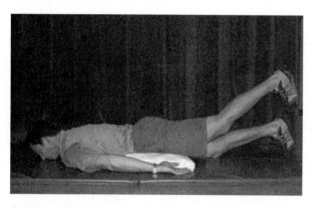

FIGURE 28-5 Prone hip extension with abdominal setting.

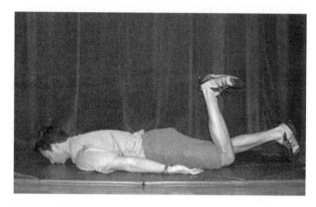

FIGURE 28-7 Prone knee flexion for femoral nerve mobilization.

worsened and can also be attributed to an increase in inflammation surrounding the nerve root. Generally, most postoperative pain will resolve with time, use of anti-inflammatory medications, and slow return to normal movement. Some patients with more severe and/or persistent pain may require modalities, such as ultrasound and TENS. Patients whose pain does not improve should be referred back to the surgeon for further workup.

The other pitfall that may be encountered during phase I is fear. Patients may be very fearful of movement during the initial phase of rehabilitation following LMD. Some patients have been unable to move normally for substantial periods of time before surgery. As a result, these patients may be resistant to move in ways that were previously painful. Patients should be reassured that movement, when performed safely, is actually beneficial to the healing process. Postural correction and instruction on body mechanics are crucial.

POSTOPERATIVE PHASE II: NEUTRAL STABILIZATION (WEEKS 6 TO 10)

The neutral stabilization phase continues to address the patient's symptoms via modalities and avoiding provocative positions, but, additionally, it attempts to address the causative factors that precipitated the herniation. Sahrmann[17] describes the patient with an LDH as having a swayback or flat back posture, greater relative flexibility of the lumbar spine in flexion compared to hip flexibility, long paraspinal muscles, and, possibly, shortened gluteus maximus or hamstring muscles. Reassessment at this point is necessary to determine muscle imbalances that may have contributed to the patient's history of herniation. Standing lumbar active ROM, quadruped rocking, and seated knee extension should be assessed to determine relative flexibility and movement patterns of the hip and lumbar spine.

According to Woolsey and Norton,[20] the lumbar spine should not complete more than 50% of its motion into

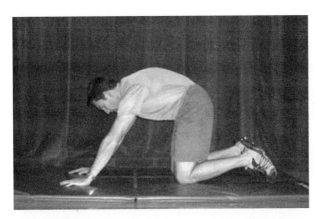

FIGURE 28-8 Quadruped rocking with excessive and early lumbar flexion.

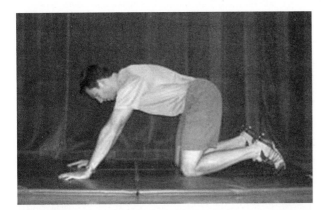

FIGURE 28-9 Quadruped rocking with neutral spine and good hip motion.

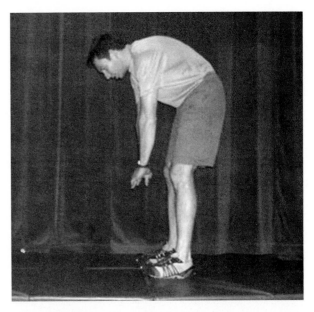

FIGURE 28-10 Forward bending with excessive lumbar flexion in the presence of long back extensors and shortened hip extensors (gluteal muscles and/or hamstrings).

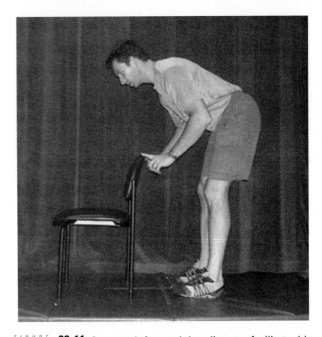

FIGURE 28-11 Corrected forward bending to facilitate hip flexion while maintaining a neutral lumbar spine.

flexion before the initiation of hip flexion. Also, those with low back pain move more in the lumbar spine than at the hips during the 30- to 60-degree phase of forward bending.[20] Therefore, it is imperative that patients be instructed in corrected forward bending in an attempt to minimize the repetitive lumbar flexion that occurs during daily activities.[15] Ultimately, the patient is at greater risk of reherniation if there is excessive lumbar flexion during forward bending and squatting activities that do not get addressed.

Initially, the patient is placed in quadruped to improve both proprioceptive awareness and the relative flexibility of the hips to the lumbar spine (Figures 28-8 and 28-9). As the patient improves, progression to corrected forward bending, wall squats, and, eventually, free-standing squats can be made (Figures 28-10 and 28-11). During wall and free-standing squats, patients will often shift away and unload the affected side. Many factors may be involved in this offsetting of weight, including pain, weakness in the hip abductors and/or hip extensors, and poor habitual motor patterns, which result from diminished lumbopelvic proprioception. If weakness is the cause, strengthening of the gluteals must be achieved before correcting squat technique (Figure 28-12). If a patient is shifting away from the affected side during squat, and there is no asymmetrical weakness in the hip abductors or extensors, then visual and manual feedback can be used to improve lumbopelvic proprioceptive awareness.

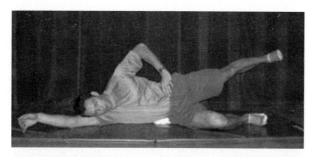

FIGURE **28-12** Hip abduction in side-lying with abdominal stabilization to strengthen gluteus medius.

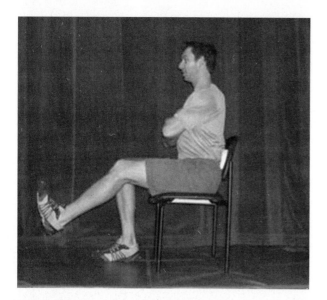

FIGURE **28-13** Seated knee extension to improve hamstring extensibility and sciatic nerve mobility while maintaining lumbar spine extension and abdominal tone.

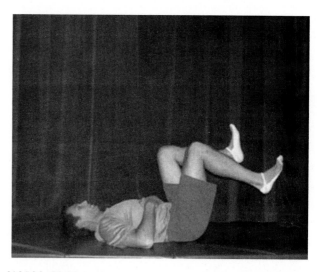

FIGURE **28-14** Lower abdominal progression level S1*A*, per Sahrmann.[17]

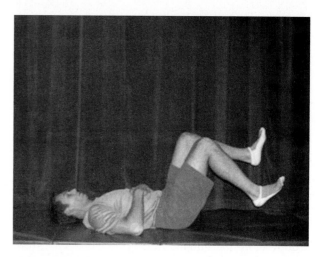

FIGURE **28-15** Lower abdominal progression level S1*B*, per Sahrmann.[17]

Seated knee extension, which assesses the relative flexibility between the hamstrings and spinal extensors, as described by Sahrmann,[17] may also be incorporated into the program at this time (Figure 28-13). The patient is given seated knee extension as an exercise within the available ROM allowed by the hamstrings. At this point, patients have been performing neural gliding for 2 to 3 weeks, which should diminish the risk of exacerbating radicular symptoms.

Patients are also progressed in an abdominal and lumbar stabilization program during phase II, as long as symptoms are not irritated and good segmental stabilization is demonstrated. Patients are instructed to perform an abdominal set and stabilize the spine while incorporating upper and lower extremity movements. Segmental stability can grossly be observed by palpating the lumbar spinous process while performing prone or quadruped exercise. Patients are encouraged to palpate the lumbar spinous processes during prone hip

extension to provide tactile feedback to limit both lumbar extension and rotation. The supine lower abdominal muscle exercise progression, described by Sahrmann,[17] is an excellent way to increase lower abdominal tone while protecting the lumbar spine (Figures 28-14 through 28-17). Patients are encouraged to palpate their anterior superior iliac spine during supine stabilization exercises to provide tactile feedback in an attempt to limit lumbar spine motion.

Initiating lumbar ROM in all directions is important during this phase because of the fear avoidance patterns of movement that may be associated with LDH. Many patients will have actively avoided specific movements for substantial periods of time before undergoing an LMD. The length, intensity, and location of symptoms before surgery often correlate with the severity of

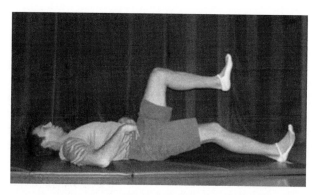

FIGURE **28-16** Lower abdominal progression level 2, per Sahrmann.[17]

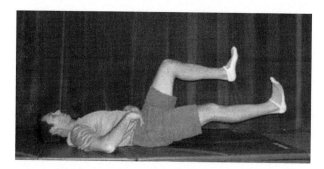

FIGURE **28-17** Lower abdominal progression level 3, per Sahrmann.[17]

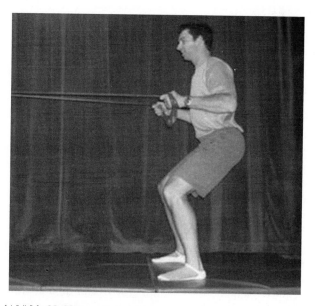

FIGURE **28-18** Standing scapular retraction with Thera-Band and abdominal setting to simulate pulling.

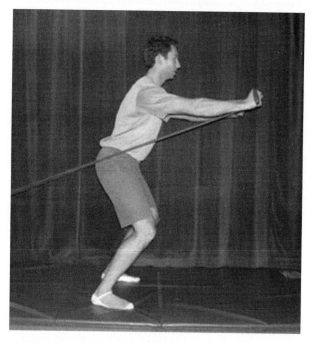

FIGURE **28-19** Standing shoulder flexion with Thera-Band, with lumbar stabilization.

joint restriction in the lumbar spine after surgery. Standing AROM of the lumbar spine will provide the clinician information, such as willingness to move in a particular direction, as well as ROM limitations that may exist. Patients who lack ROM will begin performing ROM exercises in that direction in the unloaded position first and progressing force as tolerated. For example, those patients who lack lumbar flexion will begin with single knee to chest, progressing to double knee to chest in supine and, eventually, should be able to advance to sitting and standing flexion. Patients are always encouraged to perform extension in prone following repeated lumbar flexion in an attempt to diminish any potential risks associated with repetitive flexion forces. By the end of phase II, patients should have relatively normal ROM in the lumbar spine, provided the patient has not developed a dysfunction in a particular direction. Those patients who have developed a dysfunction (as described by Mckenzie[15]) as a result of prolonged movement avoidance may require additional weeks to restore full ROM.

During phase II, exercise should be progressed from the unloaded position to more functional positions. Resistive exercises, such as scapular retraction, shoulder extension, and shoulder flexion, can be initiated in a standing position to simulate pushing and pulling

activities (Figures 28-18 and 28-19). Sagittal planes of motion are progressed to diagonal planes, if the patient is symptom free and good mechanics are observed. Patients are reminded that any activity can be a spinal stabilization exercise if an abdominal set is performed during the activity. All patients are instructed to perform a partial squat when performing these activities to facilitate proper use of the LE during ADL. Those patients who are interested in returning to a resistive training program are encouraged to review and demonstrate their routine, so postural corrections can be made before actually returning independently to the program.

Initiation of aerobic conditioning to facilitate healing via increased tissue perfusion should also be incorporated into the program at this time. Aerobic conditioning is not only beneficial physically, but also psychologically, especially for those patients who are more athletic. Generally, aerobic activities that minimize spinal flexion are encouraged; however, stationary cycling may be considered, provided the patient maintains an erect spine.

Patients are progressed to the dynamic stabilization phase when they have full pain-free AROM of the lumbar spine, demonstrate good squatting mechanics, achieve adequate LE strength (>4/5), and demonstrate the ability to maintain a neutral spine during quadruped and standing stabilization exercise.

Troubleshooting

Phase II is marked by diminished pain, decreased fear-avoidance, increased lumbar ROM, and improved segmental lumbar control. As a result, the patient's confidence during ADL improves, which often leads to increased LBP as a result of poor body mechanics. It is imperative, at this point, to reiterate and review proper body mechanics during ADL and ensure that the patient is not advancing too quickly his or her exercise program at home or in the gym.

The initiation of lumbar spine ROM may also be increasing the amount of LBP during this phase because of soft tissue tightness or postoperative scarring. Moist heat and/or ultrasound may be used to increase tissue extensibility before lumbar ROM. Another potential provocative activity is neural mobilization. If radicular symptoms are predominant, or exacerbated during this phase, the decrease in frequency and/or repetitions of neural mobilization may be necessary.

Postoperative Phase II: Neutral Stabilization (Weeks 6 to 10)

GOALS
- Patient to demonstrate improved tolerance to loaded positions (sitting, standing, and walking)
- Increase the time between peripheralization of symptoms and/or decrease frequency and intensity of pain
- Improve myotomal weakness, if present
- Patient to demonstrate proper squatting mechanics
- Patient to demonstrate good segmental lumbar control and proprioceptive awareness during unloaded lumbar stabilization exercises
- Improve muscle imbalances that contribute to patient symptoms
- Restore lumbar ROM

PRECAUTIONS
- Avoid prolonged sitting/driving or flexed postures
- Avoid activities that involve repetitive loading of the spine (i.e., jogging)

TREATMENT STRATEGIES
- Continue with repetitive movement that centralizes symptoms
- Instruct subject in proper squatting mechanics (beginning in quadruped and progressing to standing)
- Verbal/manual cueing during unsupported spinal stabilization exercise (i.e., quadruped)
- Address muscle imbalances that contribute to patient symptoms (movement imbalance principles developed by Sahrmann) (Figures 28-8 through 28-17)
- Manual techniques to improve restricted segmental ROM of the lumbar spine
- Initiate AROM lumbar spine in unloaded position (always ending with lumbar extension)
- Continue to progress supine, prone, and quadruped neutral stabilization exercise
- Standing isotonic UE and LE strengthening in cardinal planes while maintaining neutral lumbar spine (Figures 28-18 and 28-19)
- Modalities for pain control (US, TENS, Ice)
- Aerobic conditioning

CRITERIA FOR ADVANCEMENT
- Full AROM of lumbar spine
- Patient to demonstrate proper squatting mechanics
- Lower extremity strength >4/5 throughout
- Patient to demonstrate ability to maintain neutral spine during quadruped and standing stabilization exercise

Patients may not demonstrate proper squatting mechanics for a variety of reasons, including a lack of LE strength, poor proprioception, insufficient hip ROM, and/or poor relative flexibility. The therapist must focus on the restoration of normal squatting mechanics before progressing the patient to more advanced stabilization activities.

POSTOPERATIVE PHASE III: DYNAMIC STABILIZATION (WEEKS 10 TO 14)

The goals of the dynamic stabilization phase are to restore normal lower extremity strength and flexibility, and demonstrate good body mechanics during sagittal, transverse, and diagonal plane activities to prevent risk of reinjury. During this phase, patients are progressed from performing activities in a static position to performing them in a dynamic fashion, both with and without resistance. For example, in phase II, a patient may perform a sagittal plane chopping pattern with resistance while maintaining a neutral spine in a partial squat position. In phase III, the patient is progressed to performing the same sagittal plane chopping pattern, simultaneously descending and ascending from a squat.

The purpose of dynamic stabilization is to simulate, in a controlled fashion, planes of movement that occur in both ADL and sporting activities.

When performing dynamic stabilization, exercises are initiated in the sagittal plane and then progressed to the transverse plane and diagonal planes, in an attempt to facilitate motion at the lower extremity while maintaining a neutral spine.

Once a patient is able to demonstrate proper dynamic stabilization without resistance, resistance is added. The progression of resistance depends on patient tolerance and the goals for therapy. Those patients returning to sport and recreation may require more resistance training in dynamic positions than those patients returning to ADL and normal activity only. Normal lower extremity strength must be achieved before progressing to dynamic stabilization because of the increased demands associated with these higher level activities. Dynamic stabilization exercises should be performed in a slow, controlled manner. Speed and velocity can be altered to advance the demands and the difficulty of the exercises to progress the patient toward the return to sport.

Postoperative Phase III: Dynamic Stabilization (Weeks 10 to 14)

GOALS
- Patient to tolerate standing repeated motion of the lumbar spine in all planes, pain-free
- Patient to perform dynamic stabilization activities without pain
- Patient to demonstrate 5/5 lower extremity strength
- Patient to demonstrate proper body mechanics with bending/lifting and activities that involve diagonal planes of motion
- Improve muscle imbalances that contribute to patient symptoms

PRECAUTIONS
- Avoid exacerbation of symptoms

TREATMENT STRATEGIES
- Continue with repetitive movement that centralizes symptoms
- Perform dynamic stabilization exercises
- Address muscle imbalances that contribute to patient symptoms (movement imbalance principles developed by Sahrmann)
- Manual techniques to improve restricted segmental ROM of the lumbar spine
- Initiate AROM lumbar spine in loaded position (always ending with repeated motion that has been determined to centralize symptoms)
- Continue to progress supine, prone, and quadruped neutral stabilization exercise
- Standing isotonic UE and LE strengthening in cardinal planes while maintaining neutral lumbar spine, beginning on stable surfaces, progressing to unstable surfaces
- Progress aerobic conditioning

CRITERIA FOR ADVANCEMENT
- Full pain-free AROM of lumbar spine in standing
- Patient to demonstrate dynamic stabilization activities, pain-free with good body mechanics
- Lower extremity strength 5/5 throughout
- Patient to have no lower extremity neural tension signs
- Patient to demonstrate normal flexibility in bilateral LE

The demands on the trunk stabilizers also increase during this phase. Therefore, patients must also be progressed in their supine, prone, and quadruped stabilization exercises. The progression should include increasing the repetitions, increasing the hold times, performing on unstable surfaces, and adding resistance.

Aerobic conditioning can be progressed in the dynamic stabilization phase based on patient goals. With regard to aerobic conditioning, patients are encouraged to use the concept of cross-training to minimize the risk of reinjury.

Those individuals who wish to return to running can begin using the elliptical trainer if good mechanics are demonstrated. Patients are instructed to perform abdominal setting while on the elliptical trainer in an attempt to minimize lumbar spine motion. The elliptical trainer offers the runner a controlled, nonimpact means to work on aerobic conditioning before returning to running. From a rehabilitation perspective, the patient should have normal lower extremity strength, negative neural tension signs, and normal flexibility before returning to running to prevent compensation and the potential for injury.

The criteria for advancement to return to sport-specific activities are listed in the following section. Not all patients will be progressed to phase IV; however, it is imperative to stress to all patients the importance of achieving the goals in phase III.

Troubleshooting

The purpose of phase III is to ensure neutral trunk stabilization during dynamic activities. The misconception of dynamic stabilization is that it involves dynamic trunk movement during dynamic activities. The job of the physical therapist is to maximize the use of LE power while increasing trunk stiffness during such dynamic exercise. Repetition with visual and manual feedback may be required to ensure proper mechanics before progressing to phase IV. During phase III, the importance of continuing the progression of quadruped and supine neutral stabilization in the home exercise program must be stressed. The therapist is also cautioned not to add dynamic stabilization to the home exercise program until proper form is demonstrated in the clinic.

POSTOPERATIVE PHASE IV: SPORT-SPECIFIC ACTIVITIES (WEEKS 14 TO 18)

As a general rule, patients involved in recreational or competitive sports are instructed to wait until they complete phase IV of the rehabilitation protocol before returning to sports. The type and competitive level of the athlete are both factors that require consideration when returning an athlete to sports following an LMD.

Sports that involve large amounts of axial compression with lumbar flexion (i.e., football) or repetitive rotation with flexion (i.e., tennis, golf) should be initiated after the completion of phase IV; however, a sport like swimming where the axial load is relatively low may be initiated in phase II.

Running may be initiated in either phase III or IV, depending on the individual patient and the type and level of running involved. Generally, patients begin running on the elliptical trainer and progress to slow treadmill jogging, running on soft surfaces, such as dirt, and eventually returning to running on hard surfaces. The time frame for returning to running is physician-dependent but usually occurs between 12 and 16 weeks postoperatively.

In general, the inclusion of sport-specific activities following LMD should be a gradual process of initiating activities that mimic the specific sport, while correcting faulty mechanics. Sports that involve both high velocities of trunk rotation and flexion must be broken into phases to assess patient tolerance for uniplanar activities, before initiating multiplanar activities. Both golf and racquet sports involve repetitive trunk rotation with flexion and may increase the risk of reinjury. Mundt et al.[21] looked at 287 athletes with LDH to determine a relative risk compared to age-matched nonathletes. They concluded that people who participated in golf or racquet sports two or more times per week had a relative risk of 0.19 and 0.56. Each sport must be examined from a biomechanical perspective to evaluate the potential risks and safely progress the athlete back to participation.

Sport-specific plyometric activities should be incorporated into the program to reproduce the variations in speed, velocity, and direction that mimic the demands placed on the patient during competition. In addition to plyometrics, patients will also be instructed to progress weight training exercises in functional positions. Sport-specific strength and power demands must be considered when progressing the athlete in a weight training program. The goal of a weight training program is to maximize the isotonic strength and power of the extremities while minimizing spinal motion via isometric contraction of the trunk stabilizers.

Troubleshooting

If a patient is having difficulty returning to sport, the therapist must consider the specific demands of the individual sport and whether the patient has adequately met those demands. Sports that place higher loads on the spine may require longer periods of time for training before returning. Any sport that consistently provokes symptoms may need to be eliminated altogether, but this is rare and should be evaluated on an individual basis.

Postoperative Phase IV: Sport-Specific Activities (Weeks 14 to 18)

GOALS
- Patient to return pain-free to prior sport participation
- Patient to demonstrate good mechanics during functional/sporting activities so as to minimize lumbar motion
- Patient to demonstrate understanding of appropriate progression to return to sport

PRECAUTIONS
- Avoid participation in sport if symptoms exacerbated by sporting activities

TREATMENT STRATEGIES
- Perform sport-specific activities
- Continue to progress dynamic stabilization activities
- Progress cardiovascular training
- Progress upper and lower extremity strengthening

CRITERIA FOR RETURNING TO SPORT
- Patient to perform sport-specific activities pain-free
- Patient to demonstrate good mechanics during sport-specific activities

---

The following is a list of sport-specific considerations to guide the practitioner in returning patients to sport (Table 28-1):

A. Golf
  1. Total amount of rotation, approximately 90 degrees
     a) Shoulder horizontal adduction, approximately 30 degrees
     b) Thoracic spine, approximately 35 degrees
     c) Lumbar spine, approximately 5 degrees
     d) Hips, approximately 45-degree internal rotation and 45-degree external rotation
     e) Pronation/supination
  2. Address position
     a) During the address position the trunk is flexed approximately 40 degrees, most of which should occur as hip flexion
  3. Flexibility
     a) Hamstring
     b) One-joint hip flexors
     c) Hip adductors
     d) Gastrocnemius/soleus/Achilles
  4. Returning to golf (physician-dependent, approximately 14 to 18 weeks postoperatively)[22]
B. Swimming
  1. Amount of trunk ROM, dependent on type of stroke
  2. Flexibility
     a) Good pectoral and latissimus dorsi flexibility
        (1) Assess and treat relative inflexibility, as described by Sahrmann
  3. Strengthening
     a) Lower abdominal strengthening
     b) Pectoral muscles
     c) Latissimus dorsi
     d) Lower trapezius
     e) Hip flexors and extensors
C. Running
  1. Return to running (running speed dependent on prior running experience)
     a) Week 1—treadmill jogging at 5.0 m/hr, 5.5 m/hr for 1 min, then walk 1 min for approximately 3.7 m/hr. Repeat four times, 2 days in first week.
     b) Week 2—treadmill jogging 5.5 m/hr, 6.0 m/hr for 1 min, then walk 1 min for approximately 3.7 m/hr. Repeat six times, 2 days in second week.
     c) Week 3—treadmill jogging 6.0 m/hr, 6.5 m/hr for 2 min, then walk 1 min for approximately 3.7 m/hr. Repeat five times, 2 days in third week.
     d) Week 4—treadmill jogging 6.0 m/hr, 7.0 m/hr for 5 min, then walk 1 min for approximately 3.7 m/hr. Repeat two times, 2 days in fourth week, and slow jog outdoors for 10 min, 1 day in fourth week.
  2. Flexibility
     a) Hamstring
     b) Rectus femoris
     c) Gastrocnemius
     d) TFL/iliotibial band

TABLE 28-1	Progression for Return to Golf		
WEEK	MONDAY	WEDNESDAY	FRIDAY
1	10 putts 10 chips 5-min rest 15 chips	15 putts 15 chips 5-min rest 25 chips	20 putts 20 chips 5-min rest 20 putts 20 chips 5-min rest 10 chips 10 short irons
2	20 chips 10 short irons 5-min rest 10 short irons 15 medium irons (5-iron off tee)	20 chips 15 short irons 10-min rest 15 short irons 15 chips Putting 15 medium irons	15 short irons 20 medium irons 10-min rest 20 short irons 15 chips
3	15 short irons 20 medium irons 10-min rest 15 short irons 15 medium irons 5 long irons 10-min rest 20 chips	15 short irons 15 medium irons 10 long irons 10-min rest 10 short irons 10 medium irons 5 long irons 5 wood	15 short irons 15 medium irons 10 long irons 10-min rest 10 short irons 10 medium irons 10 long irons 10 wood
4	15 short irons 15 medium irons 10 long irons 10 drives 15-min rest Repeat	Play 9 holes	Play 9 holes
5	Play 9 holes	Play 9 holes	Play 18 holes

Chips = pitching wedge; short irons = wedge, 9-iron, 8-iron; medium irons = 7-iron, 6-iron, 5-iron; long irons = 4-iron, 3-iron, 2-iron; wood = 3-wood, 5-wood; drives = driver. (From Reinold, M., Wilk, K., Reed, J., Crenshaw, K., Andres, J. *Interval Sports Programs: Guidelines for Baseball, Tennis and Golf.* J Orthop Sports Phys Ther 2002;32(6):293–298, with permission.)

3. Strengthening
   a) Challenge trunk rotators isometrically in standing
   b) Hip abductor strengthening in functional positions
   c) Gluteus maximus strengthening via unilateral bridging
   d) Plyometric training to improve lower kinetic chain control

References

1. Nachemson, A. *The Load on Lumbar Disks in Different Positions of the Body.* Clin Orthop 1966;45:107–122.
2. Komori, H., Shinomiya, K., Nakai, O., Yamaura, I., Takeda, S., Furuya. *The Natural History of Herniated Nucleus Pulposus with Radiculopathy.* Spine 1996;21(2):225–229.
3. Deyo, R.A., Tsui-Wu, Y.J. *Descriptive Epidemiology of Low-back Pain and Its Related Medical Care in the United States.* Spine 1987;12(3):264–268.
4. Mooney, V. *Where Is the Pain Coming From?* Spine 1987;12:754–759.
5. Javedan, S., Sonntag, V. *Lumbar Disc Herniation: Microsurgical Approach.* Neurosurgery 2003;52(1):160–164.
6. Keskimaki, L., Seitsalo, S., Osterman, H., Rissanen, P. *Reoperations after Lumbar Disc Surgery.* Spine 2000;25:1500–1508.
7. Daneyemez, M., Sali, A., Kahraman, S., Beduk, A., Seber, N. *Outcome Analyses in 1072 Surgically Treated Lumbar Disc Herniations.* Minim Invas Neurosurg 1999;42:63–68.
8. Ito, T., Takano, Y., Yuasa, N. *Types of Lumbar Herniated Disc and Clinical Course.* Spine 2001;26:548–551.
9. Lewis, P.J., Weir, B.K., Broad, R.W., Grace, M.G. *Long Term Prospective Study of Lumbosacral Discectomy.* J Neurosurg 1987;67:49–53.
10. Weir, B.K., Jacobs, G.A. *Reoperation Rate Following Lumbar Discectomy: An Analysis of 662 Lumbar Discectomies.* Spine 1980;5:366–370.
11. Morgan-Hough, C.V., Jones, P.W., Eisenstein, S.M. *Primary and Revision Lumbar Discectomy: A 16-year Review from One Centre.* J Bone Joint Surg Br 2003;85B(6):871–874.
12. Nachemson, A. *Disc Pressure Measurements.* Spine 1981;6:93–96.
13. Ahlgren, B.D., Lui, W., Herkowitz, H.N., Panjabi, M.M., Guiboux, J.P. *Effect of Annular Repair on the Healing Strength of*

the Intervertebral Disc: A Sheep Model. Spine 2000;25(17): 2165–2170.

14. Ostelo, R.W., de Vet, H.C., Waddell, G., Kerckhoffs, M.R., Leffers, P., van Tulder, M. *Rehabilitation Following First-time Lumbar Disc Surgery: A Systematic Review Within the Framework of the Cochrane Collaboration.* Spine 2003;28(3):209–218.

15. Mckenzie, R.A. *The Lumbar Spine: Mechanical Diagnosis and Therapy.* Wright and Carmen Ltd., New Zealand, 1981, pp. 24–26.

16. Donelson, R., Murphy, K., Silva, G. *Centralisation Phenomenon: Its Usefulness in Evaluating and Treating Referred Pain.* Spine 1990;15(3):211–213.

17. Sahrmann, S.A. Diagnosis and Treatment of Movement Impairment Syndromes. In White, K. (Ed). *Movement Impairment Syndromes of the Low Back.* Mosby, St. Louis, 2002, pp. 58, 74–118, 310, 311, 403, 411, 412.

18. Hodges, P.W., Richardson, C.A. *Inefficient Muscular Stabilization of the Lumbar Spine Associated with Low Back Pain.* Spine 1996;21(22):2640–2650.

19. Yoshihara, K., Shirai, Y., Nakayama, Y., Uesaka, S. *Histochemical Changes in the Multifidus Muscle in Patients with Intervertebral Disc Herniation.* Spine 2001;26(6):622–626.

20. McClure, P.W., Esola, M., Schreier, R., Siegler, S. *Kinematic Analysis of Lumbar and Hip Motion While Rising from a Forward, Flexed Position in Patients With and Without a History of Low Back Pain.* Spine 1997;22(5):552–558.

21. Mundt, D.J., Kelsey, J.L., Golden, A.L., Panjabi, M.M., Pastides, H., Berg, A.T., Sklar, J., Hosea, T. *An Epidemiologic Study of Sports and Weight Lifting as Possible Risk Factors for Herniated Lumbar and Cervical Discs. The Northeast Collaborative Group on Low Back Pain.* Am J Sports Med 1993;21(6): 854–860.

22. Reinold, M., Wilk, K., Reed, J., Crenshaw, K., Andres, J. *Interval Sports Programs: Guidelines for Baseball, Tennis and Golf.* J Orthop Sports Phys Ther 2002;32(6):293–298.

29

Osteoporosis (Including Kyphoplasty)

HOLLY RUDNICK, PT, Cert MDT

KATALIYA PALMIERI, PT, MPT

Osteoporosis is a relatively new diagnosis, although the disease process is not. Before 1994, a clinical syndrome of low trauma fracture amongst the elderly was noted but no cause identified. In 1994 the World Health Organization (WHO) defined the threshold for the diagnosis of osteoporosis as being a bone mineral density (BMD) of more than 2.5 standard deviations below average of a normal 25- to 30-year-old Caucasian woman.[1] "Sometimes referred to as the *silent thief*, osteoporosis is a disease that robs the skeleton of its resources and causes microarchitectural deterioration of bone as people, especially post-menopausal women, age."[2] This compromised bone strength often predisposes the osteoporotic person to an increased risk of fracture. There are approximately 1.5 million osteoporosis-related fractures annually.[3] Today, in the United States, over 44 million men and women age 50 and older have low bone mass or osteoporosis, accounting for over $47 million a day spent on the medical care of osteoporosis-related fractures.[2] The primary goal for the osteoporotic patient is to prevent fracture. At the Hospital for Special Surgery (HSS), the approach to the treatment of osteoporosis is multidisciplinary and multifactorial. This chapter will outline the conservative management guideline/five-point program developed by HSS to educate and treat patients with osteoporosis, as well as the post-procedure rehabilitation following kyphoplasty for vertebral compression fractures.

ANATOMY OVERVIEW

Two types of bone are found in the body: cortical and trabecular. Cortical bone comprises 80% of the skeletal mass and is primarily responsible for skeletal strength. The cortical bone has a slow turnover rate and high resistance to bending and torsion. The trabecular bone comprises only 20% of the skeletal mass but accounts for 80% of the skeletal surface area. It has a high turnover rate and is the interior scaffolding, able to maintain skeletal shape despite compressive forces.[2,4] There are three primary types of bone cells. Osteoblasts synthesize new bone. Osteoclasts are active in resorption of bone, and the osteocytes direct bone to form where it is most needed. Bone remodeling is a continuous process of bone resorption and bone formation. Osteoporosis can result from an imbalance in the normal remodeling process.

"Both skeletal factors, such as low bone density and impaired bone quality, as well as non-skeletal factors, including poor balance and falls, play an important role in the development of osteoporosis and osteoporotic fractures. Bone density is by far the best measure of fracture risk."[2] It accounts for almost 70% of bone strength. Peak bone density is nearly attained by age 18 and fully attained by age 40.[4] Bone loss occurs at a rate of 0.5% per year and can increase up to 3% during the perimenopausal period to 7 years postmenopause and then slows down to a steady rate of 0.5% to 1% per year.[5] Bone strength is affected by changes in bone quality (impaired mineralization, increased bone turnover, and diminished trabecular microarchitecture). Because trabecular bone has high metabolic activity, it is more affected by bone turnover, resulting in greater resorption, weakening the microstructure of the bone and increasing susceptibility to fracture.[2,6]

DIFFERENTIAL DIAGNOSIS

Osteoporosis is broken down into two classifications: primary and secondary. Primary osteoporosis is age-related. It is largely caused by estrogen deficiency, which results in high turnover bone loss. Subsequently, areas that are high in trabecular bone are more affected. Vertebral, distal radius, and intertrochanteric fractures tend to be more common in this population. Secondary osteoporosis is bone loss related to chronic disease, medication therapy, or lifestyle. A wide variety of medical conditions have been linked to the development of osteoporosis, including rheumatoid arthritis, multiple myeloma, hyperparathyroidism, hyperthyroidism, inflammatory bowel disease, chronic kidney disease, and transplantation.[7] Oral glucocorticoids are by far the most common pharmaceutical associated with drug-induced osteoporosis; however, inhaled glucocorticoids, anticonvulsant medications, neuroleptic agents, methotrexate, and lithium have all been known to have detrimental effects on bone.[8,9] Secondary osteoporosis affects both cortical and trabecular bone. Therefore, femoral neck, proximal humerus, tibial, and pelvic fractures can occur in addition to vertebral, distal radius, and intertrochanteric fractures.

The diagnosis of osteoporosis is made via both laboratory tests and physical exam. Bone pain, kyphosis, loss of height, and x-ray findings are all factors that may lead to further testing to rule in or out the diagnosis of osteoporosis. The single most widely used test for diagnosing osteoporosis is bone densitometry. Several technologies are available for measuring BMD; however, central dual-energy x-ray absorptiometry (DXA) is the gold standard. Generally, the hip is the preferred site of BMD measurement and has been shown to be the best predictor of fracture risk.[10,11]

Three key pieces of information are obtained from the bone densitometry report: actual BMD, T score, and Z score. The BMD is used to determine the effectiveness of drug therapy. The T score is a comparison of the patient's measured BMD with the mean BMD of a healthy, young (25- to 30-year-old) sex matched reference population. The purpose of using a young, matched population is to compare the BMD with that of a population at peak bone mass. This number is reported as the number of standard deviations from the mean.[12] The WHO uses T scores to derive the thresholds for the diagnosis of osteopenia and osteoporosis. The T score is also used by the National Osteoporosis Foundation (NOF) to determine treatment thresholds. The Z score is the comparison of the patient's BMD to that of a healthy age- and sex-matched population that can be helpful in identifying secondary causes of osteoporosis.

REHABILITATION

PATIENT ASSESSMENT/PATIENT PROFILE

The evaluation of the osteoporotic patient should be comprehensive and include a detailed history, including prior history of fractures and falls, BMD scores, as well as any of the other risk factors that may contribute to the diagnosis of osteoporosis (Table 29-1). It is also important to obtain a detailed exercise history, paying special attention to the amount of weight-bearing activity that the patient participates in on a daily basis. The objective examination should include five major areas of assessment: patient posture and body mechanics, flexibility, strength, balance, and weight-bearing (Table 29-2). Addressing these five key areas during the evaluation and then subsequent rehabilitation is the basis of the five-point program for osteoporosis at HSS.

The severity of thoracic kyphosis has been associated with the occurrence of vertebral fractures, most likely as a result of the loss of vertebral height.[13] A measurement of the thoracic kyphosis can be taken with a FlexiCurve ruler and documented.

The measurement of strength and flexibility is fairly straightforward in this population; however, special attention should be paid to back extensor strength, in particular. Back extensor strength has been shown to be inversely proportional to both kyphosis and vertebral fracture.[13,14]

Strength measurements of hip extensors, scapular, and lower abdominal stabilizers are also important. Flexibility of the anterior chest musculature, hip flexors, and ankle plantar flexors is required to allow for correct posture and body mechanics and should be evaluated.

The assessment of balance is crucial because falls prevention in this population is a primary goal. Unilateral stance time with eyes opened and closed, functional reach (Figures 29-1 and 29-2), and "timed get-up and go test" are the tools used at HSS to measure balance, because the results can easily be correlated to falls risk.[15–18] Balance and falls risk can also be used to determine which patients are appropriate for group exercise and which may require individual instruction and

TABLE 29-2	Key Areas of Assessment for Osteoporosis

POSTURE/BODY MECHANICS
Flexicurve measurement of kyphosis

FLEXIBILITY
Hamstring (°SLR)
Quadriceps (°PKF)
Psoas (Thomas Test)
Gastrocnemius (°DFKE)
Pectoralis minor (cm from the table)
Spinal ROM

STRENGTH
UE/LE strength via MMT
Lower abdominals (Sahrmann levels 1–5)
Trunk extension (time held in secs)

BALANCE
Unilateral stance time (eyes open/eyes closed in secs)
Functional reach (average of 3 trials in inches)
Timed get-up and go (average of 3 trials in secs)

TABLE 29-1	Risk Factors Associated with Osteoporosis

Gender: women > men
Age: > with age
Body size: small frame, <127 lbs
Ethnicity: Caucasian, Asian
Family history
Personal history: fractures or falls
Dementia
Poor health/frailty
Cigarette smoking
Excessive alcohol: >2 drinks/day
Estrogen/testosterone deficiency
Low calcium intake
Sedentary lifestyle or prolonged bedrest
Use of high-risk medications

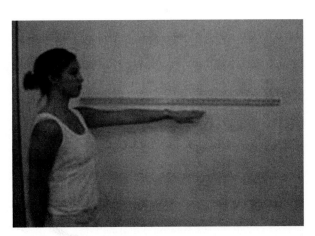

FIGURE 29-1 Assessment of functional reach starting position.

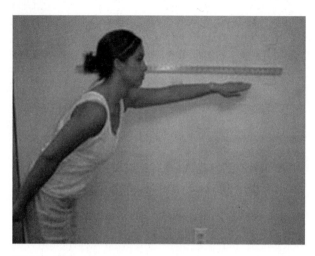

FIGURE **29-2** Assessment of functional reach final position.

balance training. At HSS, those patients who are relatively pain-free have good balance, and low falls risk are referred to a group exercise class that focuses on strengthening, flexibility, balance, posture and weight-bearing, as well as education on risk factors and fracture prevention. Any patient who has either pain or balance impairments, thereby increasing the risk of falls, should be treated in a more traditional physical therapy setting to provide individual instruction, balance training, and treatment for any pain complaint.

FIVE-POINT PROGRAM
POSTURE AND BODY MECHANICS
Posture plays an important role in spinal deformity and risk for fracture. Poor posture places high compressive loads on the spine. A young, healthy adult with normal spinal curves can resist these compressive forces. The osteoporotic spine will have difficulty resisting these postural forces, resulting in spinal changes, the most prominent being the kyphotic deformity.[19,20] Severe forward flexed posture is also associated with slowed gait and a larger base of support, as well as increasing instability.[21] To counteract these forces, a primary emphasis in rehabilitation is placed on posture and body mechanics.

Patients are taught sitting, standing, and sleeping postures to help maintain proper alignment. In a sitting position, patients are instructed to place both feet flat on the floor, with hips and knees at a 90/90 position. If a patient is of small stature and/or the chair height cannot be adjusted, a platform or stool can be placed under the feet for support. Occasionally, a patient may need a towel roll at the lumbar area to help maintain a natural lordosis or for comfort. When in a standing posture, patients are instructed to stand with legs at shoulder width apart, shoulders erect in a frontal plane, and head in a neutral posture. Some patients may feel uncomfortable in this position, so an alternative is to have their feet staggered (forward and behind) so that they may shift their weight if needed. In a sleeping position, a patient is advised to sleep with only one pillow under the head/neck, if possible. In some cases, a neck roll or ergonomic pillow may be suggested for comfort. If a person prefers to sleep in side-lying, a pillow should be placed between the legs for proper spinal alignment and, if needed, a pillow at the chest area with arms placed anteriorly to the pillow to help avoid rounded shoulders while sleeping (Figure 29-3).

Posture and Body Mechanics

GOALS
- Maintain neutral spinal posture
- Prevent vertebral fracture
- Education
- Maintain proper alignment with lifting

PRECAUTIONS
- Current fracture

TREATMENT STRATEGIES (AREAS TO FOCUS)
- Standing posture
- Sitting posture
- Hip hinge
- Sleeping position
- Lifting boxes or crates
- Golfers lift (for patients with uncompromised balance only)
- Getting out of bed (log roll)

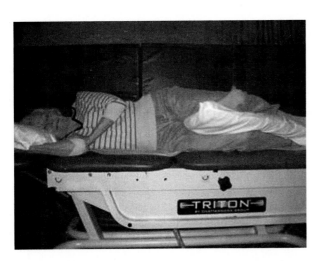

FIGURE **29-3** Corrected sleeping position in side-lying.

The most widely known precaution or contraindication for the osteoporotic patient is spinal flexion. Spinal flexion, along with rotation, has been sited as a potential risk for vertebral compression fractures.[22] The literature pertaining to this precaution is not current, and the correlation between spinal flexion and fracture risk is unclear. More recently, the differentiation between spinal flexion and *forced spinal flexion* is being considered. It is clear, however, that more research is required in this area to determine the potential risks. At this point in time, however, patients should be educated as to the possible fracture risk with flexion and, more specifically, forced flexion activities.

When assessing and teaching body mechanics, special focus is placed on getting out of bed and bending/lifting. During both of these activities, patients have a greater possibility of placing themselves into forced flexion. Many people have the tendency to flex the lumbar and thoracic spine to sit up in bed, which can place increased load on the spine. Patients should be taught to maneuver in bed using the log roll technique to maintain good spinal alignment. When getting out of bed in this manner, a patient can avoid forward flexion all together. For lifting objects, such as opening a window or lifting a heavy box, patients should give themselves a wide base of support, bend at the hips and knees, and stabilize the spine with the lower abdominal muscles. It is imperative that the patient with osteoporosis understand how to hip hinge (move from the hips vs the spine) correctly. The hip hinge allows the larger and stronger leg muscles to be used more effectively and spares the spine potentially damaging forces when bending and lifting.

FLEXIBILITY

Flexibility is the relative range of motion (ROM) of a joint when considering soft tissue (muscle, ligaments, connective tissue), boney structure, and pain. Soft tissue barriers, such as collagen changes found in ligaments and tendons, may affect flexibility. As a person ages, there is reduced extensibility of collagen, thereby decreasing flexibility of the joint.[23] Flexibility is a focus in osteoporosis treatment to assist in improved posture and enhance proper body mechanics.

Emphasis is placed on spinal extension. A patient with osteoporosis may exhibit tightness of the anterior chest muscles with thoracic kyphosis. Stretching exercises for the pectoralis major and minor are of particular focus during treatment. Exercises, such as doorway pectoralis stretch, corner stretch, and/or supine pectoralis stretch with towel roll or half foam roller placed vertically along the spine (Figures 29-4 and 29-5), can be added into the exercise program. Some stretches may require modification in the case of decreased upper extremity ROM. Also contributing to increased thoracic kyphosis is a shortened rectus abdominis. Lengthening the rectus abdominis, in conjunction with strengthening the transverse abdominis and obliques, can potentially reduce the progression of the kyphotic deformity and decrease rib splaying. Cervicothoracic flexibility is also an important component of treatment. Many patients exhibit anterior translation of the cervical spine, forward head, which can lead to tightened upper trapezius, suboccipital, and sternocleidomastoid muscles. Anterior translation of the cervical spine has been correlated to

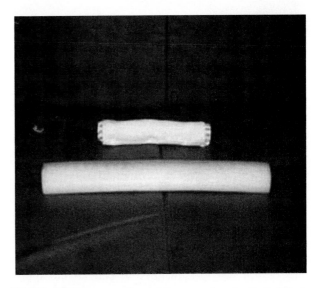

FIGURE **29-4** Foam roll used for anterior chest stretch in Figure 29-7.

Flexibility

GOALS

- Maintain ROM
- Prevent postural deformity
- Spinal extension
- Maintain extensibility of soft tissue

PRECAUTIONS

- Spinal stenosis
- Spondylolysis
- Spondylolisthesis
- Shoulder pathology
- Hip pathology

TREATMENT STRATEGIES

- Pectoralis stretch in supine or sitting
- Doorway stretch
- Corner stretch
- Prone press-up
- Quadruped rock back and forth
- AROM cervical spine
- SCM, upper trap stretching
- Dorsiflexion stretch
- STM to lumbar spine

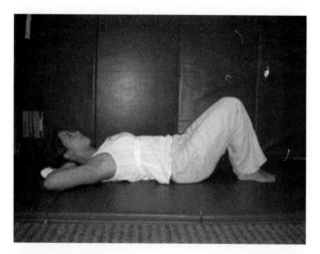

FIGURE 29-5 Supine pectoralis stretch on foam or towel roll.

increased kyphosis and fracture risk.[19] Including cervical retraction exercises and mild stretching activities to the cervicothoracic area to assist in regaining extension and normal alignment will help improve posture and may reduce potential fracture.[19] If patients are appropriate, prone press-ups can be added to improve spinal extension. Caution must be used if a patient with osteoporosis also has comorbidity of spinal stenosis, spondylolysis, or spondylolisthesis. A patient with spinal stenosis must be asymptomatic if prone press-ups are added to the therapy program.

Hip and ankle ROM can have a direct effect on lower spine movement and body mechanics for lifting and bending, as well as balance. Decreased flexibility in the posterior hip capsule and hip flexor muscles may promote posterior pelvic tilt and decreased lumbar lordosis. Exercises, such as quadruped rocking back, with proper lumbar alignment, and hip flexor stretching, with proper abdominal and pelvic stabilization, may be introduced into the treatment program to address these issues. Also, some osteoporotic patients with thoracic kyphotic deformity will present with an increased lumbar lordosis, as a result of shortened lumbar extensors and weakened lower abdominals. Some of these deformities are fixed; however, many patients benefit from soft tissue work to the lumbar paraspinals to improve the extensibility of the tissue and improve the efficacy of the flexibility exercises.

Decreased ankle ROM alters a person's ability to balance and perform lifting movements. As people age, the gastrocnemius/soleus complex becomes less elastic.[20] Dorsiflexion stretches are important not only to the osteoporotic population, but also to the aging population, in general. Dorsiflexion stretching at the wall or off a raised surface should be incorporated into the stretching program.

STRENGTHENING

Muscle strength declines by 15% per decade after age 50 and 30% after age 70.[24] Sarcopenia, loss of muscle mass, occurs more frequently in women than men, resulting in loss of muscle strength. Direct correlation exists between decreased back extensor strength in osteoporotic women and thoracic kyphosis.[13] Strengthening back extensors and abdominal stabilizers will improve posture and balance. At HSS, strengthening for patients with osteoporosis is broken down into specific levels, according to BMD.

Level I includes patients with a normal BMD measurement. Usually, these patients present with no postural deformity or pain. They may have a family history of osteoporosis, or several risk factors, and are referred to preventive therapy. Strengthening exercises should focus on mat exercises, including prone extension (Figure 29-6) and lower abdominal stabilization exercises. Closed chain exercises, including squats and lunges with free weights, are an important addition to the program. Progressive, resistive exercise with the use of dumbbells and/or exercise machines should be used as appropriate. Participation in a consistent weight–bearing-based conditioning program is encouraged.

Level II includes patients diagnosed with osteopenia (1.0 SD below normal). These patients will not have pain and probably don't have deformity; however, they most likely have postural habits that may contribute to the development of a future deformity. They may have forward head and rounded shoulders but not the actual kyphosis. Exercise at this level will include all of the previously mentioned exercises in level I, in addition to specific postural exercises to improve stature (Sahrmann[25]) (Figures 29-7 through 29-10). Scapular retraction in standing or prone, with resistance and prone lower trapezius exercises, should be a focus of treatment.

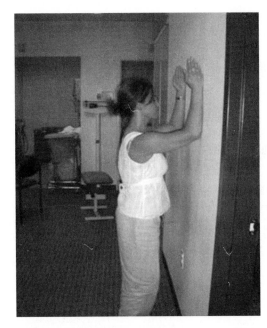

FIGURE **29-7** Shoulder flexion facing wall to improve lower trapezius performance starting position.

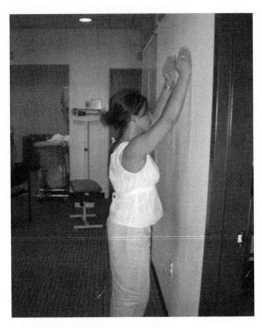

FIGURE **29-8** Shoulder flexion facing wall to improve lower trapezius performance raising arms.

Level III is designed for the patient diagnosed with osteoporosis (1.0 to 2.0 SD below normal). These patients may have deformity and pain associated with the deformity. The program at this level includes exercises from levels I and II plus mat exercises and low resistance aerobic exercise. Upper extremity proprioceptive neuromuscular facilitation (PNF) in sitting, wall slides with arc 0 to 70 degrees, and sitting/standing

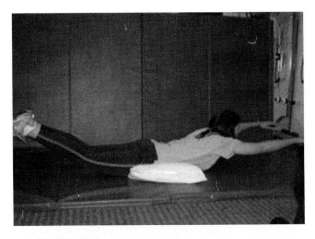

FIGURE **29-6** Prone lumbar extension over pillow.

Strengthening

GOALS

- Maintain strength
- Improve postural muscles
- Abdominal stabilization
- Improve balance

PRECAUTIONS

- Current fracture

TREATMENT STRATEGIES

Level I: Normal BMD

- Mat exercises, including prone extension, lower abdominals
- Closed chain exercises, including squats and/or lunges with free weights
- Progressive resistive exercises (PREs): dumbbells as appropriate
- Exercise machine: hoist (row, triceps, biceps, lats), total gym, multihip, treadmill, upper body ergometer (UBE), bike

Level II: Osteopenia (1.0 SD below normal)

- Level I exercises
- Postural exercises
  - Scapular retraction with Thera-Band
  - Prone scapular retraction
  - Lower traps prone
  - Latissimus dorsi
  - Cervical retraction
  - Standing lower trap

Level III: Osteoporosis (1.0 to 2.5 SD below normal)

- Postural exercises
  - Scapular retraction
  - UE PNF sitting
  - Wall slide (arc 0 to 70 degrees)
  - Sitting/standing abdominal sets with UE lift
- Mat exercises
  - Lower abdominal stabilization
  - Prone on elbows
  - Leg raises with resistance
  - Quadruped upper extremity lifts
- Low resistance aerobic
  - Bike (with resistance)
  - Treadmill

IV: Osteoporosis with fracture

- Gentle introduction to exercise
  - Abdominal setting/gluteal setting
  - Scapular retraction
  - UE PNF in sitting
  - Bent knee fallout
  - Heel slides

abdominal setting with upper extremity lifts can be added to the postural exercises. Mat exercises should include lower abdominal stabilization progression beginning at low levels (Figure 29-11), prone on elbows, leg raises with resistance, and quadruped activities, such as upper extremity lifts.

Level IV is designed for the osteoporotic patient with a fracture. These patients almost always have a deformity and usually have pain. Patients at this level may also have undergone a kyphoplasty procedure at one or more levels (refer to kyphoplasty section). Gentle exercise should be introduced into treatment to patient tolerance; however, the primary focus of treatment will be on relieving pain and preventing further fracture.

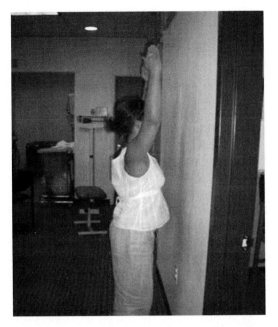

FIGURE **29-9** Shoulder flexion facing wall to improve lower trapezius performance lifting arms off wall into scaption.

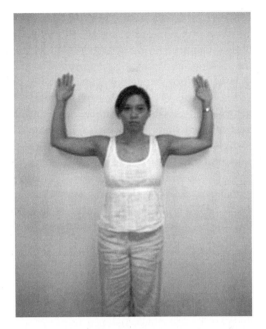

FIGURE **29-10** Posture set against wall.

WEIGHT-BEARING

Guidelines by the NOF recommend regular weight-bearing activity to reduce the risk of falls and fractures.[26] Weight-bearing and resistance training demonstrate positive effects on BMD.[28] Bone responds and adapts to the forces placed upon it. Therefore, weight-bearing activities are a crucial part of any osteoporosis treatment program. Progressive resistance training with dumbbells or machines are not necessary to provide sufficient weight-bearing. Body weight alone during closed chain activities can provide enough resistance to maintain healthy weight-bearing. The most common form of weight-bearing exercise is walking. It has been shown

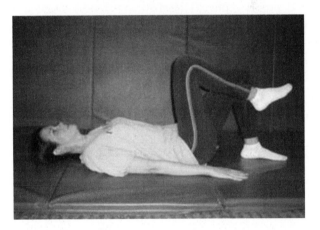

FIGURE **29-11** Lower abdominal stabilization level 1, *A* per Sahrmann.[25]

Weight-Bearing

GOALS
- Increase BMD
- Promote bone growth
- Strengthening

PRECAUTIONS
- Problematic or painful walking
- Weight-bearing status

TREATMENT STRATEGIES
- Walking program/treadmill
- Squats
- Sitting weight shifts
- Step-ups
- Sitting pushups to wall to floor
- Contralateral hip extension/abduction support to unsupported with Thera-Band

that for every 1 hour of walking per week (at an average pace), the risk of hip fracture is lowered by 6%.[29] Other examples of weight-bearing activities are jogging, stair climbing, hiking, and dancing. Swimming is not considered a weight-bearing activity because of buoyancy. Biking does not give the same resistance as walking activities; however, if true weight-bearing is problematic as a result of coexisting conditions, such as spinal stenosis, resistive cycling can be a good alternative. Closed chain weight-bearing activities can also be performed with upper extremities such as wall pushups and sitting pushups. Exercise programs should include 30 minutes to 1 hour daily of consecutive weight-bearing activities.[26]

BALANCE

Fracture risk is higher in those patients with high falls risk.[29] Aitken et al.[30] found that the primary risk for hip fracture in the elderly was increased risk of falling rather than decreased bone mass. Balance requires adequate musculoskeletal strength, flexibility, vestibular, visual, and proprioceptive/kinesthetic awareness. Decline in the previously mentioned systems occurs to varying degrees as people age. Balance exercise may decrease a person's risk for falling. Balance training also encompasses falls prevention. Patients must be aware of their environment and change potential hazards in their home, if necessary. Activities that incorporate single-limb stance, directional changes, and varying surfaces should be incorporated into a functional balance program. Teaching the patient to use balance strategies in both a controlled and open environment is essential. Patients should also be educated with how to fall and what to do in the event of a fall.

Troubleshooting

It is important to remember that with the exception of the patient who has severe deformity and/or vertebral compression fracture, osteoporosis is a painless disease. Therefore, it can be challenging to impart to a patient the necessity of performing a consistent exercise regimen and avoiding potentially harmful movements. In general, the length of treatment for a patient with the primary diagnosis of osteoporosis is 4 weeks. The patient with compression fractures may require more time, usually no longer than 6 to 8 weeks. Visits are usually no more than one to two per week.

Other considerations include the osteoporotic patient who has coexisting conditions. By far the most difficult patient to treat is the person with both osteoporosis and spinal stenosis. These two conditions are inherently contradictory. The traditional treatment for spinal stenosis

Balance

GOALS
- Decrease risk for falls
- Decease risk for fracture

PRECAUTIONS
- Environmental hazards
  - Shoes
  - Carpets
  - Nightlights
  - Inclement weather
- Physical disabilities/decreased functional mobility
- Visual deficits
- Sensory deficits
- Vestibular deficits
- Mental impairments/judgments

TREATMENT STRATEGIES
- Single-leg balance
- Heel walking
- Braiding
- Tandem walking
- Reaching
- "Timed get-up and go"
- Quick feet
- Balance board
- Obstacle course (closed and open spaces)
- Education on falls

is a flexion biased program that attempts to open posterior spaces to relieve compression.[31] As the authors have stated previously, spinal flexion has long been considered a contraindication for osteoporosis. It is crucial when treating these two conditions together, that multiple factors be taken into consideration, including the level, location, and severity of bone loss, past fracture history, severity of stenotic symptoms, presence and severity of kyphotic deformity, and general patient body mechanics and awareness.

A stenosis patient who has a relatively low to moderate and stable level of osteoporosis, with no fracture history and little to no deformity, may be appropriate for unloaded flexion, as in a single or double knee to chest. It is well documented that the majority of vertebral compression fractures occur in the mid to lower thoracic spine.[16,32] The correct performance of unloaded lumbar flexion, using greater hip flexion than spinal movement, probably presents a low fracture risk and may potentially provide significant pain relief from stenotic compression. However, a more severe level of osteoporosis (greater than level III), and certainly past fracture history, would be cause to eliminate the use of any flexion in a patient's program. These patients are best treated with a neutral stabilization program.

Choosing the most effective and least harmful exercises to strengthen the osteoporotic patient can be a challenge. It is important to have a good understanding of the biomechanics involved in performing each exercise. For example, bridging, an exercise commonly used in physical therapy to strengthen both hip and lower back extensors, may be a poor choice for this population. There is the potential for a large flexion force placed upon the thoracic spine as the patient lifts the hips off the floor, which may elevate the potential for a vertebral compression fracture to occur, especially in the level III or IV patient. A better choice for strengthening the hip and back extensors is prone leg lifts on or off a pillow. Abdominal strengthening should be limited to isometric stabilization, where the spine is relatively fixed (Figure 29-12). Abdominal crunches or curls should be avoided because they place an increased flexion load on lower thoracic and upper lumbar spine.

REHABILITATION FOLLOWING VERTEBRAL KYPHOPLASTY

The treatment of vertebral compression fractures (VCFs) has traditionally been limited to bed rest, bracing, analgesic medications, narcotic medications, and activity modification. These methods have had varying degrees of success and often require prolonged immobilization. In 1984 an innovative new technique for the treatment of VCFs was developed in France, called *percutaneous*

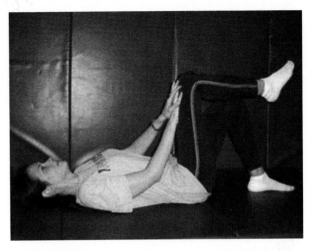

FIGURE **29-12** Isometric hip flexion with abdominal setting.

vertebroplasty. The procedure involves transpedicular, percutaneous bone cement injections into the collapsed vertebral bodies. This offers the patient reduced pain, prevention of further collapse, return to function, and eliminates the complications of bed rest.

Kyphoplasty was developed several years later as a progression of the vertebroplasty procedure. Kyphoplasty combines vertebroplasty and balloon catheter technology developed for angioplasty. It involves the placement of a cannula and inflatable bone tamp under fluoroscope into the collapsed vertebral body. The balloon is then inflated and the cavity filled with bone cement.[33] Kyphoplasty, unlike vertebroplasty, restores vertebral body height and addresses spinal deformity, as well as reduces pain and restores the patient to a normal functional level. Kyphoplasty is a relatively safe procedure; however, complications can occur. The most severe complications of kyphoplasty involve cement embolization and cement extravasation. This can happen as a result of the cement leaking into either the venous system or spinal canal.

Not all VCFs are appropriate for a kyphoplasty procedure. Fractures that are nonpainful and have minimal deformity rarely require treatment beyond activity modification. If the VCF is painful, has associated deformity, or has failed traditional nonoperative treatment, kyphoplasty may be indicated. The level and number of VCFs also play a role in determining the appropriateness of kyphoplasty.

Rehabilitation considerations following a kyphoplasty procedure are not unique. The same precautions are taken, as with any patient who has severe osteoporosis, with or without untreated VCF. Typically, rehabilitation is not initiated for a range of a few days to a week following the procedure. The post-kyphoplasty patient may have some post-procedure pain, which can be addressed with modalities; however, in general, most patients should have considerably less pain than pre-procedure. Exercise should be based upon level IV of the five-point program and tailored to the patient's functional and balance impairments, as outlined in previous sections.

REFERENCES

1. Kanis, J.A., Gluer, C.C. *International Osteoporosis Foundation: An Update on the Diagnosis and Assessment of Osteoporosis with Densitometry.* Osteoporos Int 2000;11:192–202.

2. Follin, S.L., Hansen, L.B. *Current Approaches to the Prevention and Treatment of Post Menopausal Osteoporosis.* Am J Health Sys Pharm 2003;60(9):883–901.

3. Star, V., Hochberg, M. *Osteoporosis: Treat Current Injury, Retard Future Loss.* Intern Med 1993;113(14):32–42.

4. Woolf, A.D., Dixon, A.S. *Osteoporosis: A Clinical Guide,* 2nd ed. Livery House, London, 1998.

5. Pouilles, J.M., Tremollieres, F., Ribot, C. *Effect of Menopause on Femoral and Vertebral Bone Loss.* J Bone Miner Res 1995;10: 1534–1536.

6. Delmas, P.D., Eastell, R., Garnero, P., Seibel, M.J., Stepan, J. (Committee of Scientific Advisors of the International Osteoporosis Foundation). *The Use of Biochemical Markers of Bone Turnover in Osteoporosis.* Osteoporos Int 2000;11(Suppl 6): S2–S17.

7. Fitzpatrick, L.A. *Secondary Causes of Osteoporosis.* Mayo Clin Proc 2002;77:453–468.

8. North American Menopause Society. *Management of Postmenopausal Osteoporosis: Position Statement of the North American Menopause Society.* Menopause 2002;9:84–101.

9. Tannirandorn, P., Epstein, S. *Drug-Induced Bone Loss.* Osteoporosis Int 2000;11:637–659.

10. Lipworth, B.J. *Systemic Adverse Effects of Inhaled Corticosteroid Therapy: A Systemic Review and Meta-analysis.* Arch Intern Med 1999;159:941–955.

11. Cummings, S.R., Black, D.M., Nevitt, M.C., Browner, W., Cauley, J., Ensrud, K., Genant, H.K., Palermo, L., Scott, J.,Vogt, T.M. *Bone Density at Various Sites for Prediction of Hip Fractures.* Lancet 2000;341:72–75.

12. Marshall, D., Johnell, O., Wedel, H. *Meta Analysis of How Well Measures of Bone Mineral Density Predict Occurrences of Osteoporotic Fractures.* Br Med J 1996;312:1254–1259.

13. Sinaki, M., Itoi, E., Rogers, J.W., Bergstralh, E.J., Wahner, H.W. *Correlation of Back Extensor Strength with Thoracic Kyphosis and Lumbar Lordosis in Estrogen Deficient Women.* Am J Phys Med Rehabil 1996;75:370–374.

14. Sinaki, M., Wollan, P.C., Scott, R.W., Gelczer, R.K. *Can Strong Back Extensors Prevent Vertebral Fractures in Women with Osteoporosis?* Mayo Clin Proc 1996;71(10):951–956.

15. Vellas, B.J., Wayne, S.J., Romero, L., Baumgartner, R.N., Rubenstein, L.Z., Garry, P.J. *One-leg Balance is an Important Predictor of Injurious Falls in Older Persons.* J Am Geriatr Soc 1997;45:735–738.

16. Bohannon, R.W., Larken, P.A., Cook, A.C., Gear, J., Singer, J. *Decrease in Timed Balance Test Scores with Aging.* Phys Ther 1984;64:1067–1070.

17. Duncan, P.W., Weiner, D.K., Chandler, J., Studenski, S. *Functional Reach: A Clinical Measuring of Balance.* J Gerentol Soc 1990;45:194–197.

18. Posadillo, D., Richardson, S. *The Tmied Up and Go: A Test of Basic Functional Mobility for Frail Elderly Persons.* J Am Geriatr Soc 1991;39:142–148.

19. Keller, T., Harrison, D.E., Colloca, C., Harrison, D.D., Janik, T. *Prediction of Osteoporotic Spinal Deformity.* Spine 2003;28(5): 455–462.

20. Guzick, D., Keller, T., Szpalski, M., Park, J., Spengler, D. *A Biomechanical Model of the Lumbar Spine During Upright Isometric Flexion, Extension, and Lateral Bending.* Spine 1996; 21(4):427–433.

21. Balzini, L., Vannucchi, L., Benvenuti, F., Benucci, M., Monni, M., Cappozzo, A., Stanhope, S. *Clinical Characteristics of Flexed Posture in Elderly Women.* J Am Geriatr Soc 2003;51(10):1419–1426.

22. Sinaki, M., Mikkelsen, B.A. *Postmenopausal Spinal Osteoporosis: Flexion Versus Extension Exercises.* Arch Phys Med Rehabil 1984;65:593–596.

23. Robert, M., Cavanagh, P., Evans, W., Fiatorone, M., Hagberg, J., McAuley, E., Startzell, J. *ACSM Position Stand: Exercise and Physical Activity for Older Adults.* Med Sci Sports Exerc 1998;30(6):992–1008.

24. Nied, R., Franklin, B. *Promoting and Prescribing Exercise for the Elderly.* Am Fam Phys 2002;65(3):419–426.

25. Sahrmann, S.A. *Diagnosis and Treatment of Movement Impairment Syndromes.* Mosby, St. Louis, 2002.

26. National Osteoporosis Foundation. *Physician's Guide to Prevention and Treatment of Osteoporosis.* www.nof.org. Accessed May 2004.

27. Kelly, G., Kelly, K., Vu Tran, Z. *Resistance Training and Bone Mineral Density in Women: A Meta-Analysis of Controlled Trials.* Amer J Phys Med & Rehab 2001;80:65–77.

28. Feskanich, D., Willet, W., Colditz, G. *Walking and Leisure-Time Activity and Risk of Hip Fracture in Postmenopausal Women.* Obstet Gynecol Surv 2003;58(5):327–328.

29. Kerschan, K., Alacamlioglu, Y., Kollmitzer, J., Wober, C., Kaider, A., Hartard, M. Ghanem, A., Preisinger, E. *Functional Impact of Unvarying Exercise Program in Women after Menopause.* Amer J Phys Med & Rehab 1998;July/Aug: 326–332.

30. Aitken, J.M. *Relevance of Osteoporosis in Woman with Fracture of the Femoral Neck.* Br Med J 1984;288:597–601.

31. Fritz, J.M., Erhard, R.E., Vignovic, M. *A Nonsurgical Treatment Approach to Patients with Lumbar Spinal Stenosis.* Phys Ther 1997;77:962–973.

32. Schmorl, G., Junghanns H. *The Human Spine in Health and Disease.* Grune & Stratton, New York, 1957.

33. Lieberman, I., Reinhardt, M. *Vertebroplasty and Kyphoplasty for Osteolytic Vertebral Collapse.* Clin Orthop 2003;1(415S): S176–S186.

30

Adult Lumbar Spinal Fusion

CHARLENE HANNON, PT, MBA

More than 200,000 spinal fusions are performed each year in the United States.[1]

Controversy exists as to whether spinal fusion is the treatment of choice for patients with various types of low back pain.[2] Some of the reasons for this controversy are that there is a 10% to 40% pseudarthrosis (failure of fusion) rate[1]; improved function, particularly return to work, does not always occur; and many patients experience continued postoperative pain.[2] Furthermore, in some cases, additional surgery is necessary and adds to health care costs. In the United States alone, total health care expenditures incurred by individuals with back pain reached an estimated 90.7 billion dollars, and, on average, individuals with back pain incurred 60% higher expenditures than individuals without back pain.[3] Careful patient selection and choice of the appropriate surgical procedure seem to generate the best surgical outcomes.[2] Fusions can be classified into two categories: instrumented and noninstrumented. Noninstrumented fusions do not use any hardware. They are much less commonly performed and are usually done for single-level fusions only. The two most common instrumented lumbar spinal fusion procedures are posterior lumbar interbody fusion (PLIF) and circumferential fusion. Both procedures have a very good rate of fusion. Bono and Lee[4] showed that PLIF has a fusion rate of 85%, and circumferential yielded 91% fusion.[4] For the purpose of this guideline, only the PLIF will be described. It is important, however, that the physical therapist be aware that there are many spinal fusion techniques. The principles of rehabilitation following lumbar spinal fusion remain the same, regardless of the procedure.

One of the most important concepts for the physical therapist to understand is the concept that the hardware is merely a temporary scaffold until biological healing is complete. Biological healing can be affected by many factors. Some of these factors are smoking,[5] poor surgical technique, and mechanical stress across the fusion mass (movement during the phases of healing). It is the mechanical stress with which the physical therapist is to be most concerned when developing a rehabilitation program. Careful consideration must be made of the forces generated by lever arms, such as the upper and lower extremities and their effects on the lumbar spine. Although there is a paucity of research examining the in vivo forces generated across a healing fusion site, Rohlmann et al. did show that lifting both legs in the supine position generated the highest loads on the fixation devices as compared to most other lumbar stabilization exercises.[6] Osteoporosis is a relative precaution and does not preclude complete healing from occurring.[7] Additional precautions, such as bracing, may be required in patients with osteoporosis.

In summary, the following are generally accepted indications for spinal fusion:

- When decompression (laminectomy) is warranted because of spinal stenosis, spondylosis or degenerative disc disease, and more than half of the lamina is removed, creating an unstable segment
- Without decompression to stabilize a motion segment that is unstable (defined as >4 mm excursion on bending X rays)
- To stabilize a motion segment with spondylolisthesis and thus prevent further slippage or possibly correct for slippage
- After the surgical removal of various types of bony sarcomas (this will not be addressed in this guideline)
- Intractable pain
- Neurological signs
- Failed conservative management

SURGICAL OVERVIEW

PLIF describes a technique that is indicated to treat various spinal pathologies, as listed previously. The primary goal of the technique is to provide a solid interbody fusion with decompression of the surrounding neural structures and restoration of vertebral alignment. In addition, the procedure should provide global spinal balance that protects adjacent normal segments.[8] Global spinal balance is the concept that when alignment is corrected at a given intervertebral segment, total spinal alignment is preserved. In other words, a new misalignment is not created. The PLIF is a four-stage procedure, as follows:

Stage 1: Exposure and decompression

Stage 2: Spinal instrumentation and preliminary fixation

Stage 3: Anterior column reconstruction and interbody fusion

Stage 4: Internal stabilization and completion of surgery

Stage 1: The area is decompressed, taking care to preserve normal tissues and structures at adjacent levels, particularly the posterior spinous processes and the interspinous ligaments, as well as the facet joints to prevent late adjacent segment instability. Also, care is taken so as not to denervate the paraspinal muscles.

Stage 2: The instrument system is also referred to as "hardware" and is essentially internal spinal fixation. The components may consist of rods, plates, hooks, wires, and/or screws and are available in both

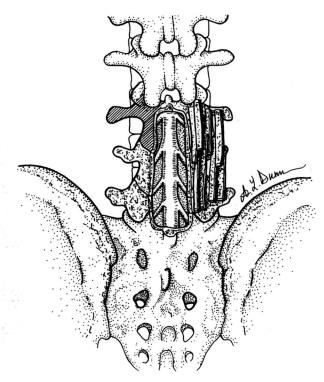

FIGURE **30-1** Posterior view of area of lumbar decompression.

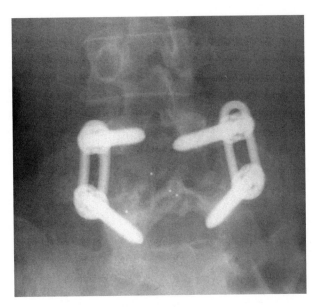

FIGURE **30-2** Posterior radiograph of fusion with hardware.

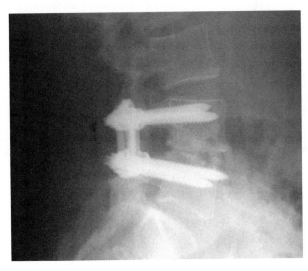

FIGURE **30-3** Lateral radiograph of fusion with hardware.

stainless steel and titanium (the main advantage of titanium is its magnetic resonance imaging [MRI] compatibility). Instrumentation is placed in the pedicles to prepare for stage 3.

Stage 3: Numerous distraction techniques may be used to restore normal disc height. Care is taken so as not to place the neural structures under excessive tension. Once the ideal height is attained, the screws on the plates are tightened to maintain the gains. Next, the disc space is prepared. A complete discectomy is performed, and the end plate is scraped to create bleeding. If bleeding becomes excessive, it must be controlled. The ultimate goal is to ensure a good bone graft to vertebral bone contact, a large surface area of bleeding bone, and no interposition of soft tissue. The bone graft is then placed. Graft material may be the bone chipped away from the decompression procedure, iliac crest bone graft, or allograft material (Figure 30-1).

Stage 4: The working hardware is replaced with the final implants, and the incision is closed. The procedure described can be repeated for multiple segments, as necessary (Figures 30-2 and 30-3).

REHABILITATION OVERVIEW

The rehabilitation program begins postoperatively at the bedside and is progressed to achieve short-term goals for discharge to the home. Patients continue a basic home exercise program for the first 4 to 6 weeks and then begin outpatient therapy. Careful consideration is given to provide a protective environment for the healing fusion. Outpatient therapy is typically provided from 6 weeks to as long as 6 months, depending on the individual and the surgeon. Generally, for a one-level procedure, fusion should occur within 4 months of the surgery. For more complex, multilevel spinal fusions biological healing of the fusion reaches a peak at 1 year but continues to mature from 1 to 2 years. Goals are set individually and are functionally based, targeting return to full activities of daily living (ADL) and return to full-time employment.

Preoperative Phase

GOALS

- Patient education: pain management, logrolling, concept of bending from the hips, and importance of avoiding lumbar movement
- Maximize strength/functional capabilities: Upper body strength becomes important for bed mobility, hamstring flexibility in the absence of neural tension signs
- General conditioning: Improvements in preoperative endurance will benefit patients in the postoperative phase

PRECAUTIONS

- Avoid movements that increase pain (patient may be flexion, neutral, or extension-biased)
- Avoid loaded positions if load-sensitive
- Avoid exercises that aggravate neural tissue in the presence of neural tension signs

TREATMENT STRATEGIES

- Neutral-biased lumbar stabilization
- Functional tests—squatting, lunging, transitions to/from floor
- Gait training (educate in progression from walker to cane)
- Home program:
  - Preoperative conditioning
  - Endurance training: stationary bicycle, treadmill, elliptical
  - Strength training: wall squats, wall push-ups
- Postoperative therapeutic exercise instruction:
  - Quadriceps sets
  - Gluteal sets
  - Abdominal sets
  - Ankle pumps
- Pain relief modalities: electrical stimulation
- Criteria for surgery:
  - Failed conservative management
  - Intractable pain
  - Neurological signs

PREOPERATIVE REHABILITATION

Ideally, before being advised to undergo a spinal fusion, patients will have received a full physical therapy program that may have included stabilization, stretching, and general conditioning exercises. In addition, patient education during the conservative phase is important to address, such as pain management, use of modalities at home, proper posture, and body mechanics. The Hospital for Special Surgery (HSS) uses a multidisciplinary preoperative educational program known as "Your Pathway to Recovery." The program has both physical therapists and nurses as instructors and uses a classroom style setting. The program is a means of providing answers to many of the most frequently asked questions and alleviating patient anxiety before surgery. Patients also have the opportunity to interact with others who are about to undergo the same or similar procedure.

POSTOPERATIVE PHASE I (DAY 1 TO 14)

During the hospital stay, patients are instructed in logrolling transfers, progressive ambulation, and stair climbing. Upon discharge, the following are the expectations for goals achieved:

- Ability to transfer in and out of bed via log rolling without assist
- Ability to ambulate with or without appropriate assistive device (usually cane)
- Ability to don and doff brace without assist if prescribed
- Ability to tolerate sitting for meals (approximately 20 minutes)
- Ability to negotiate stairs with railing

Patients are instructed in a home exercise program, which consists of the following exercises to be performed two to three times daily: quadriceps sets, gluteal sets, and ankle pumps.

Troubleshooting

The greatest obstacle during phase I is pain control. Because the majority of patients from POD 1 to 14 will be at home working independently or with home care,

Postoperative Phase I (Days 1 to 14)

USE LOGROLLING FOR TRANSFERS

- Progress from walker to cane to no device
- Balance activity with rest

GOALS

- Patient education
- Provide the most protective environment for the healing fusion
- Maximize function
- Control postoperative pain
- Independence in home therapeutic exercise program
- Improve endurance and tolerance to daily activities

PRECAUTIONS

- Avoid all lumbar movements (absolutely no lumbar flexion, extension, sidebending or rotation)
- Avoid sitting more than 20 to 30 minutes
- May or may not be wearing a brace, depending on the surgeon's advice
- No lifting more than 5 pounds (a gallon of milk is 8 pounds)
- No prone positioning or quadruped

TREATMENT STRATEGIES

- Transfer training
- Gluteal set, quadriceps set, dorsiflexion for neural gliding
- Walking in the home or community
- Pain modalities, activity modification to control pain, communication with MD regarding activity and pain medications
- Home therapeutic exercise program: as previous
- Emphasize patient compliance to home therapeutic exercise program and protective environment, body mechanics, use of assistive devices, such as reacher, elastic shoelaces, long-handled shoe horn

CRITERIA FOR ADVANCEMENT

- Pain well controlled
- Tolerating sitting for 30 minutes
- Progression to cane
- Independent in logroll transfers

---

cryotherapy and TENS may be the modalities of choice along with activity modification. Good communication with the surgeon at this time is essential. Patients with previous radicular symptoms may not have immediate relief. For patients who have a new onset of radicular symptoms, it is important to notify the referring physician and keep track of the symptoms.

Patients may have many questions regarding palpable hardware, swelling, dysesthesia, and paresthesia. It is important that the therapist educate the patient with regard to postoperative expectations.

POSTOPERATIVE PHASE II (WEEKS 2 TO 6)

Most patients do not require home or outpatient physical therapy during phase II. Although patients are at home, they are expected to increase their tolerance for upright activities and walking. Patients at this phase experience overall lack of endurance and are unable to

tolerate the sitting involved in transportation to and from therapy. Some patients may require home therapy after leaving the hospital. Indications for home physical therapy are

- Patient leaves the hospital on a walker and had not been using a walker preoperatively.
- Patient goes home alone with partial or full-time home health aide and needs therapy to problem solve for functional activities and safety.

Occasionally, patients are candidates for outpatient therapy during weeks 2 to 6. Indications for outpatient therapy are

- Patient tolerates being awake and active for 2-hour blocks of time (getting dressed, leaving the house, traveling to therapy, participating in therapy, and returning home)

Postoperative Phase II (Weeks 2 to 6)

- Use logrolling for transfers
- Continue progression from walker to cane to no device
- Progress outdoor activity

GOALS

- Patient education
- Provide the most protective environment for the healing fusion
- Maximize function: patients are usually independent in all ADL by week 6
- Control postoperative pain
- Independence in home therapeutic exercise program
- Improve endurance and tolerance to daily activities

PRECAUTIONS

- Avoid all lumbar movements (absolutely no lumbar flexion, extension, sidebending, or rotation)
- Progress sitting tolerance to between 30 and 45 minutes
- May or may not be wearing a brace, depending on the surgeon's advice
- No lifting more than 5 pounds (a gallon of milk is 8 pounds)
- No prone positioning or quadruped
- No PREs, no use of ankle cuff weights or upper extremity weights

TREATMENT STRATEGIES

- Transfer training
- Gentle submaximal abdominal sets, abdominal sets with heel slide, abdominal sets with bent knee fallout, total body extension isometric, dorsiflexion for neural gliding
- Use of stationary bicycle, treadmill
- Pain modalities, activity modification to control pain, communication with MD regarding activity and pain medications
- Home therapeutic exercise program: as previous
- Emphasize patient compliance to home therapeutic exercise program and protective environment, body mechanics, use of assistive devices, such as reacher, elastic shoelaces, long-handled shoe horn

CRITERIA FOR ADVANCEMENT

- Pain well controlled
- Tolerating sitting for 45 minutes
- Progression to ambulation without device
- Increased independence in ADL

- Patient tolerates sitting for 30 minutes
- Patient does not have home health aide or functional issues that are better solved with therapy in the home setting

For patients who attend outpatient therapy, exercises may be progressed to include abdominal setting, abdominal setting with heel slide, abdominal setting with bent knee fallout (Figure 30-4), total body isometric, use of stationary bicycle, and use of treadmill. Pain management remains an issue, and patients are decreasing medications as tolerated. For those patients who are doing well, therapists must use caution so as not to progress them too quickly. Constant reminders about body mechanics and limitations may be necessary.

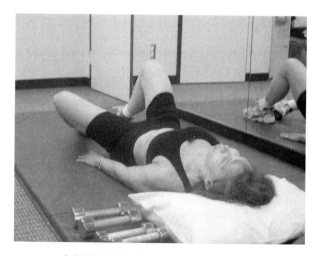

FIGURE **30-4** Supine bent knee fallout.

Troubleshooting

Whether the patient is receiving home or outpatient therapy, some of the possible pitfalls that may occur during phase II are

- Spasm at surgical site
- Persistent or new onset of radiculopathy

As mentioned in phase I, these complications are best brought to the attention of the surgeon and managed with modalities, soft tissue mobilization, and therapeutic exercise. A patient who scars heavily may experience worse postoperative pain than preoperative pain, if the scarring surrounds a nerve root. The symptomatology may actually worsen with healing rather than improve. A delicate balance of activity and neural gliding is indicated to minimize this phenomenon.

Questions often arise with regard to the use of modalities in this population (Table 30-1).

POSTOPERATIVE PHASE III (WEEKS 6 TO 14)

By weeks 6 through 8, patients generally have improved endurance, sitting tolerance, and decreased pain. At this point, most patients will be starting an outpatient program. Stabilization is the primary goal of phase III. Stabilization exercises should be first initiated in supine and progressed to prone and quadruped. When the patient is able to safely roll supine to prone, he or she can begin to exercise in prone with pillows placed at the hips to maintain a neutral spine. Quadruped activities can be initiated once the patient can transition safely to and from the floor (Figure 30-5). Transitioning into these positions is also functional for daily activities. In quadruped, the patient must demonstrate good technique in "rocking." Quadruped "rocking" is when the patient sits back on the feet with the upper extremities

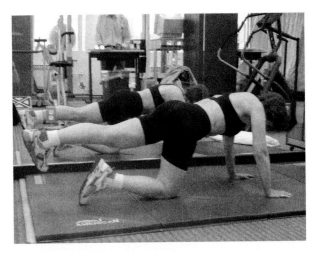

FIGURE **30-5** Quadruped stabilization: hip extension.

fully stretched forward and the spine is maintained in a neutral position. It is imperative that the patient be aware of flexing from the hips and not through the lumbar spine when performing this exercise.

Patients may be ready to progress to some resistive exercise using Thera-Band, with the spine supported in supine (Figure 30-6). Patients must demonstrate adequate lumbar control by stabilizing with abdominal muscles while performing all exercises.

During phase III, as quadriceps strength improves, it is important to continue to progress body mechanics training. Toward the latter end of phase III, if the patient has good quadriceps strength, coordination, and balance, a lunge and/or a squat can be introduced into the program. It is crucial that the patient maintain an

TABLE **30-1** The Use of Modalities in Patients with Lumbar Fusion and Instrumentation		
	NOT CONTRAINDICATED	CONTRAINDICATED
Pulsed Ultrasound	√	
Continuous Ultrasound		√
Electric Stimulation	√	
Heat	√	
Cryotherapy	√	
Traction		√

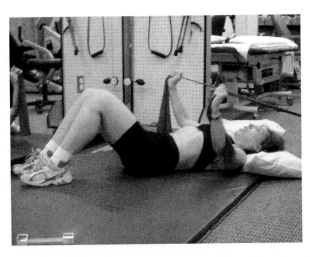

FIGURE **30-6** Supine stabilization with Thera-Band resistance.

Postoperative Phase III (Weeks 6 to 14)

- Use logrolling for transfers
- Continue progression from cane to no device
- Progress outdoor activity
- Patients getting stronger overall, progressing lumbar stabilization, improving endurance, striving toward return to work if they haven't already

GOALS

- Patient education
- Provide the most protective environment
- Maximize function: patients may return to work during this phase, depending on their occupation. Counseling and problem solving with the PT for return to work is a key component of this phase. Return part-time is ideal, if possible
- Control postoperative pain, decreasing medications, especially if returning to work
- Independence in home therapeutic exercise program
- Improve endurance and tolerance to daily activities

PRECAUTIONS

- Avoid all lumbar movements (absolutely no lumbar flexion, extension, sidebending, or rotation)
- Progress sitting tolerance to that which is necessary to perform their work
- May or may not be wearing a brace, depending on the surgeon's advice
- No lifting more than 5 pounds (a gallon of milk is 8 pounds)
- No PREs, no use of ankle cuff weights or upper extremity weights

TREATMENT STRATEGIES

- Progressive lumbar stabilization: Gentle submaximal abdominal sets, abdominal sets with heel slide, abdominal sets with bent knee fallout, total body extension isometric
- Prone on pillows protecting the neutral lumbar spine may be initiated
- Quadruped may be initiated
- Upright and loaded resistive exercises in a spine safe neutral position may be initiated if patient demonstrates good trunk control
- Use of stationary bicycle, treadmill
- Pain modalities, activity modification to control pain, communication with MD regarding activity and pain medications
- Hamstring stretching may be initiated in supine with a stretching strap
- Home therapeutic exercise program: as previous
- Emphasize patient compliance to home therapeutic exercise program and protective environment, body mechanics, use of assistive devices, such as reacher, elastic shoelaces, long-handled shoe horn

CRITERIA FOR ADVANCEMENT

- Pain well controlled
- Tolerating sitting for 45 minutes
- Return to work if indicated
- Ability to tolerate exercise in multiple positions: prone, quadruped, supine, upright
- Ability to perform resistive exercises with adequate abdominal control

erect and straight spine (Figure 30-7). Patients may also practice lifting and lowering light objects (less than 5 pounds) while demonstrating good body mechanics (Figure 30-8).

Conditioning continues during phase III, with the goal of reaching 30 minutes of continuous endurance activity, such as stationary cycling or walking on a tread-mill. Most patients do not have proper trunk control to use an elliptical machine at this point in time. Hamstring stretching is also initiated during phase III. It should not be incorporated into the program earlier because of the risk of pulling the pelvis into flexion while performing the stretch. Patients must be instructed to stabilize the abdominal region and focus

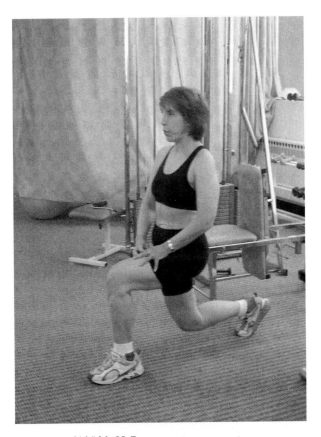

FIGURE **30-7** Lunge with erect spine.

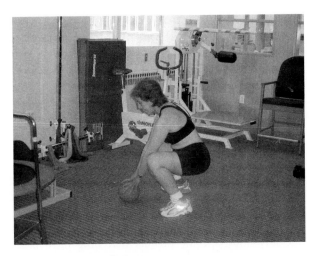

FIGURE **30-8** Lifting/Squat mechanics.

the stretch on the hamstrings only. No stretch should be felt in the lumbar spine region. If a patient has radicular symptoms, a careful assessment, including testing for the presence of neural adhesions, must be made before initiating hamstring stretching.

Troubleshooting

Some patients may not be able to position themselves in prone or quadruped for reasons unrelated to the lumbar fusion. For these patients, alternative methods of strengthening the hip and lumbar spine extensors should be used. For example, using Thera-Band in the upright position for both scapular retraction and hip extension will strengthen the extensors.

Quadruped rocking helps improve hip range of motion (ROM). Adequate hip ROM is crucial for the maintenance of correct body mechanics and limits the overuse of the lumbar spine when bending, lifting, and performing ADL. For those patients with concomitant hip pathology, the ROM required to maintain good body mechanics may not be a realistic goal and other adaptations may need to be made. For example, placing the foot on a stool and bending forward from the hips may be a reasonable alternative for tying shoelaces for those patients who do not have adequate hip flexion and external rotation.

POSTOPERATIVE PHASE IV (WEEKS 14 TO 22)

During weeks 14 to 22, patients may progress to more resistive type exercises with the spine in a loaded position, provided that they are still able to keep the spine controlled in a neutral position. Thera-Band is the safest and most effective means to add resistance to strengthening during this phase. For example, Thera-Band can be added to quadruped exercises, upright upper extremity shoulder flexion, and upright proprioceptive neuromuscular facilitation (PNF) patterns. Eventually, these exercises can be performed in single-leg stance as a progression (Figures 30-9 and 30-10). Light free weights may be used to progress function for ADL, but limits to the weights need to be specified by the surgeon. Communication with the surgeon is essential.

Regardless of the type of resistance used, the therapist must instill in the patient a sense of awareness in maintaining a neutral spine during any resistance or lifting activities.

Troubleshooting

Many patients never reach phase IV after lumbar fusion. The ability to reach this phase is dependent upon the patient's previous abilities and individual goals. For example, a patient who undergoes decompression and spinal fusion at L4–L5 because of spinal stenosis and who preoperatively walked fewer than two blocks, is unlikely to progress to a level where the control needed to perform loaded, upright, resistive exercises is achieved. However, another patient whose goals are to clean the house, lift grandchildren, and perform yard work will need to tolerate upright resistive exercises.

Postoperative Phase IV (Weeks 14 to 22)

- Use logrolling for transfers
- Continue progression from cane to no device if still using a cane
- Progress outdoor activity
- Patients getting stronger overall, progressing lumbar stabilization; most have resumed normal daily activities and will need reminders about lifting precautions
- Communicate with surgeon regarding progression and weight limits

GOALS

- Patient education
- Provide a spine-safe environment
- Maximize function: patients may return to limited gym if they demonstrate good understanding of spine-safe activity
- Independence in home therapeutic exercise program
- Improve endurance and tolerance to daily activities

PRECAUTIONS

- Avoid all lumbar movements (absolutely no lumbar flexion, extension, sidebending, or rotation)
- Progress sitting tolerance to that which is necessary to perform their work
- Wean from brace with surgeon's permission if patient is still wearing one
- Increased lifting depending on surgeon
- Light upper extremity PREs with short lever arms (biceps curls) to improve daily function, no use of ankle cuff weights

TREATMENT STRATEGIES

- Progressive lumbar stabilization: advance lower abdominal stabilization using lower extremities as longer lever arms (no cuff weights)
- Prone on pillows protecting the neutral lumbar spine
- Quadruped using resistive bands
- Use of stationary bicycle, treadmill
- Pain modalities, activity modification to control pain, communication with MD regarding activity and pain medications
- Hamstring stretching may be initiated in supine with a stretching strap
- Home therapeutic exercise program: as previous
- Set discharge goals

CRITERIA FOR ADVANCEMENT

- Pain well controlled
- Tolerating sitting for 45 minutes
- Ability to perform resisted, loaded upright exercise with good trunk control

Again, careful goal-setting at the outset and ongoing communication with the surgeon will result in the best outcome for a given patient.

POSTOPERATIVE PHASE V: RETURN TO SPORT

There is very little published information about the return to sport after spinal fusion and, therefore, much of what you will read here is anecdotal. Most surgeons recommend that patients wait at least 3 to 4 months after surgery until returning to golf and do not usually advise return to contact sports at all.[9] Most patients are already into phase V before their return to sport.

A careful evaluation should be performed to determine any sport-specific deficits that may have been overlooked in the initial evaluation. For return to sport, active range of motion (AROM) of the mobile segments needs to be assessed to determine whether there is excessive mobility at any segment and how the particular sport may impact the spine. For example, if all motion appears to come from the level adjacent to the fusion in a patient who is returning to tennis or golf, it may be beneficial to promote movement throughout several segments so that forces with each swing are more evenly distributed. For patients who are returning

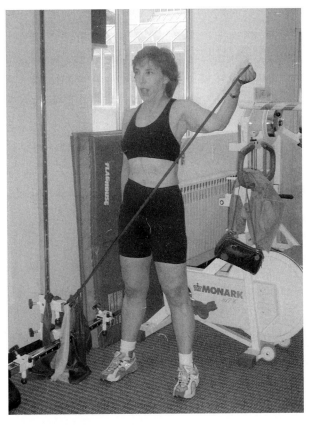

FIGURE **30-9** Standing stabilization: PNF D2 pattern with Thera-Band.

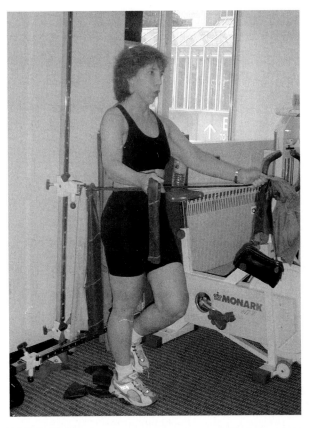

FIGURE **30-10** Standing stabilization: shoulder flexion with Thera-Band in single limb stance.

Postoperative Phase V: Return to Sport

- Use logrolling for transfers
- Patients getting stronger overall, progressing lumbar stabilization; most have resumed normal daily activities and will need reminders about lifting precautions
- Communicate with surgeon regarding gradual return to sport and progression

GOALS

- Patient education: form may need to be modified (e.g., golf swing)
- Gradual return to sport
- Independence in home therapeutic exercise program
- Minimize excessive forces at the segment adjacent to the fusion

PRECAUTIONS

- Assess AROM of nonoperated spinal segments and add gentle ROM exercises as necessary
- Surgeon may suggest wearing brace as a reminder for certain sports
- Increased lifting according to surgeon's recommendations
- Light upper extremity PREs with short lever arms (biceps curls) to improve daily function, no use of ankle cuff weights

TREATMENT STRATEGIES

- Use of equipment and resistance to simulate sport
- Upright and loaded resistive exercises in a spine safe neutral position with spinal motion, including rotation, are initiated if patient demonstrates good trunk control
- Refine discharge goals
- Maintenance of home exercise program

TABLE 30-2	Interval Return to Golf Program		
WEEK	**MONDAY**	**WEDNESDAY**	**FRIDAY**
1	10 Putts 10 chips 5-min rest 15 chips	15 putts 15 chips 5-min rest 25 chips	20 putts 20 chips 5-min rest 20 putts 20 chips 5-min rest 10 chips 10 short irons
2	20 chips 10 short irons 5-min rest 10 short irons 15 medium irons (5-iron off tee)	20 chips 15 short irons 10-min rest 15 short irons 15 chips Putting 15 medium irons	15 short irons 20 medium irons 10-min rest 20 short irons 15 chips
3	15 short irons 20 medium irons 10-min rest 15 short irons 15 medium irons 5 long irons 10-min rest 20 chips	15 short irons 15 medium irons 10 long irons 10-min rest 10 short irons 10 medium irons 5 long irons 5 wood	15 short irons 15 medium irons 10 long irons 10-min rest 10 short irons 10 medium irons 10 long irons 10 wood
4	15 short irons 15 medium irons 10 long irons 10 drives 15-min rest Repeat	Play 9 holes	Play 9 holes
5	Play 9 holes	Play 9 holes	Play 18 holes

Chips = pitching wedge; short irons = wedge, 9-iron, 8-iron; medium irons = 7-iron, 6-iron, 5-iron; long irons = 4-iron, 3-iron, 2-iron; woods = 3-wood, 5-wood; drives = driver (Borrowed from Reinold M, Wilk K, Reed J, Crenshaw K, Andres J. Interval sport program: guidelines for baseball, tennis and golf. JOSPT 2002; June: 32(6) 293–298).
These time frames vary greatly depending on the individual.

to skiing, it is important to have good motion throughout all segments so as to absorb the impact of falls more evenly throughout the spine.

Rehabilitation should be sport-specific and graduated to allow the patient to return to the sport in several increments. Constant communication with the surgeon as activities are increased is essential. With each increase there may be a slight setback. Patients are to be reminded to be aware of their symptoms and report them to their physical therapist so as not to create a chronic problem. Ice may need to be used as activity increases. Patients are ready to progress activity when they are consistently tolerating their current level of activity without exacerbation of symptoms. The interval return to golf program, described by Reinold et al.[10] is outlined in Table 30-2.

In summary, lumbar spinal fusion can lead to excellent outcomes for properly selected patients. Physical therapists play a key role in progressing patients along a comprehensive rehabilitation program. To achieve optimal outcomes, ongoing communication with the surgeon is essential. Biological healing dictates necessary precautions regarding spinal movement. Further research is necessary to study the effects of physical activity on the developing fusion.

REFERENCES

1. Boden, S.D. *Overview of the Biology of Lumbar Spine Fusion and Principles for Selecting a Bone Graft Substitute.* Spine 2002; 27(Suppl 16S):S26–S31.
2. Parker, L.M., Murrell, S., Boden, S., Horton, W. *The Outcome of Posterolateral Fusion in Highly Selected Patients with Discogenic Low Back Pain.* Spine 1996;21(16):1909–1916.
3. Luo, X., Pietrobon, R., Sun, S.X., Liu, G.G., Hey, L. *Estimates and Patterns of Direct Health Care Expenditures Among Individuals with Back Pain in the United States.* Spine 2004;29(1): 79–86.

4. Bono, C.M., Lee, C. *Critical Analysis of Trends in Fusion for Degenerative Disc Disease Over the Past 20 Years: Influence of Technique on Fusion Rate and Clinical Outcome.* Spine 2004; 29(4):455–463.

5. Glassman, S., Anagonost, S.C., Parker, A., Burke, D., Johnson, J., Dimar, J. *The Effect of Cigarette Smoking and Smoking Cessation on Spinal Fusion.* Spine 15 October 2000;25(20):2608–2615.

6. Rohlmann, A., Graichen, F., Bergmann, G. *Journal of the American Physical Therapy of Association.* 2002;82(1):44–52.

7. Hu, S. *Internal Fixation in the Osteoporotic Spine.* Spine 1997; 22(24S):43S–48S.

8. Keppler, I., Steffee, A.D., Biscup, R.S. Posterior Lumbar Interbody Fusion with Variable Screw Placement and Isola Instrumentation. In Bridwell, K., DeWald, R. (Eds). *The Textbook of Spinal Surgery,* 2nd ed., Lippincott Raven, Philadelphia, 1997.

9. Wright, A., Ferree, B., Tromanhauser, S. *Spinal Fusion in the Athlete.* Clin Sports Med 1993;12(3):599–603.

V

SPORTS MEDICINE
REHABILITATION

JOHN T. CAVANAUGH, PT, MED, ATC

31

Hip Arthroscopy

THERESA CHIAIA, PT

MATTHEW RIVERA, PT, MPT, CSCS

Hip arthroscopy has gained increased popularity over the past decade; however, it has undergone slow development compared to arthroscopy of the knee and shoulder. Knee and shoulder arthroscopy has evolved from open techniques, whereas the hip has not benefited from such early procedures. The advent of hip arthroscopy has led to improved recognition of intra-articular pathologies, which facilitated improved soft tissue diagnostic imaging techniques. This, in turn, has led to advances in hip arthroscopy techniques as a treatment for intra-articular lesions, including repair or excision of a torn labrum, removal of loose bodies, or repair of chondral lesions. Injuries to the labrum are the most common source of hip pain identified at arthroscopy.[1,2] The primary causes of these injuries are the result of femoral acetabular impingement or capsular laxity/hypermobility.[1,3] Labral injury often results from repetitive motion in sports, such as golf, hockey, and soccer.[4] Although traumatic tears are significantly less common, they are most common in high level athletes who participate in sports, such as football and skiing.[5] The rehabilitation guidelines following hip arthroscopy for a torn labrum are presented here by the Hospital for Special Surgery (HSS).

SURGICAL OVERVIEW

The labrum is a fibrocartilaginous rim that runs circumferentially around the perimeter of the acetabulum to the base of the fovea and becomes attached to the transverse acetabular ligament posteriorly and anteriorly (Figure 31-1). The labrum has many functions.[6] It creates a seal enhancing joint lubrication, reinforces the acetabular rim contributing to joint stability, and plays a role in load distribution. The labrum is distinctively thinner in the anterior inferior portion and thicker posteriorly. The majority of labral tears occurs anteri-

orly.[7] The labrum is predominately avascular, except the outermost layer that limits intrinsic healing.[8] Free nerve endings and sensory organs have been identified within the labral tissue, which contributes to nociceptive and proprioceptive input.[9]

The goal of arthroscopic debridement of a torn labrum is to relieve the pain by removing the unstable flap that causes hip discomfort and addressing the underlying pathology (Figure 31-2). The surgeon seeks to remove only torn labral tissue, leaving as much healthy intact labrum as possible. If the underlying pathology is capsular laxity, thermal capsulorrhaphy and plication is indicated, whereas with femoral acetabular impingement, bony resection is recommended.

The architectural constraints of the hip joint, as well as the proximity of the neurovascular structures, make arthroscopy of the hip more challenging than the shoulder. Recent adaptations of flexible scopes and instruments designed for the hip have led to improved safety, visualization, and accessibility of this joint. Distraction of the femoral head from the acetabulum, using 25 to 50 pounds of traction force, is necessary to visualize the articular surfaces. Typically, a three-portal approach is used (Figure 31-3). The anterolateral portal is directly off the anterosuperior portion of the greater trochanter and penetrates the gluteus medius before entering the lateral capsule. The anterior portal penetrates the sartorius and the rectus femoris and then enters the capsule. It presents the greatest risk to the lateral femoral neurovascular bundle. The posterolateral portal is posterior to the tip of the greater trochanter, placing the sciatic nerve at

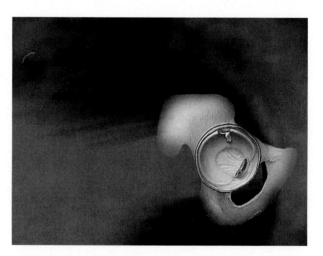

FIGURE **31-2** Drawing of an isolated anterosuperior labral tear. Note how the structure of the labrum provides depth to the acetabulum, with stability as its primary function. *(From Kelly, B.T.* Management of Non-arthritic Hip Pain. *Hospital for Special Surgery Sports Medicine Shoulder Service Core Conference, New York, 2004.)*

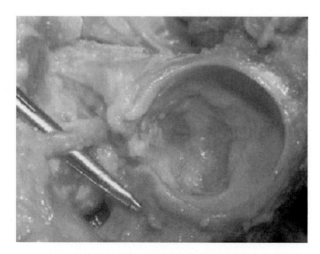

FIGURE **31-1** Photo of hip labrum.

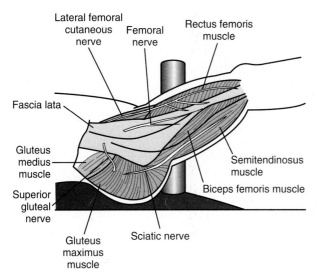

FIGURE 31-3 Schematic diagram of portal placement with anatomical reference. *(From Glick, J.M.* Hip Arthroscopy: The Lateral Approach. *Clin Sports Med 2001;4:737.)*

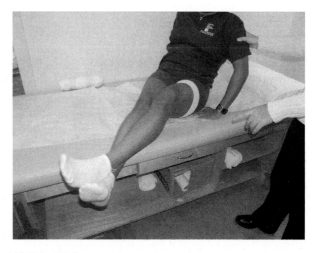

FIGURE 31-4 Transitional movements: training with the support from the opposite extremity.

risk of injury.[10] A flexible chisel is used to cut the torn labrum, then a motorized shaver is used to complete the debridement.[1] If the labrum is detached from the bone, a bioabsorbable suture anchor is placed on the rim of the acetabulum, and suture material is passed twice through the labrum. With femoral acetabular impingement, sequential removal of the osteophyte is performed, using the anterior scoping portal and distal lateral accessory portal. For capsular laxity, arthroscopic capsular plication of the iliofemoral ligament is performed following thermal modification of the capsule.[1]

REHABILITATION OVERVIEW

The rehabilitation program following hip arthroscopy for a torn labrum is initiated between 0 and 2 weeks postoperatively. The surgeon's preference, the surgical procedure, and the intraoperative findings will guide the postoperative course. The rate of progression through rehabilitation will depend on the underlying condition of the joint and the chronicity of the impairments. A period of restrictive weight-bearing with an assistive device followed by progressive weight-bearing as tolerated is recommended to allow for adequate healing, decreased inflammation, and pain control. Control of pain and inflammation through activity modification is necessary for progression of function, especially in the early phase of rehabilitation. Hip range of motion (ROM) will be progressed within the surgeon's designated parameters to allow for adequate healing and should be monitored to reduce joint compression forces and symptom provocation. The patient will follow a functionally based progression with criteria for discharge, largely depending on the goals of the patient.

The phases of rehabilitation represent a continuum rather than discrete, well-defined phases.

PREOPERATIVE REHABILITATION

Although preoperative rehabilitation is not essential for these patients, a visit before surgery is recommended for gait training, with the appropriate assistive device, and patient education in activity modification, cryotherapy, positioning, and transitional movements (Figure 31-4). Because hip arthroscopy is done as an outpatient procedure, medication, postoperative pain, and limited patient contact time in the postanesthesia care unit may affect the patient's ability to comprehend postoperative instructions. Various weight-bearing scenarios can be presented to better prepare the patient for postoperative mobility. Core stabilization, such as abdominal setting, can be introduced at this time.

POSTOPERATIVE PHASE I (DAY 1 TO WEEK 4)

This phase of rehabilitation begins on the day of surgery, and formal physical therapy should begin within the first 2 postoperative weeks. Key concepts introduced in this early rehabilitative phase act as a building block for further progression. Progression of weight-bearing, activity modification, positioning, mobility, and any precautions that are recommended by the physician are continually reinforced to minimize postoperative inflammation and thus pain. Weight-bearing, according to the surgeon's direction, is recommended to avoid overuse of the hip musculature in an attempt to suspend the limb during gait.[11] Following isolated debridement, the patient will be instructed in progressive weight-bearing with crutches to a cane, as tolerated, on level surfaces and stairs. The patient's symptoms will guide the progression. For procedures requiring bony resection, foot flat 20 pound weight-bearing will be recommended for 4 to 6 weeks and will be progressed following radiographic clearance. Partial weight-bearing for 10 to 14 days is recommended for patients who undergo a procedure involving the capsule. After the period of restrictive weight-bearing, progressive weight-bearing, as tolerated with an appropriate assistive device, will be encouraged. Progressive weight-bearing provides an environment of optimal loading to promote healing.[1] The patient will be weaned from the assistive device, as the gait is normalized and pain-free.

Following thermal modification and plication of the capsule, protection of the healing capsule is a major concern. ROM should be limited in the direction of external rotation and hyperextension. This may be achieved with the use of a night immobilization system and/or instruction in the use of pillows for positioning. Because gluteal setting and bridging for bed mobility drives the femoral head anteriorly, these exercises are not advocated, especially following procedures for anterior capsular laxity patients. The patient should be educated in deleterious effects of improper positioning, that is, allowing the operative extremity to fall into external rotation, crossing the leg with hip external rotation, or hip extension while standing in a posterior pelvic tilt.

Progression of flexion ROM following bony resection should be guided by the patient's symptoms. Flexion will be limited to 90 degrees, regardless of the procedure to avoid capsular impingement. In addition, internal rotation, flexion, and adduction may cause impingement of the soft tissues.

Straight leg raising (SLR) in supine should be avoided. Groin pain can occur with hip flexion strengthening as a result of violation of the anterior hip structures during placement of the anterior portal. Pinching in the groin occurs with active hip flexion because when the iliopsoas is weak and lengthened, it can contribute to capsular impingement.[12] Also, posterior glide of the femoral head is thought to be insufficient, exerting pressure on the anterior soft tissues of the joint.[12]

Early initiation of core control and education on correct and safe movement patterns will better prepare the patient for advanced therapeutic exercise in the weeks to come. Lower abdominal setting is initiated alone or in combination with upper extremity (UE) forward flexion and with all therapeutic exercises to begin to recruit the lower abdominals (Figure 31-5).

Balance and proprioception training, with double-limb support, are introduced with a 50% partial weight-bearing status and are performed on a proprioception board, a rocker board, or commercial balance system. Training begins with movements in the sagittal plane and progresses to the coronal plane.

Strengthening of the hip, knee, and ankle is introduced in this phase. Open chain activities such as knee extension, knee flexion in standing, and plantar flexion

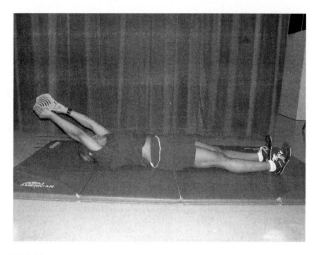

FIGURE **31-5** Initiation of core control, using upper extremity flexion.

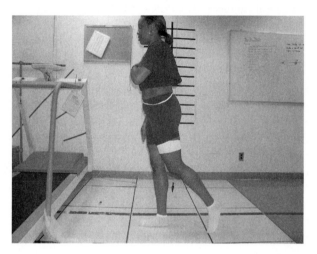

FIGURE **31-6** Strengthening: standing hip extension with core control.

with elastic bands may be initiated; however, the use of open chain hip machines should not be started until phase II. Hip strengthening can be initiated in standing (Figure 31-6). Hydrotherapy is used when there is adequate wound healing. It provides an environment of weight relief during gait training and buoyancy for hip strengthening exercises. The patient will perform hip flexion with knee flexion, hip extension to neutral with the knee flexed and also with the knee extended, abduction, and adduction. Greater buoyancy will be achieved as the extremity moves parallel to surface. Also, ipsilateral single-leg standing in water will increase joint proprioception without increasing joint reaction forces.

Troubleshooting

The patient should understand that this phase of rehabilitation sets the stage for progression of his or her rehabilitation. Emphasizing pain management and

Postoperative Phase I (Day 1 to Week 4)

GOALS

- Communication with surgeon to gain understanding of intraoperative findings of the joint and provide insight into underlying causative factors
- Provide patient with understanding of etiology
- Patient education
- Compliance with self-care, home management, activity modification
- Normalize gait with appropriate assistive device
- 0/10 pain at rest
- 0/10 pain with ambulation

PRECAUTIONS

- Capsular irritation
- Ambulation to fatigue
- Pivoting during ambulation
- Symptom provocation during ambulation, activities of daily living (ADL), therapeutic exercise
- External rotation, bridging, gluteal sets following capsular procedure
- Active hip flexion with long lever arm, such as SLR
- Weight-bearing as per surgeon's guidelines
- ROM as per surgeon's guidelines: capsular procedure

TREATMENT STRATEGIES

- Home exercise program, as instructed: abdominal setting, plantar flexion with elastic bands, gluteal setting, quadriceps setting, knee extension
- Patient education
  - Activity modification
  - Bed mobility
  - Positioning
- Gait training with appropriate assistive device on level surfaces and stairs
  - Following capsular procedure, instruct in a step to gait pattern
- Training in transitional movements with support from nonoperative leg
- Hydrotherapy when adequate wound healing for
  - Gait
  - Pain-free active-assisted range of motion (AAROM)
  - Single-leg standing
- Open chain strengthening for knee extension, flexion; gastrocnemius strengthening
- Initiate core control: heel slides, UE forward flexion, hip extension to neutral
- Balance training: double-limb support

CRITERIA FOR ADVANCEMENT

- Control of pain
- Normalized gait with appropriate assistive device

control of inflammation will allow for increased functional mobility. Postoperative pain may be better managed with an increased awareness of the body during functional activities. Symptom provocation as a result of soft tissue impingement should be avoided. For capsular procedures, protection of the healing capsule is a priority, whereas for bony procedures, protection of the healing bone is the priority.

POSTOPERATIVE PHASE II (WEEKS 5 TO 10)

Rehabilitation in the second phase emphasizes building strength, increasing ROM and flexibility, and normalizing gait without an assistive device. Continued patient education is critical to ensure adequate functional progression. The evaluation should include, but not be limited to, gait, static, and dynamic alignment, ROM, flexibility, strength, functional limitations, and core control. Core control is the ability of the lower abdominal muscles to stabilize the spine during increasingly demanding movements of the lower extremities (LEs). Expected ROM limitations include internal rotation/external rotation, flexion, and/or abduction/adduction at the hip with an empty or guarded end feel. ROM exercises may be initiated at this time following a capsular procedure, as per the surgeon's recommendations, but they must be progressed according to the patient's tolerance because of the potential for irritation of the soft tissues/joint capsule. Quadruped rocking backward

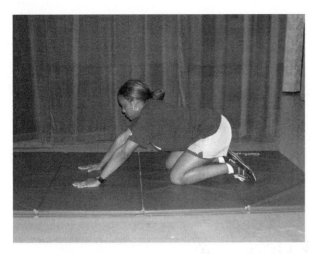

FIGURE **31-7** Hip flexion ROM, using quadruped position.

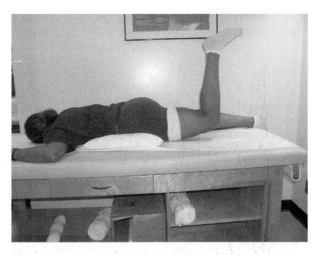

FIGURE **31-9** Gluteal strengthening: prone hip extension with knee flexion to neutral.

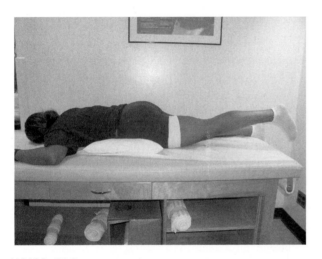

FIGURE **31-8** Strengthening: prone hip extension against gravity.

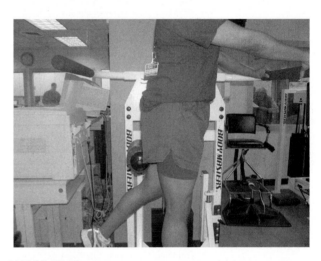

FIGURE **31-10** Hip strengthening machine with emphasis on neutral pelvis to strengthen hip extensors with knee extended and flexed.

(Figure 31-7) is used for hip flexion ROM because it stretches the hip extensors and promotes posterior and inferior glide of the femoral head.[12] Therapeutic exercises may include clam shell in side-lying and functional strengthening exercises, such as leg press, squats, and step progression. Activities such as gluteal setting, SLRs, and active hip abduction in side-lying have been shown to increase acetabular contact pressures and must be avoided if the articular surface is involved.[13] Hip strengthening exercises should progress from a gravity eliminated standing position for hip abduction, extension with knee extension (Figure 31-8), and with knee flexion to neutral to against gravity (Figure 31-9). The use of hip strengthening exercise machines is not advocated so as *not* to overload the joint and soft tissue structures. The only exception may be hip extension machines; however, the individual must demonstrate

the ability to stabilize the pelvis (Figure 31-10). Progression of exercise in an aquatic environment incorporates the effects of buoyancy (buoyancy assisting to buoyancy resisting), the length of the lever arm, and the use of floats.[14] In this phase, water can be used as a resistive medium with the phase I exercises by simply increasing the intensity and incorporating the aforementioned principles to a given exercise to further challenge the patient. Contralateral hip exercises, progressing from the sagittal to the coronal plane, can be performed to challenge balance.

Toward the latter part of this phase, muscle imbalances must be addressed. An atraumatic labral tear is a symptom of an underlying impairment. The mechanical issues that may have put the labrum at risk must be addressed. Individuals with anterior capsular laxity stand with a posterior pelvic tilt, with their hip in extension. They present with a lengthened and weakened iliopsoas, shortened hamstrings, and weak gluteals.[12] Instruction in neutral pelvic alignment, using visual and tactile feedback for postural reeducation, is incorporated (Figure 31-11). Exercises include hamstring stretching, gluteal strengthening, such as hip extension with knee flexion, quadruped leg lifts, and bridging.

Poor core control and dominance of the two-joint hip flexor musculature further irritates the hip. Stretching of the two-joint hip flexors can be introduced with active knee flexion with a stable pelvis in prone and/or standing and then progressed to passive stretching in a position where the individual can best stabilize the pelvis. Exercises for core control are progressed to include heel slides (Figure 31-12) and bent knee fallout, hip extension, and quadruped rocking backward and forward, along with all therapeutic exercises that will, ultimately, take the stress off the anterior hip. Core control is measured through visualization for overuse of the rectus abdominus, palpation of the pelvis for rocking, and when available, the Stabilizing Pressure Biofeedback Cuff (Chattanooga Group Inc., Hixson, TN). In this phase, balance is progressed from double- to single-limb support, using devices that promote an unstable surface, such as foam or a rocker board device.

Postoperative Phase II (Weeks 5 to 10)

GOALS

- Normalize gait without an assistive device
- 0/10 pain during ADL
- Ascend/descend 8-inch step with good control
- Core control during low demand exercises
- Adequate pelvic stability to meet demands of ADL
- ROM within functional limits
- Patient education and independence with home therapeutic exercise program, as instructed

PRECAUTIONS

- Premature discharge of assistive device. Continue to use assistive device until non-antalgic gait
- Symptom provocation
- Pain during ADL
- Pain during therapeutic exercise: abduction and flexion to tolerance
- Faulty movement patterns, posture
- Active hip flexion until pain subsides
- Capsular and soft tissue irritation

TREATMENT STRATEGIES

- Home exercise program, as instructed: evaluation-based
- Underwater treadmill
- Hydrotherapy: buoyancy assisting to buoyancy resisting exercises
- Hip strengthening progression
  - Multihip machine: hip extension with knee extension, knee flexion to neutral
- Functional strengthening: leg press, squats, step-ups/step-downs
- Hip ROM with a stable pelvis
  - Quadruped rocking backward
  - Bent knee fallout
  - Heel slides
- Core control progression
- Gluteal strengthening: clam shell, hip extension with knee flexion
- Postural reeducation to control at neutral pelvis
- Bicycle ergometry: progress from short crank as needed, to a standard cycle
- Proprioception and balance exercises: progress from double-limb to single-limb support
- Flexibility: evaluation-based

CRITERIA FOR ADVANCEMENT

- ROM within functional limits
- Ascend/descend 8-inch step with good pelvic control
- Good pelvic control during single-limb stance
- Normalized gait without an assistive device

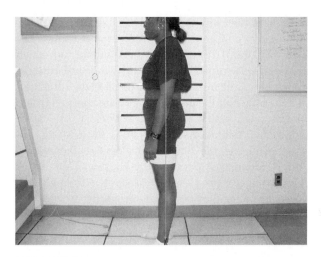

FIGURE **31-11** Postural training emphasizing neutral pelvis.

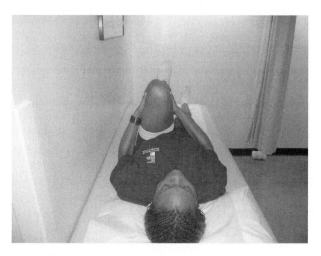

FIGURE **31-13** AAROM: hip flexion in supine.

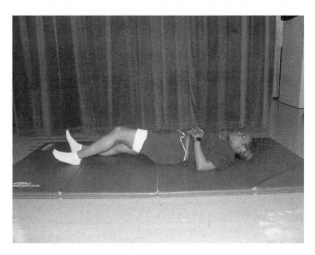

FIGURE **31-12** Heel slides.

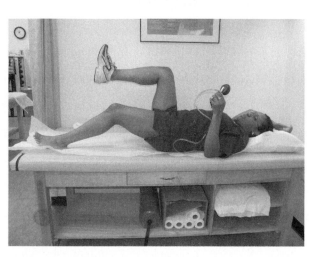

FIGURE **31-14** *A.* Core control: Sahrmann, Level II, using Stabilizing Pressure Biofeedback Cuff. *B.* Stabilizing Pressure Biofeedback Cuff.

Troubleshooting

Gains in functional mobility may be hindered if there is chronic irritation of the joint and surrounding soft tissues. Hip flexion exercises that are painful, for example, SLR, should be avoided in this phase and introduced when symptom free with a short lever arm. Educating the patient on proper activity modification continues to be the most effective tool. Patients who do not gradually increase their activities may continue to have impairments in ROM, strength, flexibility, and function, and the presence of pain or discomfort. The hip musculature becomes inhibited in the presence of pain and inflammation,[1] a response similar to that seen in the knee[15] and shoulder.[16]

POSTOPERATIVE PHASE III (WEEKS 11 TO 13)

The primary goals of this phase are to advance strengthening, optimize ROM (Figure 31-13), and improve muscular endurance for return to normal function. Other goals are for the individual to demonstrate moderate core control, such as Sahrmann level II (Figure 31-14), and to be able to perform quadruped extremity lifts (Figure 31-15). Diagonal patterns with elastic resistance can be progressed from a supported position in supine to weight transfer or weight shifting in standing during activities such as golf. Weight machines for hip strengthening can be safely incorporated in this phase. To improve endurance and optimize total aerobic output, the individual can cross-train on an elliptical trainer, bicycle, stair stepper, and/or cross-country ski machine. Balance training progresses, using a resistance cord, more dynamic movements, and unstable surfaces (Figure 31-16). Plyometric training can be introduced toward the latter part of this phase,

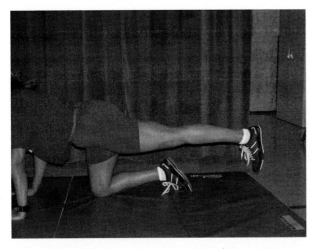

FIGURE **31-15** Core control with active hip extension.

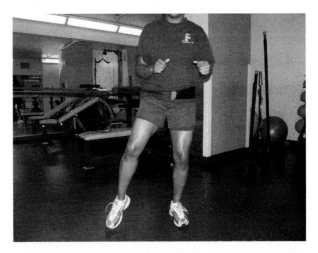

FIGURE **31-16** Resistance to challenge hip abductor strength, proprioception, and dynamic balance.

Postoperative Phase III (Weeks 11 to 13)

GOALS

- Independent home exercise program, as instructed
- Optimize ROM
- Core control: levels II–III/V, based on Sahrmann scale
- 5/5 LE strength
- Good, dynamic balance
- Pain-free ADL

PRECAUTIONS

- Symptom provocation
- Ignoring functional progression
- Sacrificing quality for quantity

TREATMENT STRATEGIES

- Home exercise program, as instructed: evaluation-based to incorporate treatment strategies
- Instruction of ROM at end range
- Demonstration of moderate level core exercises
  - Level II Sahrmann
  - Quadruped extremity lifts
  - Diagonal patterns
- Cross-training: elliptical trainer, bicycle, stair stepper, cross-country ski machine
- Initiate gym routine to include hip strengthening machines as tolerated
- Initiate plyometrics

CRITERIA FOR ADVANCEMENT

- Good, dynamic balance
- 5/5 LE strength
- Levels II–III/V core control (Sahrmann progression)
- ROM to meet demands of activities
- Pelvic control with single-limb activities is also necessary

as long as there is adequate ROM and strength to meet the demands of the activity. A solid foundation of strength, including pelvic control with single-limb activities, must precede the introduction of plyometrics because emphasis is on quality of movement and the absorption of forces. Plyometrics are introduced with

jumps onto a box and progress to jumps in place and standing jumps.

Troubleshooting

As ROM is optimized, and more challenging exercises are introduced, emphasis should continue to be on quality of movement vs quantity to avoid symptom provocation. Although symmetrical ROM may not be achieved, it is important to optimize motion to meet the level of the activity. Do not start plyometric activities that require ballistic change of direction or end ROM, unless those milestones are achieved.

POSTOPERATIVE PHASE IV (WEEKS 14 TO 16)

This phase of rehabilitation is for the patient who wants to return to higher level activities with greater demands, such as impact sports and sports requiring change of direction and/or acceleration and deceleration. Before beginning this phase, the patient must receive clearance from the orthopedic surgeon for participation in these higher level activities. Plyometric training will progress to multiple jumps on two legs to single-leg bounding, as tolerated, specific to sport pending optimal ROM and strength base. Jumping for distance, such as broad jumping, introduces shear forces to the joint, which will be tolerated in the fourth phase only. Running can be initiated when good pelvic control is demonstrated during single-limb dynamic exercises. Returning to sport involves critical evaluation before release and the following objective findings: optimal ROM, symmetry with cutting drills, adequate gluteal strength to maintain pelvic control, and greater than or equal to level III (Figure 31-17) achieved in Sahrmann's[12] abdominal progression. As with all athletes returning to sport, evaluation of endurance and quality of movement during specific activities is necessary to allow the patient to return with the best chance of success.

Troubleshooting

As the functional level continues to improve and the challenges become greater, it is important to maintain an adequate strength base. Attention must be paid to symptom provocation, even in this late stage. If the patient displays signs of breakdown in form during high level activities, factors such as total aerobic

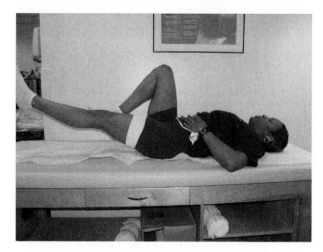

FIGURE **31-17** Core control: Sahrmann, Level III.

Postoperative Phase IV (Weeks 14 to 16)

GOALS

- Independent home exercise program, as instructed
- Minimize postexercise soreness

PRECAUTIONS

- Symptom provocation
- Ignoring functional progression
- Maintaining adequate strength base

TREATMENT STRATEGIES

- Home exercise program, as instructed: strength training and flexibility exercises
- Advance plyometric training
- Initiate running program: interval training
- Dynamic balance activities
- Cutting/agility skills
- Advance training of core
- Address muscle imbalances
- Endurance

CRITERIA FOR RETURN TO SPORT

- Gluteal strength to maintain pelvic control
- 0/10 pain with advanced activities
- Optimal ROM

endurance or strength and power must be addressed. The athlete has to continue with a strengthening and flexibility program to meet the demands of the activity.

References

1. Kelly, B., Draovitch, P., Enseki, K., Martin, R., Ernhardt, R., Philippon, M. *Hip Arthroscopy and the Management of Non-arthritic Hip Pain.* University of Pittsburgh Medical Center.
2. McCarthy, J., Barsoum, W., Puri, L., Lee, J., Murphy, S., Cooke, P. *The Role of Hip Arthroscopy in the Elite Athlete.* Clin Orthop Relat Res 2003;406:71–74.
3. Lavinge, M., Parvizi, J., Beck, M., Siebenrock, K., Ganz, R., Leunig, M. *Anterior Femoroacetabular Impingement Part I. Techniques of Joint Preserving Surgery.* Clin Orthop 2004;418:61–66.
4. Mason, J.B. *Acetabular Labral Tears in the Athlete.* Clin Sports Med 2001;4:779–790.
5. Byrd, T., Jones, K. *Hip Arthroscopy in Athletes.* Clin Sports Med 2001;4:749–778.
6. Konrath, G.A., Hamel, A.J., Olson, S.A., Bay, B., Sharkey, N.A. *The Role of the Acetabular Labrum and the Transverse Acetabular Ligament in Load Transmission in the Hip.* J Bone Joint Surg 1998;80A(12):1781–1788.
7. Baber, Y.F., Robinson, A.H., Villar, R.N. *Is Diagnostic Arthroscopy of the Hip Worthwhile? A Prospective Review of 328 Adults Investigated for Hip Pain.* J Bone Joint Surg 1999;81:600–603.
8. Kelly, B., Shapiro, G., Digiovanni, C.W., Buly, R., Potter, H., Hannafin, J.A. *Vascularity of the Hip Labrum: A Cadaveric Investigation.* Arthroscopy, 2005;21(1):3–11.
9. Kim, Y., Azusa, H. *The Nerve Endings of the Acetabular Labrum.* Clin Orthop 1995;310:60–68.
10. Byrd, T. *Hip Arthroscopy the Supine Position.* Clin Sports Med 2001;4:703–731.
11. Griffin, K. *Rehabilitation of the Hip.* Clin Sports Med 2001;20:837–850.
12. Sahrmann, S.A. *Diagnosis and Treatment of Movement Impairment Syndromes.* Mosby, St. Louis, 2002, pp. 144–147.
13. Strickland, E.M., Fares, M., Krebs, D.E., Riley, P.O., Givens-Heiss, D.L., Hodge, W.A., Mann, R.W. *In Vivo Acetabular Contact Pressures During Rehabilitation, Part I: Acute Phase.* Phys Ther 1992;10:691–699.
14. Principles of Treatment Part I—Theory. In Skinner, A.T., Thomson, A.M. (Eds). *Duffield's Exercise in Water,* 3rd ed. Bailliere Tindall, East Sussex, 1983, p. 11.
15. Spencer, J.D., Hayes, K.C., Alexander, I.J. *Knee Joint Effusion and Quadriceps Reflex Inhibition in Man.* Arch Phys Med Rehabil 1984;65:171–177.
16. Kibler, B.W. *The Role of the Scapula in Athletic Shoulder Function.* Am J Sports Med 1998;26:325–337.
17. Glick, J. *Hip Arthroscopy.* Clin Sports Med 2001;4:733–747.

32

Microfracture Procedure
of the Knee

JOHN T. CAVANAUGH, PT, MED, ATC

HEATHER WILLIAMS, DPT

Rehabilitation following articular cartilage repair continues to evolve with advances in the understanding of articular cartilage structure and function. Mechanisms of injury to articular cartilage can include direct trauma, indirect impact loading, or torsional loading at the knee joint. Injury to the articular cartilage in the knee decreases mobility and commonly causes pain with movement, eventually progressing to deformity and constant pain.[1] An awareness of acute lesions of the articular surfaces of the knee joint has increased in recent years because diagnostic application of magnetic resonance imaging (MRI) and arthroscopy techniques have improved. An estimated 385,000 procedures for repairing articular cartilage defects were performed in the United States in 1995.[2] Nonsurgical treatment may have satisfactory outcomes for some patients. However, as these defects may eventually progress to degenerative arthritis, a heightened interest among orthopedists to surgically repair these lesions has evolved. One such procedure is a microfracture chondroplasty introduced by Steadman et al.[3] The goal of this procedure is to enhance chondral resurfacing by providing an enriched environment for tissue regeneration, using the body's own healing capabilities. Indications for the microfracture procedure generally include a full-thickness articular cartilage lesion on either a weight-bearing surface (femur or tibia) or a contact lesion on either the patella or trochlear surfaces of the patellofemoral joint.[3-5] Other indications include unstable cartilage overlying subchondral bone and degenerative changes in knees that present with normal axial alignment. Contraindications for this procedure include axial misalignment, patient's potential for noncompliance, partial thickness defects, any systemic immune-mediated disease, disease-induced arthritis, or cartilage disease.[6]

SURGICAL OVERVIEW

Articular cartilage plays a crucial role in the function of the musculoskeletal system by permitting nearly frictionless motion to occur between the articular surfaces of synovial joints.[7] Its unique structure allows a joint to withstand high compressive and shear loads throughout a lifetime. Articular cartilage is avascular in nature and therefore has minimal potential to regenerate after injury.[8] Several studies[9-11] have demonstrated the medial femoral condyle to be the most common location for full-thickness focal chondral defects. These lesions are commonly found in the area that contacts the tibia between 30 and 70 degrees of flexion.[12]

"The microfracture procedure begins with an arthroscopic assessment of the articular cartilage defect (Figure 32-1). A debridement of the base of the defect is then performed to fully expose the subchondral bone with a standard arthroscopic shaver or curved curette. Any unstable cartilage is removed and a stable bound-

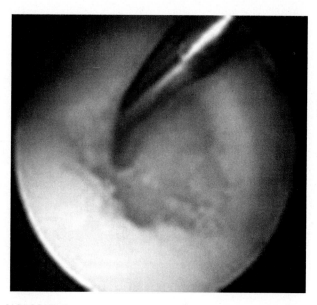

FIGURE 32-1 A 2 cm × 2 cm articular cartilage lesion of medial femoral condyle.

ary is defined. The walls of the perimeter of the defect should be perpendicular to the subchondral plate so that the marrow elements to follow will be optimally contained within the defect."[13]

Arthroscopic angled awls are then used to make multiple perforations, or microfractures, in the exposed subchondral plate. These awls produce essentially no thermal necrosis of the bone compared with hand-driven or motorized drills. The microfracture holes are approximately 3 to 4 mm apart and are typically made to a depth of 3 to 4 mm.[6,13] These perforations serve as an access channel for blood and mesenchymal stem cells from cancellous bone and the marrow cavity to migrate into the prepared defect (Figure 32-2). The eventual aim of the procedure is to establish a reparative granulation superclot that will proliferate and differentiate into a fibrous or fibrocartilage mosaic repair tissue.[6,14]

REHABILITATION OVERVIEW

Rehabilitation of the patient following any articular cartilage procedure of the knee presents a challenging task for the rehabilitation specialist. The rehabilitative process is typically several months following microfracture surgery. The rehabilitation specialist should instill the importance of compliance to the patient early in the rehabilitation period because adherence to weight-bearing restrictions and home therapeutic exercise assignments will have a direct influence on functional outcomes. The clinician should appreciate the healing response throughout the rehabilitative course by continually providing an optimal environment where the

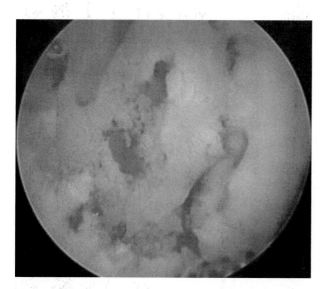

FIGURE **32-2** Microfracture holes are approximately 3 to 4 mm apart and made to a depth of 3 to 4 mm. The blood and mesenchymal stem cells will eventually form a reparative granulation superclot that will differentiate into fibrocartilage mosaic repair tissue.

articular cartilage lesion can heal. Using a working knowledge of the structure and function of articular cartilage, combined with an appreciation of the forces induced upon the articular surfaces of the knee during specific exercises and activities, will permit the clinician to protect and progress the patient toward an optimal outcome.

Communication with the surgeon throughout the rehabilitative process is important because the size and location of the lesion will have a direct effect on the rehabilitation program. A therapeutic exercise program addressing a medial femoral condyle lesion on a weight-bearing surface will differ from a non–weight-bearing femoral surface or a patellofemoral defect.

Postoperative "guidelines" should be individualized for each patient. The rehabilitative course should be advanced via a criteria-based approach. The ultimate goal of rehabilitation is to restore the range of motion (ROM), flexibility, strength, and proprioception needed for the functional demands of daily living and/or sports activity while protecting the healing cartilage and applying appropriate stresses.

POSTOPERATIVE PHASE I (WEEKS 0 TO 6)

The first phase following a microfracture procedure on the knee is the maximum protection phase. A healing environment is established by limiting weight-bearing to toe-touch (<5 pounds), with crutches for those patients with focal lesions of the femur or tibia. For patients having undergone the procedure for a patellofemoral defect, weight-bearing is initiated at 50% and then gradually progressed as tolerated. Regardless

of the location of the lesion, a postoperative brace is used. A femoral or tibial lesion is braced with the involved extremity in full extension. A patellofemoral lesion is braced, allowing for a 0- to 20-degree ROM allowance. This is to prevent placing excessive shear force on the maturing marrow clot and prevent flexion past the point where the median ridge of the patella engages the trochlear groove.[6]

Early mobilization is encouraged immediately following the microfracture procedure to achieve motion, diminish adhesion formation, and reduce pain. The goal for ROM is to achieve 0 to 120 degrees of knee motion by 6 weeks post-microfracture procedure. Research has supported early controlled motion following articular cartilage injury.[5,15–17] Suh et al.[17] demonstrated that joint motion following articular cartilage injury may facilitate healing, as long as shear forces are minimized. Excessive shear loads, therefore, should be avoided during ROM activities while the knee joint is under compression. The use of continuous passive motion (CPM) and unloaded active-assisted range of motion (AAROM) exercises are used as treatment strategies. CPM is applied immediately after surgery (Figure 32-3). ROM is begun in a 0- to 45-degree range and progressed as tolerated. Rodrigo et al.[5] concluded that the use of CPM for 6 hours daily for 8 weeks after microfracture following full-thickness cartilage defects in the knee resulted in enhanced gross healing of the lesion when evaluated by arthroscopic visualization compared with the same treatment without CPM. In conjunction to the use of CPM, the patient is instructed to perform AAROM exercises (Figure 32-4) several times per day. An early goal to be achieved during this first phase is the restoration of full passive knee extension because the development of a flexion contracture will result in gait abnormalities with resultant patellofemoral symptoms.[18–20] The patient is instructed to sit and/or lie with a towel under his or her heel, allowing gravity to apply

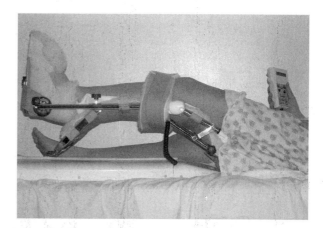

FIGURE **32-3** The CPM machine is applied immediately after surgery.

a low-load prolonged stretch into extension. This activity is performed several times per day and can be discontinued upon the achievement of full passive extension. Patellar mobilization should be performed by the rehabilitation specialist to assist in reestablishing normal patellar mobility. The patient should be instructed to incorporate this activity into his or her daily home exercise program.

Muscle strengthening during this phase is initiated by having the patient perform isometric quadriceps setting exercises. Knee position should be close to full extension because most articular cartilage lesions will not be engaged in this range. A rolled towel can be used for feedback and comfort, and a submaximal effort is encouraged. If a patient has difficulty eliciting a quadriceps contraction, a biofeedback unit or an electrical muscle stimulator can be used in conjunction with the quadriceps setting exercise to better facilitate quadriceps reeducation. Multiple angle quadriceps isometric exercises may be added later in this phase as ROM improves. The rehabilitation specialist should be careful to avoid angles that directly engage the articular cartilage lesion. This concept is especially important for patients having undergone a patellofemoral microfracture procedure. Multiple plane straight leg raises (SLRs) are begun during this phase and progressed via a progressive resistance approach for the return of normal proximal muscle strength. Proximal strengthening may also include the use of progressive resistive exercise equipment.

Stationary bicycling can be performed as range of knee motion approaches 85 degrees by using a short

---

Postoperative Phase I (Weeks 0 to 6)

GOALS

- Control postoperative pain/swelling
- ROM 0 to 120 degrees
- Prevent quadriceps inhibition
- Normalize proximal musculature muscle strength
- Independence in home therapeutic exercise program

PRECAUTIONS

- Maintain weight-bearing restrictions: postoperative brace locked at 0 degrees; 0 to 20 degrees for patellofemoral lesion
- Avoid neglect of ROM exercises

TREATMENT STRATEGIES

- CPM
- AAROM exercises (pain-free ROM)
- Towel extensions
- Patellar mobilization
- Toe-touch weight-bearing with brace locked at 0 degrees, with crutches
- Partial weight-bearing progressing to weight-bearing as tolerated; brace 0 to 20 degrees for patellofemoral lesion
- Quadriceps reeducation (quadriceps sets with electrical muscle stimulation [EMS] or electromyography [EMG])
- Multiple angle quadriceps isometrics (bilaterally to submaximal)
- Short crank ergometry to standard ergometry
- SLRs (all planes)
- Hip progressive resisted exercises
- Pool exercises
- Plantar flexion Thera-Band
- Lower extremity flexibility exercises
- Upper extremity cardiovascular exercises, as tolerated
- Cryotherapy
- Home therapeutic exercise program: evaluation-based
- Emphasize patient compliance to home therapeutic exercise program and weight-bearing restrictions

CRITERIA FOR ADVANCEMENT

- MD direction for progressive weight-bearing (week 6)
- ROM 0 to 120 degrees
- Proximal muscle strength 5/5
- SLR (supine) without extension lag

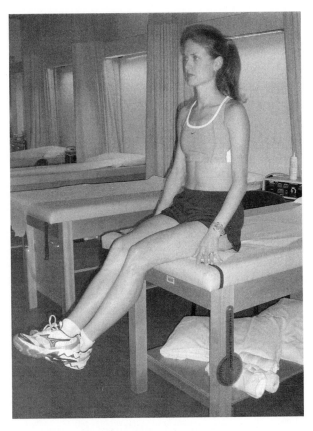

FIGURE **32-4** The patient performs active-assisted flexion and extension of the surgical knee, using the contralateral extremity for support.

crank (90 mm) ergometer.[21] As ROM progresses from 110 to 115 degrees, a standard ergometer can be used.

Deep water exercises, including use of a kick board and a flotation vest for deep water running, may be initiated at postoperative 2 to 3 weeks as quadriceps muscle control and ROM improvement are demonstrated.

Flexibility exercises for calf and hamstring musculature are incorporated into both formal and home therapeutic exercise sessions. Cryotherapy and electrical stimulation (TENS) may be used for pain control. Home therapeutic exercise programs are continually updated, and compliance is strongly encouraged.

Troubleshooting

This phase is the most challenging phase for the patient and rehabilitation specialist because strict compliance to weight-bearing limits is crucial to functional outcome. The clinician should make every attempt to make the rehabilitation process interesting by being aggressive where appropriate and adding new activities when warranted into the rehabilitation program. This will help alleviate some of the patient's psychological frustrations during this lengthy protection period.

POSTOPERATIVE PHASE II (WEEKS 6 TO 12)

This rehabilitation phase is dedicated to the restoration of normal ROM and gait as initiated. As quadriceps control is demonstrated (SLR without pain/lag), the postoperative brace is discontinued, and the patient is placed in a patella sleeve for activities of daily living (ADL). The brace serves more as a reminder to the patient than an instrument that provides structural support. For patients with patellofemoral lesions, the postoperative brace is opened gradually before it is discontinued. An unloader brace is prescribed to patients with an excessive varus or valgus misalignment (Figure 32-5).

Weight-bearing progression may vary because the size, location, and nature of the lesion dictate the aggressiveness of the treatment strategy. Typically at 6 weeks postoperative, fibrocartilage should have begun to fill in the articular defect, and a progressive weight-bearing period is inaugurated. A computerized forceplate system, NeuroCom Balance Master (NeuroCom International, Clackamas, OR), is used to assist the patient in the gradual loading of his or her involved extremity (Figure 32-6). During this activity, the patient gradually loads his or her involved limb to the prescribed percentage of body weight receiving visual feedback. This understanding is carried over into the progressive

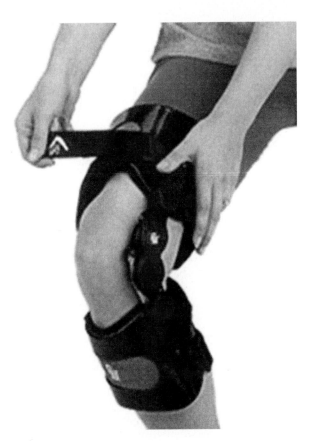

FIGURE **32-5** Generation II Unloader brace.

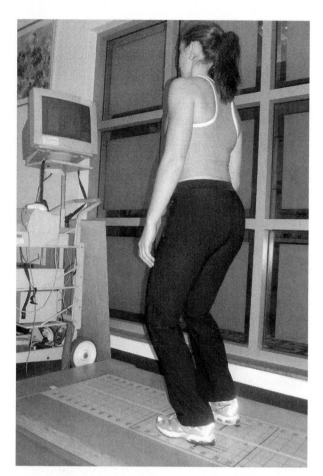

FIGURE **32-6** The patient receives feedback from the Balance Master System (NeuroCom International Inc., Clackamas, OR) for proper weight-bearing and unloading of involved extremity. Colored columns display the percentage of weight being displaced through each force plate on a computer monitor at eye level with the patient.

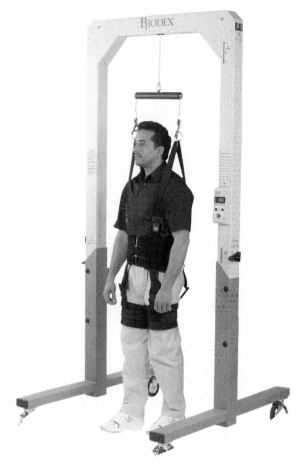

FIGURE **32-7** Biodex Deweighing System (Biodex Inc., Shirley, NY).

weight-bearing component of gait training during this phase. Treatment strategies using a deweighing system (Figure 32-7) and/or an underwater treadmill (Figure 32-8) are helpful as load is gradually introduced to the healing lesion. Walking in waist deep water results in a 40% to 50% reduction in weight-bearing, whereas walking in chest deep water results in a 60% to 75% reduction in weight-bearing.[22,23] Crutches are discontinued with demonstration of a normal gait pattern without deviations. Progression to a normal gait pattern typically takes 2 to 3 weeks to accomplish. AAROM exercises are progressed as tolerated with the goal of achieving full ROM by or before postoperative 12 weeks.

Strength development is crucial in promoting a safe progression and optimal functional outcome. A strong muscle-tendon unit may dissipate compressive force from the articular surface. The rehabilitation specialist should instruct the patient to avoid exercises that induce shear and compression forces in the range where the healing defect is articulating with the opposing joint surface. The understanding of specific compressive and shear forces induced on articular cartilage during common therapeutic strengthening exercises is limited. Research does, however, support using a combination of open kinetic chain (OKC) and closed kinetic chain (CKC) strengthening exercises in ranges that do not high load lesion site(s).[24-28] During OKC knee extension, an arc of motion from 60 to 90 degrees appears to provide the greatest amount of compressive loading at the knee joint, whereas the greatest amount of shear appears in the 40- to 0-degree range.[28] During CKC exercises, a 60- to 100-degree arc of motion appears to produce the greatest amount of shear and compression.[24,28] Palmitier et al.[26] in a biomechanical model of the lower extremity demonstrated reduced tibiofemoral shear force when a compressive force was simultaneously applied to the knee joint. Therefore, a therapeutic strengthening program is advanced during this phase, with an emphasis on CKC activities. A leg press is used inside a 60- to 0-degree arc of motion. Bilateral lower extremities are used in this activity, using a high repetition/low load

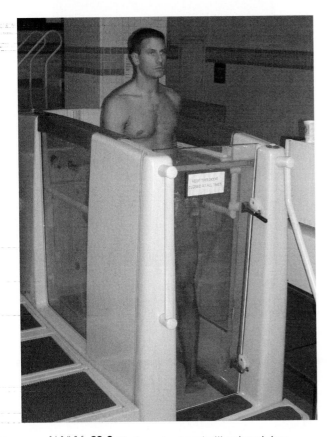

FIGURE **32-8** Underwater treadmill gait training.

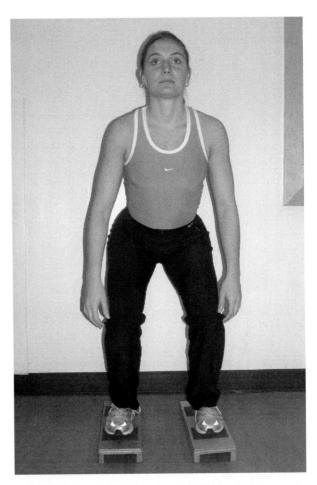

FIGURE **32-9** Mini-squat exercise performed on a medial wedge to protect area of chondral defect.

regime. ROM and weight are gradually increased. Mini-squats inside a 45- to 0-degree range are added, using a physio ball for proper technique. A progressive resistive exercise (PRE) approach is incorporated. Using a medial or lateral wedge under the involved extremity during the squatting exercise may protect the healing defect by creating a valgus or varus moment at the knee joint, thus unloading the involved compartment from compressive force (Figure 32-9). A graduated forward step-up program is introduced, beginning with a 4-inch step and progressing to an 8-inch step height (Figure 32-10).

Use of OKC knee extension exercise is used judiciously during this phase, avoiding engagement of the articular cartilage lesion. Escamilla et al.[24] have demonstrated that OKC extension exercises produce significantly greater patellofemoral forces than CKC activities at knee angles less than 57 degrees. For patients having undergone microfracture procedure for patellofemoral lesions, OKC knee extensions are withheld from the program until postoperative 3 months.

Proprioceptive and balance training is initiated as soon as the patient demonstrates the ability of 50% weight-bearing. A rocker board in sagittal and coronal planes, maintaining even weight distribution, is initiated advancing to dynamic stabilization activity on a

balance system. As strength and balance demonstrate improvement, the patient is advanced to unilateral balance/strengthening by performing contralateral elastic band exercises (Figure 32-11). Retrograde treadmill ambulation on a progressing incline is used to facilitate quadriceps strengthening.[29] Flexibility exercises throughout the involved lower extremity are continued. The addition of quadriceps stretching is added as knee ROM demonstrates improvement.

Troubleshooting

The patient is advised to avoid excessive durations of walking and standing until a sufficient strength base is attained. Progressing too rapidly in therapy and/or with normal functional ADL may result in increased effusion and pain. This is most likely related to muscular fatigue, leaving the articular surfaces unprotected against compressive forces. Therapeutic exercise programs will often need to be modified, based on daily assessment. These reevaluations are vital to ensure a consistent and safe progression of the patient's treatment plan.

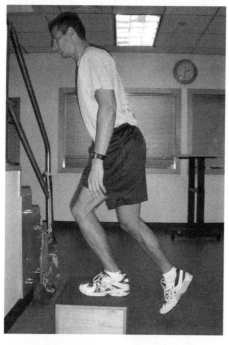

FIGURE 32-10 Forward step-up CKC exercise is gradually progressed to an 8-inch step.

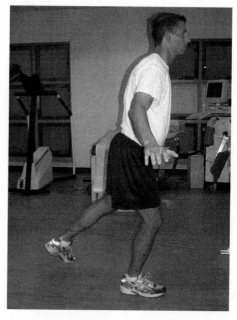

FIGURE 32-11 Contralateral hip strengthening exercise is performed using elastic bands while standing and balancing on involved limb.

Postoperative Phase II (Weeks 6 to 12)

GOALS

- ROM 0 to within normal limits (WNL)
- Normal patellar mobility
- Restore normal gait
- Ascend 8-inch stairs with good control without pain

PRECAUTIONS

- Avoid descending stairs reciprocally until adequate quadriceps control and lower extremity alignment is demonstrated
- Avoid pain with therapeutic exercise and functional activities

TREATMENT STRATEGIES

- Progressive weight-bearing/gait training with crutches
  - D/C crutches when gait is non-antalgic
- Postoperative brace discontinued as good quadriceps control (ability to SLR without lag or pain) is demonstrated
- Unloader brace/patella sleeve per MD preference
- Computerized forceplate (NeuroCom) for weight-bearing progression/patient education
- Underwater treadmill system (gait training) if incision benign
- Gait unloader device
- AAROM exercises
- Leg press (60- to 0-degree arc)
- Mini-squats/weight shifts
- Retrograde treadmill ambulation
- Proprioception/balance training
  - Proprioception board/contralateral Thera-Band exercises/balance systems
- Initiate forward step-up program
- StairMaster
- SLRs (progressive resistance)
- Lower extremity flexibility exercises
- OKC knee extension to 40 degrees (tibiofemoral lesions)—CKC exercises preferred
- Home therapeutic exercise program: evaluation-based

CRITERIA FOR ADVANCEMENT

- ROM 0 to WNL
- Normal gait pattern
- Demonstrate ability to ascend 8-inch step
- Normal patellar mobility

POSTOPERATIVE PHASE III (WEEKS 12 TO 18)

This phase of rehabilitation following knee microfracture surgery is dedicated toward the restoration of the strength required for normal functional activities. Treatment strategies used in phase II are advanced. In phase III, closed chain activities are now performed throughout a greater ROM (i.e., leg press and squatting 0 to 80 degrees). A step-down program is begun, starting with a 4-inch step, progressing to an 8-inch step as symptoms permit. Quality and control of lower extremity movement are monitored before advancement. OKC knee extension exercise is added in a range that does not engage the lesion site. Signs of pain and/or crepitus are closely monitored. A 90- to 40-degree arc of motion is used initially, progressing to full arc exercise. The rehabilitation specialist must be most cautious when implementing this activity with those patients who have undergone a microfracture procedure to the patellar/trochlear surfaces. Hamstring curls (PRE) are introduced, and proximal strengthening is progressed.

Balance/proprioception activities are progressed to include activities on multiplanar support surfaces (foam rollers, rocker boards, etc.) and perturbation training. If balance and lower extremity muscle strength demonstrate improvement, retrograde walking is progressed to retrograde running for short distances on a treadmill. A greater emphasis is now placed on lower extremity flexibility exercises in preparation for advanced functional activities to follow.

At postoperative 4 months a functional forward step-down test[30] and an isokinetic test are performed at test speeds of 180 and 300 degrees per second (Figure 32-12). These velocities are selected because they have shown to produce less compressive and shear forces than slower speeds.[31,32] The goal of 85% limb symmetry is hoped to be attained on both tests.

Upon successful achievement of set criteria, the patient is discharged from formal rehabilitation to a gym/home program or continues with the last phase of rehabilitation focused on preparation for sport activity.

Troubleshooting

Reinforcement of activity modifications needs to be instilled consistently in the patient. Developing the necessary lower extremity strength to descend stairs is a long and arduous task. The patient may therefore be limited in his or her ability to descend normal stairs (7 to 8 inches) until a sufficient strength base is demonstrated.

The rehabilitation specialist should monitor the volume of the patient's PRE program to allow for

Postoperative Phase III (Weeks 12 to 18)

GOALS
- Demonstrate ability to descend 8-inch stairs with good leg control without pain
- 85% Limb symmetry on isokinetic testing (tibiofemoral lesions) and forward step-down test
- Return to normal ADL
- Improve lower extremity flexibility

PRECAUTIONS
- Avoid pain with therapeutic exercise and functional activities
- Avoid running until adequate strength development and MD clearance

TREATMENT STRATEGIES
- Progress squat program
- Initiate step-down program
- Leg press (emphasizing eccentrics)
- OKC knee extensions 90 to 40 degrees (CKC exercises preferred)
- Advanced proprioception training (perturbations)
- Agility exercises (sport cord)
- Elliptical trainer
- Retrograde treadmill ambulation/running
- Hamstring curls/proximal strengthening
- Lower extremity stretching
- Forward step-down test (NeuroCom) at 4 months
- Isokinetic test at 4 months
- Home therapeutic exercise program: evaluation-based

CRITERIA FOR ADVANCEMENT
- Ability to descend 8-inch stairs with good leg control without pain
- 85% Limb symmetry on Isokinetic testing (tibiofemoral lesions) and forward step-down text

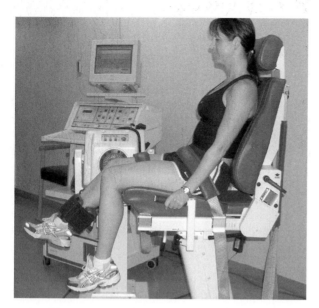

FIGURE **32-12** Isokinetic testing on Biodex System 3 (Biodex Inc., Shirley, NY).

recovery and prevent an overuse condition from developing.

POSTOPERATIVE PHASE IV: RETURN TO SPORT (WEEK 18 AND BEYOND)

This final phase is geared toward preparing the patient-athlete for return to sport. When strength (func- tional and isokinetic) in the operated extremity demon- strates less than a 15% deficit, a forward running program is initiated on a treadmill. Short distances with an emphasis on speed development is empha- sized vs longer slower distance running. Plyometric activities are then added, specific to the individual patient's desired sport. Advanced neuromuscular training activities are added to simulate game/practice conditions. A single-leg hop test and crossover hop tests are performed with the goal of achieving an 85% limb symmetry score.[33,34] The patient is observed for confi- dence and apprehension during testing and training. These observations, along with any other pertinent clinical findings, are presented to the referring ortho- pedic surgeon for the final determination of sports participation.

Troubleshooting

Monitoring volume of activity in both the formal reha- bilitation setting and daily activity is important to ensure a safe and swift return to sport participation. The rehabilitation specialist should design the therapeutic program to include days/sessions for strength develop- ment, power (plyometric) training, agility/neuromus- cular training, and rest. Criteria (ROM, flexibility, strength, power, and endurance) should be demon- strated before returning to sport participation.

Postoperative Phase IV: Return to Sport (Week 18 and Beyond)

GOALS
- Lack of apprehension with sport-specific movements
- Maximize strength and flexibility as to meet demands of individual's sport activity
- Hop test ≥85% limb symmetry

PRECAUTIONS
- Avoid pain with therapeutic exercise and functional activities
- Avoid sport activity until adequate strength development and MD clearance

TREATMENT STRATEGIES
- Continue to advance lower extremity strengthening, flexibility, and agility programs
- Forward running
- Plyometric program
- Brace for sport activity (MD preference)
- Monitor patient's activity level throughout course of rehabilitation
- Reassess patient's complaint's (i.e., pain/swelling daily—adjust program accordingly)
- Encourage compliance to home therapeutic exercise program
- Home therapeutic exercise program: evaluation-based

CRITERIA FOR DISCHARGE
- Hop test ≥85% limb symmetry
- Lack of apprehension with sport-specific movements
- Flexibility to accepted levels of sport performance
- Independence with gym program for maintenance and progression of therapeutic exercise program at discharge

REFERENCES

1. Buckwalter, J.A., Mankin, H.J. *Articular Cartilage II. Degeneration and Osteoarthritis, Repair, Regeneration and Transplantation.* J Bone Joint Surg 1997;79A(4):612–632.

2. Bobic, V. *Current Status of Articular Cartilage Repair.* E-BioMed, 2000.

3. Steadman, J.R., Rodkey, W.G., Singleton, S.B., Briggs, K.K. *Microfracture Technique for Full-thickness Chondral Defects: Technique and Clinical Results.* Oper Tech Orthop 1997;7:300–304.

4. Blevins, F.T., Steadman, J.R., Rodrigo, J.J., Silliman, J. *Treatment of Articular Cartilage Defects in Athletes: An Analysis of Functional Outcome and Lesion Appearance.* Orthopedics 1998;21:761–768.

5. Rodrigo, J.J., Steadman, J.R., Silliman, J.F., Fulstone, H.A. *Improvement of Full-thickness Chondral Defect Healing in the Human Knee after Debridement and Microfracture Using Continuous Passive Motion.* Am J Knee Surg 1994;7:109–116.

6. Steadman, J.R., Rodkey, W.G., Rodrigo, J.J. *Microfracture: Surgical Technique and Rehabilitation to Treat Chondral Defects.* Clin Orthop 2001;391(Suppl):S362–S369.

7. Buckwalter, J.A., Mankin, H.J. *Articular Cartilage. I. Tissue Design and Chondrocyte-matrix Interactions.* J Bone Joint Surg 1997;79A(4):600–611.

8. Mankin, H.J. *The Response of Articular Cartilage to Mechanical Injury.* J Bone Joint Surg 1982;64A:460–466.

9. Curl, W.W., Krome, J., Gordon, E.S., Rushing, J., Smith, B.P., Poehling, G.G. *Cartilage Injuries: A Review of 31,516 Knee Arthroscopies.* Arthroscopy 1997;13(4):456–460.

10. Hjelle, K., Austgulen, O., Muri, R. *Full-thickness Chondral Defects: A Prospective Study of 1000 Knee Arthroscopies.* Paper presented at Third International Cartilage Repair Society Symposium, April 27–29, 2000, Gothenburg, Sweden.

11. Terry, G.C., Flandry, F., van Manen, J.W., Norwood, L.A. *Isolated Chondral Fractures of the Knee.* Clin Orthop 1988;234:170–177.

12. Rosenberg, T.D., Paulos, L.E., Parker, R.D., Coward, D.B., Scott, S.M. *The Forty-five-degree Posteroanterior Flexion Weight-bearing Radiograph of the Knee.* J Bone Joint Surg 1988;70A(10):1479–1483.

13. Wright, J.M., Millett, P.J., Steadman, J.R. Osteochondral Injury: Acute Management. In Callahan, J., Rosenberg, A.G., Rubash, H.E., Simonian, P.T., Wickiewicz, T.L. (Eds). *The Adult Knee.* Lippincott, Williams & Wilkins, Philadelphia, 2003, pp. 885–893.

14. Sgaglione, N.A., Miniaci, A., Gillogly, S.D., Carter, T.R. *Update on Advanced Surgical Techniques in the Treatment of Traumatic Focal Articular Cartilage Lesions in the Knee.* Arthroscopy 2002;18(2 Suppl 1):9–32.

15. Buckwalter, J.A. *Effects of Early Motion on Healing Musculoskeletal Tissues.* Hand Clin 1996;129(10):13–24.

16. Salter, R.B., Simmonds, D.F., Malcolm, B.W., Rumble, E.J., MacMichael, D., Clements, N.D. *The Biological Effect of Continuous Passive Motion on the Healing of Full-thickness Defects in Articular Cartilage. An Experimental Investigation in the Rabbit.* J Bone Joint Surg Am 1980;62(8):1232–1251.

17. Suh, J., Aroen, A., Muzzonigro, T., DiSilvestro, M., Fu F.H. *Injury and Repair of Articular Cartilage: Related Scientific Issues.* Oper Tech Orthop 1997;7(4):270–278.

18. Benum, P. *Operative Mobilization of Stiff Knees after Surgical Treatment of Knee Injuries and Posttraumatic Conditions.* Acta Orthop Scand 1982;53:625–631.

19. Matsusue, Y., Yamamuro, T., Hama, H. *Arthroscopic Multiple Osteochondral Transplantation to the Chondral Defect in the Knee Associated with Anterior Cruciate Ligament Disruption.* Arthroscopy 1993;9(3):318–321.

20. Perry, J., Antonelli, D., Ford, W. *Analysis of Knee-joint Forces During Flexed-knee Stance.* J Bone Joint Surg 1975;57A:961–967.

21. Schwartz, R.E., Asnis, P.D., Cavanaugh, J.T., Asnis, S.E., Simmons, J.E., Lapinski, P.J. *Short Crank Cycle Ergometry.* J Orthop Sports Phys Ther 1991;13:95.

22. Bates, A., Hanson, N. The Principles and Properties of Water. In *Aquatic Exercise Therapy.* WB Saunders, Philadelphia, 1996, pp. 1–320.

23. Harrison, R.A., Hilman, M., Bulstrode, S. *Loading of the Lower Limb When Walking Partially Immersed: Implications for Clinical Practice.* Physiotherapy 1992;78:164.

24. Escamilla, R.F., Fleisig, G.S., Zheng, N., Barrentine, S.W., Wilk, K.E., Andrews, J.R. *Biomechanics of the Knee During Closed Kinetic Chain and Open Kinetic Chain Exercises.* Med Sci Sports Exerc 1998;30(4):556–569.

25. Lutz, G.E., Palmitier, R.A., An, K.N., Chao, E.Y. *Comparison of Tibiofemoral Joint Forces During Open Kinetic Chain and Closed Kinetic Chain Exercises.* J Bone Joint Surg 1993;75A:732–739.

26. Palmitier, R.A., An, K.N., Scott, S.G., Chao, E.Y. *Kinetic Chain Exercises in Knee Rehabilitation.* Sports Med 1991;11:402–413.

27. Steinkamp, L.A., Dillingham, M.F., Markel, M.D., Hill, J.A., Kaufman, K.R. *Biomechanical Considerations in Patellofemoral Joint Rehabilitation.* Am J Sports Med 1993;21:438–444.

28. Wilk, K.E., Escamilla, R.F., Fleisig, G.S., Barrentine, S.W., Andrews, J.R., Boyd, M.L. *A Comparison of Tibiofemoral Joint Forces and Electromyographic Activity During Open and Closed Kinetic Chain Exercises.* Am J Sports Med 1996;24(4):518–527.

29. Cipriani, D.J., Armstrong, C.W., Gaul, S. *Backward Walking at Three Levels of Treadmill Inclination: An Electromyographic and Kinematic Analysis.* J Orthop Sports Phys Ther 1995;22(3):95–102.

30. Cavanaugh, J.T., Stump, T.J. *Forward Step Down Test.* J Orthop Sports Phys Ther 2000;30(1):A–46.

31. Nisell, R., Ericson, M.O., Nemeth, G., Ekholm, J. *Tibiofemoral Joint Forces During Isokinetic Knee Extension.* Am J Sports Med 1989;17(1):49–54.

32. Kaufman, K.R., An, K.N., Litchy, W.J., Morrey, B.F., Chao, E.Y. *Dynamic Joint Forces During Knee Isokinetic Exercise.* Am J Sports Med 1991;19:305–316.

33. Daniel, D.M., Malcolm, L., Stone, M.L., Perth, H., Morgan, J., Richl, B. *Quantification of Knee Stability and Function.* Contemp Orthop 1982;5:83–91.

34. Barber, S.D., Noyes, F.R., Mangine, R.E., McCloskey, J.W., Hartman, W. *Quantitative Assessment of Functional Limitations in Normal and Anterior Cruciate Ligament Deficient Knees.* Clin Orthop 1990;255:204–214.

33

Patellar and Quadriceps Tendon Repair

GREG FIVES, PT, MS

PATELLAR TENDON RUPTURES

Patellar and quadriceps tendon ruptures are both rare events in the general population. The incidence of isolated patellar tendon ruptures is fairly low. Typically, this injury occurs in the male population younger than age 40.[1-4] Quadriceps tendon ruptures are also relatively infrequent, occurring more in the older population around the sixth or seventh decade of life.[5-7] Patellar tendon ruptures occurred about one-third as often as quadriceps tendon ruptures.[7,8] The mechanism of injury for both quadriceps and patellar tendon ruptures is usually a violent eccentric contraction of the quadriceps resisted by a fixed position of the leg and foot with the knee in hyperflexion.[2,4] More commonly, patellar tendon ruptures occur during sports or events that require significant extensor mechanism activation, such as basketball, volleyball, soccer, football, high jump, and gymnastics. Non–sports-related mechanisms of injury are usually the result of a trip-and-fall accident. A force of approximately 17.5 times body weight can cause a rupture of the patellar tendon.[9] Research has shown that the quadriceps tendon may be able to withstand up to 30 kg/mm of tensile force before rupturing.[6] Spontaneous patellar or quadriceps tendon rupture can occur in patients with systemic or inflammatory conditions, such as systemic lupus erythematosus, gouty arthritis, psoriatic arthritis, hyperparathyroidism, diabetes mellitus, chronic renal failure, and rheumatoid arthritis, which weakens the involved soft tissue structures.[7,10] Other risk factors include previous knee surgery, such as anterior cruciate ligament (ACL) reconstruction with patellar tendon autograft and total knee replacement.[10] Corticosteroid injections into the tendon and anabolic steroid use have also been implicated as predisposing factors to isolated patellar tendon rupture.[3,4,7] Progressive patellar tendonitis (jumper's knee) and end stage degenerative tendinopathy are also common mechanisms by which patellar tendon ruptures occur.

Some partial patellar or partial quadriceps tendon ruptures can be treated with immobilization in full extension for 4 to 6 weeks, but the treatment of choice for complete tendon rupture (quadriceps or patellar) is immediate operative repair. Immediate repair enhances postoperative outcomes for both patellar and quadriceps tendon rupture.[5,7] The deleterious effects associated with delayed diagnosis and therefore delayed repairs include knee flexion ROM deficits, quadriceps atrophy, and a decreased functional outcome for the patient.[7]

The Hospital for Special Surgery's (HSS) postoperative rehabilitation guidelines and approach to knee extensor mechanism repairs are presented here.

SURGICAL OVERVIEW

The extensor mechanism of the knee consists of the quadriceps, quadriceps tendon, patella, and patellar tendon. The quadriceps musculature is composed of the rectus femoris, vastus medialis, vastus lateralis, and vastus intermedius, which unite distally to form the common quadriceps tendon. Aponeurotic slips from both the vastus lateralis and vastus medialis form the lateral and medial retinaculi, respectively. The fibers of the quadriceps tendon traverse the anterior surface of the patella to form the patellar tendon. The patellar tendon is primarily composed of the distal central fibers of the rectus femoris, which terminate and insert into the tibial tubercle.

PATELLAR TENDON REPAIR

Most patellar tendon ruptures occur at the osteotendinous junction, where the tendon inserts at the distal pole of the patella.[11] A palpable defect is usually present below the distal pole of the patella, and the patella itself may be displaced as much as 5 cm proximally. Midsubstance patellar tendon tears are less common and can be more difficult to repair. Avulsion repairs are made by placing nonabsorbable sutures into the medial and lateral halves of the tendon. A bony trough is made across the distal patella and drill holes are made into the inferior and superior patella. The sutures are then passed through the inferior drill holes and are tied off at the superior pole of the patella (Figure 33-1, A). Midsubstance repairs can be repaired with interlocking sutures that tie the proximal and distal ends of the tendon together (Figure 33-1, B). Repairs may be reinforced or augmented, if needed, with either cerclage sutures, allograft, or surrounding knee musculature.

QUADRICEPS TENDON REPAIR

Ruptures of the quadriceps tendon may occur at the osteotendinous junction or through the midsubstance of the tendon.[6] Ruptures occur more frequently at the osteotendinous junction near the proximal pole of the patella. With this scenario, the superior pole of the patella is débrided of residual tendon, and the distal end of the rectus femoris and vastus intermedius are débrided of all chronic inflammatory tissue. A bony trough is made horizontally across the proximal pole of the patella. Drill holes are made near the base of the trough, and sutures are passed from the tendon through the drill holes to reattach the tendon (Figure 33-2). Acute midsubstance tears are made by direct repair. A midline incision is made and the proximal and distal ends are débrided. The two ends are then approximated and tied together with nonabsorbable sutures.

After quadriceps or patellar tendon repair, intraoperative ROM is assessed, as is patellar position (alta or baja) and tracking. Intraoperatively, 0-degree knee flexion should be obtained without significant stress to the repair.[12] Postoperatively, the patient's lower extremity is placed in a hinged rehabilitative brace locked at 0-

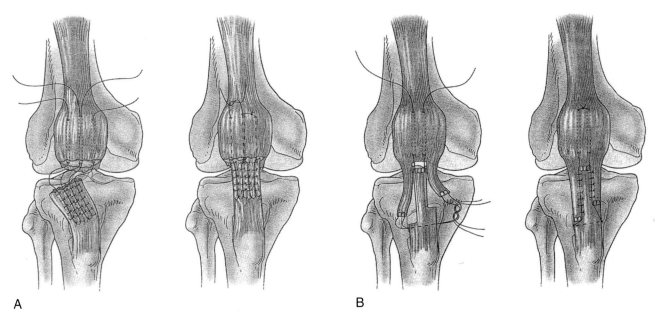

FIGURE 33-1 Patellar tendon repair. *A.* Avulsion repair. *B.* Midsubstance repair.

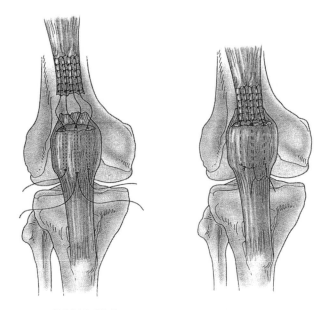

FIGURE 33-2 Acute quadriceps tendon repair.

degree extension. With an uncomplicated, acute extensor mechanism repair, patients are allowed to progressively weight-bear, as tolerated, with the brace locked in full extension.

REHABILITATION OVERVIEW

Rehabilitation after quadriceps or patellar tendon repair should be initiated soon after surgery. Communication with the referring surgeon is essential in the care of these patients. The clinician should discuss with the surgeon specific postoperative range of motion (ROM) limitations and the patient's weight-bearing status. Other

factors to be considered are the patient's age, bone and tissue quality, and the time from injury to surgery. Patient education on protection of the repair is vital and needs to be reinforced in the outpatient setting to ensure successful fixation of the repair. Also, increases in knee flexion ROM and quadriceps strengthening should be gradual during the early part of the rehabilitative process, to prevent failure of the repair.

The clinician and the surgeon need to inform the patient that the rehabilitative process is extensive following quadriceps or patellar tendon repair. The clinician should educate the patient to specific time frames and goals involved in the rehabilitative process. The patient should realize that he or she is an active participant in the rehabilitative process and not the passive recipient of care from the clinician. Also, the goals of the rehabilitation program should match those of the patient. Goals will be different for the older patient with a quadriceps tendon repair rupture as compared to the younger athlete with a patellar tendon repair. Progress is based on individualized treatment guidelines that are functional and criteria-based. Postoperative rehabilitation may also be modified if the cause of injury is secondary to any of the aforementioned underlying disease states. Postoperative precautions should be stressed to the patient.

POSTOPERATIVE PHASE I: MAXIMUM PROTECTION (WEEKS 0 TO 6)

Postoperatively, after quadriceps or patellar tendon repair the patient's lower extremity is placed in a hinged brace locked at 0-degree extension. Rehabilitation in this first phase should commence within the first week after surgery. The patient is provided with a knee continuous passive motion (CPM) machine (0 to 45 degrees, as tolerated) for home use. The CPM machine (home and clinic) can be helpful in the postoperative course, initiating early knee flexion ROM, controlling postoperative pain, the patient's need for pain medication, postoperative effusion, and, possibly, reducing the risk of arthrofibrosis.[17–19] During the first outpatient visit, patient education is strongly emphasized. Patients are instructed in the postoperative precaution of avoiding active knee extension. The patient is instructed to wear the brace, locked in extension, at all times (except when in the CPM or performing ROM exercises). The patient is taught how to don the brace with proper alignment and remove the brace as necessary for skin/incision inspection and proper application of cryotherapy modalities. Patients are also instructed in the important principles of activity modification, pain control, management of lower extremity edema, and knee joint effusion.

Gait training should focus on safe ambulation with crutches over level surfaces and stairs. Ambulation should be pain-free, and weight-bearing starts at 20% to 50% and is gradually progressed, as tolerated, with the brace locked at 0-degree extension. The use of a scale or computerized force plates can give the patient and rehabilitation specialist feedback as to initial and progressive weight-bearing levels.

One of the most common complications after quadriceps or patellar tendon repair is loss of ROM.[7,15] The deleterious effects of prolonged knee immobilization include poor cartilage nutrition, muscle atrophy, scar tissue formation, and weakened ligamentous tissue.[13,14] Traditionally, surgical protocols after extensor mechanism repair called for strict immobilization in a cast or brace for 6 weeks or more.[6,7,11,16] With improvements in surgical techniques, early mobilization under the guidance of the rehabilitation specialist has been advocated by surgeons after extensor mechanism repair.[2–4,10–12,16] Early controlled ROM can enhance reorganization, remodeling, and strengthening of collagen fibers within the repair.[12]

In general, 45-degree knee flexion should be the goal by the end of week 3, 90 degrees by 6 weeks postoperatively, and progressed as tolerated thereafter.[4,10,12] The patient and the rehabilitation specialist should know exact ROM limits/goals set by the surgeon and work toward achieving the desired ROM within specific time frames. Seated active-assisted range of motion (AAROM) knee flexion/passive extension with the assistance of the contralateral lower extremity is the first exercise taught to the patient to safely work on increasing ROM at the knee (Figure 33-3, A, B). The patient is strongly advised to avoid active extension at the knee so as to avoid tension on the repaired tissues. Short crank (90 mm) lower extremity ergometry without resistance may be initiated once 85 to 90 degrees of knee flexion has been achieved.

Quadriceps inhibition can occur secondary to increased effusion after knee trauma or surgical intervention. Spencer et al.[20] demonstrated this phenomenon by injecting saline into the joint space of the knee in 10 healthy patients. They found that the vastus medialis showed inhibition with just 20 to 30 mL of saline, and the rectus femoris/vastus lateralis muscle groups were inhibited with just 50 to 60 mL of saline. Another complication following extensor mechanism repair is extensive quadriceps weakness.[5,7,11,15,20] Siwek and Rao[7] found that 75% of their patients who underwent acute repair of the quadriceps tendon had quadriceps atrophy of 2 to 4 cm at follow-up greater than 2 years. Controlling knee effusion during all phases of rehabilitation, through the use of cryotherapy and activity modification, will enhance quadriceps function. Initial exercise instruction to improve quadriceps muscle strength includes teaching the patient submaximal quadriceps isometrics. Multiangle isometrics can be introduced as knee flexion ROM improves. Neuromuscular electrical stimulation (NMES) can also be used early on, as necessary, to improve the quadriceps contraction. When good quadriceps control is demonstrated, the patient is instructed in the supine straight leg raise (SLR) exercise, which is initially performed with the brace locked in extension.

The SLR is deferred if there is increased pain with the exercise. As quadriceps strength improves, the patient should be able to perform this exercise out of the rehabilitative brace. The ability to perform the SLR exercise without a lag is one of the main goals during this phase and a significant sign of quadriceps strength gain (Figure 33-4, A, B).

Bilateral closed chain proprioceptive exercises (in the rehabilitative brace) may be introduced in this phase once the patient achieves 50% weight-bearing. These exercises are designed to challenge the patient's sensorimotor system and help improve joint awareness. The use of computerized force plate technology can be helpful in providing visual cues to the patient during proprioceptive training. Uniplanar rocker boards are also appropriate training devices to be used during this phase (Figure 33-5).

The patient is instructed in active ankle dorsiflexion and plantar flexion, as well as ankle dorsiflexion with elastic bands to prevent calf atrophy and increase lower extremity circulation. SLR in prone and side-lying positions are performed to maintain and improve proximal hip strength.

When the incision is stable, scar mobilization is performed by the rehabilitation specialist and taught to the patient to maintain scar mobility and prevent scar formation and underlying skin adhesions.

Gentle patellar mobilizations are initiated in this phase to prevent limitation in patellofemoral joint

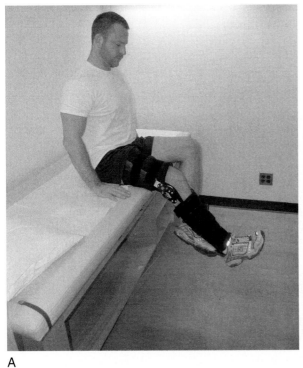

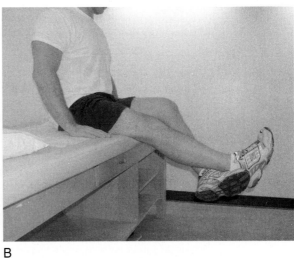

A   B

FIGURE **33-3** AAROM knee flexion in sitting. With this exercise the patient uses the contralateral lower extremity to assist in improving knee ROM. This exercise may be performed out of the rehabilitative brace if the patient respects ROM limits. *A.* The patient supports the operated leg with the contralateral lower extremity and slowly guides the knee into flexion. *B.* The patient *avoids* active knee extension by moving the operated leg with full assistance from the contralateral limb.

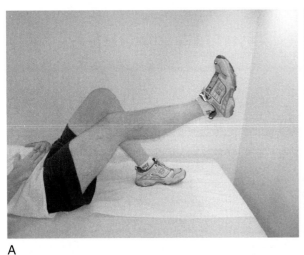

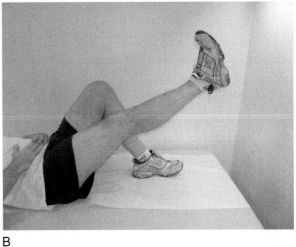

A   B

FIGURE **33-4** *A.* SLR with a lag. Inability to keep the knee in extension while performing the SLR exercise is a sign of inadequate lower extremity control and quadriceps strength. Excessive stress may be placed at the repair site if the exercise is performed in this manner. *B.* SLR without a lag.

mobility. Care should be taken to avoid stress at the repair site when performing glides in superior and inferior directions with patellar and quadriceps tendon repairs, respectively. Patellar mobilizations are also taught to the patient to perform at home.

Troubleshooting

Protection of the repair is very important. Making sure the patient is compliant with postoperative guidelines and precautions is key. Intraoperatively, the

Postoperative Phase I: Maximum Protection (Weeks 0 to 6)

GOALS

- Control postoperative pain and swelling
- Patient independent in understanding strict protection of repair
- Gradually increase knee flexion ROM (MD directed)
  Example: 0 to 45 degrees at 0 to 3 weeks, 45 to 90 degrees at 4 to 6 weeks
- Prevent quadriceps inhibition
- Independent in therapeutic home exercise program (HEP)

PRECAUTIONS

- Avoid active knee extension
- Maintain proper alignment of brace
- Avoid ambulation without brace locked at 0 degrees
- Avoid aggressive flexion; adhere to ROM limits set by MD

TREATMENT STRATEGIES

- Cryotherapy
- Patient education on brace use (locking and unlocking for ROM exercises only)
- Continuous passive motion machine (home and clinic)
- Seated active and active-assisted knee flexion exercises, passive extension
- Short crank ergometry if ROM >85 degrees
- Quadriceps reeducation (submaximal quadriceps setting with NMES or biofeedback)
- Multiangle quadriceps isometrics
- SLR (hip flexion) with brace locked at 0 degrees
- Scar mobilization
- Patellar mobilization
- Gait training—progressive weight-bearing as tolerated with crutches with brace locked in full extension, progress to WBAT with cane, brace locked in extension
- Proximal/distal strengthening, SLR other planes
- Upper body ergometry (UBE) for cardiovascular exercise as needed

CRITERIA FOR ADVANCEMENT

- ROM 0 to 90 degrees
- Good patellar mobility
- Ability to SLR without extensor lag
- Pain-free WBAT with cane, brace locked at 0-degree extension

surgeon evaluates knee flexion ROM and tension at the repair site, which will dictate postoperative ROM progression. Communication with the surgeon, via written prescription or direct contact, is essential with regard to flexion ROM progression in these patients. Long-term immobilization may still precede early ROM therapy with complex injuries, complicated repairs, delayed repairs, and unreliable patients.[10] Correct use of the postoperative rehabilitative brace needs to be stressed to the patient, and proper alignment of the hinge brace should be observed. The clinician and patient should look for inferior migration of the brace with ambulation (Figure 33-6) because a flexion moment may be created at the knee if the brace's axis of rotation is positioned inferiorly to the knee joint's center. Weight-bearing on a flexed knee will produce excessive tension and may sacrifice the repair.

Passive range of motion (PROM) and ROM exercises in the prone position are discouraged in this phase because of increased stresses imparted at the repair site (Figure 33-7).

Weight-bearing should be progressive, and consideration should be given to patients who have low pain thresholds and progress their weight-bearing too quickly. The quality of the SLR exercise is also emphasized to the patient. The clinician should be aware of signs of failure. These include the inability to perform an SLR without a lag and a palpable gap above or below the patella with quadriceps tendon or patellar tendon repairs, respectively. The rehabilitation specialist should also observe for other complications, such as infection, wound dehiscence, and increased calf tenderness/temperature, which may indicate a deep venous thrombosis (DVT).

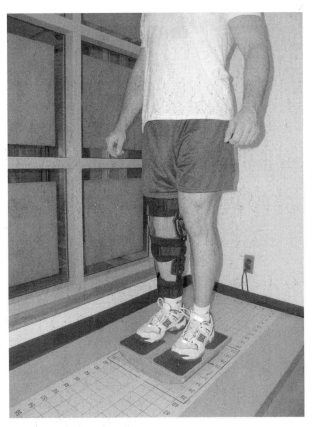

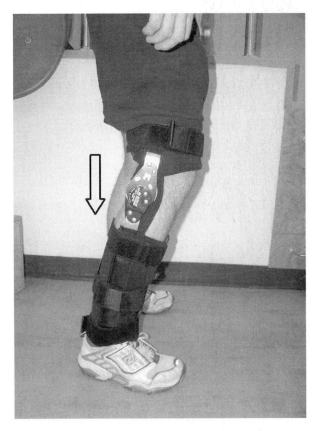

FIGURE **33-5** Proprioceptive exercises. Early bilateral proprioceptive exercise (in the rehabilitative brace) may be initiated once the patient is 50% weight-bearing. The NeuroCom Balance Master System (NeuroCom, Clackamas, OR) is useful in providing visual feedback to the patient during weight-bearing exercises and proprioceptive training. A rocker board can be used for proprioceptive training in the coronal planes.

FIGURE **33-6** Poor brace alignment. Weight-bearing on a flexed knee is contraindicated and may occur if the rehabilitative brace is allowed to migrate inferiorly.

POSTOPERATIVE PHASE II: MODERATE PROTECTIVE (WEEKS 6 TO 11)

The goals of this phase are to gradually improve and restore knee flexion ROM, improve quadriceps strength, and minimize pain and swelling. Gait and functional status will improve as these goals are attained. The patient and rehabilitation specialist should continually monitor knee edema and pain as weight-bearing, functional status, and activity levels improve. Cryotherapy and activity modification techniques help decrease pain and effusion and should be continued during this phase.

Additional exercises to improve knee flexion, which use gravity and the patient's body weight, include active-assisted supine wall slides, knee flexion stretch on a step, and seated knee flexion with the foot planted on the ground (Figure 33-8). These exercises can be added, as needed, as this phase progresses. Patellar mobilizations are continued to improve patellar mobility and tibiofemoral joint ROM and avoid abnormal tracking and increase contact stresses at the patellofemoral joint. Limited inferior glide of the patella may

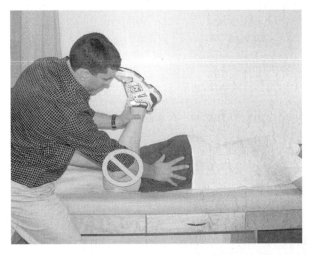

FIGURE **33-7** Avoid AAROM/PROM techniques in the prone position. Manual techniques or independent exercises to increase knee flexion in the prone position may be too aggressive and are avoided during phase I.

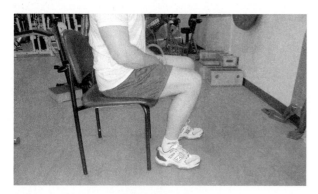

FIGURE **33-8** Seated AAROM knee flexion. During this exercise, the patient sits in a chair and bends the knee to a comfortable position, keeping the foot planted on the ground. The patient then slowly "scoots" forward on the chair, using the leverage of the upper body to assist in knee flexion ROM. The patient is informed not to aggressively perform these exercises and stop if pain is produced.

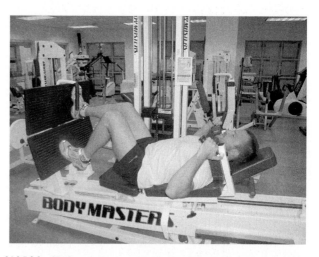

FIGURE **33-9** Eccentric leg press. The eccentric leg press (approximately 60% of the weight used with bilateral leg press exercise) is introduced as leg control improves. The patient pushes up with bilateral lower extremities and controls the descent with the affected lower extremity.

lead to difficulty in normalizing knee flexion ROM. Once the patient obtains 110 to 115 degrees of knee flexion, stationary cycling can be progressed from a short crank bike to a regular bike, with a standard crank length of 170 mm. The benefits of stationary cycling include joint motion that produces low tibiofemoral joint forces and good recruitment of the quadriceps musculature.[21,22]

Gradual progression of quadriceps strengthening activities is also a main goal of this phase. The SLR exercise is continued and performed without the brace, as long as there is no extensor lag present. Cuff weights can also be introduced to this exercise, once the patient demonstrates no difficulty with performing 3 sets of 10 repetitions. Quality of exercise must be emphasized to the patient when moving ahead in the progressive resistance exercise (PRE) program.

Gait is progressed as knee ROM and quadriceps strength improve. The dial-hinge brace can be set with a 60-degree flexion stop, and the patient can initially ambulate with axillary crutches to assist in leg control. The brace and crutches are discontinued once quadriceps control improves and a normal and symmetrical gait pattern is reestablished. Underwater treadmill systems are helpful in gait training the patient during this phase.

Closed chain exercises decrease shear force, stimulate proprioceptors, and enhance dynamic stabilization.[23] Closed kinetic chain (CKC) exercises are introduced with the patient performing the leg press machine with bilateral lower extremities. The patient should have at least 90 degrees of knee flexion ROM before performing the leg press exercise. The eccentric leg press exercise (Figure 33-9) is introduced as leg control improves and helps prepare the patient for progression to a functional step-down exercise during phase III or the latter part of phase II. As strength and ROM improve, the patient

is advanced through a functional forward step-up program with progressive step heights (4, 6, and 8 inches). A squatting program can be introduced by having the patient perform a wall slide exercise in safe and controlled arc of motion, monitoring for signs of crepitus and anterior knee pain. As lower extremity control improves, progression can be made to more dynamic ball squats.

Proprioceptive exercises are continued and progressed from bilateral lower extremity support on uniplanar rocker boards to unilateral support on multiplanar biomechanical ankle platform system (BAPS) boards or computerized balance systems. These exercises should be safely progressive and not exceed the physiological capacity of the postoperative knee. The rehabilitation specialist closely evaluates each activity for adequate lower extremity control.

Retro-ambulation is introduced with progressive speeds and inclines to enhance and facilitate lower extremity control, balance, agility, coordination, and quadriceps function.[24]

Exercises to promote strength and flexibility for proximal and distal muscle groups are incorporated and advanced during this phase. Standing calf, hamstring, and iliotibial band stretches are added to the patients HEP. Isotonic machines for the hip abductors/adductors/flexors/extensors and calf raises are appropriate to incorporate into the patient's gym program. Gentle quadriceps flexibility exercises are also added toward the latter part of this phase.

Troubleshooting

Care should be taken to monitor the volume of strengthening exercises by the patient and rehabilitation

Postoperative Phase II: Moderate Protective (Weeks 6 to 11)

GOALS

- Minimize pain and swelling
- Patient understanding of activity modification
- Restore knee flexion ROM to 125 degrees
- Normalize gait without assistive device
- Patient able to ascend 8-inch step

PRECAUTIONS

- Avoid aggressive strengthening
- Avoid excessive activity levels that increase knee effusion and pain
- Avoid aggressive flexion ROM exercises

TREATMENT STRATEGIES

- Cryotherapy
- Patient education on brace use (locking and unlocking, setting dial hinge)
- Gait training—brace unlocked with flexion stop at 60 degrees once the patient demonstrates good quadriceps control
- Discharge brace (good quadriceps control, communicate with MD)
- Pool ambulation or underwater treadmill system
- A/AAROM knee flexion exercises
- Continue patellar mobilization
- Progress to regular bike (standard crank length) as knee flexion approaches 110 to 115 degrees
- Leg press machine (bilateral); if ROM >90 degrees progress to eccentric and unilateral
- Initiate forward step-up program
- Initiate squat program—wall slide exercise within comfortable range
- Advance proprioceptive activities
- Retro-ambulation
- Progress PRE/flexibility program for proximal and distal muscle groups
- Initiate quadriceps flexibility exercises

CRITERIA FOR ADVANCEMENT

- Minimal to no joint effusion
- Knee flexion ROM to at least 125 degrees
- Normal patellar mobility
- Good LE control—*no* extensor lag present
- Able to perform 8-inch forward step-up
- Normal and symmetrical gait pattern

---

specialist. As the volume increases, the program should incorporate rest days to allow for strength gains. With ROM exercises the patient may find two or three of the exercises prescribed to be sufficient in achieving the goal of restoring knee flexion ROM. The rehabilitation specialist should observe that the patient does not experience pain with the addition of more aggressive ROM exercises.

The clinician should also observe patellar orientation. Patella baja/alta may be present after patellar/quadriceps tendon repair, respectively. Patellar joint mobilizations should be continued to normalize patellar mobility. Complaints of patellofemoral pain with exercise or daily activities should be monitored because it is a common entity encountered after extensor mechanism repair.[4,25]

Patients with a persistent knee extensor lag represent a challenging problem to the rehabilitation specialist. Postoperative knee extensor lag may be secondary to quadriceps weakness at end range knee extension, limited patellar mobility, preventing quadriceps excursion, pathological lengthening of the quadriceps secondary to overstretching, and inadequate fixation/mobilization of tissue with delayed repairs and failed repairs. Exercises, such as closed chain terminal knee extension with elastic bands and terminal knee extension on a bolster, may help improve terminal quadriceps strength (Figure 33-10, *A, B*) Because isometric exercise produces approximately a 20-degree overflow throughout the ROM,[26] multiangle isometrics, especially toward end range extension, may also be helpful in eliminating an extensor lag.

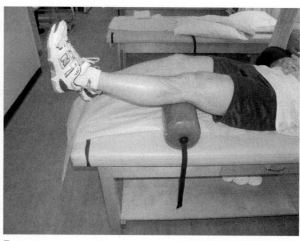

B

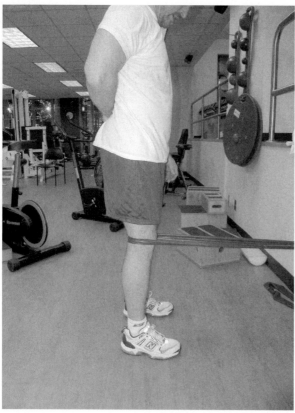

A

FIGURE **33-10** Exercises to help eliminate extensor lag. *A.* Terminal knee extension with Thera-Band. *B.* Terminal knee extension on a bolster.

POSTOPERATIVE PHASE III: EARLY FUNCTIONAL (WEEKS 11 TO 16)

This phase focuses on restoring knee flexion ROM, quadriceps flexibility, and muscle strength. Steady improvement in the patient's capacity to perform functional daily activity should be observed.

Full knee flexion ROM should be achieved during this phase. Manual techniques, such as soft tissue massage, myofascial release (MFR), and contract-relax techniques can be used by the rehabilitation specialist to assist in restoring knee flexion ROM limited by soft tissue tightness. Also during this phase the rehabilitation specialist should use muscle length testing to assess quadriceps flexibility. Measurements of prone knee flexion and the Thomas test are effective tools to implicate tightness of the quadriceps muscle group. Comparisons are made to the nonoperated lower extremity. Quadriceps flexibility exercises, with hold times of 20 to 30 seconds, are taught to the patient to help improve muscle length (Figure 33-11, *A, B*).

CKC strengthening exercises are advanced during this phase. Eccentric and bilateral leg press exercises are progressed to a unilateral leg press exercise. Squatting

exercises are advanced from ball squats to squatting with a sport cord to free squats. Advancements are made with respect to adequate lower extremity and trunk control.

Functional forward step-down exercises are introduced once the patient demonstrates improved strength and leg control (Figure 33-12). Heights are progressed from 4-inch to 6-inch to 8-inch steps.

Open kinetic chain (OKC) exercise, in the form of the leg extension machine, is introduced during this phase for isolated strengthening of the quadriceps muscle group. Full ROM should be achieved before advancing to OKC quadriceps activity. The rehabilitation specialist and patient should closely monitor this exercise for any signs of crepitus or patellofemoral pain. Pain-free arcs of motion are maintained when performing this exercise. Isokinetic exercise is also introduced as quadriceps strength improves. At HSS the authors have experienced that higher speeds (180 to 300 degrees/second) minimize stress to the patellofemoral joint and are better tolerated by the patient.

Agility exercises are incorporated into the program to improve dynamic lower extremity control. Sport cord activity is introduced gradually, starting with backward

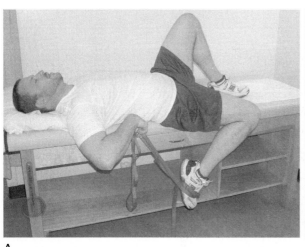 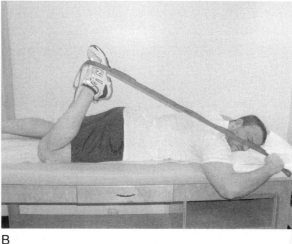

A   B

FIGURE **33-11** Quadriceps flexibility exercises. *A.* Supine quadriceps (two-joint hip flexor) stretch. *B.* Prone active-assisted quadriceps stretch.

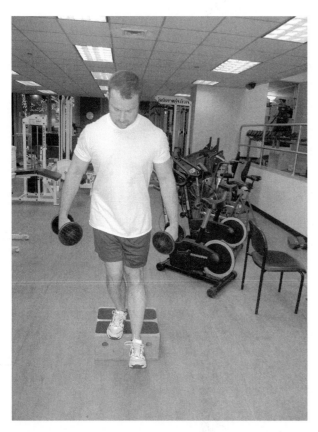

FIGURE **33-12** Forward step-down exercise. With this exercise the patient stands on top of a box or step and slowly steps down with the contralateral leg, eccentrically controlling the descent with the involved lower extremity. Verbal and visual cues (mirror) are used to optimize lower limb and trunk alignment when performing this exercise.

walking and progressed to side to side and carioca motions.

Steady improvement in the patient's functional activity is observed during this stage. Prolonged weight-bearing tolerance and ambulation distances should steadily improve without increasing knee joint effusion and pain. The weight-bearing squat test assesses functional weight-bearing deficits after knee extensor mechanism repair. A computerized force plate system (NeuroCom, Clackamas, OR) measures weight-bearing limb symmetry during varying functional squat positions (0, 30, 60, and 90 degrees) (Figure 33-13, *A, B*).

Reciprocal stair negotiation should be achieved as the patient demonstrates improved control with the prescribed step progression. The forward step down[27] test is used during this phase to evaluate functional eccentric quadriceps strength and lower extremity control. With this test the patient stands on top of an 8-inch box and is then asked to slowly step down off the box. The impact force of the descending leg is measured by the force plate, thereby measuring the ability of the stance leg to control the descent. A mean impact index of 10% body weight has been reported as normative values with this test. Eighty-five percent limb symmetry should be observed.

Retrograde running is first used before a progression to forward running is made. Adequate performance on the forward step down test is an indicator that the patient is ready to initiate retrograde running. Retrograde running is useful in improving knee extensor strength. Also, initial forefoot contact associated with retrograde running allows for the absorption of ground reaction forces, thereby limiting stress imposed upon the postoperative knee.[28]

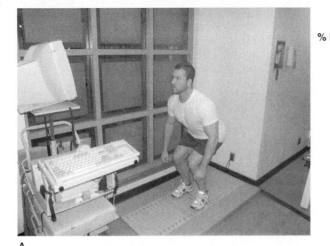

A

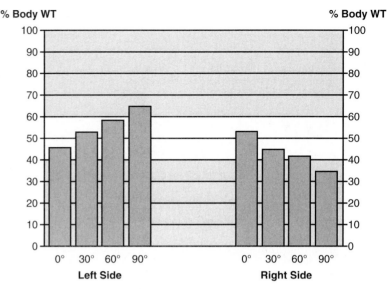

Weight-Bearing Squat Test

Left Side

Right Side

FIGURE **33-13** Weight-bearing squat test. *A.* Weight-bearing squat at 90 degrees. *B.* Results of the weight-bearing squat test. Decreased weight-bearing on the right lower extremity is demonstrated as the individual performs a squat at increasing knee flexion angles.

B

Percentage Weight-Bearing		
Angle	Left	Right
0°	47	53
30°	53	47
60°	58	42
90°	62	38

Postoperative Phase III: Early Functional (Weeks 11 to 16)

GOALS

- Full knee ROM
- Improve quadriceps and lower extremity flexibility
- Ability to descend 8-inch step with good eccentric leg control
- Return to normal ADL
- 85% limb symmetry on forward step down (FSD) test
- Independent in therapeutic home/gym exercise program

PRECAUTIONS

- Avoid pain with daily activities and therapeutic exercise
- Avoid stair descent until adequate quadriceps strength and lower extremity control
- Avoid high-level sport activity until adequate ROM, muscle strength, and flexibility is achieved

TREATMENT STRATEGIES

- Continue knee flexion ROM exercises
- Incorporate flexibility exercises for quadriceps musculature.
- Soft tissue massage, myofascial release, contract-relax techniques
- Advance closed chain exercise program—advance step program
- Initiate forward step-down program
- Progress squat program
- Incorporate OKC knee extension exercises (isokinetic/isotonic) as tolerated
- Advanced proprioception exercises
- Agility training
- Elliptical training
- Retrograde running
- FSD test (NeuroCom) at 4 months
- Patient to replicate and comply with treatment program at home/gym

CRITERIA FOR ADVANCEMENT

- Full knee ROM
- Adequate quadriceps strength and lower extremity flexibility
- Ability to descend 8-inch step with good eccentric control (85% limb symmetry on FSD test)
- No pain with ADL—ambulation, reciprocal stair negotiation
- Compliance with home/gym exercise program

Troubleshooting

The addition of multiple exercises to achieve the goals of this phase warrants close inspection of the patient's home and gym exercise program. Attention should be given to the volume (sets, repetitions, weight, and days per week) of the program to prevent overload of muscle-tendon units and an iatrogenic tendonitis from developing. Signs of patellofemoral pain should be continually monitored with the addition of OKC exercise and more advanced closed chain exercises. Patients are encouraged to perform flexibility exercises daily and to limit strengthening exercises to three or four times weekly. Continued compliance with the home/gym exercise program should be observed by the rehabilitation specialist. Patients should not be dependent on isotonic strength machines in the clinic. Patients are encouraged to exercise at a gym in addition to their home exercise program.

POSTOPERATIVE PHASE IV: LATE FUNCTIONAL/ RETURN TO SPORT (WEEKS 16 TO 24)

The main goals of this final phase of the rehabilitation program are to prepare the athlete or individual for return to sport, recreational, work, and full functional activity.

Forward running on a treadmill is initiated when the patient demonstrates improved quadriceps strength and no symptoms with retrograde running.

A lower extremity plyometric program is initiated when the following criteria are met. First, the athlete should have full ROM and good lower extremity flexibility. Second, an adequate strength base should be established. A plyometric program can be initiated if the patient can power-squat five squat repetitions in 5 seconds with a weight equal to 60% of the individual's body weight.[29] Finally, lower extremity neuromuscular control must be observed with previous proprioceptive activities. Apprehension with functional and sport-specific activities is observed and monitored by the rehabilitation specialist.

Functional and isokinetic testing should attempt to achieve greater than or equal to 85% limb symmetry and can help the rehabilitation specialist determine any strength deficits present. The one-legged hop test has been found to be a specific test to confirm lower limb asymmetry[30] and can be used in higher-level patients with extensor mechanism repairs.

Troubleshooting

The rehabilitation program is now the patient's lower extremity strengthening and conditioning program. It must be emphasized to the patient to maintain compliance with the exercise program to achieve maximum recovery and prevent reinjury when the patient returns to sport, occupational, and full functional activity.

Postoperative Phase IV: Late Functional/Return to Sport (Weeks 16 to 24)

GOALS
- Lack of apprehension with sport-specific movements
- Maximize strength and flexibility as to meet demands of individual's sport activity
- ≥85% limb symmetry with hop test and isokinetic testing
- Independent in therapeutic home/gym exercise program

PRECAUTIONS
- Avoid pain with therapeutic exercise and functional activities
- Avoid sport activity until adequate strength development and MD clearance

TREATMENT STRATEGIES
- Continue to advance lower extremity strengthening, flexibility, and agility programs
- Plyometric program
- Forward running
- Agility and sport-specific training
- Home/gym therapeutic exercise program: evaluation-based

CRITERIA FOR DISCHARGE
- ≥85% to 90% limb symmetry on functional and isokinetic tests
- Pain-free running
- Lack of apprehension with sport-specific movements
- Patient understands proper progression of home and gym exercise program

REFERENCES

1. Casey, M.T. Jr., Tietjens, B.R. *Neglected Ruptures of the Patellar Tendon. A Case Series of Four Patients.* Am J Sports Med 2001;29(4):457–460.

2. Kasten, P., Schewe, B., Maurer, F., Gosling, T., Krettek, C., Weise, K. *Rupture of the Patellar Tendon: A Review of 68 Cases and a Retrospective Study of 29 Ruptures Comparing Two Methods of Augmentation.* Arch Orthop Trauma Surg 2001; 121(10):578–582.

3. Kuechle, D.K., Stuart, M.J. *Isolated Rupture of the Patellar Tendon in Athletes.* Am J Sports Med 1994;22(5):692–695.

4. Marder, R.A., Timmerman, L.A. *Primary Repair of Patellar Tendon Rupture Without Augmentation.* Am J Sports Med 1999;27(3):304–307.

5. Kelly, D.W., Carter, V.S., Jobe, F.W., Kerlan, R.K. *Patellar and Quadriceps Tendon Ruptures—Jumper's Knee.* Am J Sports Med 1984;12(5):375–380.

6. Rasul, A.T. Jr., Fischer, D.A. *Primary Repair of Quadriceps Tendon Ruptures. Results of Treatment.* Clin Orthop 1993;289: 205–207.

7. Siwek, C.W., Rao, J.P. *Ruptures of the Extensor Mechanism of the Knee Joint.* J Bone Joint Surg Am 1981;63(6):932–937.

8. Anzel, S.H., Covey, K.W., Weiner, A.D., Lipscomb, P.R. *Disruptions of Muscles and Tendons: An Analysis of 1014 Cases.* Surgery 1959;45:406.

9. Zernicke, R.F., Garhammer, J., Jobe, F.W. *Human Patellar-Tendon Rupture.* J Bone Joint Surg Am 1977;59(2):179–183.

10. Enad, J.G., Loomis, L.L. *Patellar Tendon Repair: Postoperative Treatment.* Arch Phys Med Rehabil 2000;81(6):786–788.

11. Enad, J.G. *Patellar Tendon Ruptures.* South Med J 1999;92(6): 563–566.

12. Richards, D.P., Barber, F.A. *Repair of Quadriceps Tendon Ruptures Using Suture Anchors.* Arthroscopy 2002;18(5):556–559.

13. Enneking, W.F., Horowitz, M. *The Intra-articular Effects of Immobilization on the Human Knee.* J Bone Joint Surg 1972; 54A:973–985.

14. Laros, G.S., Tipton, C.M., Cooper, R.R. *Influence of Physical Activity on Ligament Insertions in the Knees of Dogs.* J Bone Joint Surg 1971;53A:275–286.

15. Ilan, D.I., Tejwani, N., Keschner, M., Leibman, M. *Quadriceps Tendon Rupture.* J Am Acad Orthop Surg 2003;11(3):192–200.

16. Larson, R.V., Simonian, P.T. *Semitendinosus Augmentation of Acute Patellar Tendon Repair with Immediate Mobilization.* Am J Sports Med 1995;23(1):82–86.

17. Noyes, F.R., Mangine, R.E., Barber, S. *Early Knee Motion after Open and Arthroscopic Anterior Cruciate Ligament Reconstruction.* Am J Sports Med 1987;15(2):149–160.

18. McCarthy, M.R., Yates, C.K., Anderson, M.A., Yates-McCarthy, J.L. *The Effects of Immediate Continuous Passive Motion on Pain During the Inflammatory Phase of Soft Tissue Healing Following Anterior Cruciate Ligament Reconstruction.* J Orthop Sports Phys Ther 1993;17(2):96–101.

19. O'Driscoll, S.W., Giori, N.J. *Continuous Passive Motion (CPM): Theory and Principles of Clinical Application.* J Rehabil Res Dev 2001;38(2):291.

20. Spencer, J.D., Hayes, K.C., Alexander, I.J. *Knee Joint Effusion and Quadriceps Reflex Inhibition in Man.* Arch Phys Med Rehabil 1984;65(4):171–177.

21. Ericson, M.O., Nisell, R. *Tibiofemoral Joint Forces During Ergometer Cycling.* Am J Sports Med 1986;14(4):285–290.

22. Ericson, M.O., Nisell, R., Arborelius, U.P., Ekholm, J. *Muscular Activity During Ergometer Cycling.* Scand J Rehabil Med 1985;17(2):53–61.

23. Lephart, S.M., Henry, T.J. *Functional Rehabilitation for the Upper and Lower Extremity.* Orthop Clin North Am 1995;26(3): 579–592.

24. Cipriani, D.J., Armstrong, C.W., Gaul, S. *Backward Walking at Three Levels of Treadmill Inclination: An Electromyographic and Kinematic Analysis.* J Orthop Sports Phys Ther 1995;22(3): 95–102.

25. Lancourt, J.E., Cristini, J.A. *Patella Alta and Patella Infera. Their Etiological Role in Patellar Dislocation, Chondromalacia, and Apophysitis of the Tibial Tubercle.* J Bone Joint Surg Am 1975; 57(8):1112–1115.

26. Davies, G.J. *Compendium of Isokinetics in Clinical Usage.* Simon & Schuster Publishers, LaCrosse, WI, 1984.

27. Cavanaugh, J.T., Stump, T.J. *Forward Step Down Test.* J Orthop Sports Phys Ther 2000;30(1):A–46.

28. Threlkeld, A.J., Horn, T.S., Wojtowicz, G.M., Rooney, J.G. *Kinematics, Ground Reaction Force, and Muscle Balance Produced by Backward Running.* J Orthop Sports Phys Ther 1989;11: 56–63.

29. Chu, D.A. *Jumping into Plyometrics.* Leisure Press, Champaign, IL, 1992.

30. Petschnig, R., Baron, R., Albrecht, M. *The Relationship Between Isokinetic Quadriceps Strength Test and Hop Tests for Distance and One-Legged Vertical Jump Test Following Anterior Ligament Reconstruction.* J Orthop Sports Phys Ther 1978 Jul;28(1):23–31.

34

Proximal and Distal Realignment

THERESA CHIAIA, PT

TODD CRONIN, MBA, PT

Patellofemoral pain comprises 25% of all knee patholo-gies and is the most common knee complaint in adoles-cents and young adults.[1,2] The source of pain in patients with patellofemoral disorders is multifactorial; there-fore, numerous therapeutic interventions have been advocated. They include taping, bracing, foot orthoses, quadriceps strengthening, vastus medialis oblique (VMO) strengthening, timing of muscular contractions, flexibility training, and/or proximal strengthening. Surgery for patellofemoral pain is an option only after the patient has exhausted nonoperative therapies. Sur-gical realignment has been divided into proximal and distal procedures. A *proximal realignment* is a soft tissue procedure indicated in the presence of recurrent sub-luxation/dislocation radiographic lateral patellar sub-luxation, and moderate or severe patellar tilt with minimal bony malalignment (Figure 34-1). *Distal realignment* is a bony procedure, an osteotomy of the tibial tubercle, indicated in patellofemoral arthrosis and instability (subluxation/dislocation) with underlying malalignment in a skeletally mature individual.[3] The Hospital for Special Surgery (HSS) guidelines for reha-bilitation following proximal realignment and distal realignment are presented.

SURGICAL OVERVIEW
PROXIMAL REALIGNMENT

Proximal realignment is a soft tissue balancing proce-dure that involves the lateral retinaculum and/or the medial retinaculum or the distal portion of the vastus medialis. The medial patellofemoral ligament (MPFL), a discrete component of the medial retinaculum, provides the majority of passive medial restraint to lateral dis-placement of the patella, and the distal portion of the vastus medialis (commonly referred to as the vastus

medialis oblique), through its insertion onto the medial side of the patella, is the major dynamic stabilizer of the patella.[3] A dysplastic VMO inserts more vertically near the proximal pole of the patella.[4] MPFL reconstructions utilize allograft or autograft tissue fixed at the adductor tubercle tensioned to balance the patella within the trochlea and fixed on the patellar side. In the *medial imbrication* procedure, the medial stabilizing structures (VMO and medial retinaculum) are dissected free along its insertion into the patella, leaving a small cuff of tissue and then sutured more centrally onto the patella, func-tionally tightening the redundant tissue with sutures.[3]

DISTAL REALIGNMENT

Distal realignment is an osteotomy of the tibial tubercle, with subsequent transfer of the tibial tubercle, either medially, anteriorly, anteromedially, or distally. Fulker-son Anteromedialization (AMZ) Osteotomy is a com-bination of the uniplanar tibial tubercle transfer procedures, medialization (Elmslie-Trillat Osteotomy), and anteriorization (Maquet Osteotomy).[4] The tibial tubercle is osteotomized by angling a single straight cut in anteromedial to posterolateral direction, whereby both medialization and elevation can be obtained[5] (Figure 34-2). The tibial tubercle transfer is fixed with two cortical bone screws (Figure 34-3). Complications with this procedure are related to fixation, fracture through the osteotomy or through the screw hole, wound healing, and possible deep venous thrombosis (DVT). In cases with severe patella alta, the procedure is combined with distalization. Distal transfer of the tibial tuberosity allows the articular surface of the patella to engage in the trochlea earlier in knee flexion.

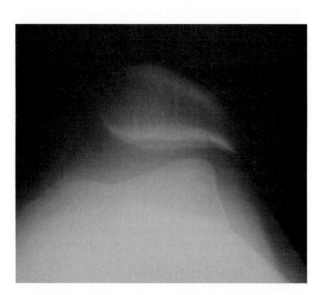

FIGURE **34-1** Radiograph showing patellar tilt. *(Courtesy of HSS Sports Medicine Service.)*

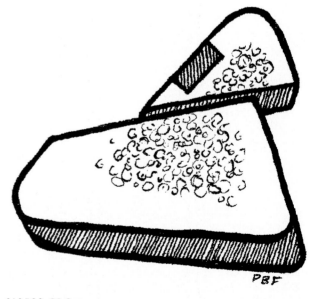

FIGURE **34-2** Schematic drawing of Fulkerson's anteromedi-alization (AMZ) osteotomy.

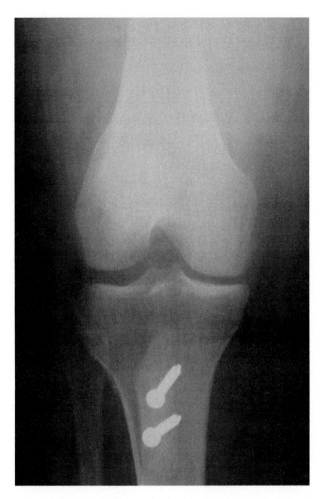

FIGURE **34-3** Radiograph of tibial tubercle transfer fixed with two cortical bone screws. *(Courtesy of HSS Sports Medicine Service.)*

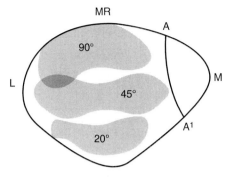

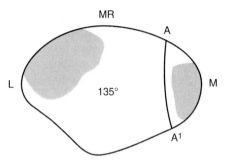

FIGURE **34-4** Patellofemoral contact pattern during knee flexion. *(From Goodfellow, J., Hungerford, D.S., Zindel, M. Patello-femoral Joint Mechanics and Pathology Functional Anatomy of the Patello-femoral Joint.* J Bone Joint Surg Br *1976;58B:287–290.)*

The tibial tubercle osteotomy is performed, freeing it up circumferentially, and then transferred distally.

Lateral retinacular release is commonly performed in combination with a proximal realignment or distal realignment.[4] It can be performed as an open procedure with an incision at the lateral border of the patella, or, more commonly, arthroscopically. The lateral retinaculum is released from the superior pole of the patella to the inferior pole. The superior geniculate vessels are located at the superior pole of the patella just deep to the retinaculum and are responsible for one of the postoperative complications: hemarthrosis in the joint.[4]

REHABILITATION OVERVIEW

Avoidance of provoking signs and symptoms, such as joint effusion, active inflammation, and pain, should guide the rehabilitation process. In the early phases, attention must be paid to the healing process of the involved structures—soft tissues following proximal realignment and bony fixation following distal realignment. No healing constraints follow release of the lateral retinaculum; however, control of postoperative

hemarthrosis is emphasized. Joint hemarthrosis is a concern with lateral retinacular release because of the proximity of the suprageniculate artery as it can lead to scarring and muscular inhibition. Bleeding in the joint will cause quadriceps inhibition, have a deleterious effect on joint proprioception, as well as the articular cartilage, and, ultimately, delay progression of rehabilitation.[6,7] Pain has also been shown to decrease muscle activity of the quadriceps.[8] Emphasis is on controlling hemarthrosis and pain, and initiating voluntary quadriceps control. Quadriceps strengthening is an essential component of patellofemoral rehabilitation and must be performed in a pain-free arc of motion. Knowledge of the location of the lesion as well as the patient's subjective complaints will help determine this range. As a result of the origin of the vasti on the linea aspera, gross quadriceps strengthening results in compressive forces through the patellofemoral joint altering contact location and pressure distribution.[9] An understanding of the biomechanics of the patellofemoral joint is essential. Articulation begins on the inferior patella with knee extension and moves proximally as the knee flexes[10] (Figure 34-4). Patellofemoral joint reaction force (PFJRF) is a measurement of compression of the patella against the femur and is dependent on the knee flexion angle and muscle tension. Another important consideration is the

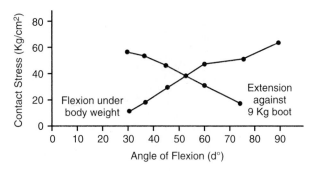

FIGURE **34-5** Unit load contact stress with knee flexion for flexion under body weight and extension against 9 kg boot resistance. *(From Hungerford, D.S., Barry, M. Biomechanics of the Patellofemoral Joint. Clin Orthop Relat Res 1979;144:9–15.)*

patellofemoral contact area. The contact load (force) divided by the contact area will determine the patellofemoral stress (stress = force/area). Quadriceps force and contact area vary according to knee flexion angles and thus has implications in prescribing quadriceps strengthening exercises. In closed chain activities, the stress increases from 0 to 90 degrees (force and contact area increase), whereas in open chain activities the stress increases as the knee extends (force increases as contact area decreases)[11,12] (Figure 34-5). Rehabilitation following these procedures is initiated immediately postoperatively. The rehabilitation potential will be dependent on the indications for surgery (instability vs arthritis) and the chronicity of the condition, premorbid status, and prior surgical history. Exercise should be performed in an optimal loading zone, the level of activity that neither overloads nor underloads the affected tissues.[13] Therapeutic exercise and activities of daily living (ADL) must be within the envelope of function, the safe range of painless loading compatible with tissue homeostasis.[14] Rehabilitation must respect the healing process and the individual knee's tolerance to imposed stresses. In short, at any given time each knee has an optimal window of function. If the knee is continually asked to work outside of this window, the window of function will become smaller. This philosophy underscores the importance of patient education. Understanding this concept will encourage compliance. The phases represent a continuum of rehabilitation rather than discrete, well-defined phases. Progression through the phases is dependent on the factors mentioned earlier, such as premorbid status and the chronicity of the condition.

POSTOPERATIVE REHABILITATION: PROXIMAL REALIGNMENT

POSTOPERATIVE PHASE I: HEALING (WEEKS 0 TO 6)

Healing constraints of the structures involved and methods of fixation must be respected and will deter-

mine weight-bearing status and range of motion (ROM) allowed. Dissection and advancement of soft tissues, as in the described proximal realignment, necessitates that precautions be taken during the initial or healing phase so as not to disrupt the repair. With advancement of the medial structures, limits with regard to knee flexion ROM are determined by the surgeon. ROM exercises include passive knee extension, with a towel under the heel in supine, and active knee flexion in sitting. The ROM goal is 0-degree knee extension to 60-degree knee flexion at 4 weeks postoperatively and 90-degree knee flexion by 6 weeks postoperatively. ROM exercises are performed with active range of motion (AROM) knee flexion and passive range of motion (PROM) knee extension in sitting.

The focus is to control effusion, inflammation, and pain, and minimize quadriceps inhibition. This is achieved through the use of cryotherapy, adherence to weight-bearing guidelines, and progression of ROM. The weight-bearing status is progressive weight bearing as tolerated (WBAT) with the brace locked in extension for 6 weeks. Improved tolerance to increased loads during gait allows the individual to progress off crutches, usually by 2 to 3 weeks. Submaximal quadriceps isometrics are performed with a towel roll under the knee to provide the patient with tactile feedback and minimize fat pad irritation. Biofeedback and/or electrical stimulation are used to facilitate a contraction. As knee flexion ROM progresses beyond 60 degrees, submaximal multiangle open chain quadriceps isometrics (Figure 34-6) and closed-chain quadriceps isometrics in sitting at 60-degree knee flexion are initiated (Figure 34-7). Proximal strengthening is initiated with straight leg raising (SLR); however, in supine the knee can be flexed to an angle of 20 degrees (Figure 34-8) to center the patella in the trochlear groove.[15] Hip abduction in sidelying is performed with hip in extension and external rotation. Proximal strengthening can progress to more advanced exercises, emphasizing the gluteals and external rotators as tolerated. Patellar mobilization within its normal ranges should be initiated in the medial direction (Figure 34-9). The patella should move a quarter of its width, exposing the lateral femoral condyle in the coronal plane, and the lateral border should lift off 20 degrees in the sagittal plane.[16] Hamstring and gastrocnemius flexibility is addressed, as needed. Triceps surae strengthening is initiated with elastic resistance. Balance and proprioceptive training is introduced at the latter part of this phase, as weight acceptance through the involved extremity improves, with double-limb support on a proprioception board, rocker board, or commercial balance system. Lower extremity alignment and a slight knee flexion posture are reinforced (Figure 34-10). Challenges can be initiated in the sagittal plane and progress to the coronal plane.

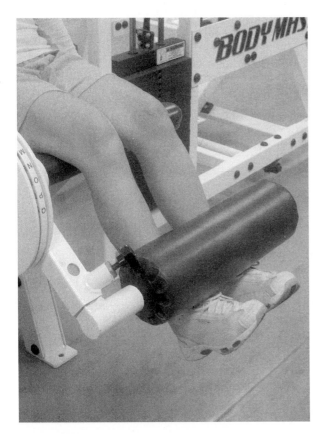

FIGURE **34-6** Submaximal multiangle open kinetic chain isometrics.

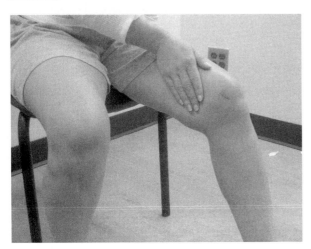

FIGURE **34-7** Closed-chain quadriceps isometrics in sitting at 60-degree knee flexion.

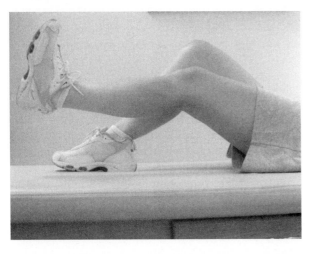

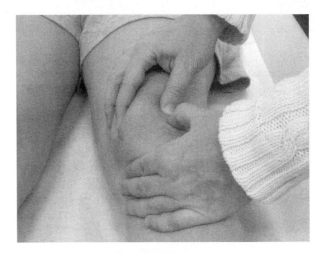

FIGURE **34-9** Patellar mobilization in the medial direction.

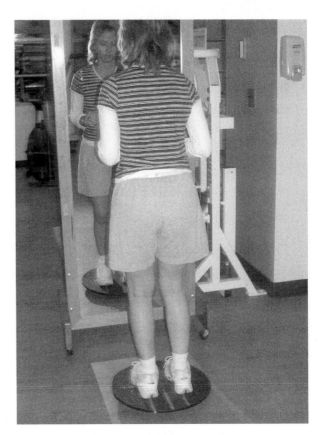

FIGURE **34-10** Lower extremity alignment and a slight knee flexion posture are reinforced on a balance board.

FIGURE **34-8** Supine hip flexion with knee flexed to 20 degrees.

Proximal Realignment
Postoperative Phase I: Healing (Weeks 0 to 6)

GOALS

- Patient education
- Control effusion
- Control pain
- ROM: 0-degree knee extension to 60-degree knee flexion (4 weeks); 90 degrees (6 weeks)
- Avoid quadriceps inhibition
- Promote healing
- Independent ambulation WBAT with brace locked in extension
- Independence in a home exercise program, as instructed

PRECAUTIONS

- Symptom provocation: quadriceps shut down, joint effusion, active inflammation
- Knee flexion ROM, as per surgeon's guidelines
- Lateralization of the patella
  - Avoid lateral patella glides
  - Terminal knee extension exercises
- Active knee extension

TREATMENT STRATEGIES

- Home exercise program, as instructed
- Educate patient
- Activity modification
- Cryotherapy
- Modalities, as needed for pain, effusion
- Quadriceps reeducation (submaximal): biofeedback, electrical stimulation, quadriceps sets performed with a towel roll, multiangle open chain isometrics, closed chain quadriceps isometrics in sitting at 60-degree knee flexion
- ROM exercises
  - PROM knee extension with a towel roll under heel
  - AROM knee flexion and PROM knee extension in sitting
- Patellar mobilization (medial direction: tilt and glide; cephalad and caudal)
- Gait training progressive WBAT, with appropriate assistive device and brace locked in extension
- Initiate proximal strengthening: SLR series; in supine, hip flexion can be performed with 20-degree knee flexion
- Address flexibility: gastrocnemius (towel stretch); hamstring stretch
- Initiate distal strengthening: elastic bands for triceps surae
- Initiate balance and proprioceptive training: double-limb support on progressively challenging surfaces

CRITERIA FOR ADVANCEMENT

- Good quadriceps contraction (pain-free)
- Good patellar mobility
- ROM: 0-degree knee extension to 90-degree knee flexion
- 0/10 pain at rest

Troubleshooting

ROM precautions must be followed. Soft tissue healing is a 12-week process. It is imperative that the patient understands that early successful completion of this phase will allow for progression in his or her rehabilitation course. Pain and effusion need to be controlled; therefore, patient compliance with activity modification, weight-bearing progression, cryotherapy, and therapeutic home exercise program is emphasized. Lateralization of the patella should be avoided; however, patellar mobility should be monitored to recognize postoperative complications (medial subluxation, lateral subluxation, suture pullout, knee flexion ROM) as a result of scarring, overtightening of the medial restraints, and/or an overzealous lateral release.

POSTOPERATIVE PHASE II: FUNCTIONAL—GAIT, MOTION, AND STRENGTHENING (WEEKS 7 TO 12)

The achievement of a good quadriceps contraction, the ability to maintain knee extension while performing an SLR, 90-degree knee flexion, and control of knee hemarthrosis and pain will allow the patient to begin the second phase of rehabilitation. Weight-bearing status is progressive weight-bearing as tolerated with an appropriate assistive device. Reintroduction of crutches, as needed, during ambulation is preferred to normalize the gait pattern. A functional brace, such as a patella cutout, is used, at the surgeon's discretion.

The emphasis in this phase is on gait training. Excessive knee extension is a common gait pattern (Figure 34-11) in these individuals. The underlying causes for this pattern must be evaluated, such as quadriceps weakness, decreased quadriceps response, habitual patterns, shortness of the gastrocnemius, and/or weakness of the hip abductors. Flexibility of the gastrocnemius and hip adductors is addressed. Gait training can be performed on a hydro-treadmill or on land with a 3% incline to encourage knee flexion. During the loading response phase of weight acceptance in the normal gait cycle, the knee is flexed for shock absorption.[17] As the gait cycle progresses into midstance, the knee extends. Decreased knee flexion in terminal stance and pre-swing phases of gait is another common gait deviation. In preparation for limb advancement, 40 degrees of knee flexion with hip extension is required. Early swing requires about 60 degrees of knee flexion.[17] Flexibility of the two-joint hip flexors can be addressed, using active knee flexion with neutral hip extension in prone and standing (Figure 34-12).

ROM can progress beyond 90 degrees with a goal of 110-degree knee flexion by postoperative week 8. Passive knee extension to 0 degrees is maintained. The bicycle ergometer is introduced as ROM allows. Short crank cycle can be initiated with 80 to 90 degrees of knee flexion. As knee flexion ROM approaches 115 degrees, progression to a standard cycle will be attainable.[18] Patella mobility continues to be monitored. Self-mobilization with the knee flexed in sitting is used so the individual can provide a low-load stretch to the retinaculum throughout the day (Figure 34-13). AROM knee extension in a 90- to 30-degree arc is begun at 8 to 10 weeks. Lieb and Perry[19] showed that a 60% increase in quadriceps force is needed to complete the last 15 degrees of knee extension.

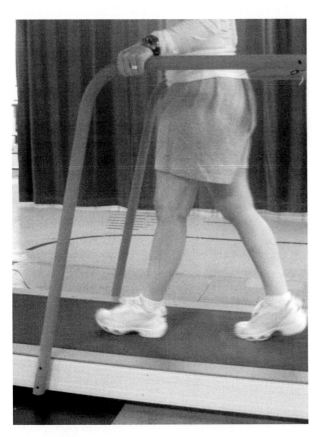

FIGURE 34-11 Evidence of a compensatory gait pattern: excessive knee extension.

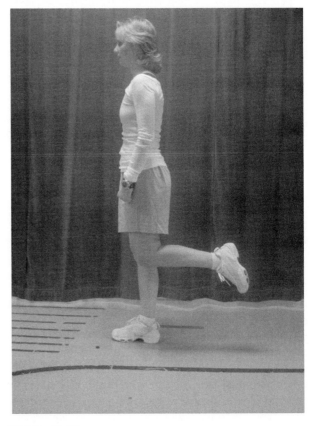

FIGURE 34-12 Active knee flexion with neutral hip extension in standing.

Proximal Realignment
Postoperative Phase II: Functional—Gait, Motion, and Strengthening (Weeks 7 to 12)

GOALS

- Patient education
- Control effusion, inflammation, and pain
- 0/10 pain with ADL, therapeutic exercise
- ROM: 0-degree knee extension to 110 degrees (8 weeks), 130 degrees (12 weeks)
- Promote healing
- Normalize gait without an assistive device
- Lower extremity postural alignment and the ability to support and control knee in single-limb stance
- Independence in a home exercise program, as instructed

PRECAUTIONS

- Sign and symptom provocation: pain, inflammation, quadriceps shutdown, joint effusion
- Knee flexion ROM, as per surgeon's guidelines through 8 weeks
- Progression of weight-bearing
- Pathological gait pattern
- "Too much, too soon" progression of strengthening exercises

TREATMENT STRATEGIES

- Home exercise program, as instructed
- Educate patient
- Activity modification
- Cryotherapy
- Quadriceps strengthening: AROM knee extension in a limited arc, bilateral leg press, forward step-up progression
- ROM exercises: progressing to AAROM knee flexion in sitting
- Patellar mobilization (medial direction: tilt and glide; cephalad and caudal)
- Cycle ergometry: progressing from short crank to standard crank
- Gait training
  - Hydro-treadmill
  - Treadmill with a low incline 3% to 5%
- Balance activities: single-limb support from stable to unstable surfaces
- Flexibility exercises: evaluation-based: gastrocnemius, AROM knee flexion with hip extension, hip adductors
- Advance proximal strengthening to include hip extension with knee flexion and closed chain activities, such as contralateral exercises

CRITERIA FOR ADVANCEMENT

- Normalized gait without an assistive device
- 0/10 pain with ADL, therapeutic exercise
- Lower extremity postural alignment and the ability to support and control knee in single-limb stance
- Able to ascend a 6-inch/8-inch step with good control
- ROM 130 degrees

Quadriceps strengthening is progressed to functional exercises, including the leg press and a forward step-up progression. Step-up training can progress from 4 to 6 to 8 inches (Figure 34-14) as strength improves. At each height, handheld weights can be added to challenge the lower extremity musculature. Quality of movement is emphasized during these functional strengthening exercises. This includes the ability to use the quadriceps without compensatory patterns. Dynamic alignment, maintaining a level pelvis with the hip, knee, and foot aligned, is monitored by using a mirror for visual feedback. Proximal strengthening is progressed, focusing on the gluteals, pelvic musculature, using the clamshell and bent knee fallout exercises, and the hip flexors (rectus femoris and iliopsoas).

Balance progresses from single-limb support on a stable surface to advanced single-limb support, paying close attention to pelvic and knee control, thereby

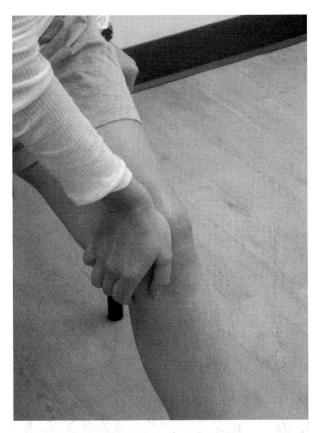

FIGURE **34-13** Self-patellar mobilization in sitting.

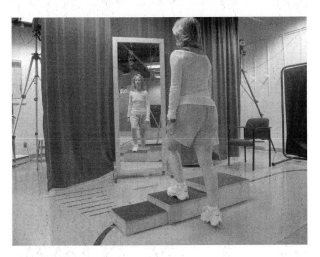

FIGURE **34-14** Forward step-up progression (4- to 6- to 8-inch step height) with visual feedback.

combining proximal strengthening. Perturbations with elastic bands, manual displacements, tapping the board, and ball tossing are added to provide additional challenge.

During this rehabilitative phase, the focus shifts toward addressing lower extremity alignment and soft tissue imbalances, in terms of length and strength. For

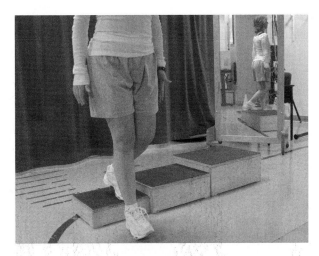

FIGURE **34-15** Forward step-down progression. Notice the lower extremity alignment.

example, are the hip abductors and external rotators weak? Subjects with patellofemoral pain demonstrated less strength than age-matched controls.[20] Does posterior calf shortness cause the foot to pronate to achieve greater dorsiflexion ROM? In other words, address proximal and distal factors that may influence the knee.

Troubleshooting

In this phase, activity modification is reinforced. Patient education continues to be important. An understanding of the rehabilitation process will encourage patient compliance and decrease the patient's frustration. With an increase in the patient's activity level, symptoms of pain and signs of joint effusion and soft tissue inflammation must be monitored. Premature discharge of the assistive device can cause the knee to enter the pain-inflammation cycle with a resultant quadriceps shutdown. It will also have a deleterious effect on the gait pattern. Over-tightening of the medial structures can make knee flexion difficult.

POSTOPERATIVE PHASE III: ADVANCED STRENGTHENING AND ENDURANCE (WEEKS 13 TO 17)

Functional ROM, a normalized gait pattern, and pelvic and knee stability in single-limb stance with control of signs and symptoms allows the patient to safely progress into the next phase of rehabilitation. Signs and symptoms must continue to be monitored as the demands on the knee continue to rise. Normal ROM is achieved using active assistive techniques in sitting, supine wall slides, and the bicycle. Patellar mobility continues to be addressed. AROM knee extension is performed through a full arc of motion. Strengthening is progressed to function and incorporates eccentric leg press, step-down progression (Figure 34-15), and squat

Proximal Realignment
Postoperative Phase III: Advanced Strengthening and Endurance (Weeks 13 to 17)

GOALS

- Patient education
- Control effusion and inflammation
- 0/10 pain with ADL, as recommended by the therapist and therapeutic exercise
- ROM: within normal limits (WNLs)
- Normalize gait
- Lower extremity postural alignment and the ability to support and control knee in single-limb dynamic balance
- Independence in a home exercise program, as instructed

PRECAUTIONS

- Sign and symptom provocation: pain and active inflammation
- Gait deviations
- "Too much, too soon" progression of strengthening exercises

TREATMENT STRATEGIES

- Home exercise program, as instructed: evaluation-based
- Educate patient
- Activity modification
- Cryotherapy
- Quadriceps strengthening
  - AROM knee extension, eccentric leg press, forward step-down progression, squat progression
- ROM exercises
  - AROM to AAROM knee flexion in sitting and supine wall slides
- Gait training
  - Retro-treadmill with a 5% to 10% incline
- Advance proximal strengthening
- Balance activities progressing to single-limb static balance to dynamic activities
- Address muscle imbalances: evaluation-based: prone figure of four, hip adduction stretch
- Cross training: elliptical trainer, bicycle, stair machine

CRITERIA FOR ADVANCEMENT

- ROM WNLs
- Normalized gait
- Ability to support control knee in dynamic single-limb stance
- Able to ascend an 8-inch step with good control
- Able to descend an 8-inch step with good control, and alignment
- Lower extremity alignment during dynamic single-limb stance

progression, as tolerated. The individual is progressed from ball squats against the wall to free squats. Alignment is stressed during these exercises. The individual is taught to unlock his or her hips to initiate the squat. Gait training continues to be emphasized so the patient does not regress into old habits, such as quadriceps avoidance. Retro-walking on a treadmill helps facilitate quadriceps control during midstance and dynamic balance[21,22] (Figure 34-16). Dynamic balance is addressed with a resistance cord, using carioca or sidestepping. Proximal strengthening is advanced, maintaining hip external rotation against an elastic band during sidestepping in a squat position. Cross training is incorporated with a bicycle and elliptical trainer. An elliptical trainer can be introduced as the individual demonstrates strength to perform a 6-inch step up (Figure 34-17). Flexibility of the hip is addressed according to evaluation findings and may include, for example, the prone figure of four[4] (Figure 34-18), hip adduction stretch, and two-joint hip flexor stretch.

Troubleshooting

Monitor the patient's knee for an active inflammatory response. Persistent gait deviations and rapid advancement of function can set the patient back. Emphasis should be on the quality of movement vs the quantity. Movement patterns will revert to pre-surgical compensatory habits, if this is not a priority.

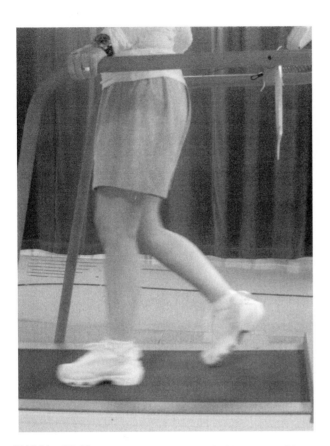

FIGURE 34-16 Retro-walking helps facilitate quadriceps control and dynamic balance.

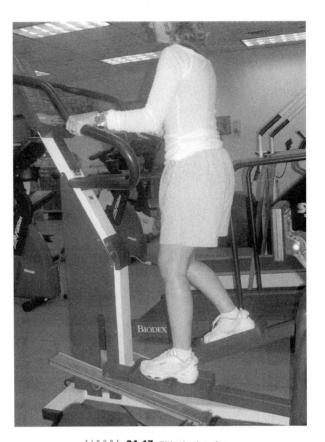

FIGURE 34-17 Elliptical trainer.

POSTOPERATIVE PHASE IV: ADVANCED FUNCTIONAL, RETURN TO SPORT (WEEKS 18 TO 25)

The rehabilitation goals for the individual patient will determine whether the patient progresses beyond the third phase. If participation in a low impact program is the goal, the emphasis will be on muscular endurance. If the goal of the patient and the surgeon is for participation in higher level activities, such as running, jumping, and cutting, this phase will prepare the individual to do so. Plyometric training will then be incorporated. A solid foundation of strength, meaning eccentric quadriceps control and pelvic control with single-limb activities, as well as adequate ROM, must precede the introduction of plyometrics. A step-down test on a force plate will measure the impact forces[23] and thus determine eccentric quadriceps control. Clinical observation will determine alignment. Plyometrics are introduced with jumps onto a box and progress to jumps in place, standing jumps, to multiple jumps on two legs, as tolerated. Plyometric exercises progress to single-leg bounding and jumping for distance, that is, broad jumps and single-leg hops. Emphasis is on quality of movement (controlling valgus) and the absorption of forces. Running is introduced with good pelvic and

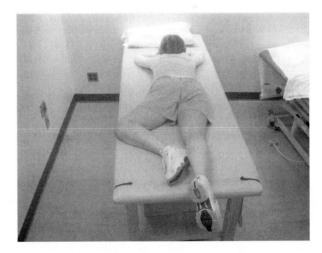

FIGURE 34-18 Prone figure of four position.

knee control during single-limb dynamic activities, beginning with retro-running at self-selected speeds. Forward running is initiated with 30-second to 1-minute intervals. Running time increases gradually. Deceleration training and change of direction are incorporated. Strength testing, isokinetics, if appropriate, and functional testing, such as single-leg hop, are used as

Proximal Realignment
Postoperative Phase IV: Advanced Functional, Return to Sport (Weeks 18 to 25)

GOALS
- Patient education
- 0/10 pain with ADL and advanced therapeutic exercise
- Muscular endurance and flexibility to meet demands of sport
- Independence in a home exercise program, as instructed
- Strength: 85% limb symmetry via testing

PRECAUTIONS
- Sign and symptom provocation
- Volume of training

TREATMENT STRATEGIES
- Home exercise program, as instructed: incorporate rest
- Educate patient
- Cryotherapy
- Continue functional quadriceps strengthening
- Patellar mobilization (medial direction: tilt and glide), as needed
- Dynamic balance activities
- Continue to address muscle imbalances: evaluation-based
- Advance proximal strengthening through functional activities
- Plyometrics training
- Initiate running program: retro to forward running intervals
- Cutting and deceleration training
- Endurance training: cross training
- Strength testing and functional testing

RETURN TO SPORT/CRITERIA FOR DISCHARGE
- 85% limb symmetry with
  - Strength testing: isokinetics, if appropriate
  - Functional testing: single-leg hop
- Muscular endurance and flexibility to meet demands of sport

criteria (85% limb symmetry) for return to sport and will help determine readiness.

Troubleshooting

Monitor the patient's signs and symptoms as high level activities are introduced. The patient must have an adequate strength base to progress to these activities, and care must be taken to follow a functional progression. High level activities must be a realistic goal. It is important to include rest/recovery days. Strength training must be continued with heavy and light days built into training. Gradual return to competition is advocated, progressing from skill drills to drills in a noncontact practice environment to contact practice drills to scrimmages and, ultimately, to games.

POSTOPERATIVE REHABILITATION: DISTAL REALIGNMENT

As compared to proximal realignment, the time frame is longer for distal realignment, as a result of the weight-bearing progression and risk of fracture.

The individual will be non–weight bearing with a brace locked in extension during the first 6 weeks to protect the bone and fixation. Radiographic evidence of healing will allow progression of the weight-bearing status and ROM. Adequate healing will allow the weight-bearing status to progress to progressive WBAT at 6 weeks with crutches. The brace will be locked in extension during ambulation for 8 weeks. Gait training is then introduced and a heel-toe gait is emphasized. An underwater treadmill can be used when wound healing is adequate. An unweighted treadmill that reduces weight-bearing forces can also be used. Retro-ambulation will assist in developing a normal gait during forward ambulation, as the knee extends concentrically. Ground reaction forces are absorbed by the calf muscles during backward walking.[24] If passive and/or active knee extension is insufficient, a flexed knee gait pattern is exhibited. This compensation will increase demands on the patellofemoral joint and quadriceps mechanism, including the patella tendon.

Patellar mobilization within its normal ranges should be initiated in the medial direction and cephalad direction. The ROM goal is 0 to 60 degrees during the first

2 weeks and progressing to 0 to 90 degrees by 6 weeks postoperatively. Prolonged immobilization has a deleterious effect on articular cartilage, bone, tendons, and ligaments. Continuous passive motion (CPM) is used immediately postoperatively to maintain joint nutrition and lubrication, regenerate articular cartilage, prevent joint stiffness, reduce hemarthrosis, and improve patient comfort.[25] ROM can progress to 120-degree knee flexion by the eighth postoperative week. The bicycle ergometer is introduced as ROM and weight-bearing allows.

As weight-bearing is limited in this phase, proximal strengthening is performed in a non–weight-bearing environment, that is, progressive resistive exercise (PRE) machines, such as a multihip machine. A straight leg series is initiated for all hip motions. The individual is monitored for postoperative complications.

Progression to higher level activities is dependent on clearance from the referring surgeon, because the risk of fracture is a major concern. Return to sport occurs at 9 to 12 months. These time frames are for 1 year. The functional strengthening phase should be about 8 weeks. The individual will continue with a home exercise program until clearance for higher level activities is received.

Distal Realignment
Postoperative Phase I (Weeks 0 to 6)

GOALS

- Patient education
- Control effusion
- Control pain
- ROM: 0-degree knee extension to 60-degree knee flexion (2 weeks); 90 degrees (6 weeks)
- Avoid quadriceps inhibition
- Promote healing
- Independent ambulation NWB with crutches and brace locked in extension on level surfaces and stairs
- Independence in a home exercise program, as instructed

PRECAUTIONS

- Symptom provocation: quadriceps shut down, joint effusion, active inflammation
- Progression of weight-bearing
- Knee flexion ROM, as per surgeon's guidelines
- Active knee extension
- Wound healing, patella position

TREATMENT STRATEGIES

- Home exercise program, as instructed
- Educate patient
- Activity modification
- Cryotherapy
- Modalities, as needed for pain, effusion
- Quadriceps reeducation: biofeedback, electrical stimulation, quadriceps sets performed with a towel roll
- Continuous passive motion
- ROM exercises
  - PROM knee extension with a towel roll under heel
  - AROM knee flexion in sitting, PROM knee extension with noninvolved extremity upon return from flexion in sitting
- Patellar mobilization: emphasize cephalad direction
- Gait training NWB with crutches and brace locked in extension
- Initiate proximal strengthening: SLR series, gluteals, comply with NWB status
- Address flexibility: gastrocnemius (towel stretch); hamstring stretch
- Initiate distal strengthening: elastic bands for triceps surae

CRITERIA FOR ADVANCEMENT

- Radiographic evidence of adequate healing
- Good quadriceps contraction
- Good patellar mobility
- ROM: 0-degree knee extension to 90-degree knee flexion
- 0/10 pain at rest

Distal Realignment
Postoperative Phase II (Weeks 7 to 14)

GOALS

- Patient education
- Control effusion, inflammation, and pain
- Establish pain-free arc of motion
- 0/10 pain with ADL, therapeutic exercise
- ROM: 0-degree knee extension to 120 degrees (8 weeks), WNL at 14 weeks
- Promote healing
- Normalize gait
- Independence in a home exercise program, as instructed

PRECAUTIONS

- Sign and symptom provocation: pain, inflammation, quadriceps shut down, joint effusion
- Knee flexion ROM as per surgeon's guidelines
- Progression of weight-bearing
- Pathological gait pattern
- Pain-free arc of motion during exercise

TREATMENT STRATEGIES

- Home exercise program, as instructed
- Educate patient
- Activity modification
- Cryotherapy
- Quadriceps strengthening
  - Submaximal multiangle closed and open chain isometrics
  - Bilateral leg press: monitor arc of motion
  - Open chain knee extension: monitor arc of motion
  - Initiate forward step-up progression
- ROM exercises
  - AAROM knee extension with noninvolved extremity upon return from flexion in sitting in a pain-free arc
  - AROM to AAROM knee flexion in sitting
- Patellar mobilization (medially and cephalad)
- Cycle ergometry: progressing from short crank to standard crank
- Gait training
  - Hydro-treadmill
  - Unweighted treadmill
- Flexibility exercises: evaluation-based: AROM knee flexion with hip extension
- Advance proximal strengthening: hip extension with knee flexion, and closed chain activities
- Initiate balance and proprioceptive training: double-limb support on progressively challenging surfaces

CRITERIA FOR ADVANCEMENT

- Normalize gait
- 0/10 pain with ADL, therapeutic exercise
- Ability to support and control knee in single-limb stance
- Able to ascend an 8-inch step with good control
- Good postural alignment during single-limb stance

Distal Realignment
Postoperative Phase III (Weeks 15 to 22)

GOALS

- Patient education
- Control effusion and inflammation
- 0/10 pain with ADL, therapeutic exercise
- ROM: WNLs
- Normalize gait
- Good single-leg dynamic balance
- Good eccentric quadriceps control
- Pelvic control during step down
- Independence in a home exercise program, as instructed

PRECAUTIONS

- Sign and symptom provocation: pain and active inflammation
- Gait deviations
- Overloading the joint

TREATMENT STRATEGIES

- Home exercise program, as instructed
- Educate patient
- Activity modification
- Cryotherapy
- Quadriceps strengthening: monitor arc of motion
  - Forward step-up progression
  - Eccentric leg press
  - Forward step-down progression
  - Squat progression
- ROM exercises
  - PROM knee extension with a towel roll under heel
  - AROM to AAROM knee flexion in sitting and supine wall slides
- Gait training
  - Treadmill
  - Retro-treadmill
- Advance proximal strengthening through functional activities
- Balance activities: single-limb static balance to dynamic activities
- Address muscle imbalances: evaluation-based
- Cross training: elliptical trainer, bicycle, stair machine

CRITERIA FOR ADVANCEMENT

- ROM WNLs
- Normalize gait
- Ability to support control knee in dynamic single-limb stance
- Able to descend an 8-inch step with good control, and alignment
- Good postural alignment during dynamic single-limb stance

Distal Realignment
Postoperative Phase IV (Weeks 36 to 44)

GOALS

- Patient education
- 0/10 pain with ADL, advanced therapeutic exercise
- Good dynamic balance
- Muscular endurance and flexibility to meet demands of ADL, and sport
- Independence in a home exercise program, as instructed
- Strength: 85% limb symmetry

PRECAUTIONS

- Sign and symptom provocation
- Volume of training

TREATMENT STRATEGIES

- Home exercise program: evaluation-based
- Educate patient
- Activity level should be within envelope of function
- Cryotherapy
- Continue functional quadriceps strengthening
- Dynamic balance activities
- Continue to address muscle imbalances: evaluation-based
- Cutting drills and deceleration training
- Endurance training: cross training
- Initiate plyometrics
- Initiate running program: retro to forward running intervals
- Strength testing and functional testing

RETURN TO SPORT/CRITERIA FOR DISCHARGE

- 85% limb symmetry with
  - Strength testing: isokinetics, if appropriate
  - Functional testing: single-leg hop
- Muscular endurance and flexibility to meet demands of ADL, and physician clearance must be obtained prior to participation in sport.

Troubleshooting

If proximal and distal realignment are performed in combination, the guideline for distal realignment is followed. Pain and effusion need to be controlled throughout the rehabilitation process; therefore, patient compliance with activity modification, weight-bearing status, cryotherapy, and therapeutic home exercise program is emphasized. Monitor the patient closely for postoperative complications. Early weight-bearing can cause complications, such as fracture, at the site of fixation. Pain during exercise will have a deleterious effect on the joint and delay progression in rehabilitation. Thus, the patient's knee is monitored for an active inflammatory response. Persistent gait deviations and rapid advancement of function can set the patient back. As the patient's daily activity level increases, exercise must be modified and prescribed accordingly. The patient must have an adequate strength base to progress to high level activities, and care must be taken to follow a functional progression. High level activities must be a realistic goal.

REFERENCES

1. Clement, D.B., Taunton, J.E., Smart, G.W. *A Survey of Overuse Running Injuries.* Phys Sportsmed 1981;9(5):47–58.
2. Devereaux, M.D., Lachmann, S.M. *Patellofemoral Arthralgia in Athletes Attending a Sports Injury Clinic.* Br J Sports Med 1984;18:18–21.
3. Shubin Stein, B.E., Ahmad, C.S. Patellofemoral Disorders in Athletes. In *Essentials of Orthopaedic Surgery Sports Medicine,* 2005.
4. Grelsamer, R.P., McConnell, J. *The Patella. A Team Approach.* Aspen Publishers, Gaithersburg, MD, 1998.
5. Fulkerson, J.P. *Anteromedialization of the Tibial Tuberosity for Patellofemoral Malalignment.* Clin Orthop 1983;177:176.
6. Spencer, J.D., Hayes, K.C., Alexander, I.J. *Knee Joint Effusion and Quadriceps Reflex Inhibition in Man.* Arch Phys Med Rehabil 1984;65:171–177.
7. deAndrade, J.R., Grant, C., Dixon, A.S. *Joint Distension and Reflex Muscle Inhibition in the Knee.* J Bone Joint Surg 1965; 47A(2):313–322.
8. Young, A., Stokes, M., Shakespeare, D.T., Sherman, K.P. *The Effect of Intra-articular Bupivacaine on Quadriceps Inhibition after Meniscectomy.* Med Sci Sports Exerc 1983;15(2):154.

9. Powers, C.M. *The Effects of Anatomically Based Multiplanar Loading of the Extensor Mechanism on Patellofemoral Joint Mechanics.* Clin Biomech 1998;13:608–615.
10. Goodfellow, J., Hungerford, D.S., Zindel, M. *Patello-femoral Joint Mechanics and Pathology: Functional Anatomy of the Patello-femoral Joint.* J Bone Joint Surg 1976;58B:291–299.
11. Hungerford, D.S., Lennox, D.W. *Rehabilitation of the Knee in Disorders of the Patellofemoral Joint: Relevant Biomechanics.* Orthop Clin North Am 1983;14(2):397–402.
12. Steinkamp, L.A., Dillingham, M.F., Market, M.D., Hill, J.A., Kaufman, K.R. *Biomechanical Considerations in Patella Femoral Joint Rehabilitation.* Am J Sports Med 1993;21(3):438–444.
13. Porterfield, J.A., DeRosa, C. *Mechanical Low Back Pain.* WB Saunders, Philadelphia, 1991.
14. Dye, S.F. *Patellofemoral Pain Current Concepts: An Overview.* Sports Med Arthrosc Rev 2001;9:264–272.
15. Doucette, S.A., Goble, E.M. *The Effect of Exercise on Patellar Tracking in Lateral Patellar Compression Syndrome.* Am J Sports Med 1992;20(4):434–440.
16. Fulkerson, J.P. *Disorders of the Patellofemoral Joint,* 3rd ed. Williams & Wilkins, Baltimore, 1997.
17. Perry, J. *Gait Analysis. Normal and Pathological Function.* New York, McGraw-Hill, 1992.
18. Schwartz, R.E., Asnis, P.D., Cavanaugh, J.T., *Short Crank Cycle Ergometry.* J Orthop Sports Phys Ther 1991;13:95.
19. Lieb, F.J., Perry, J. *Quadriceps Function. An Anatomical and Mechanical Study Using Amputated Limbs.* J Bone Joint Surg 1968;8(50A):1535–1548.
20. Ireland, M.L., Willson, J.D., Ballantyne, B.T., Davis, I.M. *Hip Strength in Females With and Without Patellofemoral Pain.* J Orthop Sports Phys Ther 2003;33(11):671–676.
21. Flynn, T.W., Soutas-Little, N.W. *Mechanical Power and Muscle Action During Forward and Backward Running.* J Orthop Sports Phys Ther 1993;17:108–112.
22. Flynn, T.W., Soutas-Little, N.W. *Patellofemoral Joint Compressive Forces in Forward and Backward Running.* J Orthop Sports Phys Ther 1995;245:277–282.
23. Cavanaugh, J.T., Stump, T.J. *Forward Step Down Test.* J Orthop Sports Phys Ther 2000;30(1):A–46.
24. Gray, G. *Chain Reaction.* New York, 1991.
25. Salter, R.S. *The Biological Concept of Continuous Passive Motion of Synovial Joints.* Clin Orthop Relat Res 1989;242:12–25.

35

Anterior Cruciate Ligament Reconstruction

JOHN T. CAVANAUGH, PT, MED, ATC

The anterior cruciate ligament (ACL) is one of the more commonly injured knee ligaments in the general population. An estimated 1 out of 3000 people will suffer an ACL injury in any given year.[1] The majority of these injuries occur during sport activities, which involve rapid change of direction and jumping (basketball, soccer, football, skiing, lacrosse). The pathomechanics of ACL injury can include contact and noncontact mechanisms. Noncontact mechanisms may account for up to 78% of all ACL injuries.[2,3] It is estimated that more than 100,000 ACL reconstructions are performed annually in the United States. Graft choices for reconstruction include autograft (patellar tendon or hamstring tendon) or allograft tissue. The Hospital for Special Surgery (HSS) ACL reconstruction guideline following autogenous patellar tendon graft is presented.

ANATOMICAL (SURGICAL) OVERVIEW

An ACL reconstruction using a patellar tendon graft is performed, using a combination of open and arthroscopic surgery. The central third of the patellar tendon is harvested along with a segment of bone from the patella above and the tibia below (Figure 35-1). The old ACL tissue is arthroscopically débrided. Drill holes are created in the tibia and femur in preparation for graft placement. The graft is passed through the tibial tunnel, through the central part of the knee joint and into the femoral tunnel. The graft is fixated by placing interference screws (one in the femur and one in the tibia) between the bone block and respective walls of the femoral and tibial tunnels (Figure 35-2). The skin incisions are reapproximated with sutures. Postoperatively, the patient is placed in a hinged brace locked at 0 degrees of extension.

REHABILITATION OVERVIEW

The rehabilitation program following ACL reconstruction is begun immediately after surgery. Care must be given by the rehabilitation specialist to protect the ACL graft substitute. The clinician must consider ACL biology throughout the progression of the postoperative rehabilitation program. Noyes et al.[4] reported that the central third of the patellar tendon was 186% of the strength of the native ACL. The graft is at its strongest at the time of reconstruction. Over time the graft undergoes periods of necrosis, revascularization, and remodeling. Graft strength decreases during the period of necrosis and gradually increases as it revascularizes and remodels.[5-8] Graft fixation techniques are an important consideration, as well as biological fixation, and replace mechanical fixation over a 3- to 6-week time frame. The patient is progressed via a criteria-based functional progression. Criteria for discharge are targeted between 4 and 6 months after surgery.

PREOPERATIVE REHABILITATION

It is recommended that reconstructive surgery be delayed until the patient's inflammation subsides and the normal range of motion (ROM), muscle function,

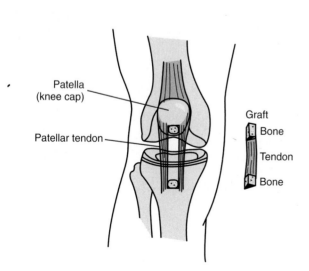

FIGURE **35-1** The central third of the patellar tendon is harvested along with a segment of bone from the patella and tibia.

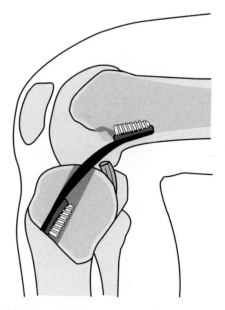

FIGURE **35-2** Bone-patella, tendon-bone graft is fixated by placing interference screws between the bone block and respective walls of the femoral and tibial tunnels.

and gait are restored. Restoring ROM preoperatively is shown to decrease the incidence of postoperative arthrofibrosis.[9] Quadriceps muscle strength is shown to return more quickly postoperatively when reconstructive surgery is delayed longer than 21 days.[10] Patients may require several weeks of therapeutic intervention to achieve preoperative goals.

An important component of the authors' preoperative program is patient education. A preoperative rehabilitation program can mentally prepare the patient/athlete for the demanding postoperative period to follow. Instruction and subsequent independence in a postoperative exercise program can expedite rehabilitation gains in the immediate postoperative period and limit complications from developing. Exercises included in

the preoperative program are passive extension with a towel rolled up under the heel, quadriceps setting, straight leg raising (SLR) with a postoperative brace locked at 0 degrees, and an active flexion/active-assisted extension (ROM 90 to 0 degrees) exercise, using the contralateral extremity (Figure 35-3, A–D). Open kinetic chain (OKC) in the terminal ranges of extension is avoided in the early postoperative period secondary to ACL strain and patellofemoral discomfort. The patient is taught self-patellar mobilizations to promote normal patellofemoral biomechanics.

The patient is measured for a postoperative brace and instructed in its management (donning/doffing). The patient is encouraged to don the postoperative brace while sleeping, ambulating, and performing a supine

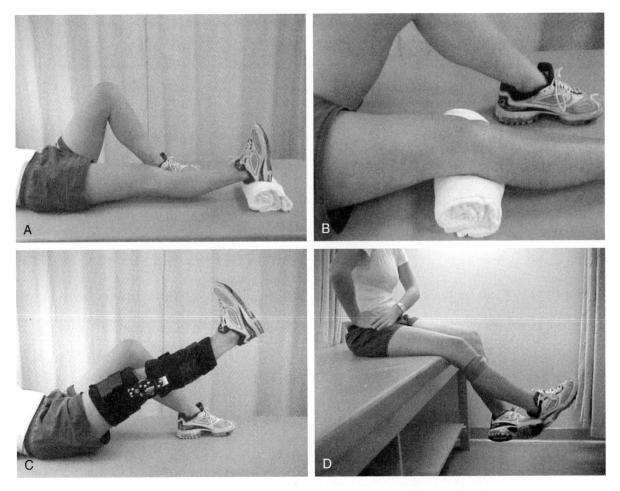

FIGURE 35-3 A. Passive knee extension, using a towel rolled up under heel to promote early full extension. B. Quadriceps setting. Towel is used for co-contraction and added comfort. Submaximal effort is encouraged. C. SLR with a postoperative brace locked at 0 degrees. D. Active flexion/active-assisted extension (ROM 90 to 0 degrees) exercise, using the contralateral extremity. Patient supports involved extremity with noninvolved limb as patient allows gravity to slowly flex involved knee. Upon feeling a stretch, the patient uses the noninvolved extremity to actively assist the involved knee to a full extension position.

SLR until told otherwise by the patient's surgeon or physical therapist. The patient is also instructed in the use of cryotherapy for postoperative pain and effusion control by using a commercial cold device (e.g., Cryo/cuff, Aircast Inc., Summit, NJ) (Figure 35-4). The patient is measured for crutches and taught to ambulate using partial (50%) weight-bearing. A KT1000 Knee ligament arthrometer test (Medmetric Corporation, San Diego) is performed to document preoperative laxity (Figure 35-5). Strength testing (isokinetic and/or functional tests) and balance testing are performed, if appropriate.

At a minimum, one preoperative physical therapy consultation is recommended. The patient is provided with a booklet, developed by the HSS rehabilitation department's staff, describing the surgery, therapeutic exercises, postoperative course, and frequently asked questions with answers.

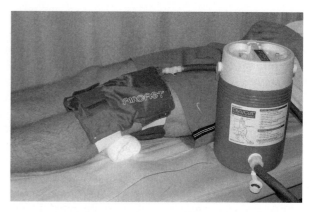

FIGURE **35-4** Cryo/cuff, commercial cold device (DJO, LLC, Vista CA).

Preoperative Rehabilitation

GOALS
- Patient education
- Restore normal ROM
- Normalize gait
- Maximize strength/functional capabilities
- Demonstrate ability to ascend/descend stairs without assistive device

PRECAUTIONS
- Avoid heat application
- Avoid prolonged standing/walking/deceleration and rotary sport activity
- Avoid valgus stress during therapeutic exercise and functional activities with concomitant medial collateral ligament (MCL) injury

TREATMENT STRATEGIES
- KT1000 exam
- Isokinetic tests/functional tests/balance test
- Measure for postoperative brace; don/doff instruction
- Cryotherapy instruction
- Gait training (progressive)
- PWB to WBAT (patella tendon) w/crutches, brace locked at 0 degrees
- Home program: postoperative therapeutic exercise instruction
  - Quadriceps sets
  - SLR (brace locked at 0 degrees)
  - Patella mobilization
  - Passive (towel) extensions
  - Active flexion/active-assisted extension 90 to 0 degrees exercise
- AROM and AAROM exercises
- Progressive resistive exercises and functional activities
- Electrical stimulation/biofeedback (muscle reeducation)

CRITERIA FOR SURGERY
- Normal ROM
- Normalize gait
- Demonstrate ability to ascend/descend stairs without assertive device
- Demonstrate independence in postoperative therapeutic exercise program

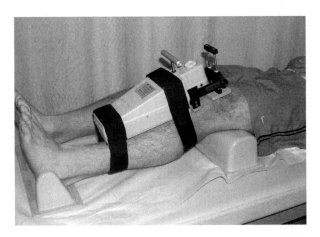

FIGURE **35-5** KT1000 Knee ligament arthrometer (Medmetric Corporation, San Diego).

POSTOPERATIVE PHASE I (WEEKS 0 TO 2)

Rehabilitation in the first phase of the postoperative program places an important emphasis on regaining full passive extension, progressive weight-bearing, control of postoperative effusion, and quadriceps reeducation. Immediate ROM is encouraged to minimize the deleterious effects of immobilization, such as articular cartilage degeneration, excessive adverse collagen formation, and pain.[11–13] Isometric graft placement allows for immediate motion without adverse loads. The patient is instructed to perform an active flexion/active-assisted extension exercise several times per day. A continuous passive motion (CPM) machine is recommended for home use, if the patient has difficulty attaining flexion ROM. Prevention of extension loss is the most crucial and important goal following ACL surgery.

Postoperative Phase I (Weeks 0 to 2)

GOALS
- Emphasis on full passive extension
- Control postoperative pain/swelling
- ROM 0 to 90 degrees
- Early progressive weight-bearing
- Prevent quadriceps inhibition
- Independence in home therapeutic exercise program

PRECAUTIONS
- Avoid active knee extension 40 to 0 degrees
- Avoid ambulation without brace locked at 0 degrees
- Avoid heat application
- Avoid prolonged standing/walking

TREATMENT STRATEGIES
- Towel extensions, prone hangs, etc.
- Quadriceps reeducation (quadriceps sets with electrical muscle simulator [EMS] or electromyography [EMG])
- Progressive weight-bearing PWB to WBAT (patella tendon) with brace locked at 0 degrees with crutches
- Patellar mobilization
- Active flexion/active-assisted extension 90 to 0 degrees exercise
- SLRs (all planes)
- Brace locked at 0 degrees for SLR (supine)
- Short crank ergometry
- Hip progressive resisted exercises
- Proprioception board (bilateral weight-bearing)
- Leg press (bilateral/70- to 5-degree arc) (if ROM >90 degrees)
- Upper extremity cardiovascular exercises as tolerated
- Cryotherapy
- Home therapeutic exercise program: evaluation-based
- Emphasize patient compliance to home therapeutic exercise program and weight-bearing precautions/progression

CRITERIA FOR ADVANCEMENT
- Ability to SLR without quadriceps lag
- ROM 0 to 90 degrees
- Demonstrate ability to unilateral (involved extremity) weight bear without pain

Loss of extension following ACL reconstruction can result in an abnormal gait, increased patellofemoral symptoms, and quadriceps weakness.[14,15] Full extension should be achieved 2 to 3 weeks following surgery. To achieve this goal the patient is instructed to sit and/or lie down with a towel under his or her heel, allowing gravity to apply a low-load prolonged stretch into extension (see Figure 35-3, A). Bracing is locked at 0 degrees for ambulation and sleeping. These activities will engage the graft in the intercondylar notch so as not to create an interval for notch scarring or arthrofibrosis to occur.

Another characteristic of the ACL reconstruction rehabilitation program is early weight-bearing. Advanced fixation techniques, such as cancellous screw bone-to-bone fixation, allow for immediate weight-bearing postoperatively. The patient is instructed to use a postoperative brace locked at 0 degrees for ambulation. Patients receiving an autogenous bone-patella tendon-bone (BPTB) graft are instructed to first partially (50%) weight-bear with crutches and then progressively bear more weight on successive days as to allow the knee joint to acclimate to increased loads. Within 1 week postoperatively the patient assumes a weight-bearing gait, as tolerated, with crutches.

Controlling postoperative effusion and quadriceps reeducation are important goals in this phase as well. The two are closely related. Spencer et al.[16] demonstrated a quadriceps inhibition in the presence of knee joint effusion. Mechanoreceptors in the joint capsule respond to changes in tension and, in turn, inhibit motor nerves supplying the quadriceps muscles. Therefore, controlling postoperative effusion will lead to decreased quadriceps inhibition, resulting in a faster return of muscle function. A commercial cold wrap device is used for 20 to 30 minutes and thereafter, 1 hour off throughout the early postoperative course. After suture removal, ice packs may be used directly for improved cooling. Quadriceps setting with an appropriate sized towel under the knee will allow for a quality/pain-free exercise for quadriceps reeducation. If a patient has difficulty eliciting a quadriceps contraction, a biofeedback unit or an electrical muscle stimulator can be used in conjunction with the quadriceps setting exercise to better facilitate quadriceps reeducation. An SLR is performed with the postoperative brace locked at 0 degrees until sufficient quadriceps control is demonstrated, that is, ability to SLR without pain and/or quadriceps lag.

Patellar mobilization should be performed by the rehabilitation specialist to assist in reestablishing normal patellar mobility. The patient can incorporate this activity into his or her daily home exercise program. The magnitude of the exercise should be graded based on the amount of inflammation present. Superior mobility of the patella is required for complete knee extension. Inferior glide of the patella is necessary for flexion.[17]

When ROM achieves 80 degrees, a short crank ergometer (Figure 35-6) can be used to develop strength, ROM, and cardiovascular conditioning. Schwartz et al.[18] have demonstrated that these therapeutic effects of stationary cycling can be attained early in the postoperative course by changing the ergometer crank from a standard 170 mm to smaller crank lengths (140 mm to 80 mm).

Proximal (hip) strengthening is initiated using a progressive resistive exercise (PRE) regime: cuff weights, isotonic exercise machines, and so forth.

Early neuromuscular training is encouraged because balance deficits have been identified following ACL reconstruction.[19–21] Balance assessment and training are started with progressive weight-bearing. A rocker board proprioception exercise can be used as soon as the patient achieves a 50% weight-bearing status (Figure 35-7).

As ROM improves ≥90 degrees and quadriceps control demonstrates improvement, a leg press exercise is incorporated into the program. This closed kinetic

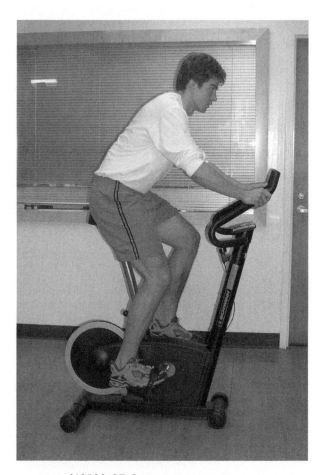

FIGURE 35-6 Short crank ergometer.

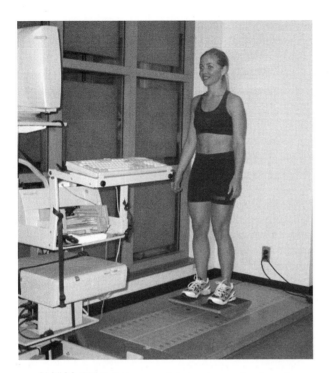

FIGURE **35-7** Balance training using rocker board.

gressed, as tolerated, using crutches. A normal gait pattern is required for discontinuing crutch ambulation. An underwater treadmill system is used to unload the involved extremity for ambulation training. Walking in chest deep water results in a 60% to 75% reduction in weight-bearing, whereas walking in waist deep water results in a 40% to 50% reduction in weight-bearing.[34,35]

The postoperative brace is changed per the surgeon's preference (off-the-shelf brace, patella sleeve, etc.). As ROM and strength improve, additional CKC exercises, such as squatting (Figure 35-8), and advanced balance activities are added to the program. Lutz et al.[23] calculated decreased posterior shear force (the resisting force to anterior drawer) during a squat vs open chain knee extension at all angles (Figure 35-9).

Balance activities are progressed to include unilateral weight-bearing, multiplanar support surfaces, and perturbation training (Figure 35-10). Activities should attempt to eliminate or alter sensory information from the visual, vestibular, and somatosensory systems so as to challenge the other systems.[36] Altering vision by having the patient close his or her eyes or catch and throw a ball while balancing will more specifically challenge the somatosensory system. Improving

chain (CKC) activity is initially performed bilaterally inside a pain-free arc (70 to 5 degrees) and, subsequently, advanced to a unilateral exercise using greater ROM in later phases. CKC exercises are used predominantly for strengthening in the early phases of the program because these activities have been shown to minimize stress to the ACL.[22-28] The patient's home therapeutic exercise program is continually updated based on evaluative findings.

Troubleshooting

Loss of motion is often cited as the most common complication following ACL reconstruction.[29-33] Full passive extension should be achieved during this phase. The patient should also strive for the attainment of 90-degree flexion. If these measurements are not attained, the rehabilitation specialist should communicate the patient's lack of progress with the referring orthopedic surgeon. Therapeutic interventions that include aggressive ROM activities, modalities to control pain and inflammation, as well as nonsteroidal anti-inflammatory drugs (NSAIDs) are implemented to achieve ROM goals. Emphasize patient compliance to home therapeutic exercise program and weight-bearing precautions/progression.

POSTOPERATIVE PHASE II (WEEKS 2 TO 6)

As quadriceps control improves, the postoperative brace is opened 0 to 50 degrees to allow for sufficient knee motion for level gait. Weight-bearing is pro-

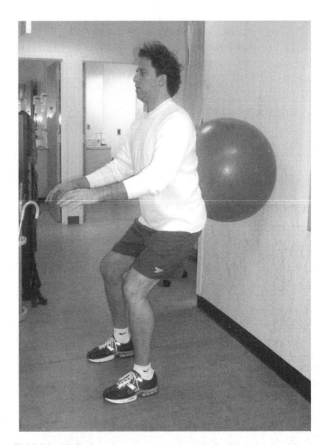

FIGURE **35-8** Squatting: CKC exercise. Patient squats down and up inside a pain-free arc of motion. Ball is used to promote proper form and balance during exercise.

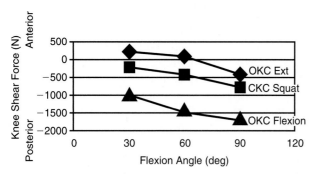

FIGURE **35-9** Graph representing anterior and posterior tibiofemoral shear forces incurred during select exercises: OKC knee flexion, CKC squat, OKC knee extension. *(Adapted from Lutz, G.E., Palmitier, R.A., An, K.N., Chao, E.Y. Comparison of Tibiofemoral Joint Forces During Open Kinetic Chain and Closed Kinetic Chain Exercises. J Bone Joint Surg 1993;75A:732–739.)*

neuromuscular reaction time to imposed loads will enhance dynamic stabilization around the knee and thus protect the static reconstructed tissue from overstress or reinjury.[37,38] As ROM improves to 110 to 115 degrees, cycling is advanced to a standard 170-mm ergometer. Fleming et al.[39] demonstrated in vivo relatively low ACL peak strain values during stationary cycling.

Unilateral CKC exercises, such as contralateral hip abduction and extension with Thera-Band, and graduated forward step-ups are added for additional strengthening and neuromuscular training. The patient is expected to demonstrate the ability to ascend an 8-inch step without pain and sufficient lower extremity control by 6 weeks postoperatively. Sequential KT1000 arthrometer examinations are performed at 6 weeks, 3 months, and 6 months postoperatively to record laxity values and substantiate progression of the postoperative

Postoperative Phase II (Weeks 2 to 6)

GOALS

- ROM 0 to 125 degrees
- Good patellar mobility
- Minimal swelling
- Restore normal gait (non-antalgic)
- Ascend 8-inch stairs with good control without pain

PRECAUTIONS

- Avoid descending stairs reciprocally until adequate quadriceps control and lower extremity alignment
- Avoid pain with therapeutic exercise and functional activities

TREATMENT STRATEGIES

- Progressive weight-bearing/WBAT (patellar tendon) with crutches brace opened 0 to 50 degrees, if good quadriceps control (good quadriceps set/ability to SLR without lag or pain)
- Discontinue crutches when gait is non-antalgic
- Brace changed to surgeon's preference (OTS brace, patella sleeve, etc.)
- Standard ergometry (if knee ROM >115 degrees)
- Leg press (80- to 0-degree arc)
- AAROM exercises
- Mini squats/weight shifts
- Proprioception training: prop board/biomechanical ankle platform system/contralateral Thera-Band exercises
- Initiate forward step-up program
- StairMaster
- AquaCiser (gait training) if incision benign
- SLRs (progressive resistance)
- Hamstring/calf flexibility exercises
- Hip/hamstring PRE
- Active knee extension to 40 degrees
- KT1000 Knee ligament arthrometer exam at 6 weeks (no max manual test)
- Home therapeutic exercise program: evaluation-based

CRITERIA FOR ADVANCEMENT

- ROM 0 to 125 degrees
- Normal gait pattern
- Demonstrate ability to ascend 8-inch step
- Good patellar mobility
- Functional progression pending KT1000 and functional assessment

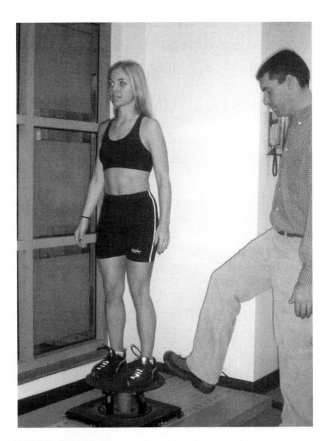

FIGURE **35-10** Perturbation training: Patient attempts to maintain balance as rehabilitation specialist taps stabilization training device.

program. Results of these examinations, along with patient progress, are shared with the referring orthopedic surgeon.

The patient's home therapeutic exercise program is continually updated based on evaluative findings.

Troubleshooting

A more common complication during this phase is the complaint of anterior knee pain. With the newfound ability to ambulate without an assistive device, patients may accelerate their activity level before they attain the sufficient lower extremity strength to meet the demands of their activity level. The patient must come to understand his or her limitations regarding standing, walking, and negotiating stairs. The rehabilitation specialist needs to individualize patient treatment, based on subjective complaints or a lack thereof as well as objective measures in progressing the patient through the criteria-based rehabilitation program. Modifications to daily findings must be considered to remediate complaints and safely continue the planned progression of the program. Compliance to prescribed or modified home therapeutic exercise as well as to activity modification in activities of daily living (ADL) should be emphasized.

POSTOPERATIVE PHASE III (WEEKS 6 TO 14)

Upon meeting the established criteria for advancement, the patient enters a phase designed to restore full ROM and improve lower extremity muscle strength and flexibility. Active-assisted range of motion (AAROM) exercises are continued and quadriceps stretching (supine and prone) are initiated. A PRE program is used during open kinetic chain (OKC) and CKC/functional exercises. A forward step-down program is introduced with progressive step heights (4, 6, and 8 inches). Retrograde treadmill ambulation on progressive percentage inclines is used to facilitate quadriceps strengthening[40] (Figure 35-11). If the 3-month knee ligament arthrometer testing proves satisfactory, isotonic knee extensions in a 90- to 40-degree arc may be implemented, monitoring patellofemoral symptoms. Advanced neuromuscular training activities are added to include sport cord agility activities, balance activities on less stable surfaces (foam rollers, rocker boards, etc.), and perturbation training.

At 3 months postoperatively a Forward Step-Down Test[41] (Figure 35-12) is performed to measure functional lower extremity muscle strength. This test entails the patient stepping down an 8-inch step onto a force plate as slowly and controlled as possible with each leg. Lower extremity control is observed for deviations. Mean impact and limb comparison are calculated and compared to the established norms of 10% body weight and 85% symmetry, respectively.[41]

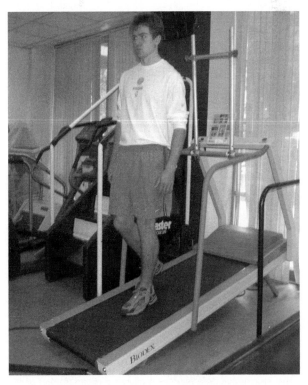

FIGURE **35-11** Retrograde treadmill ambulation.

Postoperative Phase III (Weeks 6 to 14)

GOALS

- Restore full ROM
- Demonstrate ability to descend 8-inch stairs with good leg control without pain
- Improve ADL endurance
- Improve lower extremity flexibility
- Protect patellofemoral joint

PRECAUTIONS

- Avoid pain with therapeutic exercise and functional activities
- Avoid running and sport activity until adequate strength development and surgeon's clearance

TREATMENT STRATEGIES

- Progress squat program
- Initiate step-down program
- Leg press
- Lunges
- Isotonic knee extensions 90 to 40 degrees (CKC exercises preferred)
- Advanced proprioception training (perturbations)
- Agility exercises (sport cord)
- VersaClimber
- Retrograde treadmill ambulation/running
- Quadriceps stretching
- Forward Step-Down Test (NeuroCom)
- KT1000 Knee ligament arthrometer exam at 3 months
- Home therapeutic exercise program: evaluation-based

CRITERIA FOR ADVANCEMENT

- ROM to WNL
- Ability to descend 8-inch stairs with good leg control without pain
- Functional progression pending KT1000 and functional assessment

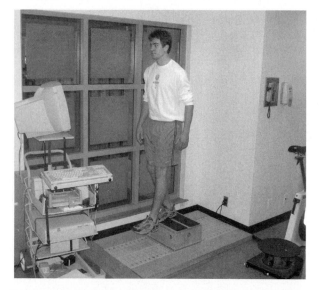

FIGURE 35-12 Forward Step-Down Test. The patient steps down an 8-inch step onto the force plate (Balance Master System, NeuroCom International Inc., Clackamas, OR) as slowly and controlled as possible on each leg. Three trials are recorded. Mean impact and limb symmetry are calculated and interpreted. Lower extremity control is observed for deviations. Normative data have established a mean impact of 10% body weight and limb symmetry of 85%.

Upon satisfactory results, a running program is initiated on a treadmill. Forward running is preceded by backward running because retro-running is shown to have decreased patellofemoral joint compression forces when compared to backward running.[42] The patient's home therapeutic exercise program is continually updated based on evaluative findings.

Troubleshooting

Now functioning at a higher level, the patient continues to need encouragement to adhere to functional limitations based on deficits in ROM, flexibility, and muscle strength. The rehabilitation specialist needs to implement treatment strategies, as described previously, to ensure that criteria are met before advancing to higher demand activities (e.g., descending an 8-inch step before initiating a forward-running program).

Patients should be advised to watch the volume of their PRE program. Altering weight training days, monitoring the number of repetitions of select strengthening exercises, and cross-training will allow for recovery and decrease the possibility of an overuse condition from developing.

POSTOPERATIVE PHASE IV (WEEKS 14 TO 22)

Upon meeting set criteria for advancement, the patient enters a phase directed at improving overall function. Also emphasized are treatment strategies designed to prepare the patient/athlete for the safe return to that individual's sport. A forward-running program (treadmill) is progressed with an emphasis on speed over shorter distances vs slower distance running. Isotonic and isokinetic knee extension exercises are progressed to a full arc. PRE and flexibility programs continue to be progressed as tolerated. Depending on the individual's sport, agility activities, that is, deceleration training, are adapted for sport-specific performance. If deemed a requirement for a specific sport, plyometric exercises are implemented. Attention should be made to also incorporate a contralateral lower extremity flexibility program to decrease overuse symptoms from developing.

The patient's home therapeutic exercise program is continually updated based on evaluative findings.

Troubleshooting

Before incorporating plyometric exercises into a treatment regime, full ROM and good flexibility should be restored. An adequate strength base should also be developed. Chu[43] has described a simple functional test to determine whether plyometric training should be initiated. Acceptable strength is demonstrated by the patient power squatting five squat repetitions in 5 seconds, with a weight equal to 60% of the patient's body weight. Plyometric training should follow a functional progression with its components of speed, intensity, load, volume, and frequency being monitored and progressed accordingly.

Activities should begin with simple drills and advance to more complex exercises (e.g., double-leg jumping) (Figure 35-13) vs box drills. The patient/athlete should be counseled to maintain variety into his or her weekly program. More specifically, the patient/athlete should dedicate 1 day to weight training, after a proper warm-up, another day for running, another day for his or her plyometric program, and, most importantly, a day of rest to allow for muscle recovery.

Postoperative Phase IV (Weeks 14 to 22)

GOALS
- Demonstrate ability to run pain-free
- Maximize strength and flexibility as to meet demands of ADL
- Hop test ≥75% limb symmetry

PRECAUTIONS
- Avoid pain with therapeutic exercise and functional activities
- Avoid sport activity until adequate strength development and surgeon's clearance

TREATMENT STRATEGIES
- Start forward-running (treadmill) program when 8-inch step-down satisfactory
- Continue lower extremity strengthening and flexibility programs
- Advance agility program/sport-specific
- Start plyometric program when strength base sufficient
- Isotonic knee extension (full arc/pain and crepitus free) (CKC exercises preferred)
- Isokinetic training (fast to moderate velocities) (CKC exercises preferred)
- KT1000 Knee ligament arthrometer exam at 3 months
- Home therapeutic exercise program: evaluation-based

CRITERIA FOR ADVANCEMENT
- Symptom-free running
- Hop test ≥75% limb symmetry
- Functional progression pending and functional assessment

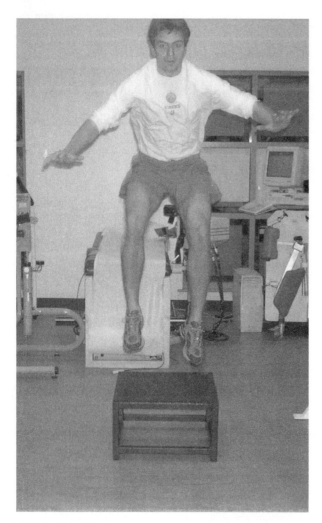

FIGURE **35-13** Plyometric training (double-leg jumping): Patient jumps up onto 10-inch step and softly lands.

POSTOPERATIVE PHASE V (WEEK 22 AND BEYOND)

This final phase of the rehabilitation program can truly be considered a return to sport phase. Particular emphasis is paid to the individual patient's sport and position in that sport. Strength and flexibility deficits are addressed. Plyometric and agility exercises are advanced to sport-specific movement. Such activities may include actual sport participation drills, with or without contact. An ACL brace is often prescribed.

Subjective complaints as well as objective observation of apprehension in sport-specific movement are recorded. Final testing to include KT1000 testing, functional hop tests, and isokinetic tests are performed to substantiate laxity, strength, and power at discharge. The goals of isokinetic and functional testing include a less than 15% deficit for quadriceps and hamstring

average peak torque and total work at test velocities of 60 and 240 degrees per second. Functional testing links specific components of function and the actual task and provides direct evidence to prove functional status. The single-leg hop test (Figure 35-14) and cross-over hop tests are performed with the goal of achieving an 85% limb symmetry score.

The results of these tests, along with any other pertinent clinical findings, are presented to the referring orthopedic surgeon for the final determination of sports participation.

Troubleshooting

In this final (return to play) phase the rehabilitation specialist should prepare the patient/athlete to meet the demands of his or her individual sport by ensuring that the criteria of ROM, flexibility, strength, power, and endurance have been restored. These criteria need to be met to decrease the possibility of reinjury. Assessment of strength and functional capacity will provide evidence as to the progress and success of the rehabilitation program.

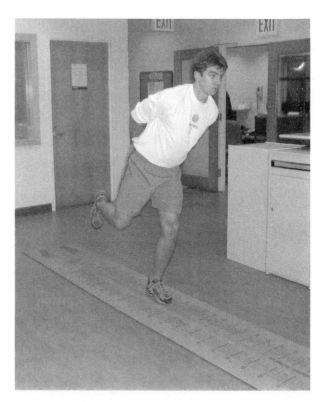

FIGURE **35-14** Hop test: Patient stands on one leg and attempts to jump as far as possible, landing on the same leg. Three trials are recorded on each extremity and averaged. Limb symmetry is calculated by dividing the involved extremity score by the noninvolved extremity score.

Postoperative Phase V (Week 22 and Beyond)

GOALS

- Lack of apprehension with sport-specific movements
- Maximize strength and flexibility as to meet demands of individual's sport activity
- Hop test ≥85% limb symmetry

PRECAUTIONS

- Avoid pain with therapeutic exercise and functional activities
- Avoid sport activity until adequate strength development and surgeon's clearance

TREATMENT STRATEGIES

- Continue to advance lower extremity strengthening, flexibility, and agility programs
- Advance plyometric program
- Brace for sport activity (surgeon's preference)
- Monitor patient's activity level throughout course of rehabilitation
- Reassess patient's complaint's (i.e., pain/swelling daily—adjust program accordingly)
- Encourage compliance to home therapeutic exercise program
- KT1000 Knee ligament arthrometer exam at 6 months
- Home therapeutic exercise program: evaluation-based

CRITERIA FOR DISCHARGE

- Hop test ≥85% limb symmetry
- Lack of apprehension with sport-specific movements
- Flexibility to accepted levels of sport performance
- Independence with gym program for maintenance and progression of therapeutic exercise program at discharge

REFERENCES

1. Miyasaka, K.C., Daniel, D.M., Stone, M.L., Hirschman, P. *The Incidence of Knee Ligament Injuries in the General Population.* Am J Knee Surg 1991;4:3–8.
2. Johnson, R.J. *The Anterior Cruciate Ligament Problem.* Clin Orthop 1983;172:14–18.
3. Noyes, F.R., Mooar, P.A., Matthews, D.S., Butler, D.L. *The Symptomatic Anterior Cruciate-deficient Knee. Part I. The Long-term Functional Disability in Athletically Active Individuals.* J Bone Joint Surg Am 1983;65:154–162.
4. Noyes, F.R., Butler, D.L., Grood, E.S., Zernicke, R.F., Hefzy, M.S. *Biomechanical Analysis of Human Ligament Grafts Used in Knee Ligament Repairs and Reconstructions.* J Bone Joint Surg 1984;66A:344–352.
5. Clancy, W.G., Narechania, R.G., Rosenberg, T.D., Gmeiner, J.G., Wisnefske, D.D., Lange, T.A. *Anterior and Posterior Cruciate Ligament Reconstruction in Rhesus Monkeys.* J Bone Joint Surg 1981;63A:1270–1284.
6. Drez, D.J., DeLee, J., Holden, J.P., Arnoczky, S., Noyes, F.R., Roberts, T.S. *Anterior Cruciate Ligament Reconstruction Using Bone-patella Tendon-bone Allografts. A Biological and Biomechanical Evaluation in Goats.* Am J Sports Med 1991;19:256–263.
7. Falcoiero, R.P., DiStefano, V.J., Cook, T.M. *Revascularization and Ligamentization of Autogenous Anterior Cruciate Ligament Grafts in Humans.* Arthroscopy 1998;14(2):197–205.
8. Rougraff, B.T., Shelbourne, K.D. *Early Histologic Appearance of Human Patella Tendon Autografts Used for Anterior Cruciate Ligament Reconstruction.* Knee Surg Sports Traumatol Arthrosc 1999;7(1):9–14.
9. Shelbourne, K.D., Wilckens, J.H., Mollabaashy, A., DeCarlo, M.S. *Arthrofibrosis in Acute Anterior Cruciate Ligament Reconstruction: The Effect of Timing of Reconstruction and Rehabilitation.* Am J Sports Med 1991;9:332–336.
10. Shelbourne, K.D., Foulk, A.D. *Timing of Surgery in Acute Anterior Cruciate Ligament Tears on the Return of Quadriceps Muscle Strength after Reconstruction Using an Autogenous Patella Tendon Graft.* Am J Sports Med 1995;23:686–689.
11. Akeson, W.H., Woo, S.L.-Y, Amiel, D. *The Connective Tissue Response to Immobilization: Biomechanical Changes in Periarticular Connective Tissue of the Immobilized Rabbit Knee.* Clin Orthop 1973;93:356–362.
12. Noyes, F.R., Mangine, R.E., Barber, S. *Early Knee Motion after Open and Arthroscopic ACL Reconstruction.* Am J Sports Med 1987;15(2):149–160.
13. Salter, R.H., Simmonds, D.F., Malcolm, B.W., Rumble, E.J., MacMichael, D., Clements, N.D. *The Biological Effect of Continuous Passive Motion on Healing of Full-thickness Defects in Articular Cartilage.* J Bone Joint Surg 1980;62A(8):1232–1251.
14. Benum, P. *Operative Mobilization of Stiff Knees after Surgical Treatment of Knee Injuries and Posttraumatic Conditions.* Acta Orthop Scand 1982;53:625–631.
15. Perry, J., Antonelli, D., Ford, W. *Analysis of Knee-joint Forces During Flexed-knee Stance.* J Bone Joint Surg 1975;57A:961–967.
16. Spencer, J.D., Hayes, K.C., Alexander, L.J. *Knee Joint Effusion and Quadriceps Inhibition in Man.* Arch Phys Med Rehabil 1984;65(4):171–177.
17. Fulkerson, J.P., Hungerford, D. *Disorders of the Patellofemoral Joint,* 2nd ed. Williams & Wilkins, Baltimore, 1990.

18. Schwartz, R.E., Asnis, P.D., Cavanaugh, J.T., Asnis, S.E., Simmons, J.E., Lasinski, P.J. *Short Crank Cycle Ergometry.* J Orthop Sports Phys Ther 1991;13:95.

19. Jerosch, J., Schaffer, C., Prymka, M. *Proprioceptive Abilities of Surgically and Conservatively Treated Knee Joints with Injuries of the Cruciate Ligament.* Unfallchirurg 1998;101(1):26–31.

20. Paterno, M.V., Gelb, I.D., Hewett, T.E., Noyes, F.R. *The Return of Neuromuscular Coordination after Anterior Cruciate Ligament Reconstruction (Abstract).* J Orthop Sports Phys Ther 1998; 27(1):96.

21. Shiraishi, M., Mizuta, H., Kubota, K., Otsuka, Y., Nagamoto, N., Takagi, K. *Stabilimetric Assessment in the Anterior Cruciate Ligament Reconstructed Knee.* Clin J Sports Med 1996;6(1): 32–39.

22. Henning, C.E., Lynch, M.A., Glick, K.R. *An In Vivo Strain Gage Study of Elongation of the Anterior Cruciate Ligament.* Am J Sports Med 1985;13(1):22–26.

23. Lutz, G.E., Palmitier, R.A., An, K.N., Chao, E.Y. *Comparison of Tibiofemoral Joint Forces During Open Kinetic Chain and Closed Kinetic Chain Exercises.* J Bone Joint Surg 1993;75A:732–739.

24. Ohkoshi, Y., Yasuda, K., Kaneda, K., Wada, T., Yamanaka, M. *Biomechanical Analysis of Rehabilitation in the Standing Position.* Am J Sports Med 1991;19(6):605–611.

25. Sawhney, R., Dearwater, S., Irrgang, J.J., Fu, F.H. *Quadriceps Exercise Following ACL Reconstruction Without Anterior Tibial Displacement.* Presented at American Physical Therapy Association annual meeting, Anaheim, CA, June 1990.

26. Wilk, K.E., Escamilla, R.F., Fleisig, G.S., Barrentine, S.W., Andrews, J.R., Boyd, M.L. *A Comparison of Tibiofemoral Joint Forces and Electromyographic Activity During Open and Closed Kinetic Chain Exercises.* Am J Sports Med 1996;24(4):518–527.

27. Wojtys, E.M., Wylie, B.B., Huston, L.J. *The Effects of Muscle Fatigue on Neuromuscular Function and Anterior Tibial Translation in Healthy Knees.* Am J Sports Med 1996;24:615–621.

28. Yack, H.J., Collins, C.E., Whieldon, T.J. *Comparison of Closed and Open Kinetic Chain Exercise in the Anterior Cruciate Ligament-deficient Knee.* Am J Sports Med 1993;21(1):49–54.

29. Johnson, R.J., Eriksson, E., Haggmark, T., Pope, M.H. *Five- to 10-year Follow-up Evaluation after Reconstruction of the Anterior Cruciate Ligament.* Clin Orthop 1984;183:122–140.

30. Kornblatt, I., Warren, R.F., Wickiewicz, T.L. *Long-term Follow-up of Anterior Cruciate Ligament Reconstruction Using the Quadriceps Tendon Substitution for Chronic Anterior Cruciate Ligament Insufficiency.* Am J Sports Med 1988;16:444–448.

31. Montgomery, K.D., Cavanaugh, J., Cohen, S., Wickiewicz, T.L., Warren, R.F., Blevens, F. *Motion Complications after Arthroscopic Repair of Anterior Cruciate Ligament Avulsion Fractures in the Adult.* Arthroscopy 2002;18(2):171–176.

32. Millett, P.J., Wickiewicz, T.L., Warren, R.F. *Motion Loss after Ligament Injuries to the Knee. Part I: Causes.* Am J Sports Med 2001;29(5):664–675.

33. Harner, C.D., Irrgang, J.J., Paul, J., Dearwater, S., Fu, F.H. *Loss of Motion after Anterior Cruciate Ligament Reconstruction.* Am J Sports Med 1992;20:499–506.

34. Bates, A., Hanson, N. The Principles and Properties of Water. In *Aquatic Exercise Therapy.* WB Saunders, Philadelphia, 1996, pp. 1–320.

35. Harrison, R.A., Hilman, M., Bulstrode, S. *Loading of the Lower Limb When Walking Partially Immersed: Implications for Clinical Practice.* Physiotherapy 1992;78:164.

36. Guskiewicz, K.M. Regaining Balance and Postural Equilibrium. In Prentice, W.E. (Ed). *Rehabilitation Techniques in Sports Medicine,* 3rd ed. WCB/McGraw-Hill, New York, 1999, pp. 107–133.

37. Johansson, H., Sjolander, P., Soojka, P. *Activity in Receptor Afferents Front the Anterior Cruciate Ligament Evokes Reflex Effects on Fusimotor Neurones.* Neurosci Res (NY) 1990;8:54–59.

38. Cavanaugh, J.T., Moy, R.J. *Balance and Postoperative Lower Extremity Joint Reconstruction.* Orthop Phys Ther Clin NA 2002;11(1):75–99.

39. Fleming, B.C., Beynnon, B.D., Renstrom, P.A., Peura, G.D., Nichols, C.E., Johnson, R.J. *The Strain Behavior of the Anterior Cruciate Ligament During Bicycling.* Am J Sports Med 1998; 26(1):109–118.

40. Cipriani, D.J., Armstrong, C.W., Gaul, S. *Backward Walking at Three Levels of Treadmill Inclination: An Electromyographic and Kinematic Analysis.* J Orthop Sports Phys Ther 1995;22(3): 95–102.

41. Cavanaugh, J.T., Stump, T.J. *Forward Step Down Test.* J Orthop Sports Phys Ther 2000;30(1):A–46.

42. Flynn, T.W., Soutas-Little, R.W. *Patellofemoral Joint Compressive Forces in Forward and Backward Running.* J Orthop Sports Phys Ther 1995;21(5):277–282.

43. Chu, D.A. *Jumping into Plyometrics.* Leisure Press, Champaign, IL, 1992.

36

Posterior Cruciate
Ligament Reconstruction

JOHN T. CAVANAUGH, PT, MED, ATC

The posterior cruciate ligament (PCL) functions as the primary restraint to posterior displacement of the tibia relative to the femur.[1] Injury to the PCL accounts for approximately 3% of all knee injuries in the general population.[2] In patients who present to trauma centers with knee injuries, the incidence has reported as high as 37%.[3] Isolated PCL injuries may occur at a rate of 40%.[4] The most frequent mechanism of injury in isolated PCL tears is a direct blow on the anterior tibia with the knee flexed position.[5] Injury to the PCL is often associated with concomitant pathology. Additional knee structures may be injured as a result of hyperextension, hyperflexion, or rotational mechanisms associated with valgus/varus stress.[5,6] Management following PCL injury remains controversial. Some investigators have reported successful outcomes in patients treated without surgery who have developed excellent quadriceps strength.[7–11] Other long-term follow-up studies of PCL injuries treated conservatively have demonstrated degenerative changes accompanied by pain in the patellofemoral joint and the medial compartment of the tibiofemoral joint.[4,12,13] Whether reconstruction of the PCL will alter the natural history of the PCL-deficient knee continues to be studied. Clinical results following PCL reconstruction have not been as predictable as those after anterior cruciate ligament reconstruction.[12]

Posterior cruciate ligament reconstructions may be performed using various surgical techniques and graft substitutes. Traditional techniques use a transtibial technique, whereas, more recently, PCL reconstructions have used the posterior inlay technique as well as a two-femoral tunnel (double bundle) procedure. Achilles tendon allograft and bone-patella, tendon-bone autografts are commonly used as graft substitutes. The technique of choice at the Hospital for Special Surgery (HSS) is a transtibial fixation double-bundle PCL reconstruction with an Achilles tendon allograft. The rehabilitation program following this procedure is presented.

SURGICAL OVERVIEW

The PCL is the stronger and larger of the cruciate ligaments. The ligament has a broad, fan-shaped femoral attachment and a narrower insertion to the posterior tibia.[13] The PCL is composed of two separate bundles: the anterolateral and posteromedial (Figure 36-1). The anterolateral bundle is taut when the knee is flexed, and the posteromedial bundle is taut when the knee is near extension.[14] The anterolateral bundle is stronger, stiffer, and has a higher ultimate load to failure than the posteromedial bundle.[15,16] Traditionally, the anterolateral bundle has been the focus of PCL reconstructive surgery. In recent years, a double-bundle PCL reconstruction

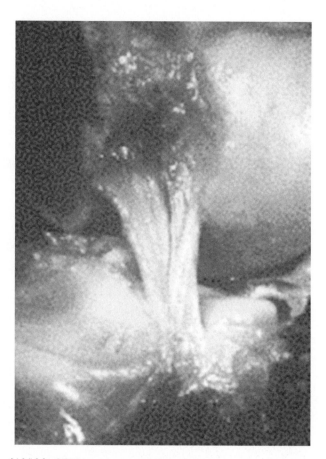

FIGURE **36-1** Posterior cruciate ligament. *(Photo courtesy HSS Sports Medicine Service.)*

has been used to better replicate knee anatomy and biomechanics.[17–19]

The transtibial fixation double-bundle PCL reconstruction is performed using an all arthroscopic technique. A split Achilles tendon allograft is used as the graft substitute because it allows for excellent tibial fixation with the bone block and sufficient soft tissue for two femoral bundles (Figure 36-2). The bundles are split to make bundles of 8 mm (anterolateral) and 7 mm (posteromedial). The tibial tunnel is prepared first for the transtibial fixation. A PCL tibial guide is placed through an anteromedial portal and the tibial tunnel is then reamed. The femoral tunnels are then created after an anteromedial incision is made for exposure of the anteromedial femoral condyle (Figure 36-3). A double femoral tunnel guide is used to place the guide pins for the two tunnels. The tunnels are drilled using an outside-in technique. The two bundles are then passed up the tibial tunnel and pulled through their respective femoral tunnels and tensioned appropriately. A metal interference screw placed between the bone block and the tunnel is used for tibial fixation. The individual bundles are fixated into the femoral tunnels, using bioabsorbable

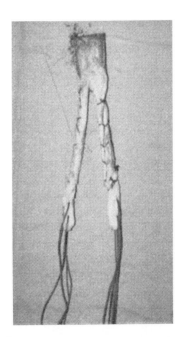

FIGURE **36-2** Split Achilles tendon allograft prepared for passage. *(Photo courtesy HSS Sports Medicine Service.)*

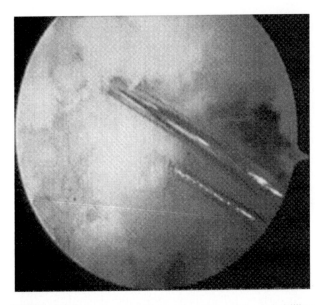

FIGURE **36-3** K-wires positioned for femoral tunnel drilling on the anteromedial femoral condyle during double-bundle PCL reconstruction. *(Photo courtesy HSS Sports Medicine Service.)*

interference screws and an outside-in technique. Postoperatively, the patient is placed in a double upright hinged brace locked at 0 degrees of extension.

REHABILITATION OVERVIEW

The rehabilitation program following PCL reconstruction is designed to progressively restore knee range of motion (ROM) and lower extremity strength while at the same time protect the graft replacement and fixation from deleterious forces. The rehabilitation specialist needs to consider and apply his or her knowledge of knee biomechanics and the altered biomechanics inherent of the PCL-deficient and reconstructed knee throughout the rehabilitative process. Communication between the surgeon and rehabilitation specialist is vital. Additional structural involvement identified during surgery will have a direct effect on program design and progression. The patient is progressed via a criteria-based functional progression. The patient should be made aware of his or her role in the rehabilitative process. The patient's compliance to prescribed therapeutic exercises and activity modifications is vital for a successful outcome.

PREOPERATIVE REHABILITATION

Before undergoing a PCL reconstruction, restoring normal knee ROM and lower extremity muscle function is recommended. Normalization of gait and the ability to reciprocate stairs are also goals of a preoperative rehabilitation program. At least one formal preoperative rehabilitation session is recommended. Patient education is emphasized during preoperative sessions. Instruction and subsequent independence in a postoperative exercise program can accelerate rehabilitation gains in the immediate postoperative period and limit complications from developing. Therapeutic exercises include passive extension with a pillow placed under the involved calf to promote full extension quadriceps setting, straight leg raise (SLR) with a postoperative brace locked at 0 degrees, and an active-assisted range of motion (AAROM) exercise where concentric and eccentric control of the involved quadriceps muscles are used. Active knee flexion is avoided during the early phases following PCL reconstruction. High forces on the graft substitute and fixation site have been demonstrated with this activity.[20-22] The patient is also taught self-patellar mobilizations to prevent postoperative adhesion formation. The patient is measured for a postoperative double-hinged brace and instructed in its management (donning/doffing). The patient is encouraged to don the postoperative brace while sleeping, ambulating, and performing a supine SLR. The patient is measured for crutches and taught to ambulate using toe-touch weight-bearing on all surfaces. A KT1000 Knee ligament arthrometer test (Medmetric Corporation, San Diego) is performed to document preoperative laxity. Strength testing (isokinetic and/or functional tests) and balance testing are performed if appropriate for baseline measures. The patient is encouraged to administer cryotherapy for postoperative pain and effusion control. Portable commercial cold devices (e.g., Cryo/cuff, Aircast Inc., Summit, NJ) are often prescribed by the patient's surgeon.

Posterior Cruciate Ligament Reconstruction: Preoperative Phase

GOALS

- Patient education
- Restore normal ROM
- Normalize gait
- Maximize strength/functional capabilities and demonstrate ability to ascend/descend stairs without assistive device
- Independent with postoperative therapeutic exercise program
- Independent with crutches toe touch weight bearing on all surfaces

TREATMENT STRATEGIES

- Knee ligament arthrometer exam
- Isokinetic test/functional tests/balance testing as appropriate
- Measure for postoperative brace; don/doff instruction
- Cryotherapy instruction
- Gait training: TTWB w/crutches, brace locked at 0 degrees
- Therapeutic exercise instruction
  - Passive (pillow under calf) extensions
  - Quadriceps sets
  - SLR (brace locked at 0 degrees)
  - Patellar mobilization
  - Active-assisted knee extension/passive flexion exercise (ROM 0 to 70 degrees)

POSTOPERATIVE PHASE I (WEEKS 0 TO 6)

Rehabilitation following PCL reconstruction is begun immediately postoperatively. Early mobilization of the surgical knee is encouraged. Early motion has been shown to minimize the deleterious effects of immobilization, such as articular cartilage degeneration, excessive collagen formation, and pain.[23-25] ROM exercises are performed in sitting, with the goal of achieving 70-degree flexion by 4 weeks and 90-degree flexion at 6 weeks. The patient is taught to passively flex the involved knee with the support of the noninvolved extremity (eccentric quadriceps contraction). The knee is then active-assistively extended to 0 degrees via concentric contractions of the bilateral quadriceps muscles (Figure 36-4). Achieving full passive extension is seldom a complication following PCL reconstructive surgery, but it must be addressed and achieved in the early postoperative period to ensure proper patellofemoral mechanics. Extension ROM is facilitated by having the patient rest his or her involved calf on a pillow, allowing gravity to assist in regaining extension (Figure 36-5). Patellar mobilization is an important intervention during this phase because flexion is restricted to protect the graft substitute (Figure 36-6). Normal inferior glide of the patella is necessary for knee flexion.[26] This treatment is performed by the rehabilitation specialist and taught to the patient to perform at home.

Weight-bearing with crutches progresses from toe-touch weight-bearing for the first 2 weeks to partial weight-bearing (50%) by week 4 and (75%) weight-bearing by week 6. The brace is kept locked at 0 degrees extension for ambulation during this period as to minimize posterior tibial shear forces created by hamstrings activation. Morrison[27] reported a posterior tibiofemoral shear force of 0.4 times body weight during level walking. Quadriceps strengthening is a central component for PCL reconstruction programs because the quadriceps serve as a dynamic stabilizer in preventing posterior tibial translation.[28] Quadriceps setting with an appropriate sized towel under the knee will allow for a quality/pain-free exercise for quadriceps reeducation. Electrical stimulation and/or biofeedback used in conjunction with this exercise is useful in deterring quadriceps inhibition and atrophy.[29,30] An SLR is performed with the postoperative brace locked at 0 degrees until sufficient quadriceps control is demonstrated, that is, the ability to SLR without pain and/or quadriceps lag.

To further aid in lower extremity strength development, select open kinetic chain (OKC) and closed kinetic chain (CKC) exercises are implemented into the program. Supported by research, these activities aim to build lower extremity strength without placing undo stress on the maturing graft substitute.[21,22,31,32] OKC multiple angle quadriceps isometrics inside a 60- to 30-degree arc of motion are used bilaterally with submaximal effort. As ROM improves, a CKC leg press is introduced inside a 60- to 0-degree arc of motion (Figure 36-7). When ROM achieves 80-degree flexion, short crank ergometry is incorporated into the program to develop strength, ROM, and cardiovascular conditioning.[33]

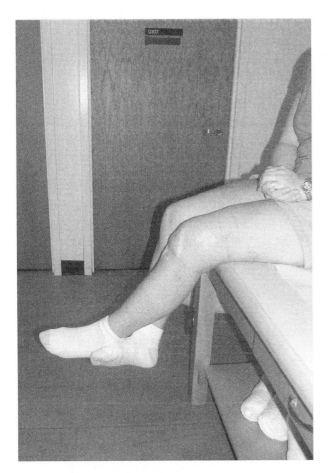

FIGURE **36-4** AAROM exercise. The uninvolved extremity supports the involved extremity as gravity assists in flexing the involved knee until a stretch is felt. The noninvolved quadriceps then assists the involved quadriceps in returning the involved knee to full extension. Concentric and eccentric controls of both quadriceps are used.

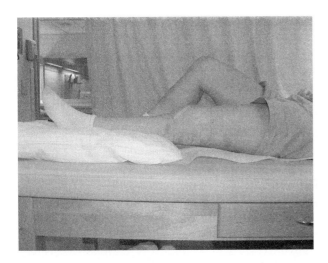

FIGURE **36-5** Passive extension with a pillow placed under the involved calf to promote extension.

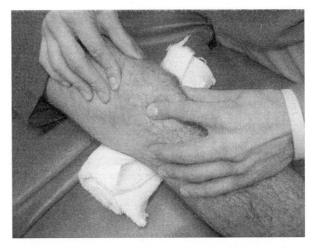

FIGURE **36-6** Patellar mobilization.

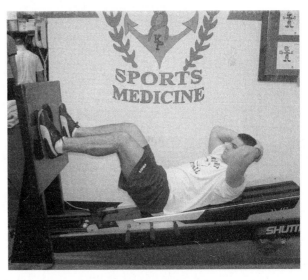

FIGURE **36-7** Closed kinetic chain leg press. Arc of motion 60 to 0 degrees.

Neuromuscular training is initiated as a 50% weight-bearing status is achieved. Balance training in cardinal planes is performed using a rocker board. A computerized force plate system is incorporated into the program to provide the patient with visual feedback. Proximal (hip) strengthening is initiated with multiple plane SLRs, progressing to a progressive resistive exercise (PRE) regime, using cuff weights. Isotonic exercise machines are added to further challenge the proximal musculature.

Flexibility exercises are performed for the hamstring and calf musculature. Knee joint effusion and quadriceps inhibition are closely related.[34] Controlling postoperative swelling, therefore, will lead to a faster return of muscle function. To assist in this goal, the patient is encouraged to avoid prolonged standing, maintain

Postoperative Phase I (Weeks 0 to 6)

GOALS

- Control postoperative pain/swelling
- ROM 0 to 90 degrees
- Prevent quadriceps inhibition
- Improve patellar mobility
- Independence in home therapeutic exercise program

PRECAUTIONS

- Avoid active knee flexion
- Avoid heat application
- Avoid ambulation without brace locked at 0 degrees
- Avoid exceeding ROM and weight-bearing limitations
- Avoid pain with therapeutic exercise and functional activities

TREATMENT STRATEGIES

- Passive extension (pillow under calf)
- Quadriceps reeducation (quadriceps sets with electrical muscle stimulator [EMS] or electromyography [EMG])
- Gait: weight-bearing TTWB with brace locked at 0 degrees with crutches
  - Progressive weight-bearing at weeks 2 to 6 to 75%
- Patellar mobilization
- Active-assisted knee extension/passive flexion exercise (ROM 0 to 70 degrees)
  - Progress to 90 degrees, as tolerated, weeks 4 to 6
- SLRs (supine/prone), brace locked at 0 degrees
- SLRs (all planes)/progressive resistance
- Multiple angle quadriceps isometrics (ROM 60 to 20 degrees)
- Leg press (ROM 60- to 0-degree arc) (bilaterally)
- Proximal (hip) strengthening PREs
- Proprioception training (bilateral weight-bearing)
- Hamstring/calf flexibility exercises
- Short crank ergometry
- Cardiovascular exercises (UBE, Airdyne, etc.), as tolerated
- Cryotherapy
- Emphasize patient compliance to home therapeutic exercise program and weight-bearing precautions

CRITERIA FOR ADVANCEMENT

- ROM 0 to 90 degrees
- Ability to bear 75% weight on involved extremity
- Ability to SLR without quadriceps lag
- Continued improvement in patellar mobility and proximal strength

proper weight-bearing restrictions, and apply some form of cryotherapy to the involved knee several times per day based on symptoms. Throughout phase I, the patient's home therapeutic exercise program is continually updated. Compliance to this program is encouraged.

Troubleshooting

During this maximal protective phase of rehabilitation, the patient will need encouragement to adhere to weight-bearing and ROM restrictions. Graft fixation needs time to mature, and excessive weight-bearing or flexion ROM may compromise long-term outcome. Communication between the rehabilitation specialist and the referring orthopedic surgeon is vital during

this phase. Compliance to rehabilitation and progress, or lack thereof, serves as important information for the physician in his or her endeavor to direct the program.

POSTOPERATIVE PHASE II (WEEKS 6 TO 12)

The second phase of rehabilitation following PCL reconstruction is directed toward progressive improvement in knee ROM, the normalization of gait and improved ability to perform activities of daily living (ADL).

AAROM exercises are performed with the goal of achieving 130 degrees of flexion by the twelfth postoperative week. As ROM improves to 110 to 115 degrees, cycling is advanced to a standard 170-mm ergometer. At 6 weeks postoperatively, the postoperative brace is changed per the surgeon's preference (OTS-PCL brace, patellar sleeve, etc.).

Weight-bearing is progressed, as tolerated, using crutches. Upon demonstrating a normal gait pattern, crutches are discontinued. To assist the patient in the transition off crutches, an underwater treadmill system is used. Gait sequencing is aided by the unloading properties of the water.[35,36]

Strengthening programs are advanced, with specific attention paid to the forces generated during therapeutic exercises. A CKC leg press, squats, and OKC knee extensions are performed inside a 0- to 60-degree ROM. Wilk et al.[32] demonstrated increased posterior forces with OKC knee extension, CKC squat, and leg press at flexion angles greater than 60 degrees. Lutz et al.[21] demonstrated posterior shear forces during a CKC squat exercise, but the forces were significantly less than those produced during OKC knee flexion. Quadriceps strengthening is further developed by having the patient retrograde ambulate on a treadmill at progressive inclines.[37] Isolated OKC hamstring strengthening is avoided for the first 5 postoperative months (Figure 36-8). Toutoungi et al.[22] calculated that during isokinetic/isometric flexion exercises, peak PCL loads occur at approximately 90-degree knee flexion and that these loads may exceed four times body weight. Careful attention must be paid to the patellofemoral joint during strengthening exercises. Loaded arcs of motion that present with pain and/or crepitus should be avoided. Skyhar et al.[38] studied the effects of sectioning the PCL on medial compartment and patellofemoral contact pressures. The group reported a 16% increase in patellofemoral contact pressure when the PCL was sectioned, with the most significant increases occurring at 60 degrees of knee flexion. As ROM and lower extremity muscle strength demonstrate improvement, functional activities, such as graduated step-ups (4, 6, and 8

inches) and step-downs are later introduced to the program. The goals for this phase include having the patient demonstrate the ability to ascend an 8-inch step and descend a 6-inch step by the twelfth postoperative week (Figure 36-9).

Neuromuscular control activities are used to aid in the development of dynamic stabilization. Balance activities are progressed to include unilateral weight-bearing on less stable support surfaces (foam rollers, rocker boards, multiplanar surfaces, etc.), contralateral elastic band exercises, and perturbation training. Improving neuromuscular reaction time is intended to enhance dynamic stabilization around the knee and thus protect the static reconstructed tissue from overstress or reinjury.[39]

Lower extremity flexibility exercises are continued, with the addition of quadriceps stretching, as the involved knee attains 120 degrees of flexion. Daily application of cryotherapy, compliance to home therapeutic exercises, and activity modification in ADL are emphasized.

At 3 months postoperatively, a KT1000 Knee ligament arthrometer test (Medmetric Corporation, San Diego) is performed to document laxity. These results and patient's progress to date are communicated with the referring surgeon.

Troubleshooting

After being on crutches for 6 or more weeks, patients are often anxious to resume their normal ADL. The

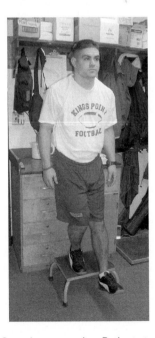

FIGURE 36-9 Step-down exercise. Patient steps down slowly from a step and controlled leading with his or her noninvolved extremity. Deviations from limb alignment and subjective complaints from the patient are considered before progressing to a higher step.

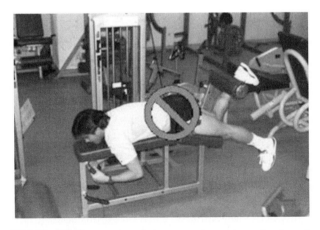

FIGURE 36-8 Isolated OKC hamstring strengthening is avoided for the first 5 postoperative months.

Postoperative Phase II (Weeks 6 to 12)

GOALS

- ROM 0 to 130 degrees
- Restore normal gait
- Demonstrate ability to ascend 8-inch stairs with good leg control without pain
- Demonstrate ability to descend 6-inch stairs with good leg control without pain
- Improve ADL endurance
- Improve lower extremity flexibility
- Protect patellofemoral joint

PRECAUTIONS

- Avoid exceeding ROM limitations in therapeutic exercises
- Avoid resistive knee flexion exercises
- Avoid pain with therapeutic exercise and functional activities
- Monitor activity level (prolonged standing/walking)

TREATMENT STRATEGIES

- Discontinue crutches when gait is non-antalgic (weeks 6 to 8)
- Brace changed to surgeon's preference (OTS brace, patellar sleeve, unloader brace, etc.)
- Standard ergometry (if knee ROM >115 degrees)
- Leg press/mini-squats (ROM 60- to 0-degree arc)
- AAROM exercises
- Proprioception training: multiplanar support surfaces
  - Progress to unilateral support/contralateral exercises (elastic band)
  - Perturbation training
- Forward step-up program
- Step machine
- Underwater treadmill system/pool (gait training)
- Retrograde treadmill ambulation
- Active knee extension: PRE (OKC) 60 to 0 degrees (monitor patellar symptoms)
- NO active (OKC) hamstring exercises
- Initiate step-down program when appropriate
- Knee ligament arthrometer exam at 3 months

CRITERIA FOR ADVANCEMENT

- ROM 0 to 130 degrees
- Normal gait pattern
- Demonstrate ability to ascend 8-inch step
- Demonstrate ability to descend a 6-inch step
- Functional progression pending knee ligament arthrometer exam and functional assessment

rehabilitation specialist needs to encourage the patient during this phase to avoid excessive standing and walking. The patient needs to be aware of the strength requirements yet to be demonstrated or achieved regarding normal ADL, for example, stair negotiation. Modifications in rehabilitation programs need to be made based on daily reassessment of symptoms. Compliance to home therapeutic exercises and activity modifications is crucial to meeting the set criteria for advancement into the next phase of rehabilitation.

POSTOPERATIVE PHASE III (WEEKS 12 TO 20)

Based on meeting the criteria for advancement from the previous phase, the patient enters a phase designed to restore full ROM and improve lower extremity muscle strength, flexibility, and dynamic stability.

Knee ROM exercises are continued. Normal ROM should be achieved during this phase. Flexibility exercises take on a greater emphasis during this phase in preparation for the higher demand/sport-specific activities that will follow. Prone quadriceps stretching is added (Figure 36-10).

Lower extremity strengthening in advanced leg press, squats, and OKC knee extension ROM is advanced to an 80- to 0-degree arc of motion. Advanced neuromuscular training activities are added to include sport cord agility activities, ball toss/catch on an unstable surface (Figure 36-11), and unilateral balance activities on multiplanar support surfaces with perturbation

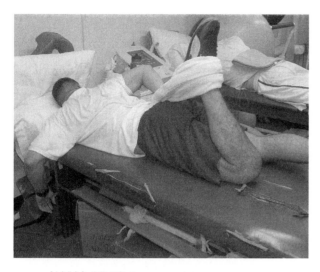

FIGURE 36-10 Prone quadriceps stretching.

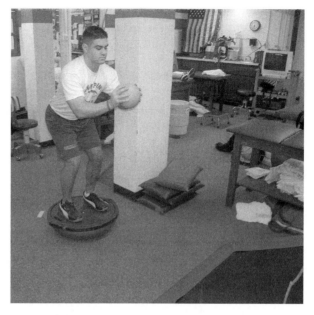

FIGURE 36-11 Ball toss/catch against a Plyoback while balancing on drum.

Postoperative Phase III (Weeks 12 to 20)

GOALS

- Restore full ROM
- Demonstrate ability to descend 8-inch stairs with good leg control without pain
- Improve ADL endurance
- Improve lower extremity flexibility
- Protect patellofemoral joint

PRECAUTIONS

- Avoid descending stairs reciprocally until adequate quadriceps control and lower extremity alignment
- Avoid resistive knee flexion exercises
- Avoid pain with therapeutic exercise and functional activities
- Monitor activity level (prolonged standing/walking)

TREATMENT STRATEGIES

- Leg press/squats (ROM 80- to 0-degree arc)
- AAROM exercises
- Proprioception training: unilateral balance on multiplanar surfaces
  - Perturbations
- Lunges
- Agility exercises (sport cord)
- Step machine
- Retrograde treadmill running
- Forward running
- Lower extremity PRE and flexibility programs
- Forward Step-Down Test (NeuroCom, Clackamas, OR)
- Active knee extension—PRE (OKC) to ROM 80 to 0 degrees
- NO resistive (OKC) hamstring exercises

CRITERIA FOR ADVANCEMENT

- ROM to WNL
- Demonstrate ability to descend an 8-inch step with good leg control without pain
- Functional progression pending functional assessment
- Improved flexibility to meet demands of running and sport-specific activities

training. Advanced balance activities include altering sensory information from the visual, vestibular, and somatosensory systems during training activities so as to challenge the other systems.[40]

At 4 months postoperatively, a Forward Step-Down Test[41] is performed to measure functional lower extremity muscle strength. The goals of this test are to attain an 85% limb symmetry and/or a 10% mean impact score on the involved extremity. Upon satisfactory results of this test a running program is initiated on a treadmill. Forward running is preceded by backward running. Introduction to impact loading is best initiated by retro-running as decreased patellofemoral joint compression forces are generated when compared to forward running.[42]

When full ROM is achieved and lower extremity strength is demonstrated as described previously, a plyometric training program is initiated. Plyometric training during this phase includes jumping activities in which the patient jumps up and lands softly on progressive box heights and bilateral pattern jumps (Figure 36-12).

The patient's home therapeutic exercise program is continually updated based on evaluative findings.

Troubleshooting

The rehabilitation specialist is encouraged to progress the patient through the criteria-based progression, as

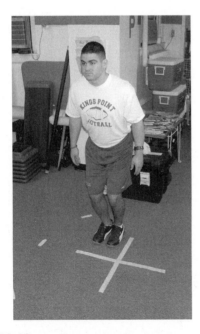

FIGURE 36-12 Plyometric bilateral jumps in a "square" pattern. Patient jumps and lands continuously into each quadrant. Four jumps clockwise are followed by four jumps counterclockwise.

defined. Demonstration of knee ROM and lower extremity strength criteria are required for safe return to higher demand activities, for example, running and jumping. Because the patient is now functioning at a higher level, attention should be given to the patient's volume of PREs as well as increased ADL. Adequate recovery must be implemented to avoid an overuse condition from developing.

POSTOPERATIVE PHASE IV (WEEKS 20 AND BEYOND)

The last phase of rehabilitation following PCL reconstruction is dedicated to prepare the patient/athlete for a safe return to his or her sport. Advancement criteria from phase III need to have been met to meet the demands of sport-specific activities used in phase IV.

Lower extremity strengthening continues to be advanced via a PRE program. The exercise arc for the leg press, squat, and OKC isotonic knee extension exercise is increased to 0 to 90 degrees. Isokinetic training for quadriceps and hamstrings musculature is initiated, using moderate to fast velocities. Training speeds are gradually lowered as tolerated.

Dynamic stability is continued to be challenged by advanced neuromuscular training. Flexibility exercises are continued as part of an exercise sessions warm-up and cool-down.

Forward running is progressed with an emphasis on speed over shorter distances vs slower distance running. Sport-specific exercises are incorporated into the program based on that sports requirements, for example, deceleration training, cutting, and change of direction.

Plyometric exercises are progressed as appropriate, for example, bilateral box jumps, unilateral pattern jumps, box jumps, and depth jumps.

Final testing includes a KT1000 test, functional hop tests, and an isokinetic test. These tests are performed to substantiate laxity, strength, power, and endurance at discharge. The goals of isokinetic testing include a less than 15% deficit for quadriceps and hamstring average peak torque and total work at test velocities of 60 and 240 degrees per second. Single-leg hop tests[43] and crossover hop tests[44] (Figure 36-13) are performed with the goal of achieving an 85% limb symmetry score. The rehabilitation specialist should also document any apprehension during sport-specific movement.

The results of these tests, along with any other pertinent clinical findings, are presented to the referring orthopedic surgeon for the final determination of sports participation. A custom-built or off-the-shelf PCL brace is often prescribed for sport participation in the first year following PCL reconstruction.

Postoperative Phase IV (Weeks 20 and Beyond)

GOALS

- Hop test ≥85% limb symmetry
- Isokinetic testing ≥85% limb symmetry
- Lack of apprehension with sport-specific movements
- Maximize strength and flexibility to meet demands of individual's sport activity

PRECAUTIONS

- Avoid pain with therapeutic exercise and functional activities
- Protect patellofemoral joint
- Avoid sport activity until adequate strength development and surgeon's clearance

TREATMENT STRATEGIES

- Continue lower extremity strengthening, leg press, squat, OKC extension 0- to 90-degree arc
- Lower extremity flexibility program
- Advance proprioception training
- Advance forward running program
- Advance plyometric program (sport-specific)
- Sport-specific agility activities
- Isokinetic training/testing
- Functional testing
- Knee ligament arthrometer exam at 6 months
- Home therapeutic exercise program: evaluation-based

CRITERIA FOR DISCHARGE

- Hop test ≥85% limb symmetry
- Isokinetic test ≥85% limb symmetry
- Lack of apprehension with sport-specific movements
- Flexibility to accepted levels for sport performance
- Independence with gym program for maintenance and progression of therapeutic exercise program at discharge

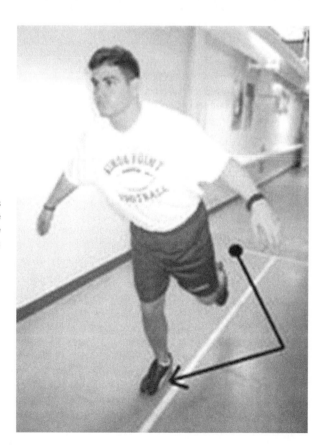

FIGURE **36-13** Crossover hop for distance test. Patient performs three consecutive jumps on one leg, crossing over the drawn line with each jump. Total distance jumped is recorded. Three trials are performed on each leg and averaged. Limb symmetry is then calculated.

Troubleshooting

Before advancing the patient into higher level plyometric and sport-specific activities, the rehabilitation specialist should be sure that adequate flexibility and strength are restored. Variety should be implemented into the patient's/athlete's program. Weight training, running, agility activities, and plyometrics should not all be performed on the same training day. Special attention should be paid to proper warm-up and cool-down segments of the rehabilitation program. Emphasis should be placed on flexibility during this phase. Continued training may be needed if the patient/athlete does not meet stated criteria for return to sport. By ensuring that criteria have been met, the rehabilitation team can be confident that a safe return to athletic participation is, in fact, suitable.

REFERENCES

1. Butler, D.L., Noyes, F.R., Grood, E.S. *Ligamentus Restraints to Anterior-Posterior Drawer in the Human Knee. A Biomechanical Study.* J Bone Joint Surg 1980;62A:259–270.
2. Miyasaka, K.C., Daniel, D.M., Stone, M.L., Hirschman, P. *The Incidence of Knee Ligament Injuries in the General Population.* Am J Knee Surg 1991;4:3–8.
3. Fanelli, G.C. *Posterior Cruciate Ligament Injuries in Trauma Patients.* Arthroscopy 1993;9:291–294.
4. Clancy, W.G. Jr. Repair and Reconstruction of the Posterior Cruciate Ligament. In Chapman, M.W. (Ed). *Operative Orthopaedics.* JB Lippincott, Philadelphia, 1988, pp. 1651–1666.
5. Kannus, P., Bergfeld, J., Jarvinen, M., Johnson, R.J., Pope, M., Renstrom, P., Yasuda, K. *Injuries to the Posterior Cruciate Ligament of the Knee.* Sports Med 1991;12(2):110–131.
6. Cooper, D.E., Warren, R.F., Warner, J.P. *The PCL and Posterolateral Structures of the Knee: Anatomy, Function, and Patterns of Injury.* Instr Course Lect 1991;40:249–270.
7. Cross, M.J., Powell, J.F. *Long-term Follow-up of Posterior Cruciate Ligament Rupture: A Study of 116 Cases.* Am J Sports Med 1984;12:292–297.
8. Dejour, H., Walsh, G., Peyrot, J. *The Natural History of Rupture of the PCL.* J Orthop Surg 1988;2:112–120.
9. Fowler, P.J., Messieh, S.S. *Isolated Posterior Cruciate Ligament Injuries in Athletes.* Am J Sports Med 1987;15:553–557.
10. Parolie, J.M., Bergfeld, J.A. *Long-term Results of Nonoperative Treatment of Isolated Posterior Cruciate Ligament Injuries in the Athlete.* Am J Sports Med 1986;14(1):35–38.
11. Torg, J.S., Barton, T.M. *Natural History of the Posterior Cruciate Deficient Knee.* Clin Orthop 1989;246:208–216.
12. Bach, B.R. Jr. *Graft Selection for Posterior Cruciate Ligament Surgery.* Oper Tech Sports Med 1993;1:104–109.
13. Van Dommelen, B.A., Fowler, P.J. *Anatomy of the Posterior Cruciate Ligament. A Review.* Am J Sports Med 1989;17:24–29.
14. Girgis, F.G., Marshall, J.L., Al Monajem, A.R. *The Cruciate Ligaments of the Knee Joint: Anatomical, Functional and Experimental Analysis.* Clin Orthop 1975;106:216–231.
15. Harner, C.D., Xerogeanes, J.W., Livesay, G.A., Carlin, G.J., Smith, B.A., Kusayama, T., Kashiwaguchi, S., Woo, S.L. *The Human Posterior Cruciate Ligament Complex: An Interdisciplinary Study. Ligament Morphology and Biomechanical Evaluation.* Am J Sports Med 1995;23:736–745.
16. Race, A., Amis, A.A. *The Mechanical Properties of the Two Bundles of the Human Posterior Cruciate Ligament.* J Biomech 1994;27:13–24.
17. Clancy, W.G. Jr., Bisson, L.J. *Double Tunnel Technique for Reconstruction of the Posterior Cruciate Ligament.* Oper Tech Sports Med 1999;7:110–117.
18. Harner, C.D., Höher, J. *Evaluation and Treatment of Posterior Cruciate Ligament Injuries.* Am J Sports Med 1998;26:471–482.
19. Race, A., Amis, A.A. *PCL Reconstruction: In Vitro Biomechanical Comparison of "Isometric" Versus Single and Double-bundle "Anatomic" Grafts.* J Bone Joint Surg 1998;80B:173–179.
20. Höher, J., Harner, C.D., Vogrin, T.M. *Hamstring Loading Increases In Situ Forces in the PCL.* Trans Orthop Res Soc 1998;23:48.
21. Lutz, G.E., Palmitier, R.A., An, K.N., Chao, E.Y. *Comparison of Tibiofemoral Joint Forces During Open Kinetic Chain and Closed Kinetic Chain Exercises.* J Bone Joint Surg 1993;75A:732–739.
22. Toutoungi, D.E., Lu, T.W., Leardini, A., Catani, F., O'Connor, J.J. *Cruciate Ligament Forces in the Human Knee During Rehabilitation Exercises.* Clin Biomech (Bristol, Avon) 2000;15(3):176–187.
23. Akeson, W.H., Woo, S.L., Amiel, D. *The Connective Tissue Response to Immobilization: Biomechanical Changes in Periarticular Connective Tissue of the Immobilized Rabbit Knee.* Clin Orthop 1973;93:356–362.
24. Noyes, F.R., Mangine, R.E., Barber, S. *Early Knee Motion after Open and Arthroscopic ACL Reconstruction.* Am J Sports Med 1987;15(2):149–160.
25. Salter, R.H., Simmonds, D.F., Malcolm, B.W., Rumble, E.J., MacMichael, D., Clements, N.D. *The Biological Effect of Continuous Passive Motion on Healing of Full-thickness Defects in Articular Cartilage.* J Bone Joint Surg 1980;62A(8):1232–1251.
26. Fulkerson, J.P., Hungerford, D. *Disorders of the Patellofemoral Joint,* 2nd ed. Williams & Wilkins, Baltimore, 1990.
27. Morrison, I.B. *The Biomechanics of the Knee Joint in Relation to Normal Walking.* J Biomech 1970;3:51–61.
28. Hirokawa, S., Solomonow, M., Lu, Y., Lou, Z.P., D'Ambrosia, R. *Anterior-posterior and Rotational Displacement of the Tibia Elicited by Quadriceps Contraction.* Am J Sports Med 1992;20:299–306.
29. Eriksson, E., Haggmark, T. *Comparison of Isometric Muscle Training and Electrical Stimulation Supplementing Isometric Muscle Training in the Recovery after Major Knee Ligament Surgery.* Am J Sports Med 1979;7:169–171.
30. Wigerstad-Lossing, I., Grimby, G., Jonsson, T., Morelli, B., Peterson, L., Renstrom, P. *Effects of Electrical Muscle Stimulation Combined with Voluntary Contractions after Knee Ligament Surgery.* Med Sci Sports Exerc 1988;20(1):93–98.
31. Jurist, K.A., Otis, J.C. *Anteroposterior Tibiofemoral Displacements During Isometric Extension Efforts. The Roles of External Load and Knee Flexion Angle.* Am J Sports Med 1985;13:254–258.
32. Wilk, K.E., Escamilla, R.F., Fleisig, G.S., Barrentine, S.W., Andrews, J.R., Boyd, M.L. *A Comparison of Tibiofemoral Joint Forces and Electromyographic Activity During Open and Closed Kinetic Chain Exercises.* Am J Sports Med 1996;24(4):518–527.
33. Schwartz, R.E., Asnis, P.D., Cavanaugh, J.T., Asnis, S.E., Simmons, J.E., Lasinski, P.J. *Short Crank Cycle Ergometry.* J Orthop Sports Phys Ther 1991;13:95.
34. Spencer, J.D., Hayes, K.C., Alexander, L.J. *Knee Joint Effusion and Quadriceps Inhibition in Man.* Arch Phys Med Rehabil 1984;65(4):171–177.

35. Bates, A., Hanson, N. The Principles and Properties of Water. In *Aquatic Exercise Therapy.* WB Saunders, Philadelphia, 1996, pp. 1–320.
36. Harrison, R.A., Hilman, M., Bulstrode, S. *Loading of the Lower Limb When Walking Partially Immersed: Implications for Clinical Practice.* Physiotherapy 1992;78:164.
37. Cipriani, D.J., Armstrong, C.W., Gaul, S. *Backward Walking at Three Levels of Treadmill Inclination: An Electromyographic and Kinematic Analysis.* J Orthop Sports Phys Ther 1995;22(3):95–102.
38. Skyhar, M.J., Warren, R.F., Ortiz, G.J., Schwartz, E., Otis, J.C. *The Effects of Sectioning of the Posterior Cruciate Ligament and the Posterolateral Complex on the Articular Contact Pressures Within the Knee.* J Bone Joint Surg Am 1993;75(5):694–699.
39. Cavanaugh, J.T., Moy, R.J. *Balance and Postoperative Lower Extremity Joint Reconstruction.* Orthop Phys Ther Clin N Am 2002;11(1):75–99.
40. Guskiewicz, K.M. Regaining Balance and Postural Equilibrium. In Prentice, W.E. (Ed). *Rehabilitation Techniques in Sports Medicine,* 3rd ed. WCB/McGraw-Hill, New York, 1999, pp. 107–133.
41. Cavanaugh, J.T., Stump, T.J. *Forward Step Down Test.* J Orthop Sports Phys Ther 2000;30(1):A–46.
42. Flynn, T.W., Soutas-Little, R.W. *Patellofemoral Joint Compressive Forces in Forward and Backward Running.* J Orthop Sports Phys Ther 1995;21(5):277–282.
43. Daniel, D.M., Malcolm, L., Stone, M.L., Perth, H., Morgan, J., Riehl, B. *Quantification of Knee Stability and Function.* Contemp Orthop 1982;5:83–91.
44. Barber, S.D., Noyes, F.R., Mangine, R.E., McCloskey, J.W., Hartman, W. *Quantitative Assessment of Functional Limitations in Normal and Anterior Cruciate Ligament Deficient Knees.* Clin Orthop 1990;255:204–214.

37

Meniscal Repair and Transplantation

JOHN T. CAVANAUGH, PT, MED, ATC

COLEEN T. GATELY, PT, DPT, MS

Meniscal cartilage plays a significant role in the function and biomechanics of the knee joint. The meniscus functions in load bearing, load transmission, shock absorption, joint stability, joint lubrication, and joint congruity.[1-3] The meniscus can fail from either mechanical or biochemical (degenerative) causes.[4] The most common mechanism of injury to the menisci involves noncontact forces.[2] Stress across the knee joint from a sudden acceleration or deceleration movement, in conjunction with a change in direction, can trap the menisci between the tibia and femur, resulting in a tear. As a result of these traumas, the patient may present with pain, effusion, locking, and persistent focal joint line tenderness. If conservative treatment proves to be unsuccessful, surgical intervention is often necessary. Meniscal tear pattern, geometry, site, vascularity, size, stability, tissue viability or quality, as well as associated pathology, are all taken into account when determining whether to resect or repair a meniscal lesion.[5] The literature has demonstrated that removal of the meniscus leads to degenerative changes of the knee joint.[6-8] Partial meniscectomy when compared with total meniscectomy, reduces the degeneration of articular cartilage. However, results of stresses on the underlying cartilage following partial meniscectomy have been reported to be higher than normal.[9-11] Therefore, attempts to preserve the injured meniscus are made whenever possible.

The first reported meniscal repair was reported by Annandale[12] in 1885. The goal of a meniscus repair is to allow the torn edges of the meniscus to heal once they have been fixated with sutures. Meniscal repair techniques have evolved from the placement of sutures across the torn meniscus through arthrotomy to using arthroscopy. Published meniscal repair results have supported favorable success at extended follow-up in over 70% to 90% of patients.[13-16]

As a means to address symptomatic meniscal-deficient patients, the meniscal transplantation procedure was introduced by Milachowski and colleagues[17] in 1984. Ideal candidates for this procedure include patient's whose knees are normally aligned, stable, and demonstrate little degenerative changes. Meniscal transplantation may also be indicated during concomitant anterior cruciate ligament reconstruction, because absence of the meniscus could preclude satisfactory stabilization.[5,18-20] Contraindications for meniscal transplantation include advanced articular cartilage wear (especially on the flexion weight-bearing zone of the condyle), axial misalignment, and flattening of the femoral condyle.[19] Reports from 2002 suggest that more than 4000 meniscal transplants have been performed since 1991, with an estimated 800-plus menisci implanted annually.[18] When properly indicated and performed, transplantation leads to good results in over 90% of patients.[19]

Rehabilitation following these procedures are crucial toward the attainment of optimal functional outcome.

In this chapter we will discuss the Hospital for Special Surgery's (HSS) clinical guidelines following meniscal repair and transplantation.

SURGICAL OVERVIEW

The menisci are wedge-shaped crescents of fibrocartilage found between the femur and tibia (Figure 37-1). The menisci allows for a more congruous articulation between the already incongruent femoral condyle and tibial plateau. The lateral meniscus is O-shaped, whereas the medial meniscus is C-shaped. The lateral meniscus picks up 70% of the load transmitted across the lateral compartment, whereas the medial meniscus and articular cartilage share the load.[21] Each meniscus is divided anatomically into horizontal thirds: the posterior horn, mid-body, and anterior horn. Menisci are divided into vertical thirds when looking at blood supply. The outer edge of each meniscus has a rich blood supply from the medial and lateral genicular arteries.[22] Vascularization decreases approaching the inner portion of the meniscus and becomes dependent upon diffusion.[23] Because of the poor blood supply, tears that approach the inner avascular area have a more difficult time with healing. Arnoczky and Warren[22] have reported that to allow meniscal tears to heal, the tear needs to be in contact with the peripheral vascular area (Figure 37-2).

The surgical management of repairing meniscal tears varies. In relatively stable tears, the literature has reported the use of rasping and trephination.[24-26] Arthroscopic meniscal repair techniques can be divided into three techniques, based upon suture placement. They include an inside-out repair, outside-in repair,

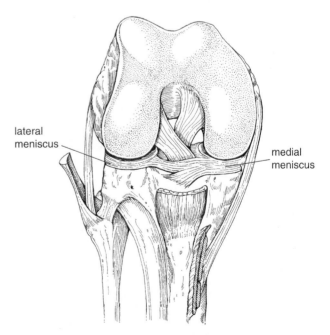

lateral meniscus

medial meniscus

FIGURE **37-1** The menisci are wedge-shaped crescents of fibrocartilage found between the femur and tibia.

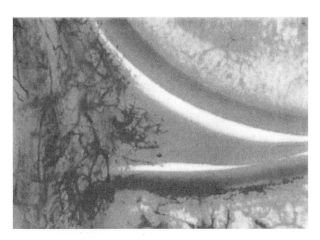

FIGURE **37-2** Menisci are divided into vertical thirds when looking at blood supply. Branching radial vessels from the perimeniscal capillary plexus penetrate the peripheral third of the medial meniscus. *(From Arnoczky, S.P., Warren, R.F. Microvasculature of the Human Meniscus. Am J Sports Med 1982;10:90–95, with permission.)*

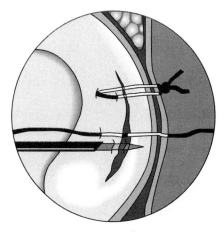

FIGURE **37-3** The arthroscopic inside-out surgical technique involves the placement of sutures across the meniscus inside the joint, and the sutures are then tied down outside the joint capsule.

and all-inside repair. The arthroscopic inside-out surgical technique involves the placement of sutures across the meniscus inside the joint, and the sutures are then tied down outside the joint capsule (Figure 37-3).[27] This technique has been successful with tears to the middle one-third and, to some degree, tears of the posterior horns.[5,28]

The arthroscopic outside-in surgical technique involves the placement of a suture with a Mulberry knot to one side of the meniscal tear inside the joint, and then sutures are tied on the joint capsule (Figure 37-4).[29] This technique has been advocated in repairing tears to the mid-one-third and anterior horn regions.[30] The arthroscopic all-inside surgical technique involves the placement of a suture, screws, and/or darts through an arthroscopic portal to stabilize the tear (Figure 37-5).[31] Because it does not make use of any incisions, the all-inside technique is favorable in decreasing the risk of iatrogenic neurovascular damage. This technique has favorable results for posterior horn tears.[32,33]

Meniscus allograft transplant (MAT) has evolved into a primarily arthroscopic technique in which a cadaveric meniscus is inserted into a meniscus deficient knee. The cadaveric meniscus is supplied by a tissue bank. Although there are no set standards, most tissue banks determine implant size through estimates made from radiographs.[34,35] Following a diagnostic arthroscopy of the knee, the native meniscus is removed.[36] Different techniques have evolved in transplanting medial or lateral menisci. With a medial meniscus replacement, two bone plugs, one to the anterior horn and another to the posterior horn, are inserted in their respective tibial tunnels while sutures along the rim hold the graft in place[36–39] (Figure 37-6). With lateral meniscus transplantation, a rectangular bone trough is created between

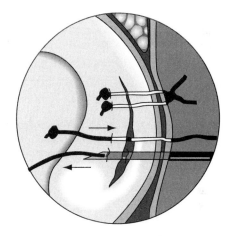

FIGURE **37-4** The arthroscopic outside-in surgical technique involves the placement of a suture with a Mulberry knot to one side of the meniscal tear inside the joint, and then sutures are tied on the joint capsule.

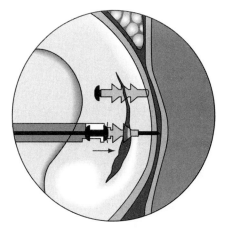

FIGURE **37-5** The arthroscopic all-inside surgical technique involves the placement of a suture, screws, and/or darts through an arthroscopic portal to stabilize the tear.

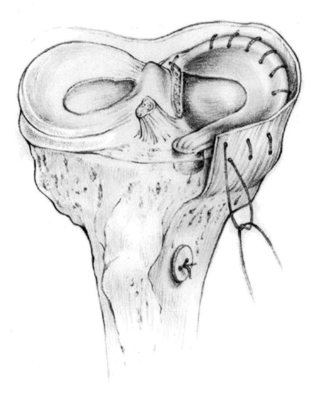

FIGURE **37-6** In medial meniscus replacement, two bone plugs, one to the anterior horn and another to the posterior horn, are inserted in their respective tibial tunnels while sutures along the rim hold the graft in place. *(From Noyes, F.R., Barber-Westin, S.D., Rankin, M. Meniscal Transplantation in Symptomatic Patients Less Than Fifty Years Old. J Bone Joint Surg Am 2004;86A(7):1392–1404, with permission.)*

the anterior and posterior lateral meniscal attachment sites[36–39] (Figure 37-7). Suture placement holds the meniscus in place.

REHABILITATION OVERVIEW

Rehabilitation programs following meniscal repair and transplantation should reflect an optimal environment for healing. Surgical technique, type of repair fixation, location of the repair, concomitant procedures, and surgeon's preference will have a direct influence on weight-bearing status, range of motion (ROM) restrictions, and treatment progressions. Therefore, communication between the surgeon and rehabilitation specialist, particularly in the early protective phases of rehabilitation, is vital.

Customarily, following meniscal repair and transplantation procedures, immediate ROM is encouraged. Early motion has been shown to minimize the deleterious effects of immobilization, such as articular cartilage degeneration, excessive adverse collagen formation, and pain.[40–42]

Weight-bearing following meniscal repair will be typically progressive throughout the early postoperative

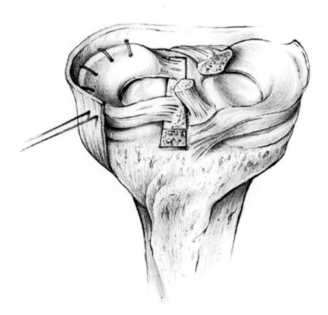

FIGURE **37-7** In lateral meniscus transplantation a rectangular bone trough is created between the anterior and posterior lateral meniscal attachment sites. Suture placement holds the meniscus in place. *(From Noyes, F.R., Barber-Westin, S.D., Rankin, M. Meniscal Transplantation in Symptomatic Patients Less Than Fifty Years Old. J Bone Joint Surg Am 2004;86A(7):1392–1404, with permission.)*

period. Weight-bearing following meniscal transplantation and meniscal repairs involving complex or radial tears will be limited to toe-touch ambulation for the first 4 weeks. The involved knee is maintained in full extension, donning a double-upright hinged brace locked at 0 degrees during the designated protection phase, regardless of which meniscal procedure was performed.

The pre-surgical status of the patient, any associated pathology, and a comprehensive evaluation will each play an important factor in designing an individualized rehabilitation program for each patient.[43] An elite athlete may progress faster as a result of greater preoperative muscle strength as compared to a nonathlete in weak physical condition. Patients with degenerative joint disease may need a slower weight-bearing progression. Patients with patellofemoral disorders may or may not be candidates for certain isotonic or isokinetic knee extension exercises. Subjective complaints and physical findings ascertained during evaluations and continual reassessments will direct the rehabilitation program to the proper speed and direction.

The realistic goals of the patient, surgeon, and rehabilitation specialist should be discussed and defined early in the postoperative course. The patient should be brought to understand the magnitude of his or her surgery and the timetable for recovery. Goals should be specific and functional to the individual needs of the patient. The patient should be made aware of his or her role in the rehabilitative process. The patient's compliance to activity modifications and home therapeutic exercises is vital for a successful outcome. Postoperative guidelines following these procedures abide by a criteria-based progression. ROM and strength requirements are to be met before advancement to subsequent phases.

POSTOPERATIVE REHABILITATION: MENISCAL REPAIR GUIDELINES

POSTOPERATIVE PHASE I (WEEKS 0 TO 6)

Following meniscal repair the patient is placed in a double-upright knee brace that is locked in full extension. This brace is used exclusively for ambulation and sleeping for the first 4 to 6 postoperative weeks. Rehabilitation following meniscal repair is initiated immediately postoperatively. Communication with the surgeon regarding the anatomical site of the repair (vascular vs nonvascular) and location within the meniscus (anterior or posterior) will directly affect the postoperative regimen.

The patient is instructed in ROM exercises to attain full extension and the recommended degree of flexion. Extension appears to reduce the meniscus to the capsule, while flexion causes posterior horn tears to displace from the capsule.[44] Thompson et al.[45] demonstrated that menisci translate posteriorly during flexion but that meniscal movement was minimal below 60 degrees of flexion. Active-assisted range of motion (AAROM) exercises are performed, with flexion restricted to 90 degrees during the initial (4 to 6 weeks) protection phase (Figure 37-8). Repairs to the posterior horn are limited to 70 degrees for the first 4 weeks then progressed, as tolerated. Active or resisted knee flexion is avoided during this phase because of the attachment of the semimembranosus muscle on the medial meniscus and the popliteus muscle on the lateral meniscus.[46]

The patient is encouraged to progressively weight-bear with a double-upright brace locked in full extension, using crutches. Bucket-handle and longitudinal repairs may be closed by compressive loads with the knee in extension. Weight-bearing will be limited to toe-touch for radial or more complex repairs for 4 to 6 weeks because compressive loading may cause distraction of these repairs.[30] Weight-bearing with the knee in progressive flexion is avoided until 4 to 6 weeks because the meniscus is subjected to greater stress in this position.[21] At 4 to 6 weeks postoperatively the hinged brace is opened to 60 degrees to allow for ROM during gait. Gait training, using a pool or underwater treadmill, is used to unload the involved extremity. Crutches are discharged when a non-antalgic gait is demonstrated.

Quadriceps reeducation is addressed on postoperative day 1, with the patient instructed to perform

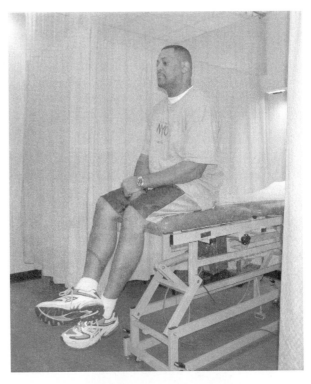

FIGURE **37-8** Following a meniscal repair, AAROM exercises are performed with flexion restricted to 90 degrees during the initial (4 to 6 weeks) protection phase.

quadriceps setting exercises with a rolled towel under the surgical knee. In the formal rehabilitation setting, electrical stimulation and/or biofeedback can be used if the patient demonstrates quadriceps inhibition (Figure 37-9). A straight leg raise (SLR) in multiple planes is encouraged for the development of proximal strength. Weights, a progressive resistive exercise (PRE), are added to these exercises when tolerated, along with exercise machines to further advance proximal

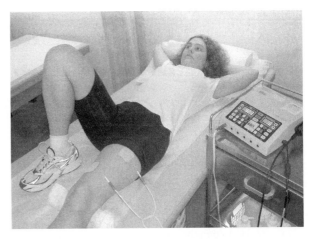

FIGURE **37-9** Electrical stimulation can be used to facilitate quadriceps reeducation.

strengthening (Figure 37-10). Proprioceptive and balance training is started as soon as the patient demonstrates the ability to bear 50% of his or her weight. A rocker board is used, starting in a sagittal plane, and then progressed to a more challenging coronal plane. A computerized balance platform can be used for patient feedback (Figure 37-11).

As ROM demonstrates improvement greater than 85 degrees, select open kinetic chain (OKC) and closed kinetic chain (CKC) exercises are introduced to the therapeutic exercise program. Bilateral leg press and mini-squats are performed inside a 60- to 0-degree arc of motion (Figure 37-12). Quadriceps isometrics are performed submaximally at 60 degrees of flexion (Figure 37-13). Stationary bicycling is added to the rehabilitation

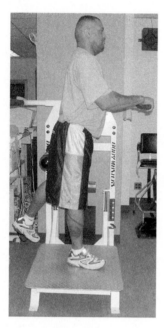

FIGURE **37-10** Exercise machines can be used to further advance proximal strengthening. Above the multihip is used to strengthen the hip extensor musculature.

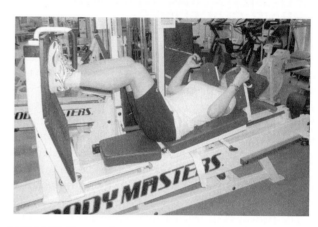

FIGURE **37-12** Bilateral leg press, a CKC exercise, is performed inside a 60- to 0-degree arc of motion.

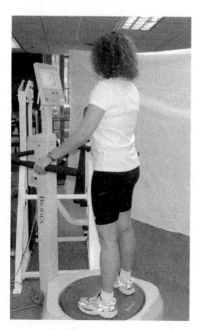

FIGURE **37-11** A computerized balance platform can be used for patient feedback while performing proprioceptive and balance training activities.

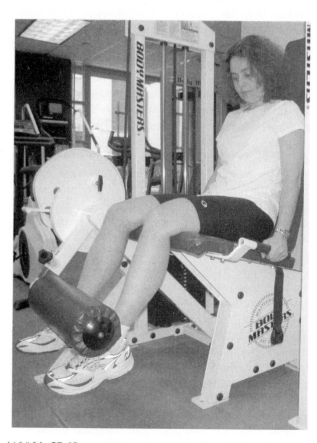

FIGURE **37-13** Quadriceps isometrics, an OKC exercise, are performed submaximally at 60 degrees of flexion.

Meniscal Repair Guidelines
Postoperative Phase I (Weeks 0 to 6)

GOALS

- Emphasis on full passive extension
- Control postoperative pain/swelling
- ROM to 90-degree flexion
- Regain quadriceps control
- Independence in home therapeutic exercise program

PRECAUTIONS

- Avoid active knee flexion
- Avoid ambulation without brace locked at 0 degrees before 4 weeks
- Avoid prolonged standing/walking

TREATMENT STRATEGIES

- Towel extensions, prone hangs, and so on
- Quadriceps reeducation (quadriceps sets with electrical muscle stimulator [EMS] or electromyography [EMG])
- Progressive weight-bearing PWB to WBAT with brace locked at 0 degrees with crutches
- Toe-touch weight-bearing for complex or radial tears
- Patellar mobilization
- Active-assisted flexion/extension 90- to 0-degree exercise
- SLRs (all planes)
- Hip PREs
- Proprioception board (bilateral weight-bearing)
- Aquatic therapy—pool ambulation or underwater treadmill (weeks 4 to 6)
- Short crank ergometry (if ROM >85 degrees)
- Leg press (bilateral/60- to 0-degree arc) (if ROM >85 degrees)
- OKC quadriceps isometrics (submaximal/bilateral at 60 degrees) (if ROM >85 degrees)
- Upper extremity cardiovascular exercises as tolerated
- Hamstring and calf stretching
- Cryotherapy
- Emphasize patient compliance to home therapeutic exercise program and weight-bearing and ROM precautions/progression

CRITERIA FOR ADVANCEMENT

- Ability to SLR without quadriceps lag
- ROM 0 to 90 degrees
- Demonstrate ability to unilateral (involved extremity) weight-bear without pain

---

program by using a short crank (90 mm) ergometer.[47] Hamstring and calf stretching exercises are added into both formal and home therapeutic exercise programs. Cryotherapy and electrical stimulation (TENS) may be used for pain control. Home therapeutic exercise programs are continually updated.

Troubleshooting

It is imperative that the prescribed weight-bearing status and ROM allowance be enforced during this critical maximum protective phase. These precautions need to be reinforced continually to the patient to provide the optimal environment for meniscal healing. Compliance to home therapeutic exercises should also be emphasized so as to better meet the desired goals at the end of this phase.

POSTOPERATIVE PHASE II (WEEKS 6 TO 14)

The second phase following meniscal repair is dedicated to restoring normal ROM to the involved knee and improving muscle strength to the level needed to perform activities of daily living (ADL).

The demonstration of a normal gait pattern is an early goal of this phase. Treatment interventions using an underwater treadmill or pool ambulation for gait training will continue to be used. AAROM exercises are progressed as tolerated with the goal of attaining full ROM by the end of this phase (Figure 37-14). As ROM improves to 110 to 115 degrees, cycling is advanced to a standard 170-mm ergometer. Quadriceps stretching is added as ROM improves to greater than 120 degrees (Figure 37-15).

Strengthening programs continue to emphasize a CKC approach. Leg press exercise will progress to eccentric and, eventually, unilateral training using greater ROM (<90 degrees). A squat program with progressive resistance is initiated using a physio ball for support and comfort inside a 60- to 0-degree arc of motion. A forward step-up program is begun on suc-cessive step heights (4, 6, and 8 inches). StairMaster and the elliptical machine are incorporated as symptoms allow. Retrograde treadmill ambulation on progressive percentage inclines is used to facilitate quadriceps strengthening.[48] Isotonic knee extensions in a pain/crepitus-free arc may be implemented monitoring patellofemoral symptoms. This OKC activity should be performed with light weight, using bilateral lower extremities and progressed carefully. A forward step-down program is initiated on successive height increments (4, 6, and 8 inches) (Figure 37-16). The functional strength goal at the end of this phase is for the patient to demonstrate pain-free descent from an 8-inch step with adequate lower extremity control without deviations. At 14 weeks postoperatively a Forward Step-Down Test[49] is performed to assist in objectively measuring functional lower extremity muscle strength.

Neuromuscular training is advanced to include unilateral balance activities, for example, contralateral elastic band exercises, and balance systems training. As these activities are mastered, the rehabilitation specialist can incorporate less stable surfaces (foam rollers, rocker boards, etc.) as well as perturbation training to these activities to further enhance neuromuscular development (Figure 37-17).

The patient's home therapeutic exercise program is continually updated based on evaluative findings and functional level.

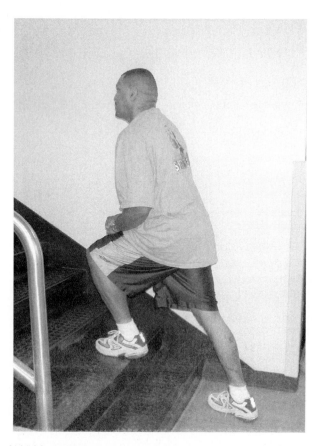

FIGURE **37-14** The stair stretch, an AAROM exercise, is progressed as tolerated with the goal of attaining full knee ROM.

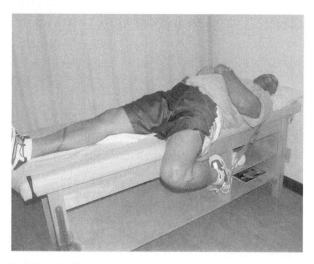

FIGURE **37-15** Quadriceps stretching is added as ROM improves to greater than 120 degrees.

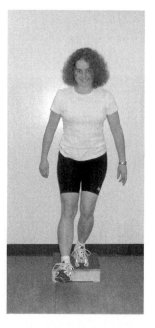

FIGURE **37-16** A forward step-down program is initiated on successive height increments (4, 6, and 8 inches). Patient is performing a 6-inch forward step-down. The left leg is the involved leg.

Meniscal Repair Guidelines
Postoperative Phase II (Weeks 6 to 14)

GOALS

- Restore full ROM
- Restore normal gait (non-antalgic)
- Demonstrate ability to ascend and descend 8-inch stairs with good leg control without pain
- Improve ADL endurance
- Improve lower extremity flexibility
- Independence in home therapeutic exercise program

PRECAUTIONS

- Avoid descending stairs reciprocally until adequate quadriceps control and lower extremity alignment
- Avoid pain with therapeutic exercise and functional activities
- Avoid running and sport activity

TREATMENT STRATEGIES

- Progressive weight-bearing/WBAT with crutches/cane (brace opened 0 to 60 degrees), if good quadriceps control (good quadriceps set/ability to SLR without lag or pain)
- Aquatic therapy—pool ambulation or underwater treadmill
- Discontinue crutches/cane when gait is non-antalgic
- Brace changed to surgeon's preference (OTS brace, patellar sleeve, etc.)
- AAROM exercises
- Patellar mobilization
- SLRs (all planes) with weights
- Proximal PREs
- Neuromuscular training (bilateral to unilateral support)
- Balance apparatus, foam surface, perturbations
- Short crank ergometry
- Standard ergometry (if knee ROM >115 degrees)
- Leg press (bilateral/eccentric/unilateral progression)
- Squat program (PRE) 0 to 60 degrees
- OKC quadriceps isotonics (pain-free arc of motion) (CKC preferred)
- Initiate forward step-up and step-down programs
- StairMaster
- Retrograde treadmill ambulation
- Quadriceps stretching
- Elliptical machine
- Forward Step-Down Test (NeuroCom)
- Upper extremity cardiovascular exercises as tolerated
- Cryotherapy
- Emphasize patient compliance to home therapeutic exercise program

CRITERIA FOR ADVANCEMENT

- ROM to WNL
- Ability to descend 8-inch stairs with good leg control without pain

Troubleshooting

Restoration of knee active range of motion (AROM) and strength is crucial during phase II. Attainment of these goals is necessary to allow for a safe advancement through this and subsequent phases. Pain while performing ROM and strengthening exercises is the best indicator in knowing when to modify treatment choices. Patellofemoral symptoms should be monitored during this phase. Exercises should be modified accordingly so as to avoid anterior knee pain. During this phase a nor-malized gait pattern is achieved. Patients will progress from using crutches to using one crutch and/or a cane. It is critical that patients realize there is a weaning process with assistive device use rather than a finite end date. A pain-free normalized gait pattern will determine when the uses of assistive devices while ambulating are no longer needed. The patient is also encouraged to modify his or her functional activities to the present strength level. Reciprocally descending stairs, for example, should be avoided until a sufficient lower extremity strength base is demonstrated. As in the pre-

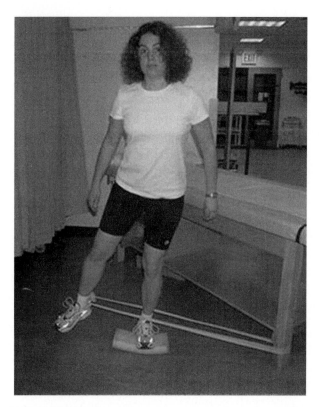

FIGURE **37-17** Neuromuscular training is advanced to include unilateral balance activities, for example, contralateral elastic band exercises with an unstable surface (foam roller). The left leg is the involved extremity.

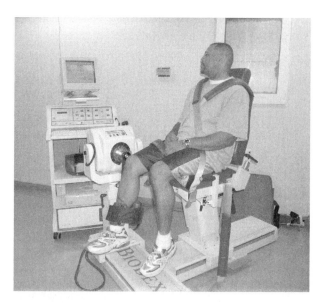

FIGURE **37-18** Isokinetic training is initiated using higher velocities and is progressed to moderate and slower velocities over time.

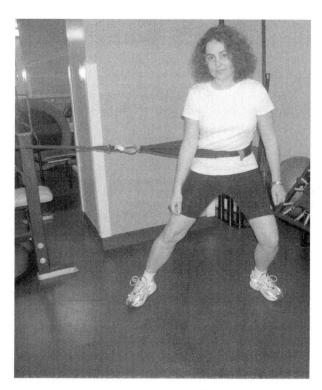

FIGURE **37-19** A sports cord can be used for agility activities. Deceleration, cutting, and sprinting movements can be simulated based upon specific return to sports demands.

vious phase, compliance with a home exercise program is always encouraged.

POSTOPERATIVE PHASE III (WEEKS 14 TO 22)

As criteria are met in the preceding phase, the patient then enters a phase directed at optimizing functional capabilities and preparing the patient/athlete for a safe return to sport activity.

At 4 months postoperatively a running program on a treadmill is initiated. Retrograde running is preceded by forward running. An initial emphasis on speed over shorter distances vs slower distance running is recommended.

Lower extremity strengthening and flexibility programs are continued. Advanced strengthening activities, including isokinetic and plyometric training, are introduced. Isokinetic training is initiated using higher velocities and progressed to moderate and slower velocities over time (Figure 37-18). Patient feedback regarding symptoms, or lack thereof, of anterior knee discomfort is crucial during this progression. Plyometric training should follow a functional sequence with the components of speed, intensity, load, volume, and frequency being monitored and progressed accordingly. Activities begin with simple drills and advance to more complex exercises (e.g., double-leg jumping vs box drills).

Agility exercises are introduced with the demands of the individual's sport taken into consideration, for example, deceleration, cutting, and sprinting (Figure 37-19).

Meniscal Repair Guidelines
Postoperative Phase III (Weeks 14 to 22)

GOALS

- Demonstrate ability to run pain-free
- Maximize strength and flexibility as to meet demands of ADL
- Hop test ≥85% limb symmetry
- Isokinetic test >85% limb symmetry
- Lack of apprehension with sport-specific movements
- Flexibility to accepted levels of sport performance
- Independence with gym program for maintenance and progression of therapeutic exercise program at discharge

PRECAUTIONS

- Avoid pain with therapeutic exercise and functional activities
- Avoid sport activity until adequate strength development and surgeon's clearance

TREATMENT STRATEGIES

- Progress squat program <90-degree flexion
- Lunges
- Retrograde treadmill running
- Start forward running (treadmill) program at 4 months postoperatively if 8-inch step down satisfactory
- Continue lower extremity strengthening and flexibility programs
- Agility program/sport-specific (sports cord)
- Start plyometric program when strength base is sufficient
- Isotonic knee flexion/extension (pain- and crepitus-free arc)
- Isokinetic training (fast to moderate to slow velocities)
- Functional testing (hop test)
- Isokinetic testing
- Home therapeutic exercise program: evaluation-based

CRITERIA FOR ADVANCEMENT

- Symptom-free running and sport-specific agility
- Hop test ≥ 85% limb symmetry
- Isokinetic test > 85% limb symmetry
- Lack of apprehension with sport-specific movements
- Flexibility to accepted levels of sport performance
- Independence with gym program for maintenance and progression of therapeutic exercise program at discharge

The rehabilitation specialist should be certain to observe any apprehension during the agility activity progression.

To quantify strength and power both isokinetic and functional testing are performed. The goals of isokinetic testing include a less than 15% deficit for quadriceps and hamstring average peak torque and total work at test velocities of 60 and 240 degrees per second. Functional testing links specific components of function and the actual task and provides direct evidence to prove functional status. The single-leg hop test[50] and crossover hop test[51] are performed with the goal of achieving an 85% limb symmetry score.

The results of these tests, along with any other pertinent clinical findings, including the lack of apprehen-sion with sport-specific movements, are presented to the referring orthopedic surgeon for the final determination of sports participation.

Troubleshooting

During phase III, if needed, goals from the previous phase continue to be addressed. The rehabilitation specialist should be sure that recommended criteria are met to ensure a safe progression. A return to optimal function and sports will be strongly based on the restoration of full knee ROM, normal lower extremity strength, and adequate flexibility to meet the demands of the individual's sport. These criteria are needed before the initiation of higher level plyometric, agility, and sport-

Meniscal Transplantation Guidelines
Postoperative Phase I (Weeks 0 to 6)

GOALS

- Emphasis on full passive extension
- Control postoperative pain/swelling
- ROM to 90-degree flexion
- Regain quadriceps control
- Independence in home therapeutic exercise program

PRECAUTIONS

- Avoid active knee flexion
- Avoid ambulation without brace locked at 0 degrees before 4 weeks
- Avoid prolonged standing/walking

TREATMENT STRATEGIES

- Towel extensions, prone hangs, and so on
- Quadriceps reeducation (quadriceps sets with EMS or EMG)
- Toe-touch weight-bearing with brace locked at 0 degrees, with crutches for 4 weeks
- Progressive weight-bearing PWB to WBAT, weeks 4 to 6
- Patellar mobilization
- CPM machine
- Active-assisted flexion/extension 90- to 0-degree exercise
- SLRs (all planes)
- Hip PREs
- Proprioception board (bilateral weight-bearing)
- Aquatic therapy—pool ambulation or underwater treadmill (weeks 4 to 6)
- Short crank ergometry (if ROM >85 degrees)
- Leg press (bilateral/60- to 0-degree arc) (if ROM >85 degrees) (weeks 4 to 6)
- OKC quadriceps isometrics (submaximal/bilateral at 60 degrees) (if ROM >85 degrees)
- Upper extremity cardiovascular exercises as tolerated
- Hamstring and calf stretching
- Cryotherapy
- Emphasize patient compliance to home therapeutic exercise program and weight-bearing and ROM precautions/progression

CRITERIA FOR ADVANCEMENT

- Ability to SLR without quadriceps lag
- ROM 0 to 90 degrees
- Demonstrate ability to unilateral (involved extremity) weight-bear without pain

specific activities. The clinician should be observant to any apprehension with sport-specific movement. This finding will assist the physician in determining whether and/or when a return to sport is appropriate.

POSTOPERATIVE REHABILITATION: MENISCAL TRANSPLANTATION GUIDELINES

Rehabilitation programs following meniscal transplantation are dependent upon surgical technique, concomitant procedures, pathology, and the surgeon's preference. The principles used for rehabilitation after meniscal repair are used with some variation. The loads placed on the healing meniscal allograft during rehabilitation activities are unknown. Because meniscal transplants are thought to be under higher stresses in a joint with early degenerative changes, a more conservative guideline is followed than the meniscal repair guideline previously described in this chapter. Weight-bearing following meniscal transplantation is limited to toe-touch ambulation with the involved knee maintained in full extension for the first 4 weeks (Figure 37-20). Gradual progression to full weight-bearing occurs by 6 weeks postoperatively. A double-upright

Meniscal Transplantation Guidelines
Postoperative Phase II (Weeks 6 to 14)

GOALS

- Restore full ROM
- Restore normal gait (non-antalgic)
- Demonstrate ability to ascend 8-inch stairs with good leg control without pain
- Improve ADL endurance
- Improve lower extremity flexibility
- Independence in home therapeutic exercise program

PRECAUTIONS

- Avoid descending stairs reciprocally until adequate quadriceps control and lower extremity alignment
- Avoid pain with therapeutic exercise and functional activities
- Avoid running and sport activity

TREATMENT STRATEGIES

- Progressive weight-bearing/WBAT with crutches/cane (brace opened 0 to 60 degrees), if good quadriceps control (good quadriceps set/ability to SLR without lag or pain)
- Aquatic therapy—pool ambulation or underwater treadmill
- D/C crutches/cane when gait is non-antalgic
- Brace changed to surgeon's preference (OTS brace, patellar sleeve, etc.)
- AAROM exercises
- Patellar mobilization
- SLRs (all planes) with weights
- Proximal PREs
- Neuromuscular training (bilateral to unilateral support)
- Balance apparatus, foam surface, perturbations
- Short crank ergometry
- Standard ergometry (if knee ROM >115 degrees)
- Leg press (bilateral/eccentric/unilateral progression)
- Squat program (PRE) 0 to 45 degrees
- OKC quadriceps isotonics (pain-free arc of motion) (CKC preferred)
- Initiate forward step-up program
- StairMaster
- Retrograde treadmill ambulation
- Quadriceps stretching
- Elliptical machine
- Upper extremity cardiovascular exercises as tolerated
- Cryotherapy
- Emphasize patient compliance to home therapeutic exercise program

CRITERIA FOR ADVANCEMENT

- Rom to WNL
- Ability to descend 8-inch stairs with good leg control without pain

---

hinged brace is used during this designated protection phase. Meniscal transplantation protection during this phase is supported by a rabbit study in which alterations in stiffness and viscoelasticity were found in the early postoperative period, with gradual recovery over time.[52]

Immediate ROM is encouraged. The goal during the first phase is to achieve full extension and 90 degrees of knee flexion. Flexion is limited to 90 degrees for the first 6 weeks as progressive knee flexion subjects the meniscus to greater stress.[44,45,21] A continuous passive motion (CPM) machine, AAROM exercises, and towel extensions are used as treatment interventions in the initial phase to achieve these goals.

ROM is progressed, as tolerated, at 6 weeks with the goal of achieving full ROM by 14 weeks postoperatively. Treatment strategies for strengthening and neuromuscular training, though more conservatively applied, are similar to those used following meniscal repair. Squatting is limited to 45 degrees for the first 3 months, 60 degrees for 5 months, and 90 degrees for 6 months. Running is not recommended before 6 months. Return

Meniscal Transplantation Guidelines
Postoperative Phase III (Weeks 14 to 22)

GOALS

- Maximize strength and flexibility as to meet demands of ADL
- Demonstrate ability to descend 8-inch stairs with good leg control without pain
- Isokinetic test >75% limb symmetry
- Independence with gym program for maintenance and progression of therapeutic exercise program at discharge

PRECAUTIONS

- Avoid pain with therapeutic exercise and functional activities
- Avoid sport activity until adequate strength development and surgeon's clearance

TREATMENT STRATEGIES

- Progress squat program <60-degree flexion
- Continue lower extremity strengthening and flexibility programs
- Initiate forward step-down program
- Forward Step-Down Test (NeuroCom)
- Isotonic knee flexion/extension (pain- and crepitus-free arc)
- Isokinetic training (fast to moderate to slow velocities)
- Isokinetic testing
- Home therapeutic exercise program: evaluation-based

CRITERIA FOR ADVANCEMENT

- Isokinetic test > 75% limb symmetry
- Ability to descend 8-inch stairs with good leg control without pain

Meniscal Transplantation Guidelines
Postoperative Phase IV (Weeks 22 to 30)

GOALS

- Demonstrate ability to run pain-free
- Maximize strength and flexibility as to meet demands of recreational activity
- Isokinetic test >85% limb symmetry
- Lack of apprehension with recreation-type sport movements
- Independence with gym program for maintenance and progression of therapeutic exercise program at discharge

PRECAUTIONS

- Avoid pain with therapeutic exercise and functional activities
- Avoid sport activity until adequate strength development and surgeon's clearance

TREATMENT STRATEGIES

- Progress squat program <90-degree flexion
- Retrograde treadmill running
- Start forward running (treadmill) program at 6 months postoperatively if 8-inch step-down satisfactory
- Continue lower extremity strengthening and flexibility programs
- Isotonic knee extension (pain- and crepitus-free arc)
- Isokinetic training (fast to moderate to slow velocities)
- Isokinetic testing
- Home therapeutic exercise program: evaluation-based

CRITERIA FOR ADVANCEMENT

- Symptom-free running (if appropriate)
- Isokinetic test > 85% limb symmetry
- Flexibility to accepted levels of recreational activity
- Independence with gym program for maintenance and progression of therapeutic exercise program at discharge

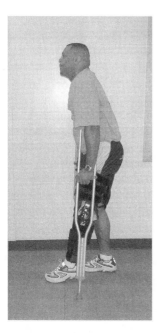

F I G U R E **37-20** Weight-bearing following meniscal transplantation is limited to toe-touch ambulation with the involved knee maintained in full extension for the first 4 weeks.

to high-load activities involving cutting, jumping, and pivoting is not currently recommended after meniscal transplantation.[19]

Troubleshooting

Rehabilitation following meniscal transplantation follows a more conservative guideline than that of meniscal repair. Patients typically present for this surgery with early degenerative changes necessitating a more protective postoperative environment. Adjustments must be made to the postoperative guideline for patients who have undergone concomitant articular cartilage surgery. Examples include a longer restricted weight-bearing period and the use of an unloader brace for ADL.

Following meniscal transplantation, weight-bearing and ROM restrictions need to be reinforced to optimize functional outcome based on present scientific realizations. Loads placed on a transplanted meniscus during ADL and rehabilitation exercises are presently unknown. The failure strength of meniscal horn fixation in a drill tunnel in the tibia is also unknown. Kobayashi[52] in a meniscal transplantation study on rabbits found alterations in meniscus stiffness and viscoelasticity in the early postoperative period, with gradual recovery over time. Supplementary basic science research is needed to provide evidence for a more accelerated rehabilitation guideline.

References

1. Kurosawa, H., Fukubayashi, T., Nakajima, H. *Load-bearing Mode of the Knee Joint: Physical Behavior of the Knee Joint with or without Menisci.* Clin Orthop 1980;149:283–290.
2. Levy, I.M., Torzilli, P.A., Warren, R.F. *The Effect of Medial Meniscectomy on Anterior-Posterior Motion of the Knee.* J Bone Joint Surg Am 1982;64A(6):883–888.
3. Wirth, C.J., Peters, G. **Meniscus** Injuries of the Knee Joint: Pathophysiology and Treatment Principles. In *Baillière's Clinical Orthopedics: Baillière Tindall.* London, 1997, pp. 123–144.
4. Radin, E.L. Factors Influencing the Progression of Osteoarthrosis. In Ewing, J.W. (Ed). *Articular Cartilage and Knee Joint Function.* Raven Press, New York, 1990, pp. 301–309.
5. Sgaglione, N.A., Steadman, J.R., Shaffer, B., Miller, M.D., Fu, F.H. *Current Concepts in Meniscus Surgery: Resection to Replacement.* Arthroscopy 2003;19(Suppl 1):161–188.
6. Allen, P.R., Denham, R.A., Swan, A.V. *Late Degenerative Changes after Meniscectomy. Factors Affecting the Knee after Operation.* J Bone Joint Surg Br 1984;66(5):666–671.
7. Fairbank, T.J. *Knee Joint Changes after Meniscectomy.* J Bone Joint Surg Br 1948;30B(4):664–670.
8. Jorgensen, U., Sonne-Holm, S., Lauridsen, F., Rosenklint, A. *Long-term Follow-up of Meniscectomy in Athletes. A Prospective Longitudinal Study.* J Bone Joint Surg Br 1987;69B(1):80–83.
9. Ferkel, R.D., Davis, J.R., Friedman, M.J., Fox, J.M., DelPizzo, W., Snyder, S.J., Berasi, C.C. *Arthroscopic Partial Medial Meniscectomy: An Analysis of Unsatisfactory Results.* Arthroscopy 1985;1(1):44–52.
10. McGinty, J.B., Geuss, L.F., Marvin, R.A. *Partial or Total Meniscectomy. A Comparative Analysis.* J Bone Joint Surg Am 1977; 59:763–766.
11. Northmore-Ball, M.D., Dandy, D.J., Jackson, R.W. *Arthroscopic Open Partial and Total Meniscectomy. A Comparative Study.* J Bone Joint Surg Br 1983;65(4):400–404.
12. Annandale, T. *An Operation for Displaced Semilunar Cartilage.* Br Med J 1885;1:779.
13. Belzer, J., Cannon, W. *Meniscal Tears: Treatment in the Stable and Unstable Knee.* J Am Acad Orthop Surg 1993;1(1):41–47.
14. Gillquist, J., Messner, K. *Long-term Results of Meniscal Repair.* Sports Med Arthrosc 1993;1:159–163.
15. Cannon, W.D., Vittori, J.M. *The Incidence of Healing in an Arthroscopic Meniscal Repairs in ACL-Reconstructed Knees Versus Stable Knees.* Am J Sports Med 1992;20(2):176–181.
16. Sommerlath, K., Gillquist, J. *Knee Function after Meniscus Repair and Total Meniscectomy: A 7-year Follow-up Study.* Arthroscopy 1987;3(3):166–169.
17. Milachowski, K.A., Weismeier, K., Wirth, C.J. *Homologous Meniscus Transplantation. Experimental and Clinical Results.* Int Orthop 1989;13(1):1–11.
18. Allen, C.R., Wong, E.K., Livesay, G.A., Sakare, M., Fu, F.H., Woo, S.L. *The Importance of the Medial Meniscus in the Anterior-Cruciate Ligament-Deficient Knee.* J Orthop Res 2000; 18(1):109–115.
19. Rodeo, S. *Meniscal Allografts—Where Do We Stand?* Am J Sports Med 2001;29(2):246–261.
20. van Arkel, E.R., deBoer, H.H. *Human Meniscal Transplantation. Preliminary Results at 2- to 5-year Follow-up.* J Bone Joint Surg Br 1995;77(4):589–595.
21. Walker, P.S., Erkman, M.J. *The Role of the Menisci in Force Transmission Across the Knee.* Clin Orthop Relat Res 1975; 109:184–192.

22. Arnoczky, S.P., Warren, R.F. *Microvasculature of the Human Meniscus.* Am J Sports Med 1982;10(2):90–95.

23. Day, B., Mackenzie, W.G., Shim, S.S., Leung, G. *The Vascular and Nerve Supply of the Human Meniscus.* Arthroscopy 1985; 1(1):58–62.

24. Zhang, Z., Arnold, J.A., Williams, T., McCann, B. *Repair by Trephination and Suturing of Longitudinal Injuries in the Avascular Area of the Meniscus in Goats.* Am J Sports Med 1995; 23(1):35–41.

25. Okuda, K., Ochi, M., Shu, N., Uchio, Y. *Meniscal Rasping for Repair of Meniscal Tear in the Avascular Zone.* Arthroscopy 1999;15(3):281–286.

26. Uchio, Y., Ochi, M., Adachi, N., Kawasaki, K., Iwasa, J. *Results of Rasping of Meniscal Tears with and without Anterior Cruciate Ligament Injury as Evaluated by Second-look Arthroscopy.* Arthroscopy 2003;19(5):463–469.

27. Henning, C.E. *Arthroscopic Repair of Meniscal Tears.* Orthopedics 1983;6:1130–1132.

28. Scott, G.A., Jolly, B.C., Henning, C.E. *Combined Posterior Incision and Arthroscopic Intra-articular Repair of the Meniscus. An Examination of Factors Affecting Healing.* J Bone Joint Surg Am 1986;68(6):847–861.

29. Morgan, C.D., Casscells, S.W. *Arthroscopic Meniscus Repair: A Safe Approach to the Posterior Horns.* Arthroscopy 1986;2(1):3–12.

30. Rodeo, S.A. *Arthroscopic Meniscal Repair with Use of the Outside-in Technique.* J Bone Joint Surg Am 2000;82(1):127–141.

31. Cannon, W.D. Jr., Morgan, C.D. *Meniscal Repair. Part II: Arthroscopic Repair Techniques.* J Bone Joint Surg 1994;76A: 294–311.

32. Albrecht-Olsen, P., Kristensen, G., Burgaard, P., Joergensen, U., Toerholem, C. *The Arrow Versus Horizontal Suture in Arthroscopic Meniscus Repair. A Prospective Randomized Study with Arthroscopic Evaluation.* Knee Surg Sports Traumatol Arthrosc 1999;7(5):268–273.

33. Morgan, C.D. *The "All-inside" Meniscus Repair.* Arthroscopy 1991;7(1):120–125.

34. Shaffer, B., Kennedy, S., Klimkiewicz, J., Yao, L. *Preoperative Sizing of Meniscal Allografts in Meniscus Transplantation.* Am J Sports Med 2000;28(4):524–533.

35. Pollard, M.E., Kang, Q., Berg, E.E. *Radiographic Sizing for Meniscal Transplantation.* Arthroscopy 1995;11(6):684–687.

36. Stone, K.R., Rosenberg, T. *Surgical Technique of Meniscal Replacement Arthroscopy.* J Arthrosc Relat Surg 1993;9(2):234–237.

37. Cole, B.J., Carter, T.R., Rodeo, S.A. *Allograft Meniscal Transplantation: Background, Techniques, and Results.* Instr Course Lect 2003;52:383–396.

38. Chen, M.I., Branch, T.P., Hutton, W.C. *Is It Important to Secure the Horns During Lateral Meniscal Transplantation? A Cadaveric Study.* Arthroscopy 1996;12(2):174–181.

39. Noyes, F.R., Barber-Westin, S.B., Rankin, M.D., Rankin, M. *Meniscal Transplantation in Symptomatic Patients Less Than Fifty Years Old.* J Bone Joint Surg 2004;86A(7):1392–1404.

40. Akeson, W.H., Woo, S.L., Amiel, D., Coutts, R.D., Daniel, D. *The Connective Tissue Response to Immobility: Biomechanical Changes in Periarticular Connective Tissue of the Immobilized Rabbit Knee.* Clin Orthop 1973;93:356–362.

41. Noyes, F.R., Mangine, R.E., Barber, S. *Early Knee Motion after Open and Arthroscopic ACL Reconstruction.* Am J Sports Med 1987;15(2):149–160.

42. Salter, R.B., Simmonds, D.F., Malcolm, B.W., Rumble, E.J., MacMichael, D., Clements, N.D. *The Biological Effect of Continuous Passive Motion on the Healing of Full-thickness Defects in Articular Cartilage. An Experimental Investigation in the Rabbit.* J Bone Joint Surg 1980;62A(8):1232–1251.

43. Cavanaugh, J.T. Rehabilitation Following Meniscal Surgery. In Engle, R.P. (Ed.) *Knee Ligament Rehabilitation.* Churchill Livingstone, New York, 1991, pp. 59–69.

44. Morgan, C.D., Wojtys, E.M., Casscells, C.D., Casscells, S.W. *Arthroscopic Meniscal Repair Evaluated by Second-look Arthroscopy.* Am J Sports Med 1991;19(6):632–637.

45. Thompson, W.O., Thaete, F.L., Fu, F.H., Dye, S.F. *Tibial Meniscal Dynamics Using Three-dimensional Reconstruction of Magnetic Resonance Images.* Am J Sports Med 1991;19(3):210–215.

46. Fritz, J.M., Irrgang, J.J., Harner, C.D. *Rehabilitation Following Allograft Meniscal Transplantation: A Review of the Literature and Case Study.* J Orthop Sports Phys Ther 1996;24(2):98–106.

47. Schwartz, R.E., Asnis, P.D., Cavanaugh, J.T., Asnis, S.E., Simmons, J.E., Lasinski, P.J. *Short Crank Cycle Ergometry.* J Orthop Sports Phys Ther 1991;13(2):95–100.

48. Cipriani, D.J., Armstrong, C.W., Gaul, S. *Backward Walking at Three Levels of Treadmill Inclination: An Electromyographic and Kinematic Analysis.* J Orthop Sports Phys Ther 1995;22(3):95–102.

49. Cavanaugh, J.T., Stump, T.J. *Forward Step Down Test.* J Orthop Sports Phys Ther 2000;30(1):A46–A47.

50. Daniel, D.M., Malcolm, L., Stone, M.L., Perth, H., Morgan, J., Riehl, B. *Quantification of Knee Stability and Function.* Contemp Orthop 1982;5:83–91.

51. Barber, S.D., Noyes, F.R., Mangine, R.E., McCloskey, J.W., Hartman, W. *Quantitative Assessment of Functional Limitations in Normal and Anterior Cruciate Ligament Deficient Knees.* Clin Orthop Relat Res 1990;255:204–214.

52. Kobayashi, K. *Visco-elasticity of Transplanted Menisci in Rabbits. A Correlative Histological and Hydrodynamic Study [in Japanese].* Nippon Ika Daigaku Zasshi 1995;62(4):377–385.

38

Achilles Tendon Repair

ROBERT MASCHI, PT, DPT, CSCS

HEATHER M. CLOUTMAN, PT, MSPT, CSCS

NICOLE FRITZ, DPT

The incidence of Achilles tendon rupture is increasing in Western society where lifestyles are sedentary and interest in athletic activities has increased.[1-4] Acute ruptures are commonly associated with white-collar professional men in the third or fourth decades of life who are involved in recreational athletics. The majority of injuries occur during racquet or ball sports, which involve acceleration/deceleration mechanisms, sprint starts and jumping.[2,3,5-8] Traumatic injury is another common cause of acute Achilles tendon rupture, including falling from a height, falling down stairs, or slipping into a hole.[6] Operative repair of an Achilles tendon rupture combined with early rehabilitation enables the patient to return to preinjury functional level, achieve normal ankle range of motion (ROM), and decrease the risk of rerupture.[2,3,9] The Hospital for Special Surgery (HSS) Achilles tendon repair rehabilitation guideline is presented.

SURGICAL OVERVIEW

Open repair of the Achilles tendon is accomplished by exposing the tendon via an incision on the posterior aspect of the leg. The paratenon is opened and the tendon ends are juxtaposed and sutured together. Many different suture techniques can be used, and these vary among surgeons (Figure 38-1).

If the tendon ends are frayed where the Achilles has ruptured often a circumferential suture is used as well. The repair can be reinforced with the plantaris tendon grafts. The paratenon is closed and then the skin is closed and covered with a sterile dressing. A plantar splint is placed at this time to prevent dorsiflexion, which could disrupt the repair. Some surgeons prefer to use a cast or an anterior splint. A Cam walker boot can also be used after sutures are removed in 10 to 14 days, which allows for examination of the wound and early mobilization (Figure 38-2). Meticulous soft tissue handling and closure of the paratenon are key elements of the procedure.

REHABILITATION OVERVIEW

The rehabilitation program following Achilles tendon repair begins 2 to 6 weeks postoperatively. Special attention must be given by the rehabilitation specialist to protect the repair. For example, it is imperative that passive heel cord stretching is avoided until at least 12 weeks postoperatively. In addition, weight-bearing should be progressed incrementally and guided by communication with the surgeon. The clinician must consider the four phases of tendon healing (inflammation, proliferation, remodeling, and maturation) throughout the progression of the postoperative rehabilitation program. The tendon is weakest during the first 6 weeks of healing (inflammation and proliferation phases) and then slowly increases in strength over the next 6 weeks to 12 months (remodeling and maturation phases).[5,19,20] The patient is progressed via criteria-based functional progression.

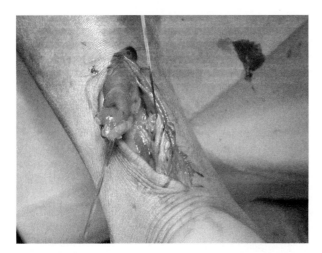

FIGURE **38-1** An approach along either border to the Achilles tendon in a straight-line fashion will demonstrate the lateral sural nerve and the flexor hallucis longus in the depth of the wound. This gives good exposure of the Achilles tendon. In both cases, there is a Bunnell stitch in both ends of the tendon. The tendon ends are prepared to be tied together for the repair. (*Photo courtesy of Robert Marx, MD, Hospital for Special Surgery.*)

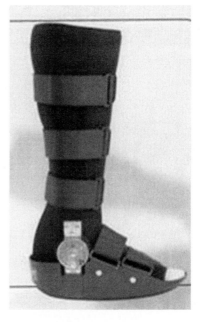

FIGURE **38-2** Cam walker boot. Used for protection of the healing repaired Achilles tendon.

POSTOPERATIVE PHASE I: PROTECTION AND HEALING (WEEKS 1 TO 6)

Rehabilitation in the first phase of the postoperative program places an important emphasis on protecting the repair, controlling effusion and pain, minimizing scar formation, and promoting ROM. Postoperative weight-bearing status and orthosis type or cast is physician directed. Weight-bearing status may range from non-weight-bearing in an orthosis or cast to partial weight-bearing or weight-bearing as tolerated in an orthosis. Protected weight-bearing precautions range from 2 to 8 weeks postoperatively. With the evolution of surgical and rehabilitation techniques, the current approach is commonly to place the patient in a Cam walker boot and observe partial weight-bearing with the use of crutches.

Early mobilization and protected weight-bearing are the most important treatment interventions in the first postoperative phase. Tendon healing and strength are promoted by weight-bearing and ROM while also preventing the negative effects of immobilization (muscle atrophy, joint stiffness, degenerative arthritis, adhesion formation, and deep vein thrombosis).[10,11]

The patient is instructed to perform active range of motion (AROM) dorsiflexion, plantar flexion, inversion, and eversion several times a day. Active dorsiflexion ROM is limited to 0 degrees (neutral) when the knee is flexed at 90 degrees (Figure 38-3, A and B). Passive range of motion (PROM) and stretching is avoided to protect the healing tendon from excessive lengthening and rerupture.

When the patient is partial to full weight-bearing, a stationary bike with low resistance is added to the program. The patient is instructed to weight-bear through the hind-foot (or heel) and avoid pressure through the forefoot while cycling. Scar massage and gentle joint mobilizations are used to promote healing and avoid adhesions and joint stiffness.

Cryotherapy and elevation of the involved extremity are used to control pain and effusion. The patient is instructed to elevate the involved extremity throughout the day and avoid long periods in the gravity-dependent position. A cold pack several times a day for 20 minutes is also advised.

Proximal hip and knee exercises are initiated using a progressive resistive exercise (PRE) regime. Open chain

---

Postoperative Phase I: Protection and Healing (Weeks 1 to 6)

GOALS

- Protect repair
- Control edema and pain
- Minimize scar formation
- Improve ROM of dorsiflexion to neutral (0 degrees)
- Increase proximal lower extremity musculature 5/5 in all planes
- Progressive weight-bearing—surgeon directed
- Independence in home exercise program

PRECAUTIONS

- Avoid passive heal cord stretching
- Limit active dorsiflexion ROM to neutral (0 degrees) with knee flexed at 90 degrees
- Avoid heat application
- Avoid prolonged dependent position

TREATMENT STRATEGIES

- Progress weight-bearing status in the Cam boot with crutches or cane—surgeon directed
- AROM dorsiflexion/plantar flexion/inversion/eversion
- Scar massage
- Joint mobilizations
- Proximal musculature strengthening
- Modalities
- Cryotherapy

CRITERIA FOR ADVANCEMENT

- Pain and edema controlled
- Weight-bearing status—surgeon directed
- ROM dorsiflexion to neutral (0 degrees)
- Proximal lower extremity muscle strength 5/5

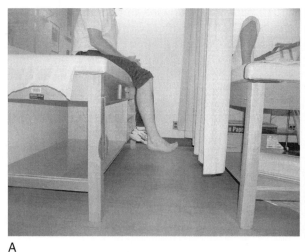 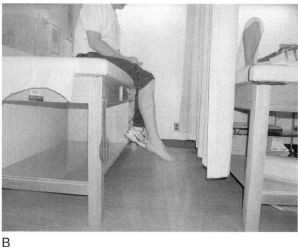

A   B

FIGURE **38-3** *A.* AROM with the knee flexed in the direction of dorsiflexion and *(B)* plantar flexion.

exercises and isotonic machines are used for the patient with weight-bearing precautions.

Troubleshooting

Poor wound healing and infection are the most common cited complications following Achilles tendon repair. Frequent inspection of the incision site by the rehabilitation specialist and the patient is critical in the first postoperative phase. The physician is notified by the rehabilitation specialist or the patient at the first sign of poor healing or infection.

Effusion of the involved leg is the other common complication following Achilles tendon repair. Emphasize patient compliance with weight-bearing precautions, elevation of the involved leg (limited time in the dependent position), AROM exercises, and the use of a cold pack several times a day.

POSTOPERATIVE PHASE II: EARLY MOBILIZATION (WEEKS 6 TO 12)

The second postoperative phase marks a change in weight-bearing status, increasing mobilization of the involved extremity, and gentle strengthening. The patient is first progressed to full weight-bearing in the orthosis with crutches and then advanced to full weight-bearing in a shoe without crutches. A heel lift placed in the shoe allows for an easier transition from the orthosis (which is often plantar flexed 20 to 30 degrees). The size of the heel lift can be gradually decreased as ROM improves. The heel lift is removed when the patient achieves a normal gait pattern. A normal gait pattern is the prerequisite for discontinuing crutch ambulation.

If the incision is well healed, gait training in an underwater treadmill system is used to unload the involved extremity. Walking with water at chest level provides a reduction in weight-bearing of 60% to 75%, whereas waist level water provides a reduction of 40% to 50%.[12]

AROM in all planes is continued without limits, whereas PROM is avoided. Normal ambulation will help facilitate functional ROM. Stretching should not be needed to achieve normal ROM; however, at this stage ROM is expected to return to normal.

Gentle inversion and eversion isometrics begin during this phase, with progression to elastic bands later in the phase. Strengthening is progressed using a multiaxial device while the patient draws letters from the alphabet using his or her ankle joint (Figure 38-4). When adequate ROM is achieved, strengthening of the two main plantar flexor muscles of the calf (gastrocnemius

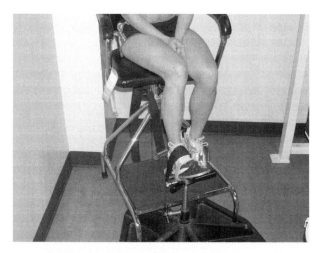

FIGURE **38-4** Drawing alphabets to increase ankle strength using a multiaxial device. *(Multi Axial Ankle Exerciser, Multi-axial, Inc., Lincoln, RI.)*

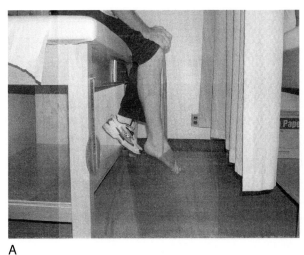
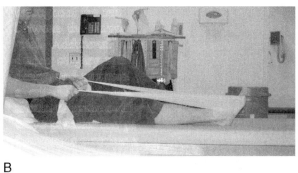

A   B

FIGURE **38-5** *A.* PREs using an elastic band to strengthen the planter flexors with the knee flexed and *(B)* with the knee straight.

and soleus) begins. At week 6 resistive plantar flexion is performed with the knee flexed to 90 degrees (Figure 38-5, *A*). By week 8, the resistive plantar flexion is done with the knee extended at 0 degrees (Figure 38-5, *B*).

Plantar flexion on the leg press and plantar flexion using a leg curl machine are also added at this time (Figure 38-6, *A* and *B*). Stationary bike continues with increasing weight-bearing through the forefoot.

A retrograde treadmill ambulation program is introduced to facilitate eccentric plantar flexion control. These patients usually find retroambulation comfortable because it eliminates the need to push off.[13] A

forward step-up program is introduced with progressive heights (4, 6, and 8 inches).

Early neuromuscular training and ROM is encouraged using a biomechanical ankle platform system (BAPS) board in the seated position and progressed to a standing position. In addition, bilateral weight-bearing activities on a NeuroCom Balance Master System (NeuroCom International Inc., Clackamas, OR) or similar force plate system is used for developing proprioception, neuromuscular training, and balance. Activities begin bilaterally and progress to unilateral activities as balance and strength continue to improve (Figure 38-7). Scar massage, modalities, and gentle joint mobilizations are continued as needed.

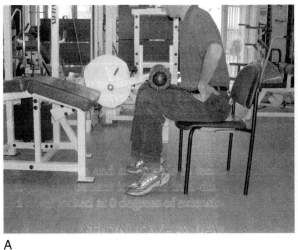
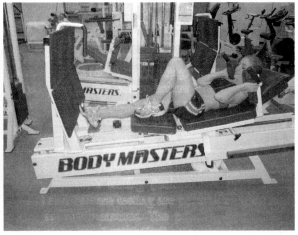

A   B

FIGURE **38-6** PREs for the plantar flexor muscles using *(A)* the leg curl machine and *(B)* leg press.

Postoperative Phase II: Early Mobilization (Weeks 6 to 12)

GOALS

- Normalize gait
- Restore full functional ROM necessary for normal gait (15-degree dorsiflexion) and for ascending stairs (25 degrees)
- Normalize dorsiflexion, inversion, and eversion ankle strength 5/5

PRECAUTIONS

- Avoid pain with therapeutic exercise and functional activities
- Avoid passive heal cord stretching

TREATMENT STRATEGIES

- Gait training WBAT to FWB with/without orthoses or assistive device
  - d/c crutches when gait is non-antalgic
- Underwater treadmill system for gait training
- Heel lift in shoe to assist nonapprehensive and normalized gait
- AROM dorsiflexion/plantar flexion/inversion/eversion
- Proprioception training: BAPS
- Isometrics/isotonics: inversion/eversion
- Week 6: PREs plantar flexion/dorsiflexion with knee flexed to 90 degrees
- Week 8: PREs plantar flexion/dorsiflexion with knee extended 0 degrees
- Plantar flexor strengthening using a leg press and leg curl machine
- Bike
- Alphabet drawing using multiaxial plate
- Retro treadmill
- Modalities
- Scar massage
- Forward step-up program

CRITERIA FOR ADVANCEMENT

- Normal gait pattern
- Full PROM dorsiflexion, 20 degrees
- Manual muscle test grade of 5/5 for dorsiflexion, inversion, and eversion

PREs for the proximal musculature of the involved extremity are advanced.

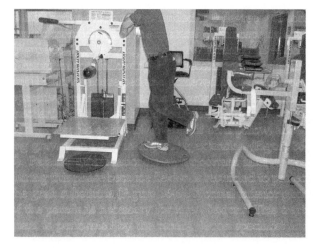

FIGURE 38-7 Unilateral ROM and neuromuscular training, using a BAPS.

Troubleshooting

Achilles tendonitis and/or general Achilles pain is a more common complication of phase II. Patients often increase their activity level when they no longer have to ambulate with crutches or wear a Cam boot. In turn, the healing tendon becomes painful and inflamed because it does not yet have the strength to meet the demands of the patient's new activity level. The patient must be made aware of his or her limitations with activities of daily living (ADL) and instructed to modify behavior to pain-free activities. Similarly, a rehabilitation program that progresses ROM and strengthening exercises too quickly can also cause Achilles pain and inflammation. The patient's subjective complaints and objective measures are considered by the rehabilitation specialist when progressing the treatment plan. Compliance to the home exercise program should also be emphasized.

POSTOPERATIVE PHASE III: EARLY STRENGTHENING (WEEKS 12 TO 20)

Upon meeting the established criteria for advancement, the patient enters this phase designed to restore full AROM, normalize plantar flexor strength, and improve balance and neuromuscular control.

Normal plantar flexor strength is demonstrated by the patient's ability to perform 10 unilateral heel raises.[15] However, the patient must first demonstrate bilateral heel raise on a flat surface without apprehension followed by the progression shown in the following diagram.

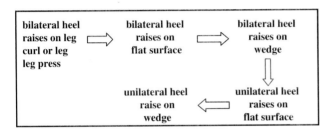

Higher level endurance equipment is added to the program to work on both strength and endurance (i.e., StairMaster, VersaClimber) when the previous tasks are performed with good technique and without apprehension.

A forward step-down program is introduced with progressive heights (4, 6, and 8 inches). Balance activities are progressed to include unilateral weight-bearing, multiplanar support surfaces (trampoline, rocker boards, foam rollers, etc.), and perturbation training (Figure 38-8, A and B).

Isokinetic training is used to further improve strength and endurance of ankle musculature. Isokinetics have a fixed speed with accommodating resistance. Therefore, maximal dynamic loading of the muscle is accomplished through the full ROM at a preset speed.[16]

Once the patient achieves a normal gait pattern, full PROM, and normal strength, running in water at chest height is introduced. An underwater treadmill system uses the property of buoyancy to lessen the load placed on the Achilles tendon.

The patient's home therapeutic exercise program is continually updated based on reevaluative findings.

Phase III: Early Strengthening (Weeks 12 to 20)

GOALS
- Restore full AROM
- Normalize plantar flexion strength 5/5
- Normalize balance (tested using NeuroCom or Biodex Balance System)
- Return to functional activities without pain
- Ability to descend stairs

PRECAUTIONS
- Avoid pain with therapeutic exercise and functional activities
- Avoid high loading the Achilles tendon (i.e., aggressive stretching in dorsiflexion with body weight or jumping)

TREATMENT STRATEGIES
- Inversion/eversion isotonics/isokinetics
- Bike, StairMaster, VersaClimber
- Proprioception training: Prop board/BAPS/foam rollers/trampoline/NeuroCom
- Aggressive plantar flexion PREs (emphasize eccentric activity)
- Submaximal sport-specific skill development
- Progress proprioception program
- Running in underwater treadmill system
- Progress proximal strengthening of lower extremities (PREs)
- Isokinetic PF/DF
- Flexibility as needed for activity
- Forward step-down program

CRITERIA FOR ADVANCEMENT
- No apprehension with ADL
- Normal flexibility
- Adequate strength base shown by ability to perform 10 unilateral heel raises
- Ability to descend stairs reciprocally
- Symmetrical lower extremity balance

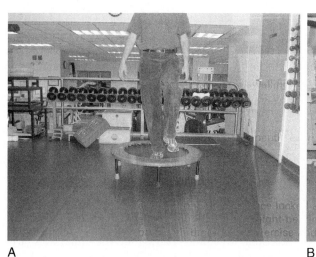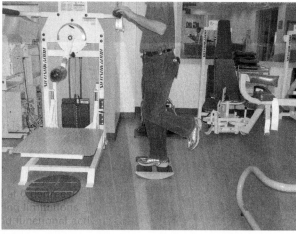

A   B

FIGURE **38-8** Unilateral balance activities, using *(A)* a trampoline and *(B)* rocker board.

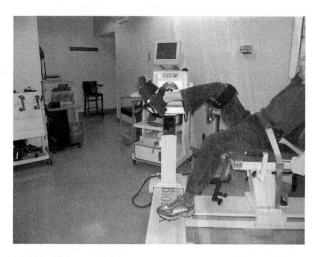

FIGURE **38-9** Using a Biodex machine for isokinetic strengthening of the ankle plantar flexors. *(BIODEX Inc., Shirley, NY.)*

Balance is assessed in comparison to the contralateral limb, using the NeuroCom or a Biodex Balance System (Figure 38-9). Symmetry is expected by the end of this phase.

Troubleshooting

The patient needs continued encouragement to adhere to activity modification based on remaining deficits in ROM and/or muscle strength. A more common complication during this phase is the complaint of muscle soreness or tendonitis with the newfound ability to perform higher level activities. Patients may attempt to progress their activity level (i.e., stair negotiation) without sufficient lower extremity strength. The rehabilitation specialist must continue to educate the patient about his or her limitations. If the patient has returned

to a gym to perform his or her home program, he or she needs to follow the therapy program and not advance independently.

POSTOPERATIVE PHASE IV: LATE STRENGTHENING (WEEKS 20 TO 28)

As calf strength normalizes and activity level increases, the patient enters a phase designed specifically to return to higher level dynamic activity. Treatment strategies are incorporated to prepare the patient/athlete for the safe return to the individual's sport.

At 20 weeks postoperatively an isokinetic test is performed on ankle plantar flexors, dorsiflexors, inverters, and everters. Isokinetic assessment allows a more accurate assessment of dynamic strength than does isometric manual muscle testing. Isokinetic testing affords the clinician objective criteria and provides reproducible data to assess and monitor a patient's status.[16] The objective data obtained will determine whether calf muscle strength, power, and endurance have normalized. If the results are within 75% of the opposite limb, and the patient demonstrates the ability to perform 10 unilateral heel raises, a running program may be initiated on a treadmill. A forward treadmill running program is progressed with an emphasis on short distances, low to moderate speeds, and subjective reports from the patient indicating pain-free motion.

Isokinetic strengthening is continued to improve the strength and endurance of dorsiflexors, plantar flexors, inverters, and everters.

PRE and flexibility programs continue to be progressed as tolerated, and agility activities based on the individual's sport are added. Running and sport drills should begin in straight planes and then progress to more demanding activities, such as crossovers, braiding, cutting, figure eights, acceleration, and deceleration

Postoperative Phase IV: Late Strengthening (Weeks 20 to 28)

GOALS

- Demonstrate ability to run forward on a treadmill symptom-free
- Average peak torque of 75% with isokinetic testing
- Maximize strength and flexibility as to meet all demands of ADL
- Return to functional activity without limitation
- Higher level dynamic activity with lack of apprehension with sport-specific movements

PRECAUTIONS

- No apprehension or pain with dynamic activity
- Avoid running or sport activity until adequate strength and flexibility is achieved

TREATMENT STRATEGIES

- Start forward treadmill running
- Isokinetic testing and training
- Continue lower extremity strengthening and flexibility program
- Advance proprioception training with perturbation
- Light plyometric training (bilateral jumping activities)
- Continue aggressive plantar flexion PREs (emphasize eccentric activity)
- Submaximal sport-specific skill development drills
- Progress bike, StairMaster, VersaClimber
- Continue to progress proximal strengthening of lower extremities (PREs)

CRITERIA FOR ADVANCEMENT

- Pain-free running
- Average peak torque of isokinetic test = 75%
- Normal flexibility
- Normal strength (5/5 throughout ankle)
- Sport-specific drills with no apprehension

---

training. These activities can be further progressed by adding the resistance of a sport cord.

A large focus is put on balance activities, such as those mentioned during phase III. However, now perturbation training is used in conjunction with balance activities to challenge the muscle control and strength of the ankle. Perturbation can be given to the patient while the patient balances on a trampoline, rocker board, foam roller, and so on.

Introduction of light plyometric activities begins in this phase. Plyometrics are strengthening exercises using the stretch-shortening cycle to enhance performance.[16] It is essential that the patient has full ROM, flexibility, and normal strength to perform these activities without pain or apprehension. Plyometric activity can be initiated using bilateral activities, such as jumping in place on two feet. Impact can be minimized by jumping up onto a box with both feet. As the patient progresses, more demanding bilateral activities can be used, such as side-to-side jumps and quadrant jumping (Figure 38-10).

The patient's home therapeutic exercise program is continually updated based on reevaluative findings and functional level.

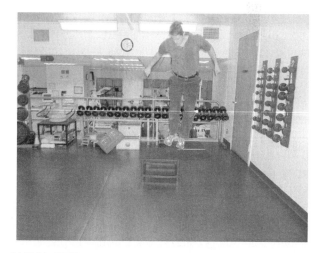

FIGURE **38-10** Bilateral plyometric training, using lateral box jumping.

Troubleshooting

The patient still requires continued encouragement to adhere to activity modification based on remaining deficits. The rehabilitation specialist must pay close attention to signs of apprehension with the introduction

Postoperative Phase V: Return to Full Sport (Week 28 to Year 1)

GOALS

- Lack of apprehension with sports activity
- Maximize strength and flexibility to meet demands of individual sport activity
- 85% limb symmetry with vertical jump test
- 85% limb symmetry for average peak isokinetic torque (PF/DF/INV/EV)

PRECAUTIONS

- Avoid pain with therapeutic, functional, and sport activity
- Avoid full sport activity until adequate strength and flexibility

TREATMENT STRATEGIES

- Advanced functional exercises and agility exercises
- Plyometrics
- Sport-specific exercises
- Isokinetic testing
- Functional test assessment, such as vertical jump test

CRITERIA FOR DISCHARGE

- Flexibility and strength to accepted levels for sports performance
- Lack of apprehension with sport-specific movements
- 85% limb symmetry with functional tests
- 85% limb symmetry for average peak isokinetic torque (PF/DF/INV/EV)
- Independent performance of gym/home exercise program

---

of treadmill running and agility activities. In many cases, the patient/athlete is enthusiastic about his or her return to a running program and may try to continue, despite discomfort. The clinician must carefully observe signs of weakness and fatigue and adjust the running program appropriately. Focus should be directed on short distance running at slow speeds, progressing to moderate distances/long distances at the patient's normal speed. In addition, the patient should be advised to monitor his or her PRE program, allowing for adequate recovery. This will decrease the risk of an overuse condition developing. The volume of running done should be kept to a minimum, using cross-training (swimming, biking) to avoid reinjury or tendonitis.

POSTOPERATIVE PHASE V: RETURN TO FULL SPORT (WEEK 28 TO YEAR 1)

The final phase of rehabilitation may take from 28 weeks up to a full year, depending on the patient's desired activity level and physical status. During this phase, any remaining deficits in strength and flexibility should be addressed. Sport-specific drills, advanced plyometrics, and agility exercises should be used, which reproduce the functional demands of the desired sport.

Isokinetic training continues with the goal of returning endurance to normal levels required for sport activities. Plyometric drills may be progressed in this phase to more demanding unilateral activities, such as single-leg jumps and hops, single-leg side-to-side jumps and

quadrant jumping. Functional testing, such as the vertical jump test, can be used to determine the patient's ability to perform under dynamic conditions as the patient prepares to return to full sport activity. The vertical jump test has been demonstrated to be a valid measure of leg muscle power and is capable of detecting functional limitations of the lower limb.[17,18] It is desired that the patient demonstrates 85% limb symmetry and has clearance from the referring physician before a complete return to sport.

Troubleshooting

Care should be taken in this phase to ensure that the patient has an adequate strength base, ROM, and flexibility to participate in higher level activities, such as plyometrics and sport-specific training drills. The patient should also demonstrate a lack of apprehension with lower level activities before being progressed to higher level, more demanding activities and, eventually, returned to sport. The chosen functional tests should reproduce the specific demands of the athlete's sport to ensure safe return to full activity.

REFERENCES

1. Myerson, M.S. *Achilles Tendon Ruptures.* Instr Course Lect 1999;48:219–230.
2. Schepsis, A.A., Jones, H., Haas, A.L. *Achilles Tendon Disorders in Athletes.* Am J Sports Med 2002;30(2):287–305.

3. Aoki, M., Ogiwara, N., Ohta, T., Nabeta, Y. *Early Motion and Weightbearing After Cross-Stitch Achilles Tendon Repair.* Am J Sports Med 1998;26(6):794–800.

4. Motta, P., Errichiello, C., Pontini, I. *Achilles Tendon Rupture. A New Technique for Easy Surgical Repair and Immediate Movement of the Ankle and Foot.* Am J Sports Med 1997;25(2): 172–176.

5. Mandelbaum, B., Gruber, J., Zachazewski, J. *Rehabilitation of the Postsurgical Orthopedic Patient: Achilles Tendon Repair and Rehabilitation.* Mosby, St. Louis, 2001.

6. Maffulli, N. *Current Concepts Review: Rupture of the Achilles Tendon.* J Bone Joint Surg 1999;81:1019–1036.

7. Nicholas, J.A., Hershman, E.B. *The Lower Extremity and Spine in Sports Medicine,* 2nd ed. Mosby, St. Louis, 1995.

8. Soldatis, J.J., Goodfellow, D.B., Wilber, J.H. *End-to-end Operative Repair of Achilles Tendon Ruptures.* Am J Sports Med 1997;24(1):90–95.

9. Cetti, R., Christensen, S.E., Ejsted, R., Jensen, N.M., Jorgensen, U. *Operative Versus Nonoperative Treatment of Achilles Tendon Rupture: A Prospective Randomized Study and Review of the Literature.* Am J Sports Med 1993;21(6):791–799.

10. Maffuli, N., Tallon, C., Wong, J., Lim, K.P., Bleakney, R. *Early Weightbearing and Ankle Mobilization after Open Repair of Acute Midsubstance Tears of the Achilles Tendon.* Am J Sports Med 2003;31(5):692–700.

11. Mandelbaum, B.R., Myerson, M.S., Forester, R. *Achilles Tendon Ruptures. A New Method of Repair, Early Range of Motion, and Functional Rehabilitation.* Am J Sports Med 1995;23:392–395.

12. Bates, A., Hanson, N. The Principles and Properties of Water. In *Aquatic Exercise Therapy.* WB Saunders, Philadelphia, 1996, pp. 1–320.

13. Threlkeld, J., Horn, T.S., Wojtowicz, G.M., Rooney, J.G., Shapiro, R.S. *Kinematics, Ground Reaction Force, and Muscle Balance Produced by Backward Running.* J Orthop Sports Phys Ther, American Physical Therapy Association, 1989.

14. Norkin, C.C., Levangie, P.K. *Joint Structure and Function: A Comprehensive Analysis.* FA Davis, Philadelphia, 1992.

15. Kendall, F., McCreary, E. *Muscles Testing and Function,* 4th ed., chap 7. Williams & Wilkins, Baltimore, 1993.

16. Davies, G. *Open Kinetic Chain Assessment and Rehabilitation, Athletic Training.* Sports Health Care Perspect 1995;1(4):347–370.

17. Thomas, M., Fiatarone, M., Fielding, R. *Leg Power in Young Women: Relationship to Body Composition, Strength, and Function.* Med Sci Sports Exerc 1996;28(10):1321–1326.

18. Petschnig, R., Baron, R., Albrecht, M. *The Relationship Between Isokinetic Quadriceps Strength Tests and Hop Tests for Distance and One-Legged Vertical Jump Test Following ACL Reconstruction.* J Orthop Sports Phys Ther 1998;28(1):23–31.

19. Curwin, S. Tendon Injuries: Pathology and Treatment. In Zachazewski, J.E., Magee, D.J., Quillen, W.S. (Eds). *Athletic Injuries and Rehabilitation.* WB Saunders, Philadelphia, 1996.

20. Leadbetter, W.B. *Cell Matrix Response in Tendon Injury.* Clin Sports Med 1992;11(3):533.

39

Lateral Ankle
Reconstruction

JAIME EDELSTEIN, PT, MSPT, CSCS

DENNIS J. NOONAN, ATC, CMT

The lateral ligaments of the ankle are the most commonly injured structures in the body of an athlete.[1] The ligaments involved in this injury are the anterior talofibular ligament (ATFL), calcaneofibular ligament (CFL), and posterior talofibular ligament (PTFL). The etiology of a lateral ankle sprain is related specifically to sports involving running or jumping, such as soccer, basketball, and dance.[2] Eighty percent to 85% of acute ankle sprains are treated successfully with conservative treatment.[3,4] Research has shown that those who have sustained an ankle sprain are approximately 10% to 20% more susceptible to develop chronic instability, pain on exertion, or recurrent swelling.[2,5,6]

Chronic lateral ankle instability is defined as instability and associated symptoms for greater than 6 months.[2,7] These signs and symptoms are caused by either mechanical or functional instability. Mechanical instability, referred to as *laxity*, is defined as ankle movement beyond the physiological limit of the ankle's range of motion (ROM).[8] True mechanical instability may be demonstrated using clinical tests, including the anterior drawer, the talar tilt, or diagnostically using a wide variety of radiographic tests, including stress radiography, magnetic resonance imaging (MRI), computed tomography (CT scan), and bone scan.[9] The presence of mechanical instability alone does not correlate to a need for surgical repair. *Functional instability*, a term first defined by Freeman et al.,[10] is a subjective feeling of "giving way" or evidence of recurrent, symptomatic ankle sprains. As well documented, mechanical instability is not a reliable indicator of a functionally unstable ankle.[6,11–13] Studies have shown that joint position sense and kinesthesia are greatly diminished in individuals with chronic ankle instability (CAI), which, in turn, leads to repetitive lateral ankle sprains.[3,4] Other proprioceptive deficits may be accountable for these levels of instability. Additional contributing factors leading to functional instability include deficits in center of pressure excursion measures, postural stability, ROM, and invertor and evertor muscles strength.[6,13,14] The focus of conservative rehabilitation for this population has been placed on challenging and regaining postural-control strategies, in addition to strengthening, flexibility, and regaining ROM.

The 10% to 20% of individuals who have functional instability, with or without true mechanical instability, may require surgical intervention.[15] These individuals have failed conservative treatment with guided physical therapy and are still having subjective complaints and recurrent incidents of instability. More than 50 surgical procedures have been described to treat lateral ankle instability. The surgical procedures for treating this pathology may be described as anatomical or nonanatomical. The preferred surgical procedure at the Hospital for Special Surgery (HSS) is the modified Broström-Gould Procedure, an anatomical procedure. The rehabilitation guidelines for this procedure are described in this chapter.

SURGICAL OVERVIEW

The ATFL resists inversion of the talus within the ankle mortis (talar tilt). The CFL acts as a restraint against subtalar inversion and thereby indirectly acts as a restraint for talar tilt.[16] Without these restraints the ankle will be mechanically unstable. Anatomical repairs involve the ATFL and the CFL being imbricated and sutured. In cases where the ATFL and CFL tissues are obliterated, ligament augmentation may also be performed, using fascia lata, plantaris tendon, Achilles tendon, or allograft.[2,9,17–20] The nonanatomical procedures are checkrein and tenodesis procedures using the peroneus brevis tendon.[9,19,20]

Nonanatomical surgical procedures have been developed and modified by multiple surgeons.[5,9,16,19,21] All of these physicians developed surgical variations using the peroneus brevis to reconstruct and stabilize the lateral ankle. A tenodesis is the procedure of choice when an individual has general ligamentous laxity, has failed a modified Broström-Gould procedure, is an obese individual, or a direct repair is not possible because of chronic, repetitive trauma.[15,17,19] Because all of these tenodesis procedures somewhat change the biomechanics of the subtalar joint, instability may be a complication for any of the tenodesis surgical procedures. Subjective complaints of instability following anatomical procedure tend to be less prevalent (0% to 3%).[22]

In 1966, Broström[7,23] repaired the ATFL and CFL by attenuating and shortening the ATFL and CFL ligaments (Figure 39-1). This allowed for isometry of the ligaments as well as full ROM at the talocrural and subtalar joints. However, this procedure had a high rate of subtalar instability.[16,22] In 1980, Gould et al.[24] addressed this instability by developing the modified Broström procedure, whereby the extensor retinaculum was sutured to the anterior aspect of the fibula (Figure 39-2). The surgical procedure entails the foot being placed in a vertical or slightly internally rotated position. A curvilinear incision is made anteriorly to the distal fibula, stopping at the peroneals. Care must be taken because the sural nerve lies just below this incision over the peroneal tendons. The joint capsule is dissected along the anterior border of the lateral malleolus. The ATFL lies within the joint capsule, and the CFL lies deep to the capsule. Once both structures are identified, the repair can be made. The final phase is to attach the posterior portion of the extensor retinaculum to the distal fibula via sutures passed through holes in the fibula.[25] This type of procedure reinforces the repair as well as limits inversion. This limitation of inversion is considered an acceptable outcome of the procedure given that instability was the initial pathology being corrected. The patient is placed in a short leg cast or bivalve cast and is non–weight-bearing following surgery. Outcome studies have reported at least an 85% success rate.[7,15,22]

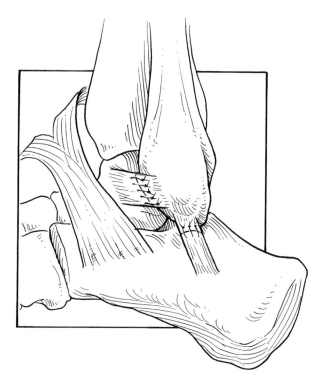

FIGURE **39-1** Broström procedure: original procedure developed to reconstruct the lateral ankle.

REHABILITATION OVERVIEW

Rehabilitation following a modified Broström procedure begins immediately postoperatively with gait training, patient education, and a home exercise program. The individual is initially non–weight-bearing following surgery. The ankle is in a neutral position in the cast. Once active range of motion (AROM) is allowed, special care must be taken in limiting forces into inversion through the earliest phase of the healing process. Excessive tensile forces on the repair could potentially disrupt the repair. Formal physical therapy is initiated 6 weeks following surgery. The patient bears weight as tolerated in an Aircast and uses either a cane or crutches as an assistive device. Initial rehabilitation will focus on review of the home exercise program and continued patient education and progression of ROM into all planes. During the initial physical therapy outpatient evaluation, it is necessary to assess for intrinsic mechanical factors, including hind foot varus or generalized ligamentous laxity, because this will affect postoperative stresses on the repair as well as overall treatment approaches. The format for progression in rehabilitation is functionally based. It is important to note that most of the research and literature supporting this proposed guideline is relative to functional ankle instability (FAI). Lateral ankle reconstruction and FAI are comparable in their philosophies. Proprioceptive training is very important with this population as well as strengthening of the evertors and the invertors. Return to full activity or to sport is expected to occur at approximately 3 months. Objective measures and subjective reports, however, will outweigh a rehabilitation timeline. Understanding the goals and abilities of the population

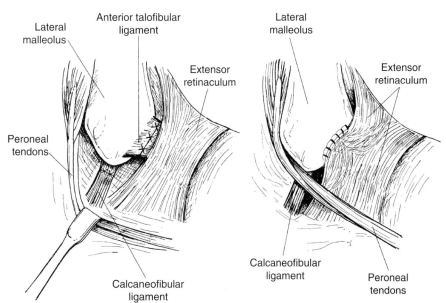

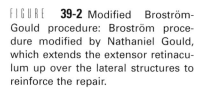

FIGURE **39-2** Modified Broström-Gould procedure: Broström procedure modified by Nathaniel Gould, which extends the extensor retinaculum up over the lateral structures to reinforce the repair.

being instructed is vital. Athletes returning to play will be expected to participate initially with a lace-up ankle brace or taping for 4 to 6 months.

IMMEDIATE POSTOPERATIVE INSTRUCTIONS AND HOME EXERCISE PROGRAM (WEEKS 0 TO 6)

Immediately following surgery, the patient is instructed in procedures for reducing edema, including elevation of the involved lower extremity in both sitting and supine positions. Before discharge from the hospital, the individual is instructed in proper non–weight-bearing gait training with an appropriate assistive device. Particularly for the athletic population, it is vital to instruct the individual in proximal strengthening exercises for a home exercise program as well as aerobic conditioning (i.e., upper body ergometry) and strength training for the core and upper body. The goal of these activities is to prevent overall deconditioning and develop proximal strength in preparation for weight-bearing loads. A deconditioned patient may have compensatory movement patterns as a result of lack of strength in another muscle group. For example, the patient may be firing evertors when trying to perform hip abduction, especially if he or she has posterior gluteus medius weakness.

The patient is progressed at 2 weeks following surgery from non–weight-bearing to progressive weight-bearing as tolerated in a CAM walker using an appropriate assistive device. The physician encourages AROM of the ankle at 4 weeks postoperatively as a home program. ROM is limited at this time from neutral into dorsiflexion and neutral into eversion, because motion into plantar flexion and inversion is protected until the 6-week mark. Submaximal isometrics for all musculature surrounding the ankle joint may also be initiated at 4 weeks with proper instruction. Six weeks following surgery, the patient is placed into an Aircast, further normalizing his or her gait and weight-bearing status.

POSTOPERATIVE PHASE I (WEEKS 6 TO 8)

Research has repeatedly proven that the proliferation phase of tissue healing overlaps with the maturation phase at 21 days following insult.[26-28] The maturation phase of soft tissue healing is complete at 42 days. Therefore, plantar flexion and inversion must be restricted to 0 degrees until 6 weeks following surgery because the CFL is stressed into inversion and dorsiflexion, and the ATFL is taut in plantar flexion. After 6 weeks, ROM in all planes may be progressed without limitations. It is shown that cyclical loads of well-controlled stresses on a ligament scar will promote proliferation and strength of the healing tissue.[29] The patient should initially perform AROM into straight

planes and then progress into multiplanar movements. Having the patient work with a BAPS board while seated is an effective means of facilitating ROM and introducing proprioception. Aquatic therapy, using a pool or underwater treadmill, is also a safe and functional means of regaining ROM and normalizing the gait pattern. Isometrics should have already been initiated in the home program. Isotonic strengthening may be initiated in this phase once 50% pain-free ROM into the plane has been achieved. These exercises may be performed through the use of elastic bands, ankle weights, or motion against gravity. All patients should be progressed as tolerated without pain or residual edema.

Wilkerson[30] has shown that an increase in capsular swelling leads to a decrease in proprioception and kinesthetic awareness. Therefore, edema reduction using various modalities will assist in regaining ROM as well as limiting the loss of proprioception. A contrast bath is just one example of a safe and useful modality for these individuals. It uses the theory of vasodilation and vasoconstriction to provide a milking effect to the joint to rid the area of edema. It is recommended to initiate with a cold bath of 50°F to 60°F followed by a warm bath of 93°F to 98°F for time ratios of 1 : 3-minute spans. Four repetitions are performed, ending with the cold bath.[31]

The idea of initiating proprioception exercises as early as possible in the rehabilitation process is considered rudimentary. In the 1960s, Freeman[11,12,28,32] was the first to investigate the existence of mechanoreceptors in the ankle ligaments. His belief was that deficits in proprioception would lead to symptoms of giving way and additionally affect postural control. Multiple studies have been performed investigating the concept of reaction time of peroneals versus proximal musculature reaction time. The results in comparing these studies have been inconclusive.*

Ryan[11] investigated the mechanical stability of the talocrural joint, the strength of the evertors and invertors, and the dynamic control of the ankle. He found that 50% of individuals had no significant difference in grades of talar tilt between extremities. This supported the low correlation of mechanical instability to functional instability.[11] A summary of all of these findings indicated that (1) decreased postural control may be inconclusively associated with functional instability, (2) mechanical instability has no correlation to functional instability, and (3) a deficit in the central motor control, and not solely of peripheral proprioception, is associated with functional instability.

Riemann[12] further investigated the link between CAI and postural instability. This study concluded that it is still unknown whether postural control is disrupted by

---

*References 2, 5, 6, 11, 13, 14, 33.

ankle instability because increased hip strategies may enable individuals to demonstrate normal equilibrium with CAI. This evidence has highlighted the importance of peroneal dynamic stability and strength exercises as well as the proprioceptive challenge of the entire kinematic chain in returning the individual to the highest level of performance possible. This concept is relevant, regardless of whether the patient has CAI or is in postoperative phase following lateral ankle reconstruction.

As a result, bilateral proprioception exercises are initiated immediately in this first phase of rehabilitation.

Initially, the proprioceptive program should begin on a relatively stable surface like a rocker board in sagittal and coronal planes and progress to more challenging surfaces, including multiplanar wobble boards. Multiplane challenges should be graded in difficulty in accordance with the ROM and pain limitations of the patient. The Biodex Balance System (Shirley, NY), if available, offers multiple variations in settings to train and assess proprioceptive deficits and improvements. Within the progression of these challenging surfaces, there should be a variation of visual afferent input to increase vestibular and proprioceptive input.

Postoperative Phase I (Weeks 6 to 8)

GOALS

- Patient education, wound recognition, infection avoidance
- Edema control
- Regaining ROM, progressing motion into inversion and plantar flexion. Achieve 75% functional ROM
- Prevent deconditioning
- Pain reduction
- Reduce scar adhesions/myofascial restriction
- Normalized gait without assistive device on level surfaces

PRECAUTIONS

- Avoid standing or walking for extensive periods of time
- Excessive tensile force into plantar flexion or inversion. No active assist or passive stretching into these planes of motion

TREATMENT STRATEGIES

- Edema control: cryotherapy, contrast baths, elevation, IFC electrical stimulation, retrograde massage
- ROM:
  - AROM into eversion (EV), plantar flexion (PF), inversion (INV)
    - Straight plane movements, circles, alphabets A to Z
  - Sitting: BAPS board, rocker board, foam roll
- Flexibility: gastrocnemius and soleus
  - Towel/strap stretch, manual stretch by therapist
- Cross training: pool, UBE, core stabilization
- Gait training
  - Use mirror for feedback, assistive device as needed
  - Pool/AquaCiser
- Strengthening:
  - Foot intrinsics: towel grab, marble pick-up
  - Isometrics: evertors, invertors, dorsiflexion, and plantar flexors
  - PREs: elastic band, ankle weights, manual resistance
  - Proximal strengthening: open chain hip, light leg press/ball squats
- Mobilization: soft tissue
  - Scar
  - Plantar fascia, lumbricals
- Proprioception: bilateral
  - Rocker board, proprioception board, Biodex Balance System

CRITERIA FOR ADVANCEMENT

- Normalized gait, pain-free without assistive device
- Pain-free eversion with 4/5 strength throughout full ROM
- ROM: PF 15 degrees

Troubleshooting

During this phase of rehabilitation, it may be difficult to regain ankle ROM after having been immobilized. It is important to address fascial restrictions, in addition to accessory joint mobilization. If there is a limitation into dorsiflexion, it may be the result of an anterior restriction in the anterior crural compartment and extensor retinaculum fascia.[34] Performing the appropriate myofascial release may be useful. A clear understanding of the type of surgical procedure performed and communication with the physician will set the parameters for the ability to perform joint mobilization techniques as needed. A talocrural joint distraction is extremely effective for addressing pain.[35] Regarding soft tissue limitations, attention should be given to gastrocnemius length and flexibility. Tight gastrocnemius can be a predisposing factor to ankle sprains, and this is a soft tissue limitation that should be investigated following surgery.

The nonanatomical reconstruction using the peroneus brevis requires attention when progressing isometrics and progressive resistance exercises (PREs) because of the anatomical displacement of the structure. Work within the individual's limits of discomfort. Limitation into inversion is expected following the modified Broström procedure. Postoperative stiffness is not the only potential complication associated with lateral ankle reconstruction procedures. Numerous reports have indicated that nerve and wound complications occur more often with the tenodesis procedures. Nerve dysfunction has been reported to be as high as 52%, with varying ranges of severity, particularly to the sural nerve.[20,22,33]

POSTOPERATIVE PHASE II (WEEKS 8 TO 12)

Ankle ROM should be fully restored within 8 to 10 weeks postoperatively. Following surgery it is common for the subject to have complaints of stiffness into inversion and plantar flexion, and goniometric measurements may prove some loss of motion. The goal is for the patient to have pain-free, functional ROM. ROM required to descend is 25-degree dorsiflexion and to ascend stairs is 20-degree plantar flexion.[36] Limitations into dorsiflexion are usually not an issue unless the patient has not been compliant with his or her home exercise program of performing gastrocnemius and soleus flexibility exercises.

Strengthening exercises have traditionally focused on the evertors for individuals with FAI as well as for individuals who have undergone a lateral ankle reconstruction. A question has been raised as to whether the evertors or the invertors are more weakened with FAI. Normal data for torque and total work have shown the isokinetic ratio of evertors to invertors (E/I) to be 1.0 to

1.3.[37] Ryan et al.[11] discovered that evertor weakness was not a significant finding in those with unilateral functional instability, but, surprisingly, invertor weakness was significant. They attributed this weakness to the concept of reflexive inhibition, whereby the muscle shuts down to protect against further injury. The study also theorized the possibility of neural injury to the deep peroneal and tibial nerves, creating weakness. Similar findings of E/I ratios of significantly greater than one in individuals with FAI have also been supported by Wilkerson and colleagues.[38] It may be theorized that over the 6-month course of rehabilitation, physical therapy may have emphasized eversion strengthening at the expense of inversion. The end result is a relative weakness of the invertors. During the rehabilitation following a lateral ankle reconstruction, it is vital to focus not only on evertor strength but also on the invertors. This concept should also hold true for strengthening the plantar flexors and dorsiflexors. The strengthening program should challenge the muscles eccentrically and concentrically, using isotonics as well as isokinetics. Open chain exercises allow for particular muscles to be isolated during these types of strengthening exercises. Tools for isotonic strengthening include the use of elastic bands, weights, and manual resistance. Manual resistance exercises should begin at 60% effort and work from neutral out into one plane of motion. The resistance may then be increased, and the joint should be brought through a full ROM passing through neutral. For example, begin with the foot in full inversion and provide resistance all the way through the end range of eversion and then reverse the motion. Isokinetic training begins at speeds of 60 and 90 degrees per second to focus on improving strength. Using the isokinetic machine at a higher velocity (180 degrees per second for DF/PF and 120 degrees per second for INV/EV) will assist in improving endurance.

Isolated muscular strength should not be the only focus. Development of a muscle balance around all of the lower extremity joints should be examined closely and treated appropriately. Closed chain exercise is a functional and appropriate means of creating a co-contraction and working all musculature surrounding the joint. The co-contraction created assists in joint protection. The leg press is a closed chain exercise, whereby weight-bearing down through the ankle joint may be modified so that the exercise is performed without pain or apprehension. The leg press may be progressed by increasing weight and changing to an antigravity exercise like ball or wall squats and then further advanced to free squats. The bilateral calf raise is another closed chain exercise that is initiated early on in phase II as pain and strength gains allow.

Proprioceptive exercises are progressed from bilateral to unilateral challenges through this phase of rehabili-

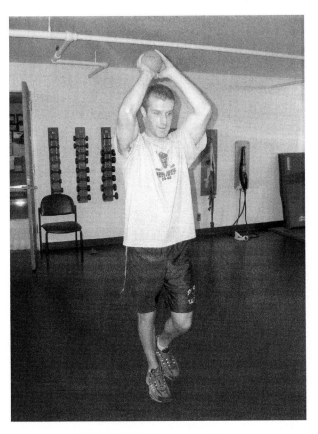

FIGURE **39-3** Unilateral ball toss.

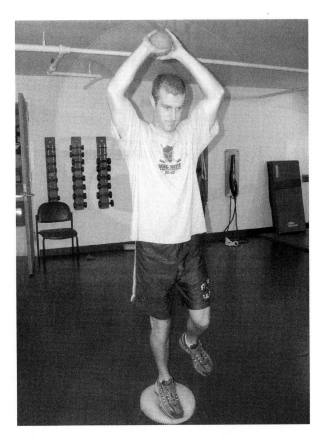

FIGURE **39-4** Unilateral ball toss on disc.

tation. The patient is progressed from a stable surface to a more unstable surface, like the rocker board and wobble board. Removing visual input, adding external perturbation, elastic band resistance, or tossing a ball, further challenges proprioception (Figures 39-3 through 39-5). At this time, proprioception and closed chain exercises combine to yield a series of dynamic stabilizing exercises, which optimizes the goal of developing a functionally based rehabilitation program. Contralateral elastic band exercises, first developed by Tomaszewski,[39] are an effective means of dynamically challenging the entire lower extremity in multiple planes and on multiple surfaces (Figure 39-6). It is strongly encouraged to perform these types of exercises with the knee on the affected side, which is the stabilizing leg, extended as well as flexed. Knee flexion will facilitate dynamic stability throughout the lower extremity. Performing the same exercise with knee extension places greater emphasis on the ankle musculature to provide distal stability[40] (Figure 39-7). This activity may as well be advanced by placing the individual on an unstable surface (Figure 39-8). Activities should be functionally based, as in kicking a soccer ball where indicated (Figure 39-9). Any attempt to bring the individual outside of his or her base of support may be useful in increasing his or her proprioception. This concept should be carried throughout the kinematic chain. One example is to perform a squat while standing on a half dome (Figure 39-10). This challenges strength and stability of the lower extremities and core. Toward the end of phase II, the individual should be performing unilateral calf raises. One activity to further engage the ankle evertors would be to place an elastic band around a stable surface, causing a constant pull into inversion while the individual performs unilateral calf raises. This should be done for the invertors as well (Figure 39-11). Another means of facilitating all ankle stabilizers in a closed chain exercise would be to place an elastic band around the ankles and have the individual perform a side-stepping exercise. This is done for approximately a 20-foot distance for six repetitions (Figure 39-12). Maintaining a squat position throughout this exercise promotes hip and core stabilization as well.

Once the patient has full ROM and is able to exhibit 10 unilateral eccentric calf raises (up with 2, controlling down with the involved one) with good control and no apprehension or pain, plyometric exercises may be introduced. To allow for appropriate healing time for the ligaments, the initiation of plyometrics should be held until earliest at week 11. Plyometrics should be

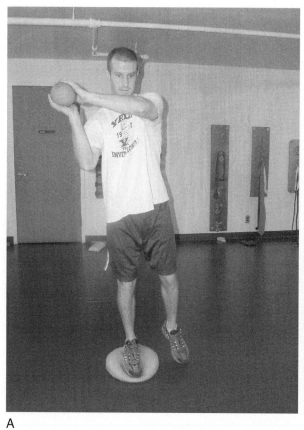

A

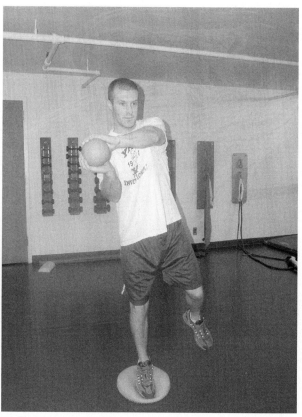

B

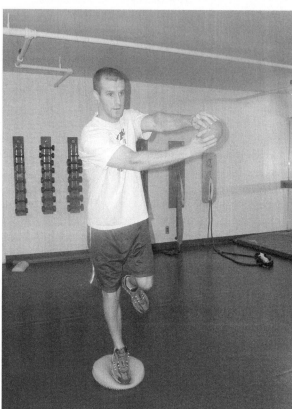

C

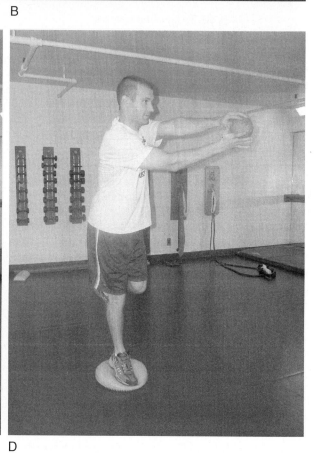

D

FIGURE **39-5** Change direction of toss and force.

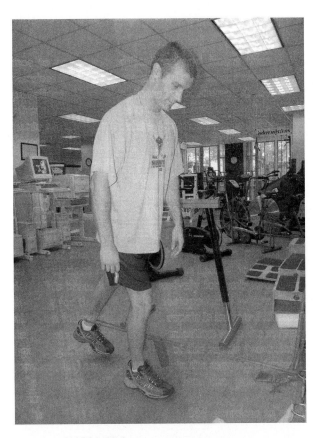

FIGURE **39-6** Contralateral Thera-Band.

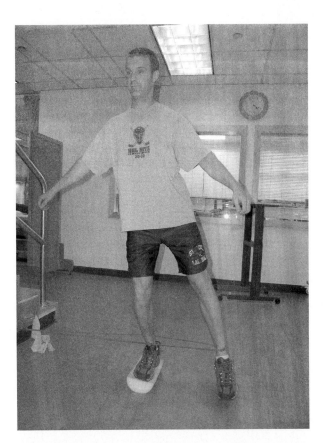

FIGURE **39-8** Contralateral Thera-Band on foam roll further challenges balance and stability, adding to the level of difficulty from standing on a stable surface.

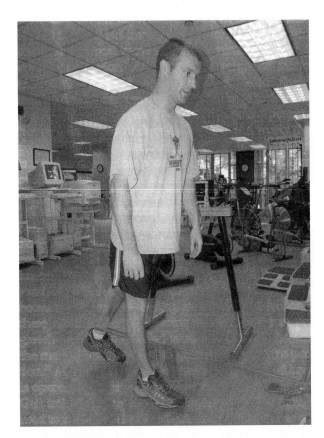

FIGURE **39-7** Contralateral Thera-Band with knee extension places emphasis on the use of the muscles surrounding the muscle to work as dynamic stabilizers.

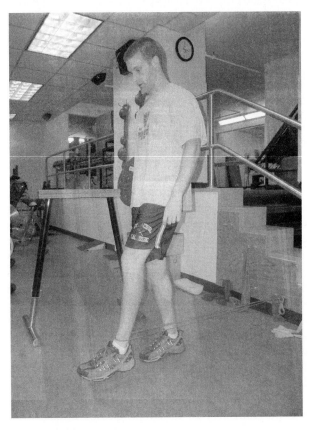

FIGURE **39-9** Thera-Band with functional simulation to a soccer kick.

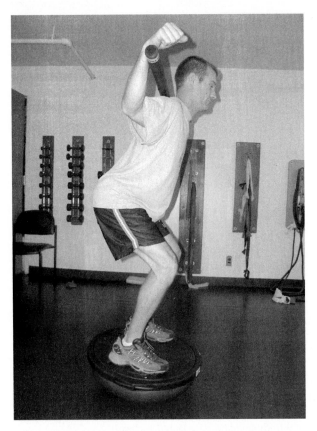

FIGURE **39-10** Squats on a half dome require stabilization of the core and lower extremities as well as being a proprioceptive challenge.

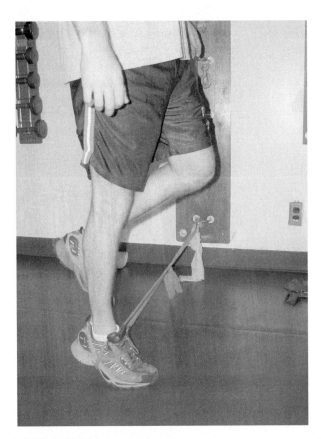

FIGURE **39-11** Unilateral plantar flexion with pull into eversion. This should be performed pulling the foot into inversion as well.

initiated on a horizontal leg press in which, ideally, the body is the mobile segment not the platform. The weight should be set at 30% of the individual's body weight, and bilateral jumps can be performed with the force controlled and gravity partially eliminated. This activity is progressed by jumping up bilaterally onto a 4- to 6-inch platform. Jumping up onto a surface decreases the vertical distance traveled in the landing and therefore less impact force on the ankle. The focus of this exercise is on proper landing technique, and it is essential to reinforce a soft absorptive landing. These activities should be guided by level of discomfort or clinical findings of post-activity edema. Any indication of pain or apprehension signifies that the individual is not ready to participate at that level. A full progression of plyometric advancement is shown in Table 39-1.

The ability to perform 15 unilateral calf raises is a good indication that a running program may be initiated. It is suggested that the program begin on a treadmill at a 0% incline at the patient's comfortable speed for 30 seconds for three intervals. If the patient has no complaints of pain and the gait pattern is symmetrical, this program may be slowly progressed in 30-second increments.

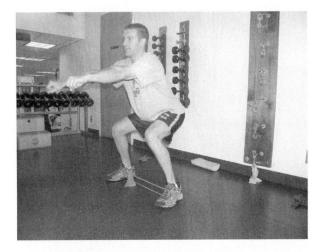

FIGURE **39-12** Thera-Band side-stepping requires recruitment of the core and hip musculature to perform the task.

The home exercise program, at this time, should consist of maintaining flexibility in the gastrocnemius and soleus, unilateral proprioception exercises, closed chain dynamic stability with an elastic band, isotonic exercises using an elastic band, and calf raises. All proximal strengthening and cardiovascular exercises should be continued. A program may be devised for both at home and at the gym. Once plyometric exercises have begun, it is important to educate the patient not to overload his or her program. Plyometrics should be performed two to three times a week. On these days the clinician and patient should be sensitive to the volume of strength exercises. The criteria for the completion of phase II are indicated by the individual's ability to return to his or her activities of daily living (ADL) without apprehension, pain, or residual edema unless the work is extremely physically demanding. The

Postoperative Phase II (Weeks 8 to 12)

GOALS

- Restore full ROM
- Patient independent in donning brace
- No edema post-activity
- Normalized, non-antalgic gait on stairs and inconsistent surfaces
- Maintain full body conditioning
- Unilateral calf raise 10 repetitions (5/5 strength)
- Initiate plyometrics
- Initiate jogging to running

PRECAUTIONS

- Patient education to continue activity modification

TREATMENT STRATEGIES

- Protection: Aircast, semi-rigid support
- Edema control: cryotherapy
- ROM: full ROM (by latest 12 weeks); focus on multiplanar movements
  - Standing/weight-bearing BAPS board
  - Mobilizations: joint mobilizations, Mulligan techniques
- Flexibility:
  - Standing gastrocnemius and soleus stretching
  - Soft tissue mobilization and myofascial release (MFR) to posterior contractile tissues and fascia
    - Gastrocnemius, soleus, tibialis posterior
- Proprioception:
  - Unilateral standing: eyes open, eyes closed
  - Dynamic neuromuscular training with Biodex Balance Master system
  - Unilateral stance on proprioception board, rocker/wobble board, foam block
  - Add perturbation or other modes of dynamic stability/multitasking
    - Ball toss, reaching
- Strengthening: focus on invertors and evertors as well as all muscle groups that support the ankle
  - Rhythmic stabilization
  - Concentric and eccentric
  - Open chain
    - Thera-Band, manual resistance, isokinetics training
  - Closed chain
    - Side step with elastic band, contralateral elastic band activity (KE and HE), leg press, step up/step down, sports cord (retro, side to side, carioca)
  - Muscle endurance: StairMaster, Elliptical
- Plyometrics
  - Bilateral jumps
  - Unilateral jumps
- Treadmill
- Cardiovascular: Elliptical, StairMaster, VersaClimber

CRITERIA FOR ADVANCEMENT

- Full ROM
- No residual edema after activity
- No pain after activity
- Non-antalgic, no apprehension with treadmill jog

TABLE 39-1	Plyometric Progression: Phase II of Rehabilitation

- Horizontal leg press jumps
- Bilateral jumps:
  - Up to a 4-inch box then to a 6-inch box
  - Vertical jumps in place
  - Jumps up to and down from first a 4-inch box then to a 6-inch box
  - Vertical jumps in series
  - Depth jumps up and down from 8-inch and 12-inch boxes
- Lateral jumping bilaterally over a line
  - Up and over a 4-inch box
  - Jumps in series in multiple planes, that is, four-quadrant box jumps
- Unilateral jumps may then be initiated in the same progression pattern

individual will not be able to perform high level jumping skills, full speed running, or return to sport activities. A brace should be worn for physically demanding work and recreation. The semi-rigid stirrup should be used earlier postoperatively for its stability vs the lace-up, which should be used in more functional activity because the stirrup is bulkier, less comfortable, and does not accommodate footwear as well as the lace-up.

Troubleshooting

Residual edema and lateral ankle pain are two problems faced in this phase. It is vital throughout the rehabilitation process to continually educate the patient on activity modification and be wary of any pain or edema following the treatment session. Once the plyometric regimen has begun, it is very important not to overload these activities. If there is any discomfort associated with initial plyometric exercises, the patient is not ready. Working through such pain can cause irritation or additional injury and set progression back. Begin with 10 repetitions of one activity, then progress to performing up to three of the plyometric activities for maximum of two sets of 10 repetitions. Plyometrics should be performed at the beginning of treatment following an active warm-up. Do not overload the patient with high repetitions of plyometrics and then a full regimen of strengthening on the same day. This could also potentiate irritation or injury. Make sure that there is a safe balance of these activities for day-to-day treatment.

POSTOPERATIVE PHASE III (WEEKS 12 TO 16)

The goals of phase III are to progress those individuals who plan to return to some level of physical labor or organized athletics. This is achieved by progressing the patient though a series of advanced plyometrics, dynamic stability, strengthening, agility drills and work, or sport-specific activities.

Multiple studies have indicated that strengthening, balance, and proprioception are all effective tools when combined for regaining function.[11,13,37,41] However, with regard to returning an individual to play, there is a dearth of information on the specifics of the number of treatments and the volume or combination of exercises required to efficiently and effectively meet the end goals. It is very important that needs be specific to the functional requirements of the individual.

Functional assessment should include performance testing and recording of limb symmetry. In 1982, Daniel et al.[42] investigated the knee and described the single-leg hop for distance to determine limb symmetry. Normal limb symmetry, focusing on the knee, was defined as greater than or equal to 85%.[43] In 1990, Barber et al.[43] described four knee functional hop tests: the single-legged hop, triple hop for distance, crossover triple hop for distance, and one-legged timed hop. The literature has yet to determine the validity and reliability of functional tests in detecting ankle performance deficits. No literature to date has investigated the efficacy of functional testing following lateral ankle reconstruction. Worrell et al.,[44] in 1994, reported that no significant difference existed using the hop test in individuals with CAI. Munn et al.[45] looked at the triple-crossover hop for distance and the shuttle run and was unable to discriminate between the injured and uninjured limbs of individuals with CAI. Reports of subjective instability in CAI were more reliable for determining functional ability than most of the functional tests.[28,44,45] Therefore, it is vital to develop a functional performance program for the patient, one that is specific to his or her needs and then receive subjective feedback regarding pain or apprehension. However, these tests are still used as benchmarks of functional progression. Ideally, with respect to the ankle, the goal is to achieve 85% symmetry between lower extremities in the results of these tests.

Isokinetic testing is an objective means of measuring strength and endurance gains. The normal E/I ratios (1.0 to 1.3), as described previously, should be the goal. Eighty-five percent limb symmetry is also expected in the results of these isokinetic tests. Data should be recorded throughout the rehabilitative process, when isokinetics are being used in treatment for the invertors, evertors, plantar flexors, and dorsiflexors. Testing should then be performed upon discharge to provide objective measures.

The Specific Adaptations to Imposed Demands (SAID) Principle, developed by Allman,[46] is a useful guide for functional training. This principle creates a program relevant to the sport and demands placed on the individual. At this stage of rehabilitation, the focus should be on optimizing power, endurance, and agility in multiple planes of movement throughout the entire kinematic chain to maximize performance and minimize the potential for future injury. This progression is based on a sequence through uniplanar movements and then multiplanar movements. The addition of speed and various degrees of direction change will further challenge the athlete and assimilate the demands of the sport (Table 39-2). The rehabilitation specialist must recognize the energy systems involved in particular sports and apply this concept to the rehabilitation regimen. For example, a cross-country runner will require different training tactics than a volleyball player, based on their aerobic vs anaerobic output and the demands on the body.

Ankle bracing for return to play is highly encouraged. The role of bracing is to provide mechanical stability as

Postoperative Phase III (Weeks 12 to 16)

GOALS

- Running to sprinting
- Multiplane activities
- Regain full cardiovascular and muscular endurance
- Strength ≥85% limb symmetry through isokinetic testing
- No apprehension with high level activity, direction change
- Functional testing: 85% limb symmetry
- Skill progression, no pain, no apprehension
- Return to full sport, high level activity

PRECAUTIONS

- Continue to wear ankle brace during sports for 6 months
- Apprehension or pain with return to sport
- Volume awareness with high intensity activities and drills

TREATMENT STRATEGIES

- Protection: lace-up ankle brace for activities
- Strengthening
  - Testing: isokinetic, dynamometry, functional testing
  - Increase workload, resistance, and intensity in PREs
- Endurance
  - Jumping rope: bilateral skip, alternating skip, then unilateral skip
  - Isokinetics
- Proprioception
  - Single-leg stance on change of surfaces (most stable to least stable)
  - Add perturbation or other modes of dynamic stability/multitasking, visual input changes
  - Ball toss, reaching, walking, jogging with variation in speed of movement and intensity of perturbation
  - Introduction of sport-specific skills
- Plyometrics: advanced
  - Depth pumps, jumps in series, dot drills
- Return to sport functional progression and testing

SPORT-SPECIFIC ACTIVITIES

- Single skill activities (e.g., shooting baskets from stationary stance)
- Add multitasking skills (e.g., dribble and shot drills; running, throwing, and catching ball)
  - Progress from linear movement to change of direction
- Add defensive player/coach to drill
- Practice drills with team
- Scrimmage with team
- Return to play

CRITERIA FOR DISCHARGE

- Regain full cardiovascular and muscular endurance
- Strength ≥85% limb symmetry through isokinetic testing
- No apprehension with high level activity, direction change
- Functional testing: 85% limb symmetry
- Skill progression, no pain, no apprehension
- Return to full sport, high level activity

TABLE 39-2	Return to Sport Functional Progression and Clinical Testing

1. Retro-jog
2. Side shuffles
3. Carioca
4. Bilateral bounding (A–P then lateral)
5. Run
6. Unilateral quadrant jumps
7. Jog-sprint-jog
8. Sprint-jog
9. Sprint-stop
10. Figure eights
11. Unilateral bounding (A–P then lateral)
12. 45-degree cuts
13. Single-leg hop test for time and distance
14. 90-degree cuts
15. Shuttle run test

well as proprioceptive stimulation. Ankle braces should be of a lace-up or stirrup variety. Rovere et al.,[47] using an ASO lace-up brace, and Sitler et al.,[48] using a semi-rigid stirrup (Aircast), have shown that bracing reduced the rate of recurrent ankle sprains. An additional study by Bocchinfuso et al.[49] found that ankle bracing resulted in no performance deficits when investigating speed, agility, or vertical jumps. Compliance with brace wear is dependent on the brace being comfortable, aesthetically pleasing, durable, an easy fit into footwear, and financially feasible.

Troubleshooting

The purpose of the surgery was to correct for a chronically unstable ankle. It is not uncommon for patients to have complaints of residual ankle stiffness even at discharge. This is an acceptable outcome.

It is highly encouraged that the individual continue to wear a brace or some sort of protective wrap for up to 4 to 6 months following surgery while engaging in higher levels of activity. This provides additional structural support, in addition to proprioceptive feedback. Despite some symptoms of stiffness and the need to use a brace, the prognosis for full return to sports is very good following this surgery, and the patients are pleased with the final result.

REFERENCES

1. Garrick, J.G. *The Frequency of Injury, Mechanism of Injury, and Epidemiology of Ankle Sprains.* Am J Sports Med 1977;5(6):241–242.
2. Karlsson, J., Eriksson, B.I., Bergsten, T., Rudholm, O., Sward, L. *Comparison of Two Anatomic Reconstructions for Chronic Lateral Instability of the Ankle Joint.* Am J Sports Med 1997;25(1):48–53.
3. Karlsson, J., Lansinger, O. *Lateral Instability of the Ankle Joint. Non-surgical Treatment Is the First Choice, 20% Need Ligament Surgery.* Lakartidnengen 1991;88:1399–1402.
4. Konradsen, L., Holmer, P., Sondergaard, L. *Early Mobilizing Treatment for Grade III Ankle Ligament Injuries.* Foot Ankle 1991;12(2):69–73.
5. Louwerens, J.W., Snijders, C.J. Lateral Ankle Instability: An Overview. In Ranawat, C.S., Positano, R.G. (Eds). *Disorders of the Heel, Rearfoot, and Ankle,* chap 24. Churchill Livingstone, New York, 1999, pp. 341–353.
6. Bernier, J.N., Perrin, D.H. *Effect of Coordination Training on Proprioception of the Functionally Unstable Ankle.* J Orthop Sports Phys Ther 1998;27(4):264–275.
7. Messer, T.M., Cummins, C.A., Ahn, J., Kelikian, A.S. *Outcome of the Modified Brostrom Procedure for Chronic Lateral Ankle Instability Using Suture Anchors.* Foot Ankle Int 2000;21(12):996–1003.
8. Tropp, H. *Commentary: Functional Ankle Instability Revisited.* J Athl Train 2002;37:512–515.
9. Clanton, T.O. Lateral Ankle Sprains. In Coughlin, M.J., Mann, R.A. (Eds). *Surgery of the Foot and Ankle,* 7th ed., vol 2. Mosby, St. Louis, 1999, pp. 1891–1210.
10. Freeman, M.A., Dean, M.R., Hanham, I.W. *The Etiology and Prevention of Functional Instability of the Foot.* J Bone Joint Surg Br 1965;47:678–685.
11. Ryan, L. *Mechanical Stability, Muscle Strength and Proprioception in the Functionally Unstable Ankle.* Aust J Physiother 1994;40(1):41–47.
12. Riemann, B.L. *Is There a Link Between Chronic Ankle Instability and Postural Instability?* J Athl Train 2002;37(4):386–393.
13. Tropp, H. *Pronator Muscle Weakness in Functional Instability of the Ankle Joint.* Int J Sports Med 1986;7:291–294.
14. Riemann, B.L., Caggiano, N.A., Lephart, S.M. *Examination of Clinical Method of Assessing Postural Control During a Functional Performance Task.* J Sports Rehabil 1999;8:171–183.
15. Baumhauer, J.F., O'Brien, T. *Surgical Considerations in the Treatment of Ankle Instability.* J Athl Train 2002;37(4):458–462.
16. Hollis, J.M., Blasier, R.D., Flahiff, C.M., Hofmann, O.E. *Biomechanical Comparison of Reconstruction Techniques in Simulated Lateral Ankle Ligament Injury.* Am J Sports Med 1995;23(6):678–682.
17. Girard, P., Anderson, R.B., Davies, W.H., Isear, J.A., Kiebzak, G.M. *Clinical Evaluation of the Modified Broström-Evans Procedure to Restore Ankle Stability.* Foot Ankle Int 1999;20(4):246–252.
18. Hamilton, W.G., Thompson, F.M., Snow, S.W. *The Modified Brostrom Procedure for Lateral Ankle Instability.* Foot Ankle 1993;14(1):1–7.
19. Sammarco, G.J., Idusuyi, O.B. *Reconstruction of the Lateral Ankle Ligaments Using a Split Peroneus Brevis Tendon Graft.* Foot Ankle Int 1999;20(2):97–103.
20. Rosenbaum, D., Engelhardt, M., Becker, H.P., Claes, L., Gerngro, H. *Clinical and Functional Outcome after Anatomic and Nonanatomic Ankle Ligament Reconstruction: Evans Tenodesis Versus Periosteal Flap.* Foot Ankle Int 1999;20(10):636–639.
21. Schmidt, R., Cordier, E., Bertsch, C., Eils, E., Neller, S., Benesch, S., Herbst, A., Rosenbaum, D., Claes, L. *Reconstruction of the Lateral Ligaments: Do the Anatomical Procedures Restore Physiologic Ankle Kinematics?* Foot Ankle Int 2004;25(1):31–36.
22. Sammarco, V.J. *Complications of Lateral Ankle Ligament Reconstruction.* Clin Orthop Relat Res 2001;391:123–132.

23. Broström, L. *Sprained Ankles.* Acta Orthop Scand 1966;132(6): 551–565.

24. Gould, N., Seligson, D., Gassman, J. *Early and Late Repair of Lateral Ligament of the Ankle.* Foot Ankle 1980;1(2):84–89.

25. Hamilton, W.G. Ankle Instability Repair: The Broström-Gould Procedure. In Johnson, K.A. (Ed). *The Foot and Ankle.* Raven Press, Ltd., New York, 1994, pp. 437–446.

26. Woo, S.L., Hildebrand, K., Watanabe, N., Fenwick, J.A., Papageorgiou, C.D., Wang, J.H. *Tissue Engineering of Ligament and Tendon Healing.* Clin Orthop Relat Res 1999;1(367S):S312–S323.

27. Martinez-Hernandez, A., Amenta, P.S. Basic Concepts in Wound Healing: Clinical and Basic Science Concepts. In Leadletter, W.B., Buckwalter, J.A., Gordan, S.L. (Eds). *Sports-Induced Inflammation.* American Association of Orthopaedic Surgeons, Park Ridge, IL, 1990, pp. 55–102.

28. Mattacola, C.G., Dwyer, M.K. *Rehabilitation of the Ankle after Acute Sprain or Chronic Instability.* J Athl Train 2002;37(4):413–429.

29. Frank, C.B. *Ligament Injuries: Pathophysiology and Healing.* WB Saunders, Philadelphia, 1996.

30. Wilkerson, G.B. *Mechanical Versus Functional Ankle Instability.* Paper presented at National Athletic Trainers Association, 48th Annual Meeting and Clinical Symposium, June 18–21, 1997, Salt Lake City, UT.

31. Cooper, D.W., Fair, J. *Contrast and Pressure Treatments of Lateral Ankle Sprains.* Phys Sports Med 1979;7:143.

32. Freeman, M.A. *Instability in the Foot after Injuries to the Lateral Ligament of the Ankle.* J Bone Joint Surg 1965;47B: 678–685.

33. Kleinrensink, G.J., Snijders, C.J., Stoeckart, R. The Chronically Unstable Ankle: Anatomic, Biomechanical, and Neurological Considerations. In Ranawat, C.S., Positano, R.G. (Eds). *Disorders of the Heel, Rearfoot, and Ankle,* chap 25. Churchill Livingstone, New York, 1999, pp. 354–360.

34. Myers, T.W. *Anatomy Trains: Myofascial Meridians for Manual and Movement Therapists.* Churchill Livingstone, New York, 1995.

35. Prentice, W.E. *Rehabilitation Techniques in Sports Medicine,* 3rd ed. McGraw-Hill, Boston, 1999.

36. Norkin, C.C., Levange, P.K. *The Ankle-Foot Complex,* 2nd ed., chap 12. FA Davis, Philadelphia, 1992.

37. Davies, G.J., Wilk, K.E., Ellenbecker, T.S. *Assessment of Strength,* 3rd ed. Mosby, St. Louis, 1997.

38. Wilkerson, G.B., Pinerola, J.J., Caturano, R.W. *Invertor vs. Evertor Peak Torque and Power Deficiencies Associated with Lateral Ankle Ligament Injury.* J Orthop Sports Phys Ther 1997;26(2):78–86.

39. Tomaszewski, D. *"T Band Kicks" Ankle Proprioception Program.* Athletic Trainer: J Natl Athl Train Assoc 1991;26:216, 217, 219, 227.

40. Bernier, J.N. *Ankle Proprioception and Neuromuscular Control.* Paper presented at National Athletic Trainers Association: 51st Annual Clinical Symposia, 2000, Nashville, TN.

41. Wilkerson, G.B. *Functional Rehabilitation. A Protocol for Management of the Lateral Ankle Sprain.* Rehab Manag 1996;9(4): 54–60.

42. Daniel, D., Malcom, L., Stone, M., Perth, H., Morgan, J., Riehl, B. *Quantification of Knee Stability and Function.* Contemp Orthop 1982;5:83–91.

43. Barber, S., Noyes, F., Mangine, R., McCloskey, J., Hartman, W. *Quantitative Assessment of Functional Limitations in Normal and Anterior Cruciate Deficient Knees.* Clin Orthop Relat Res 1990; 225:204–214.

44. Worrell, T.W., Booher, L.D., Hench, K.M. *Closed Kinetic Chain Assessment Following Inversion Ankle Sprain.* J Sports Rehabil 1994;3:197–203.

45. Munn, J., Beard, D.J., Refshauge, K.M., Lee, R.W. *Do Functional Performance Tests Detect Impairment in Subjects with Ankle Instability?* J Sports Rehabil 2002;11:40–50.

46. Allman, F.L. *Sports Medicine.* Academic Press, New York, 1974.

47. Rovere, G.D., Clarke, T.J., Yates, C.S., Burley, K. *Retrospective Comparison of Taping and Ankle Stabilizers in Preventing Ankle Injuries.* Am J Sports Med 1988;16:228–233.

48. Sitler, M., Ryan, J., Wheeler, B. *The Efficacy of a Semirigid Ankle Stabilizer to Reduce Acute Ankle Injuries in Basketball. A Randomized Clinical Trial at West Point.* Am J Sports Med 1994; 22:454–461.

49. Bocchinfuso, C., Sitler, M.R., Kimura, I.F. Effects of Two Semirigid Prophylactic Ankle Stabilizers on Speed, Agility, and Vertical Jump. J Sports Rehabil 1994;3:125–134.

40

Rotator Cuff Repair: Arthroscopic and Open

ROBERT MASCHI, PT, DPT, CSCS

GREG FIVES, PT, MS

Rotator cuff pathology is a significant cause of pain and disability in the general population.[1] Rotator cuff tears may occur as the result of trauma, degeneration secondary to repetitive microtrauma, or a combination of both. Rotator cuff repair is a common intervention used by surgeons to improve the function and pain level in this population. Different surgical techniques are used to repair the torn rotator cuff. In 1911, Codman[2] first described open surgical repair of the supraspinatus. Since then, rotator cuff repair techniques have evolved significantly, and the introduction of shoulder arthroscopy in 1980 dramatically changed the way rotator cuff repairs are performed.[3] Surgical techniques progressed from open to arthroscopic-assisted mini-open repair techniques during the early to mid-1990s.[1] The trend now seems to be the progression to an all-arthroscopic surgical technique. The advantages associated with an all-arthroscopic rotator cuff repair are deltoid preservation; smaller skin incisions; better visualization and evaluation of the glenohumeral joint and rotator cuff defect; improved ability to mobilize and release the rotator cuff; decreased postoperative pain and stiffness; and improved rehabilitation potential.[1,3-6] Some disadvantages include bone-tendon fixation and the technical difficulty of performing the procedure.[3,4] Overall, the results of arthroscopic repairs appear to be very promising.[5,7-9] Wolf et al.[6] showed good to excellent results in 94% of patients who underwent arthroscopic rotator cuff repair. Factors, such as choice of technique, size and location of the tear, and quality of the tissue involved, will influence the timing of therapeutic interventions and the progression of rehabilitation. The Hospital for Special Surgery (HSS) postoperative guidelines and approach to rehabilitation following arthroscopic rotator cuff repair is presented in this chapter.

SURGICAL OVERVIEW

The muscles of the rotator cuff consist of the subscapularis, supraspinatus, infraspinatus, and teres minor. All of the tendons of the cuff blend with and reinforce the glenohumeral joint capsule. The primary function of the rotator cuff is to balance the force couples about the glenohumeral joint during active elevation of the upper extremity.[10] With this in mind, the primary goal of rotator cuff repair surgery is to restore, as closely as possible, the anatomical cuff configuration and these biomechanical force couples.

Surgery initially involves positioning the patient in the lateral decubitus or upright beach chair position.[4,11,12] Bony landmarks are identified and marked, and the arthroscope is placed into the joint space via posterior, anterior, and lateral portals. The glenohumeral joint is then inspected via the arthroscope to help identify possible concomitant intra-articular pathologies. The tear is

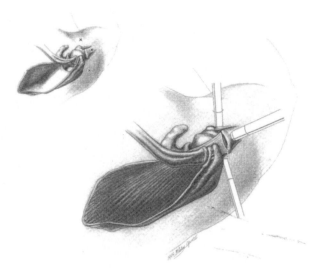

FIGURE **40-1** Arthroscopic rotator cuff repair.

located and evaluated in regard to its size and shape. The amount of retraction of the rotator cuff is assessed, as is cuff mobility, using grasper hooks. If present, adhesions are released to improve cuff mobility. Excursion of the cuff is determined to identify the exact area of bony preparation and the anatomical "footprint" of the cuff.[4,6] The torn tendon edges are débrided of devascularized tissue, and sutures are placed through the torn edges. The cuff is fixated with anchors placed into the tuberosity, if an anatomical repair is possible (Figure 40-1). Acromioplasty and/or subacromial decompression may not be needed at the time of rotator cuff repair if the acromion does not compromise the subacromial space and/or if the cuff tear is secondary to trauma or intrinsic tendinopathy caused by eccentric tendon overload.[1,11,13]

Patients are placed in a postoperative sling or abduction brace to immobilize and protect the repair and discharged home on the day of surgery.

REHABILITATION OVERVIEW

The rehabilitation program following rotator cuff repair must take into account the healing time of surgically repaired tissue. The program should balance the aspects of tissue healing and appropriate interventions to restore range of motion (ROM), strength, and function. Factors that influence the rate at which a patient can be progressed through the program include surgical technique, quality of the tissue repaired, size of the tear, and location of the tear.

Good tissue quality will allow a secure repair, which may allow for a faster rehabilitation than a more tenuous repair of poorer quality tissue. Tissue quality can be influenced by conditions, such as rheumatoid arthritis, diabetes, and by the chronicity of the tear, previous surgery, repeated injections, or chronic steroid use. These can increase the risk of suture pull-out.[3]

Also, functional outcome is directly related to the size of the tear.[14-18] Tear size, not age, is more of a factor in predicting a successful outcome after rotator cuff repair.[19,20] Larger tears involve more tissue and are often retracted, which requires greater mobilization of the tissue to achieve closure. Therefore, in larger tears tissue trauma is greater, which requires a more conservative postoperative rehabilitation course.[18]

The location of the tear will also affect interventions. For example, a small tear of the supraspinatus may allow for early activation of the internal and external rotators, whereas a tear extending into the infraspinatus and teres minor or the subscapularis will delay strengthening of the corresponding musculature. The therapist must take into account what structures are involved to avoid disruption of healing tissues in the early phases of rehabilitation. Communication with the referring surgeon is essential to determine this information.

One must keep in mind that the information in this chapter should serve as a guideline only and that progression through the rehabilitative course will vary, depending on all points previously mentioned.

PREOPERATIVE EDUCATION

Preoperative rehabilitation should educate the patient on expectation regarding the length of the rehabilitative process and inform the patient of postoperative activity restrictions. The patient is also educated in proper posture and sleeping positions and instructed in proper donning and doffing of the postoperative sling/immobilizer.

At HSS the authors have designed a one-time preoperative visit for patients who have not had formal conservative or preoperative therapy. Patients are given a booklet that informs them of the different aspects of the pre- and post-surgical process. Sections include a general description of the surgical procedure, with corresponding precautions and information on regional anesthesia. Other sections include cryotherapy instruction, postoperative exercise instruction, pain management, and a list of frequently asked questions. The booklet is multidisciplinary and contains input from all members of the health care team, including the surgeon, therapist, nurses, and anesthesiologists.

POSTOPERATIVE PHASE I: MAXIMUM PROTECTION (WEEKS 0 TO 3)

During the initial assessment, the rehabilitation specialist should note the type of repair performed. The surgeon's physical therapy prescription should provide the therapist with information pertaining to the type of repair, ROM limitations, and other postoperative precautions. At this time, the therapist should communicate

directly with the surgeon to determine the specific surgical procedure performed and variables previously discussed that may affect postoperative rehabilitation. Communication with the surgeon is necessary to achieve consensus on the treatment plan and the expected postoperative outcome for the patient.

The primary goal of this phase of rehabilitation is to establish a healing environment for the patient's shoulder. Both the surgeon and the therapist should convey to the patient the importance of activity modification and strict protection of the repair. Patients are taught not to actively use the operated extremity for activities of daily living (ADL) and to avoid sudden movements. Excessive tensioning at the tendon-bone reattachment site can lead to a failed rotator cuff repair and a diminished functional outcome for the patient.[21] Patients are instructed in proper donning/doffing of the sling and to wear it at all times, except when performing their home exercise program (HEP). Sleeping postures are discussed with the patient. When sleeping, patients are instructed to lie supine and place a pillow or towel under the posterior aspect of the brachium to provide support to the shoulder. The patient usually finds this position to be most comfortable and provide pain relief. The patient is discouraged from lying on the operated side.

The patient is instructed to use cryotherapy extensively during the day for 10 to 20 minutes on and 1 hour off. The proposed benefits of cryotherapy include decreased pain, decreased inflammation, and decreased muscle spasm.[22-24]

ROM is assessed within prescribed limits, and the patient is instructed in exercises to help gradually restore deficits in motion. Care is taken to maintain specific ROM limits set by the surgeon. The patient is taught Codman/pendulum exercises to help improve motion and relieve pain. Care is taken to ensure that this exercise is done passively with the body initiating and driving small arcs of shoulder motion in various planes. Patients are instructed not to actively move the arm and to avoid pain with this exercise.

Wand exercises to increase both external and internal rotation ROM are shown to the patient within pain-free and prescribed ROM limits (Figure 40-2, *A* and *B*). Supine active-assisted range of motion (AAROM) forward elevation in the plane of the scapula is taught to the patient (Figure 40-3). During this exercise, patients generally have pain upon guiding the arm back down from the elevated position secondary to inability to control the arm against the effect of gravity. The therapist should reinforce to the patient to control the descent with full support of the contralateral arm. When teaching the patient supine AAROM forward elevation, it is helpful for the rehabilitative specialist to first perform this exercise on the patient, so the patient

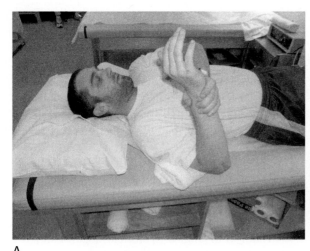
A

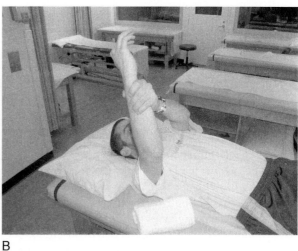
B

FIGURE **40-2** PROM forward elevation in the scapular plane. With this exercise, the patient uses the contralateral upper extremity to initiate PROM in the operated shoulder. The patient should firmly grasp the opposite wrist and passively elevate the arm. *A. Start position:* A towel is placed under the arm to provide comfort and a base of support to the shoulder. The patient's upper extremity is abducted away from the body 30 to 45 degrees. *B. Elevation:* Patient elevates operated extremity with full support from the contralateral limb. Verbal and manual cues are given to ensure this exercise is performed as passively as possible.

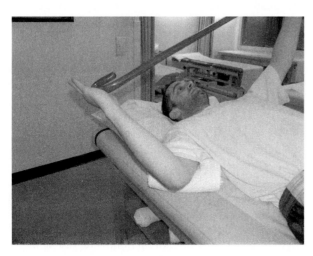

FIGURE **40-3** PROM, with wand in external scapular plane.

understands the concept of controlled AAROM. Patients are instructed to perform ROM exercises three to five times daily, and it is emphasized to the patient to avoid pain when performing these activities. A family member or friend can be taught to perform passive range of motion (PROM) exercises on the patient if the patient has difficulty independently performing AAROM exercises. Active-assisted pulley exercises and arm elevation with a wand have been shown to have high levels of muscle activation and *are not* initiated during this phase.[25] Distal ROM exercises include hand gripping (with and without a theraball), wrist flexion/extension,

forearm supination/pronation, and elbow flexion/extension. Elbow extension ROM is emphasized to prevent a flexion contracture at the elbow joint secondary to sling immobilization.

During the initial assessment, the rehabilitation specialist should also assess sitting posture and scapula position. Increased scapula protraction, usually seen with thoracic kyphosis and forward head posture, can narrow the subacromial space and lead to subacromial impingement of the rotator cuff tendons.[26] Patients are taught gentle scapula retraction exercises and proper postural awareness techniques. Poor scapula mechanics, or "scapula dyskinesis," may be noted after injury or postoperatively.[27] Therefore, early scapula rehabilitation is essential following rotator cuff repair.

Early strengthening exercises include teaching the patient submaximal deltoid isometrics into forward flexion, abduction, and extension. These exercises should be initiated with the elbow flexed to 90 degrees to provide a short lever arm, which avoids excessive muscle force being produced at the shoulder. The rehabilitation specialist should manually instruct the patient to perform shoulder isometric exercises into his or her hand to ensure that the exercises are performed submaximally (Figure 40-4).

Manual therapy techniques to be used during this phase include guided scapula mobilization, in the side-lying position, with and without manual resistance (Figure 40-5). Gentle scapula distraction may also be used to improve scapula mobility. Gentle PROM provided by the rehabilitation specialist is also helpful to

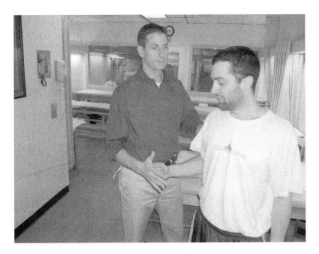

FIGURE **40-4** Short lever submaximal deltoid isometrics. Anterior deltoid: The therapist instructs the patient in the concept of submaximal isometric exercise.

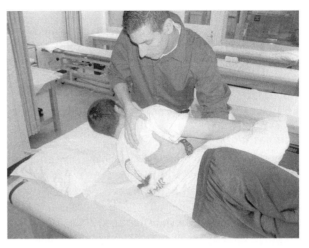

FIGURE **40-5** Side-lying manual scapular mobilization/resistance. The patient is positioned in the side-lying position with a pillow under the arm for support. The rehabilitation specialist guides the patient to actively move the scapula into the protracted/retracted, elevated/depressed positions. As mobility improves, gentle manual resistance may be added to this activity.

Postoperative Phase I: Maximum Protection (Weeks 0 to 3)

GOALS

- Protect surgical repair
- Decrease pain/inflammation
- Gradually increase shoulder ROM (surgeon directed) external rotation (ER) to 45 degrees, internal rotation (IR) to 45 degrees, and forward flexion (FF) to 120 degrees
- Improve proximal (scapula) and distal strength and mobility
- Independence in an HEP

PRECAUTIONS

- Maintain sling immobilization when not performing exercises
- NO active movements at the operated shoulder joint other than gentle self-care activity below shoulder level
- Avoid exceeding ROM limitations set by surgeon
- Avoid pain with ROM and isometric exercises

TREATMENT STRATEGIES

- Sling immobilization (surgeon directed)
- Patient education: sleeping postures, activity modification
- Cryotherapy (Cryo/cuff, gel packs, ice)
- Pendulum exercises
- AAROM/PROM exercises
  - PROM by the rehabilitation specialist
  - AAROM forward flexion in supine with contralateral upper extremity
  - Supine wand ER/IR in scapular plane
  - Continuous passive motion (CPM) for ER if needed
- Active range of motion (AROM) exercises
  - Elbow/forearm/wrist/hand
- Scapula stabilization exercises—side-lying (progress to manual resistance)
- Submaximal deltoid isometrics in neutral as ROM improves (short lever arm)
- Progress and update HEP

CRITERIA FOR ADVANCEMENT

- Normal scapular mobility
- Full AROM distal to shoulder
- Shoulder ROM to within surgeon's set goals

increase ROM at the shoulder. The patient should be comfortable with the shoulder well supported, and PROM should be introduced gradually so as to avoid pain and reflex muscle contraction. Gentle joint mobilization techniques (grades I and II) can also be used to neuromodulate and decrease the patient's pain, thereby facilitating gains in PROM.[28]

Troubleshooting

During the initial treatment sessions, it is important for the rehabilitative specialist to get a sense of the patient's expectations and goals following rotator cuff repair. The patient's goals will determine the goals of the rehabilitative program. The patient should be informed of postoperative limitations and the purpose of postoperative exercises. The patient should also be given adequate verbal and written instruction to help understand the precautions and exercises prescribed during this phase and the subsequent phases of rehabilitation. In addition to verbal and hands-on instruction, computerized exercise programs, digital photos with instructions, and even videos are all excellent mediums to aid in making the patient independent in therapeutic exercise performance and postoperative precautions. Compliance in regard to the patient's HEP as well as his or her adherence to activity restrictions is assessed and monitored throughout the rehabilitative process. The patient is encouraged to ask questions regarding exercise performance and postoperative limitations and restrictions. Successful outcome after rotator cuff repair involves making the patient an active participant in the rehabilitative process.

POSTOPERATIVE PHASE II: MODERATE PROTECTION (WEEKS 3 TO 7)

This phase of rehabilitation will continue to focus on improving ROM, decreasing postoperative pain, and initiating gentle activation of the rotator cuff musculature. ROM should continue to progress in the directions of forward flexion and external rotation, abduction, and gentle internal rotation.

As strengthening progresses in this phase, the patient can begin AAROM exercises to initiate gentle, controlled activation of the deltoid and rotator cuff muscles. This is best done supine with wand-assisted elevation in the scapular plane (Figure 40-6). The patient can assist elevation, using the contralateral arm.

If the patient demonstrates adequate elevation (greater than approximately 120 degrees), pulleys can be initiated. The rehabilitation specialist must be careful to monitor for compensations, including trunk side bending and hiking of the involved shoulder. Also, the patient should not have pain while performing the pulley exercise. If this occurs, the exercise should be deferred to when the patient can perform it without pain.

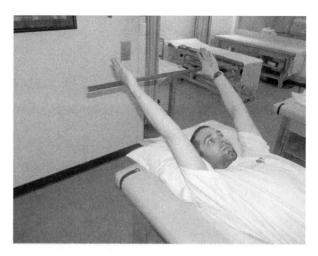

FIGURE 40-6 AAROM supine forward flexion, with wand in scapular plane.

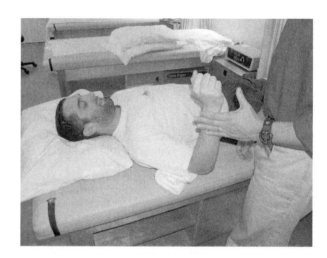

FIGURE 40-7 Rhythmic stabilization (supine): Gentle resisted motion is applied manually in alternating directions, eliciting a submaximal isometric contraction of the rotator cuff muscles.

In the presence of postoperative edema, the rotator cuff muscles must be gently activated to minimize rotator cuff inhibition.[18] During this phase, the therapist can begin manually resisted rhythmic stabilization exercises to begin gentle activation of the rotator cuff muscles (Figure 40-7). In this manner, the therapist can control the amount of resistance applied and thus the amount of tension generated in the rotator cuff muscles.

When the patient is able to tolerate activation of the rotator cuff without pain, he or she can begin independent submaximal isometric exercises in a modified neutral position. When performing isometric exercises, a towel roll or small pillow can be placed between the trunk and elbow to place the arm in slight abduction (modified neutral). This position places less tension on the supraspinatus and may improve vascular flow compared to the fully adducted (0 degrees) position.[29] Also, patients often find this position most comfortable. Contractions should be 20% to 30% of maximum and should be done without pain. Resistance can be given manually or by use of a stationary object (wall) (Figure 40-8).

When incisions are completely closed, a hydrotherapy program can begin. Motion should initially take place below the surface of the water at slow speeds. At slow speeds, the buoyancy of the water creates an active-assisted exercise. At faster speeds, the movement becomes a resistive exercise.[30] The early active-assisted effect of the water will allow patients to elevate the arm (below the surface) in the pool, long before they could perform the same exercise on dry land against gravity.

Toward the latter end of this phase, the patient should begin to use active exercise, such as an upper

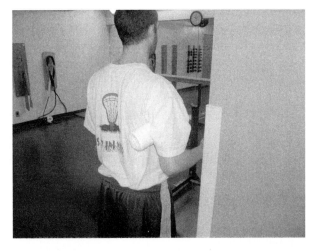

FIGURE **40-8** Rotator cuff isometrics in modified neutral: submaximal isometrics, using the wall with towel roll at elbow to put shoulder in modified neutral position.

Postoperative Phase II: Moderate Protection (Weeks 3 to 7)

GOALS

- Protect surgical repair
- Decrease pain/inflammation
- Improve ROM 80% to 100% forward flexion and external rotation
- Improve proximal scapula strength and stability
- Improve scapulohumeral rhythm and neuromuscular control
- Decrease rotator cuff inhibition

PRECAUTIONS

- Avoid pain with ADL
- Avoid active elevation of arm
- No maximal cuff activation
- Avoid pain with ROM/therapeutic exercise
- Avoid exceeding ROM limitations

TREATMENT STRATEGIES

- Continue exercises in phase I, progressing ROM as tolerated
- Discontinue sling (surgeon directed)
- AAROM exercises
  - Supine forward flexion with wand (scapula plane)
  - Continue wand ER/IR
  - Joint mobilization techniques
  - Initiate pulleys as ROM and upper extremity control improves
  - Airdyne ergometer
  - Initiate hydrotherapy (pool) program
- Physio ball scapular stabilization (below horizontal)
- Isometric exercises
  - ER/IR (submaximal) at modified neutral
  - Progress deltoid isometrics to long lever arm in neutral
- Isotonic exercises
- Scapula, elbow
- Begin humeral head stabilization exercises as ROM improves (>90 degrees)
- Modalities as needed
- Modify HEP

CRITERIA FOR ADVANCEMENT

- Ability to activate cuff and deltoid without pain
- Tolerates arm out of sling
- ROM 80% or greater for forward flexion and external rotation

body ergometer (Airdyne) for warm-up before ROM exercises.

Scapular strengthening can progress if the patient demonstrates adequate scapular mobility and active scapular control. Scapular isotonics (retraction with resistance tubing) and scapular stabilization exercise below the horizontal (physio ball) can be used (Figure 40-9).

The sling is discontinued between weeks 3 and 6, based on the surgeon's direction. The patient must still take care to avoid active overhead elevation of the involved arm and lifting of heavy objects because these may disrupt the healing repair.

Troubleshooting

This is a phase during which surgical pain can start to diminish, and the patient may feel as though he or she is able to perform activities, such as lifting and reaching. The patient must be educated regarding the healing process and modification of his or her activities to prevent injury during this phase. It is important that motion is facilitated and not forced. Painful ROM can result in more inflammation and pain and create a ROM problem. Use of gentle mobilization techniques is appropriate at this time. It is important to keep in mind that patients with preoperative limitations may have difficulty restoring shoulder ROM in the postoperative course of rehabilitation because postoperative ROM is directly proportional to preoperative ROM.[31]

During the performance of isometric exercises, the rehabilitation specialist should frequently question the patient regarding the amount of pressure being exerted and whether the exercise is painful. The isometrics should be submaximal and pain-free. Pushing too hard can create pain and slow progress.

POSTOPERATIVE PHASE III: EARLY FUNCTIONAL/STRENGTHENING (WEEKS 7 TO 13)

This phase of rehabilitation focuses on restoring full shoulder ROM, gradually progressing with shoulder strengthening exercises and returning the patient to light, functional activity below 90 degrees of elevation. Within the time frames associated with this phase, increases in ROM, strength, and functional activity may vary, depending on the type of repair and the surgeon's preference. Again, communication with the surgeon through written or direct communication is essential when progressing the patient's shoulder ROM, strength, and functional activity.

Restoring full PROM at the glenohumeral joint is accomplished by continuing wand exercises for forward flexion, external, and internal rotation. Wand exercises to increase external rotation at 90 degrees of shoulder abduction are added at this time (Figure 40-10). This is especially practical if the patient participates in an overhead athletic sport that requires rotational ROM in elevated positions, such as swinging a tennis racquet, throwing a football or baseball, and swimming. Active-assisted pulley exercises are continued during this phase. Functional ROM exercises are also taught to the patient later in this phase. These exercises include reaching behind the back with assist from a strap or the opposite hand and a towel pass behind the back. The rehabilitative specialist should monitor for capsular tightness. Grades III and IV glenohumeral joint mobilizations may be used to address capsular tightness. Posterior capsule tightness may lead to anterosuperior migration of the humeral head, which can lead to impingement of the healing tendons.[32] Self active-assisted movement into horizontal adduction may help

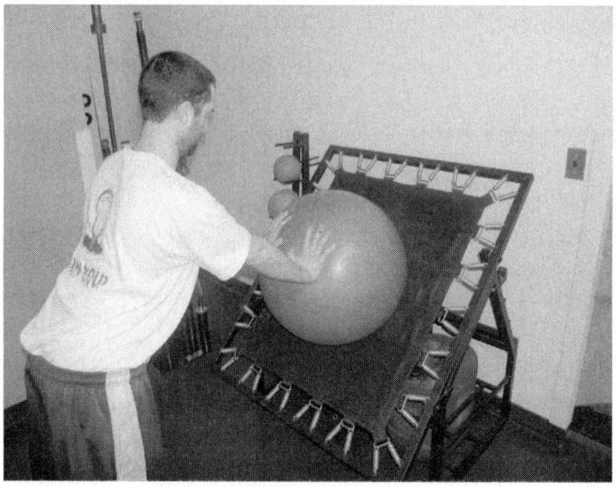

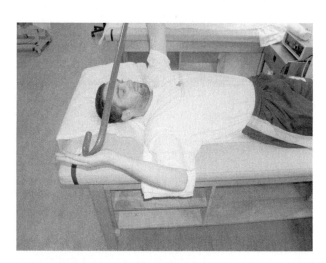

FIGURE 40-9 Closed-chain shoulder stabilization exercises: bilateral upper extremity support on ball below the horizontal.

FIGURE 40-10 Wand exercise to increase external rotation and at 90 degrees of shoulder abduction.

address a tight posterior capsule, if present, and can help increase internal rotation ROM (Figure 40-11).

Scapular rehabilitation is continued and progressed during this phase. Progressive strengthening of the periscapular muscles is essential to normalizing scapular function and overall scapulohumeral rhythm. Scapular retraction and shoulder extension exercises with Thera-Band elastic help to strengthen the posterior deltoid, latissimus dorsi, rhomboids, and middle trapezius muscle groups and are progressed during this phase.

The serratus anterior and lower trapezius appear to be affected by muscle inhibition after shoulder injury.[27] The supine punch with weight isotonically trains the serratus anterior and helps promote dynamic control around the shoulder.

Adequate scapular stability should be achieved before rotator cuff strengthening exercises are advanced because the scapula is the base from which the rotator cuff muscles activate. Strengthening of the repaired rotator cuff musculature must be progressed slowly and with care. Isotonic side-lying external rotation, in modified neutral, can be initiated first and isometrics discontinued if adequate strength and ROM are present and the exercise is performed without pain. Progression should then be made to isotonic ER/IR with elastic bands in modified neutral (Figure 40-12, *A* and *B*). Isotonic cuff exercise should be performed with low weight and high repetitions because these are mainly endurance-type muscles.[33]

Progression of closed-chain exercises should take place during this phase as scapular control and cuff strength improve. Closed chain ball exercises may be progressed from bilateral upper extremity support to unilateral support and from activities below the horizontal to shoulder level (Figure 40-13, *A* and *B*).

Isotonic exercises for the biceps and triceps brachii, as well as the forearm and wrist musculature, are advanced as tolerated to help improve strength of the distal musculature.

Active elevation (plane of scapula) to 90 degrees in the supine position can be initiated and gradually progressed to the standing position as rotator cuff strength

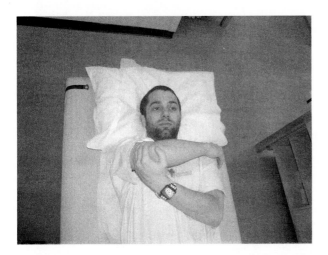

FIGURE **40-11** Posterior capsule stretch (supine): This exercise is performed in the supine position to stabilize the scapula, thereby avoiding excessive scapular protraction, and isolate the stretch to the posterior capsule.

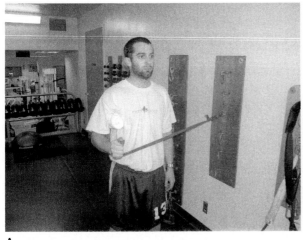

A

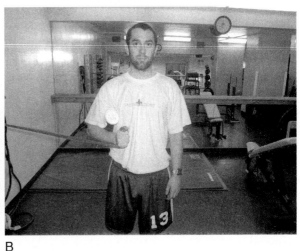

B

FIGURE **40-12** External and internal rotation in modified neutral, using elastic bands. During these exercises, the rehabilitation specialist should be aware of compensatory patterns, such as trunk rotation and scapular retraction/protraction with external and internal rotation, respectively. *A. External rotation:* A towel is placed under the axilla. *B. Internal rotation:* Patient uses pure rotary movement and should avoid scapular protraction and horizontal adduction.

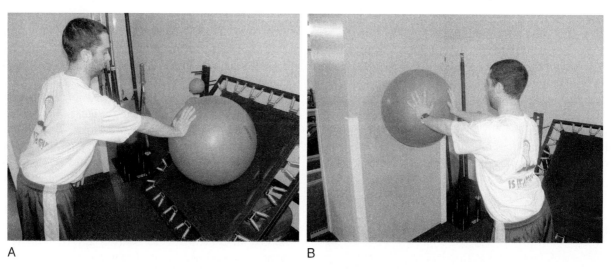

FIGURE **40-13** Advanced closed-chain scapular stabilization exercises. *A.* Unilateral upper extremity support below the horizontal. *B.* Bilateral upper extremity support at shoulder level.

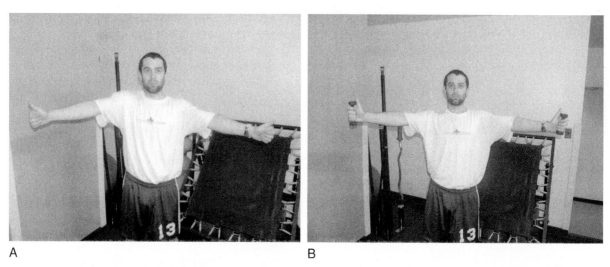

FIGURE **40-14** Forward flexion in the scapular plane. *A.* Poor scapulohumeral rhythm: The patient may exhibit a "shrug sign" when attempting upper extremity elevation. *B.* Good scapulohumeral rhythm.

and neuromuscular control improve. Upon initiation of active elevation against gravity (to 90 degrees), the rehabilitation specialist needs to assess scapulohumeral rhythm and be aware of excessive activation of the shoulder girdle musculature (upper trapezius) and a compensatory "shrug sign" (Figure 40-14, *A* and *B*). This may lead to impingement of subacromial tissues, including the repaired cuff, and should be avoided with active exercise.

Manual techniques should also be continued and advanced during this phase. Glenohumeral joint mobilization techniques are continued and progressed, based on assessment of accessory joint motions. Grades III and IV glenohumeral joint mobilizations in the inferior, ante-

rior, and posterior directions can help facilitate ROM gains into elevation, external, and internal rotations.[28] Limitations in external rotation ROM are generally the result of capsular restrictions and tightness of the internal rotators. If limitations are the result of subscapularis tightness, soft tissue mobilizations to "release" the subscapularis, along with gentle contract-relax techniques, have been shown to improve ROM into external rotation.[34] Rhythmic stabilization exercises are continued and advanced toward the end of this phase. Angles are progressed out of the balanced position of 100- to 110-degree elevation, as described by Wilk,[35] to more difficult flexion angles of 30, 60, and higher than 110 degrees. Patient position can also be advanced from supine to the

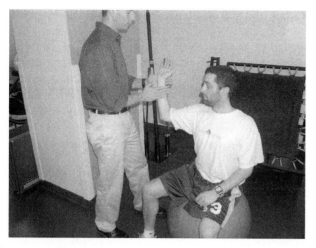

FIGURE **40-15** Rhythmic stabilization in the seated position.

seated position to sitting on an unstable surface, such as a physio ball (Figure 40-15).

Troubleshooting

A significant number of new exercises are added during this phase. The rehabilitation specialist must monitor and update the patient's written HEP. The patient needs to understand the purpose and rationale for each exercise. Flexibility and ROM exercises should be performed three to five times daily. Overzealous patients may attempt to perform strengthening activities on a daily basis, which may lead to pain and inflammation of healing structures and an overuse tendonitis. The rehabilitation specialist should closely monitor the progression of isotonic cuff exercises because these are the muscles that have been surgically influenced and

Postoperative Phase III: Early Strengthening (Weeks 7 to 13)

GOALS

- Eliminate/minimize pain and inflammation
- Restore full PROM
- Improve strength/flexibility
- Restore normal scapulohumeral rhythm below 90-degree elevation
- Gradual return to light ADL below 90-degree elevation

PRECAUTIONS

- Monitor activity level
- Limit overhead activity
- Avoid shoulder "shrug" with activity and exercise
- Patient to avoid jerking movements and lifting heavy objects

TREATMENT STRATEGIES

- Activity modification, continue cryotherapy PRN
- Continue wand exercises for external/internal rotation and flexion
- Continue joint mobilization techniques—progress to grades III and IV
- Flexibility exercises, horizontal adduction (posterior capsule stretching)
- Progress to functional ROM exercises (IR behind back, towel pass)
- Periscapular isotonic strengthening
  - Scapular protraction
  - Progress to scapular retraction exercises
  - Shoulder extension with elastic bands
  - Dumbbell rowing
- Rotator cuff isotonic strengthening exercises
  - AROM, side-lying ER
  - ER/IR at modified neutral with elastic bands, if sufficient scapular strength base developed
- Functional strengthening exercises
  - AROM supine forward flexion (scapular plane)
  - Progress to standing forward flexion
- Progress to rhythmic stabilization exercises
- Progress to closed-chain exercises
- Upper body ergometer (UBE) as ROM and strength improve

CRITERIA FOR ADVANCEMENT

- Minimal pain and/or inflammation
- Full PROM
- Improved rotator cuff and scapular strength
- Normal scapulohumeral rhythm with shoulder elevation below 90 degrees
- Independence with current HEP

repaired. Patients should be informed both verbally and through the written HEP that strengthening exercises should be performed once daily, three to four times per week, as the intensity of strengthening exercises is progressed.

Adequate scapular rehabilitation needs to occur before advanced rotator cuff and strengthening activities are incorporated into the program. The rehabilitation specialist should continually monitor improvements in muscle function and scapulohumeral rhythm to safely progress to more advanced strengthening activity. Poor scapulohumeral rhythm/mechanics ("shrug sign"), secondary to compensatory muscle patterns (upper trapezius), muscle weakness, and poor movement patterns/habits may lead to superior migration of the humeral head and impingement of the subacromial tissues.

POSTOPERATIVE PHASE IV: LATE STRENGTHENING (WEEKS 14 TO 19)

The goals of this phase are to normalize strength and flexibility and prepare the patient to return to all ADL, including return to sport for appropriate individuals. All remaining impairments in ROM, flexibility, and strength should be addressed.

Use of more challenging isotonic devices, such as the chest press and row machines, is initiated. Internal and external rotation isokinetics can be used to develop strength power and endurance in the rotator cuff during this phase.

Emphasis should be placed on reestablishment of normal scapulohumeral rhythm by focusing on correcting any muscle imbalance in the force couples directing shoulder motions. More advanced exercises that strengthen the lower trapezius and serratus anterior, such as prone arm elevation, dynamic hug, and diagonal exercises,[36] are used in this phase. Proximal scapular stability in the overhead positions should be adequate before progressing to more demanding distal activities.

In patients who are returning to overhead or throwing sports, plyometric activity is begun below the horizontal to develop power and coordination. Plyometrics are performed, only if the patient is nonapprehensive, pain-free, and has good proximal stability in this range.

Flexibility exercises can be advanced during this phase. Patients may develop tightness in the posterior capsule or posterior rotator cuff, as a result of immobilization and trauma of the surgery. As the patient's ROM improves, these deficits may become more apparent and need to be addressed. The posterior cuff can be stretched in the side-lying position by the rehabilitation specialist or by the patient as part of the home program (Figure 40-16).

Troubleshooting

If patients attempt to progress to overhead activity without proper flexibility and proximal stability, the patient may develop compensatory movement patterns. They may also complain of shoulder pain with more demanding activities. This should be an indication that they are not adequately prepared for these advanced activities. Pain and quality of movement should be monitored closely. A common problem encountered in

---

Postoperative Phase IV: Late Strengthening (Weeks 14 to 19)

GOALS
- Improve strength to 5/5 for scapula and shoulder musculature
- Improve neuromuscular control
- Normalize scapulohumeral rhythm throughout the full ROM

PRECAUTIONS
- Progress to overhead activity only when proper proximal stability is attained

TREATMENT STRATEGIES
- Continue to progress isotonic strengthening for periscapular and rotator cuff musculature
  - Latissimus pull-down (LPD)
  - Row machine
  - Chest press
- Continue flexibility—side-lying posterior capsule stretch
- Progress scapular stabilization program
- Initiate isokinetic strengthening (IR/ER) in scapular plane
- Initiate plyometric exercises below horizontal, if sufficient strength base (surgeon directed)

CRITERIA FOR ADVANCEMENT
- Normal scapulohumeral rhythm throughout the full ROM
- Normal strength 5/5 manual muscle test (MMT) of scapular and humeral muscles

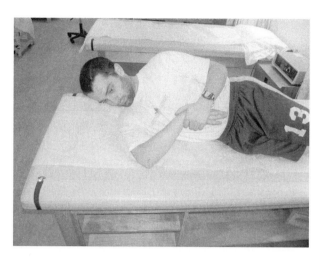
FIGURE **40-16** Side-lying posterior capsule stretch.

this phase is lack of flexibility of the posterior capsule and posterior rotator cuff. These deficits must be addressed before progressing to a higher level and more demanding activity.

POSTOPERATIVE PHASE V: RETURN TO SPORT (WEEKS 20 TO 24)

The last phase focuses on restoring normal strength and flexibility in preparation for the patient to meet the demand of daily activities and return to sport activity.

For overhead athletes, it is imperative to have adequate strength, flexibility, and neuromuscular control before returning to sport. Flexibility exercises are encouraged and continued during this phase, especially if the individual is an overhead athlete. Patients are encouraged to independently continue strengthening and flexibility exercises to facilitate gains in shoulder function and overall muscle strength. The HEP should be thoroughly reviewed and updated before the patient is discharged from a supervised exercise program.

Upper extremity plyometrics are progressed to activities above the horizontal. Plyometric exercise should be individualized and match the activities to which the athlete is returning. Progression should be safe, gradual, and criteria-based. Bilateral ball throws from the side can be progressed to bilateral overhead throws to a one-arm overhead throwing motion. Progression should be made from total body motions to isolated joint motions.

Isokinetic testing is conducted at this time to evaluate ER/IR strength ratios and upper extremity limb symmetry. Core control and lower extremity strength are essential and should be evaluated and incorporated into the program, if the individual is returning to an overhead sport.

Return to sport is based on communication with the surgeon, the individual patient, and the type of surgery. A gradual progression should be made with regards to

Postoperative Phase V: Return to Sport (Weeks 20 to 24)

GOALS
- Maximize flexibility, strength, and neuromuscular control to meet demands of sport, return to work, recreational, and daily activity
- Isokinetic testing: 85% limb symmetry
- Independent in home and gym therapeutic exercise programs for maintenance and progression of functional level at discharge

PRECAUTIONS
- Avoid pain with therapeutic exercises and activity
- Avoid sport activity until adequate strength, flexibility, and neuromuscular control
- Surgeon's clearance needed for sport activity

TREATMENT STRATEGIES
- Continue to progress isotonic strengthening for periscapular and rotator cuff musculature
- Isokinetic training and testing for external and internal rotators
- Continue flexibility and stabilization programs
- Individualize program to meet demands of sport-specific requirements
- Plyometrics (above horizontal)
- Interval training program for pitchers and overhead athletes
- Periodization training

CRITERIA FOR DISCHARGE
- Isokinetic testing close to normal ER/IR ratios (66%), 85% symmetry
- Independence with home/gym program at discharge for maintenance and progression of flexibility, strength, and neuromuscular control

the specific sport to which the individual is returning. The overhead thrower should initiate an interval throwing program. The tennis player can initiate ground strokes first and gradually progress to overhead serves. Golfers are encouraged to drive the golf ball with less intensity and first use smaller swings. Swimmers should monitor the intensity and volume of their individual activity sessions.

Troubleshooting

The rehabilitation specialist should understand the biomechanics of the sport to which the individual is returning. Faulty biomechanics may put the athlete at risk for reinjury. Interval training programs should be initiated in the athlete's program before a full return to play.

The volume of the patient's exercise program needs to be monitored to avoid overuse syndromes from developing. If the individual is an overhead athlete, periodization should be incorporated into the individual's exercise program to allow for adequate control of the shoulder activity during in-season sport participation.

The rehabilitation program is now the patient's upper extremity strength and conditioning program and needs to be continued independently by the patient to promote optimal shoulder function. The patient should understand how to safely progress strengthening exercises to maximize gains in muscle strength and upper limb performance.

References

1. Wahl, C.J., Wickiewicz, T.L. *Surgical Treatment of Rotator Cuff Tears.* Curr Opin Orthop 2002;13(4):281–287.
2. Codman, E.A. *Complete Rupture of the Supraspinatus Tendon. Operative Treatment with Report of Two Successful Cases.* Boston Med Surg J 1911;164:708–710.
3. Yamaguchi, K., Levine, W.N., Marra, G., Galatz, L.M., Klepps, S., Flatow, E.L. *Transitioning to Arthroscopic Rotator Cuff Repair: The Pros and Cons.* Instr Course Lect 2003;52:81–92.
4. Baker, C.L., Whaley, A.L., Baker, M. *Arthroscopic Rotator Cuff Tear Repair.* J Surg Orthop Adv 2003;12(4):175–190.
5. Gartsman, G.M., Khan, M., Hammerman, S.M. *Arthroscopic Repair of Full-thickness Tears of the Rotator Cuff.* J Bone Joint Surg Am 1998;80:832–840.
6. Wolf, E.M., Pennington, W.T., Agrawal, V. *Arthroscopic Rotator Cuff Repair: 4- to 10-year Results.* Arthroscopy 2004;20(1):5–12.
7. Burkhart, S.S., Danaceau, S.M., Pearce, C.E. Jr. *Arthroscopic Rotator Cuff Repair: Analysis of Results by Tear Size and by Repair Technique-margin Convergence Versus Direct Tendon-to-bone Repair.* Arthroscopy 2001;17:905–912.
8. Severud, E.L., Ruotolo, C., Abbott, D.D., Nottage, W.M. *All-Arthroscopic Versus Mini-open Rotator Cuff Repair: A Long-term Retrospective Outcome Comparison.* Arthroscopy 2003;19:234–238.
9. Tauro, J.C. *Arthroscopic Rotator Cuff Repair: Analysis of Technique and Results at 2- and 3-year Follow-up.* Arthroscopy 1998; 14:45–51.
10. Lo, I.K., Burkhart, S.S. *Current Concepts in Arthroscopic Rotator Cuff Repair.* Am J Sports Med 2003;31(2):308–324.
11. Gartsman, G.M. *All Arthroscopic Rotator Cuff Repairs.* Orthop Clin North Am 2001;32(3):501–510.
12. Galatz, L.M., Ball, C.M., Teefey, S.A., Middleton, W.D., Yamaguchi, K. *The Outcome and Repair Integrity of Completely Arthroscopically Repaired Large and Massive Rotator Cuff Tears.* J Bone Joint Surg Am 2004;86A(2):219.
13. Goldberg, B.A., Lippitt, S.B., Matsen, F.A. III. *Improvement in Comfort and Function after Cuff Repair Without Acromioplasty.* Clin Orthop 2001;390:142–150.
14. Debeyre, J., Patte, D., Elmelik, E. *Repair of Ruptures of the Rotator Cuff of the Shoulder with a Note on Advancement of the Supraspinatus Muscle.* J Bone Joint Surg 1965;47B:36–42.
15. Gore, D.R., Murray, M.P., Sepic, S.B., Gardner, G.M. *Shoulder Muscle Strength and Range of Motion Following Surgical Repair of Full Thickness Rotator Cuff Tears.* J Bone Joint Surg Am 1986;69:266–272.
16. Post, M., Sliver, R., Singh, M. *Rotator Cuff Tears: Diagnosis and Treatment.* Clin Orthop 1983;173:78–91.
17. Watson, M. *Major Ruptures of the Rotator Cuff: The Result of Surgical Repair in 89 Patients.* J Bone Joint Surg Br 1985;67: 618–624.
18. Wilk, K.E., Crockett, H.C., Andrews, J.R. *Rehabilitation after Rotator Cuff Surgery.* J Shoulder Elbow Surg 2000;0:1–18.
19. Yel, M., Shankwiler, J.A., Noonan, J.E. Jr., Burkhead, W.Z. Jr. *Results of Decompression and Rotator Cuff Repair in Patients 65 Years Old and Older: 6- to 14-year Follow-up.* Am J Orthop 2001;30:347–352.
20. Grondel, R.J., Savoie, F.H. III, Field, L.D. *Rotator Cuff Repairs in Patients 62 Years of Age or Older.* J Shoulder Elbow Surg 2001;10:97–99.
21. Waltrip, R.L., Zheng, N., Dugas, J.R., Andrews, J.R. *Rotator Cuff Repair. A Biomechanical Comparison of Three Techniques.* Am J Sports Med 2003;31(4):493–497.
22. McMaster, W.C., Liddle, S., Waugh, T.R. *Laboratory Evaluation of Various Cold Therapy Modalities.* Am J Sports Med 1978;6: 291–294.
23. Meeusen, R., Lievens, P. *The Use of Cryotherapy in Sports Injuries.* Sports Med 1986;3:398–414.
24. Osbahr, D.C., Cawley, P.W., Speer, K.P. *The Effect of Continuous Cryotherapy on Glenohumeral Joint and Subacromial Space Temperatures in the Postoperative Shoulder.* Arthroscopy 2002; 18(7):748–754.
25. Dockery, M.L., Wright, T.W., LaStayo, P.C. *Electromyography of the Shoulder: An Analysis of Passive Modes of Exercise.* Orthopedics 1998;21(11):1181–1184.
26. Solem-Bertoft, E., Thuomas, K.A., Westerberg, C.E. *The Influence of Scapular Retraction and Protraction on the Width of the Subacromial Space. An MRI Study.* Clin Orthop 1993;296:99–103.
27. Kibler, W.B. *The Role of the Scapula in Athletic Shoulder Function.* Am J Sports Med 1998;26(2):325–337.
28. Edmond, S.L. *Manipulation and Mobilization: Extremity and Spinal Techniques.* Mosby–Year Book, St. Louis, 1993.
29. Rathbun, J.B., Macnab, I. *The Microvascular Pattern of the Rotator Cuff.* J Bone Joint Surg Br 1970;52(3):540–553.
30. Kelly, B.T., Roskin, L.A., Kirkendall, D.T., Speer, K.P. *Shoulder Muscle Activation During Aquatic and Dry Land Exercises in Nonimpaired Subjects.* J Orthop Sports Phys Ther 2000;30(4): 204–210.

31. Cofield, R.H., Parvizi, J., Hoffmeyer, P.J., Lanzer, W.L., Ilstrup, D.M., Rowland, C.M. *Surgical Repair of Chronic Rotator Cuff Tears. A Prospective Long-term Study.* J Bone Joint Surg Am 2001;83A:71–77.

32. Harryman, D.T. II, Sidles, J.A., Clark, J.M., McQuade, K.J., Gibb, T.D., Matsen, F.A. III. *Translation of the Humeral Head on the Glenoid with Passive Glenohumeral Motion.* J Bone Joint Surg Am 1990;72(9):1334–1343.

33. Berger, R.A. *Applied Exercise Physiology.* Lea & Febiger, Philadelphia, 1982.

34. Godges, J.J., Mattson-Bell, M., Thorpe, D., Shah, D. *The Immediate Effects of Soft Tissue Mobilization with Proprioceptive Neu-romuscular Facilitation on Glenohumeral External Rotation and Overhead Reach.* J Orthop Sports Phys Ther 2003;33(12):713–718.

35. Malone, T.R. *Orthopedic and Sports Physical Therapy,* 3rd ed. Mosby–Year Book, St. Louis, 1997.

36. Ekstrom, R.A., Donatelli, R.A., Soderberg, G.L. *Surface Electromyographic Analysis of Exercises for the Trapezius and Serratus Anterior Muscles.* J Orthop Sports Phys Ther 2003;33(5):247–258.

41

Subacromial Decompression

LEE ROSENZWEIG, MSPT, CHT

ADAM PRATOMO, PT, MSPT

Impingement of the rotator cuff tendons and bursae in the subacromial space is the most common cause of shoulder pathology.[1,2] The pathophysiology of the impingement process involves repetitive encroachment and subsequent microtrauma to these structures as a result of narrowing of the space between the humeral head and acromion.[3] The indications for surgical management of impingement are pain or weakness that interferes with work, sports, or activities of daily living (ADL). Neer[4] first described the pathology of shoulder impingement syndrome in 1972. Neer performed the first open anterior acromioplasty, which was the standard surgical procedure for stages II and III impingement lesions through the 1980s. During this time, Ellman[5] began to perform an arthroscopic technique for subacromial decompression (SAD), and this type of procedure has now become widely accepted. The objectives of arthroscopic SAD are the same as those for open decompression: removal of the structures that are creating impingement within the confines of the subacromial space.

SAD is typically recommended to patients who have failed a 6- to 12-month course of rehabilitation.[6-8] The success rate of patients who have undergone arthroscopic SAD has been reported to be from 43% to 90%.[9-22] The chapter will present the Hospital for Special Surgery's (HSS) surgical approach and treatment guidelines for managing patients who have undergone SAD.

SURGICAL OVERVIEW

Anatomically, the subacromial space is considered an interstitial pseudo-articulation among the proximal humerus, coracromial arch, acromioclavicular joint, superficial surface of the rotator cuff, and the subacromial and subdeltoid bursa. The acromioclavicular joint lies in the anteromedial most aspect, and its anterior wall is composed of the coracoacromial ligament going from the anterior aspect of the acromion to the coracoid process.[23,24] The normal subacromial space is 7 to 14 mm, and narrowing of this space has been associated with rotator cuff pathology[25] (Figure 41-1).

The first reported arthroscopic SAD was performed by Ellman in 1983.[5] In the procedure, a mechanical suction shaver is used to initially perform a bursectomy to establish visualization within the subacromial space. The coracoacromial ligament is released with a surgical electrode, and electrocautery is used to release adhesions. Osteophytes along the undersurface of the acromioclavicular joint are removed with a motorized burr.

Proper decompression includes (1) extensive complete subacromial bursectomy, (2) coracoacromial ligament resection, (3) resection of the undersurface of the anterior acromion, and (4) removal of impinging

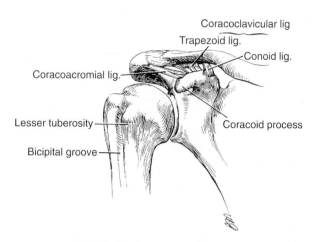

FIGURE **41-1** Subacromial space.

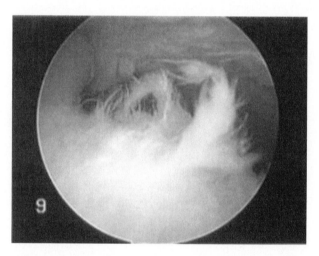

FIGURE **41-2** Arthroscopic view of the subacromial space with frayed supraspinatus tendon before SAD.

acromioclavicular joint osteophytes[26] (Figures 41-2 and 41-3).

REHABILITATION OVERVIEW

Rehabilitation begins immediately after surgery, and the patient is typically released from the hospital on the same day. A sling is used based on patient comfort for the first 2 to 7 days, but early mobilization is encouraged. The patient is instructed in a series of range of motion (ROM) exercises to prevent stiffness and promote mobility.

Patients are advanced when they meet the goals and criteria defined in each phase of rehabilitation. Individual progression is also based on the level of pain during activity. Exercise should emphasize forward flexion, internal/external rotation, posterior capsule flexibility, and scapular stability. ROM exercises should be performed daily until full range is achieved. As ROM

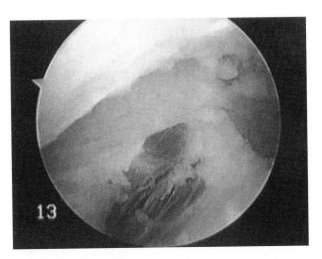

FIGURE **41-3** Arthroscopic view of subacromial space following SAD and débridement of tendon.

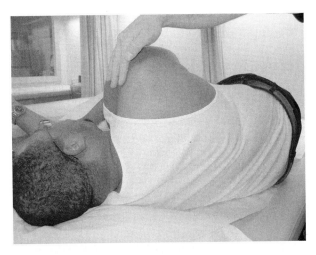

FIGURE **41-4** Manually resisted scapular strengthening is begun in side-lying.

improves, strengthening exercises can be incorporated, with an emphasis on muscular balance of the scapulohumeral and scapulothoracic muscles. The rehabilitation specialist must carefully assess flexibility, scapulohumeral rhythm, and posture. Poor posture during exercise can affect the congruency of the shoulder joint and place the musculature in a poor mechanical position. Correct positioning during exercise will permit the glenohumeral muscles to work within the ideal length–tension relationship. Proper scapulothoracic function is also important to allow a stable base for glenohumeral rotation. The scapular muscles must work in unison to maximize congruency between the humeral head and the glenoid during movement. Once sufficient scapular stability exists, rotator cuff strengthening is incorporated.[27,28]

Impingement commonly occurs when rotator cuff strength is insufficient to stabilize the humeral head during elevation, causing insufficient space for the rotator cuff tendons.[29] Superior translation of the humeral head of up to 1.5 mm occurs when the arm reaches 120 degrees of elevation. Abduction with insufficient rotator cuff strength can also result in sharp increases in this superior translation.[30] All exercises should be initially kept below the horizontal until sufficient rotator cuff and scapular strength are established to prevent impingement. Patients progress to overhead activity when they demonstrate pain-free ROM in conjunction with adequate strength. Appropriate patients progress to sport-specific activities, depending on the requirements of the sport. It is important to emphasize activity modification throughout the course of rehabilitation to avoid causing inflammation and delayed recovery. Treatment goals are to restore full ROM, strength, flexibility, neuromuscular control, and return to previous level of function.

POSTOPERATIVE REHABILITATION PHASE I (DAYS 0 TO 14)

During phase I of rehabilitation, the sling is removed several times daily for exercise. Initial exercises include Codman's/pendulums, forward flexion using the contralateral arm, and external rotation using a cane with a towel roll under the arm. This position allows the humeral head to rest in the plane of the scapula, which minimizes stress to the anterior capsular ligaments and is the most functional position for the upper extremity.[31] Initial scapular exercises can be started in side-lying, including manual scapular mobilization, active scapular retraction, protraction, elevation, and depression. Strengthening the serratus anterior and lower trapezius muscles is important because the muscles work together to produce upward rotation of the scapula during humeral elevation. They also work to provide a stabilizing influence for the scapula against the thoracic wall to prevent winging and loss of control.[27] Active scapular retraction progresses from the side-lying position to the seated or standing position. Active range of motion (AROM) then advances to manually resisted scapular strengthening, which also begins in side-lying (Figure 41-4). Distal AROM is also initiated. Patients are instructed to elevate the arm above the heart in supine, using a pillow during distal ROM exercises or when sleeping to minimize edema. Isometric exercises for the deltoid and rotator cuff muscles begin, as long as the patient has met appropriate ROM and pain criteria. As strength improves, exercises progress to (1) forward flexion using a cane in supine and (2) scapular strengthening in sitting or standing with light weights or elastic bands. Cryotherapy is used following each session, and transcutaneous electric nerve stimulation (TENS) is an additional tool that may be used to control pain.

Postoperative Rehabilitation Phase I (Days 0 to 14)

GOALS

- Control postoperative pain and swelling
- Forward flexion ROM to 120 degrees
- External rotation to 60 degrees
- Independent with home exercise program
- Independent with light ADL, dressing
- Precautions:
  - Pain with exercises
  - Overhead activity
  - Carrying heavy objects

TREATMENT STRATEGIES

- Instruction in home exercise program
- Codman's/pendulums
- Supine forward flexion AAROM, AROM
- Cane external rotation with a towel under the elbow (scapular plane)
- Scapular mobilization in side-lying
- Scapular AROM in side-lying (retraction, protraction, elevation, depression)
- Manually resisted scapular strengthening in side-lying
- Standing scapular retraction with elastic bands
- Deltoid and rotator cuff isometrics
- Distal strengthening (wrist and elbow)
- Modalities (TENS, cryotherapy)

CRITERIA FOR ADVANCEMENT

- Forward flexion ROM, 120 degrees
- External rotation to 60 degrees
- Independent with home exercise program
- Controlled pain

Troubleshooting

Early mobilization is essential in the postoperative management of SAD. Poor patient compliance will result in a delay in achieving functional goals. It is helpful to know a patient's preoperative ROM and level of function to set appropriate goals. Limited ROM, muscle weakness, or preoperative functional impairment have been found to adversely affect outcomes following SAD.[32] Therapeutic intervention for the patient failing to progress continues to focus on gentle ROM, scapular strengthening, isometrics, and modalities. All patients will advance at different paces, with some exhibiting greater muscle inhibition than others. It is crucial that the patient meet the specific criteria for advancement before progressing to the next phase. This is what allows the rehabilitation program to be individualized and meet the characteristics of each person's recovery.

POSTOPERATIVE REHABILITATION PHASE II (WEEKS 2 TO 6)

As pain and inflammation subside, the rehabilitation program continues to emphasize ROM, with the goal to achieve full ROM by 6 weeks postoperatively.

Hydrotherapy is incorporated once the incision has healed. The essential benefit of hydrotherapy is the buoyancy that the water provides the upper extremity, which allows for greater comfort and security during active exercises.[33] The patient is instructed to perform forward flexion in the plane of the scapula while standing in water at shoulder height. This exercise is a good transition for a patient who is able to elevate his or her arm on land against gravity but has some minor compensatory shoulder shrugging or scapular motion as a result of muscular weakness. Hydrotherapy can also be used to provide resistance to movement. Resistive exercises, such as rowing, shoulder extension, and internal and external rotation, can be done under the water with handheld resistive paddles. Pulley exercises to increase elevation ROM are added when the patient achieves 110 degrees of forward flexion and improved humeral head control. Posterior capsule stretching and joint mobilization are initiated to facilitate increased ROM.

Rehabilitation continues to focus on scapular strengthening. Closed kinetic chain exercises that emphasize muscular co-contraction and dynamic shoulder stabilization are incorporated. Closed kinetic chain exercises also have the added benefit of proprioceptive

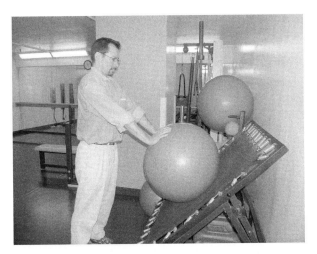

FIGURE **41-5** Closed kinetic chain exercise against a Plyoback.

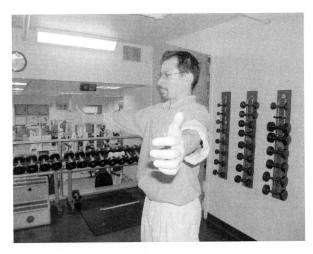

FIGURE **41-6** Forward flexion in the scapular plane.

stimulus. Proprioceptive exercises that increase kinesthetic awareness are important in restoring full function following shoulder surgery. An early closed kinetic chain exercise for the scapula would entail making small circles with a physio ball against a Plyoback at 60 degrees of elevation while bearing weight through extended arms (Figure 41-5). As scapular strength improves, the exercise is advanced by increasing the angle of elevation to 90 degrees and then progressing to a single arm. Scapular protraction exercises begin in supine, initially without weights, and are advanced by gradually incorporating weights. Closed chain scapular protraction can be performed in a standing position as part of a wall push-up. Rotator cuff isometrics begin by standing with the arm in neutral and a small towel roll under the arm to facilitate exercise in the scapular plane. This position will allow for the ideal length–tension relationship of the shoulder musculature.[34] Rotator cuff exercises are advanced to isotonic exercises, using elastic bands or weights when the patient is pain-free with isometrics, has at least 60 degrees of external rotation ROM, and demonstrates at least 4/5 internal and external rotator strength on a manual muscle test.

Distal strengthening advances in phase II to include the use of progressive resistance exercises for the biceps and triceps muscles. Biceps are important because they have been found to assist the rotator cuff with glenohumeral joint stabilizing and humeral head depression actions.[36] Upper body ergometry can be incorporated for endurance. Forward flexion in the scapular plane with thumbs pointed up (scaption or "full can" exercise) is initiated when the patient is able to actively elevate the arm to 90 degrees against gravity without compensatory motion (Figure 41-6). Increased electromyography (EMG) activity of the anterior deltoid, supraspinatus,

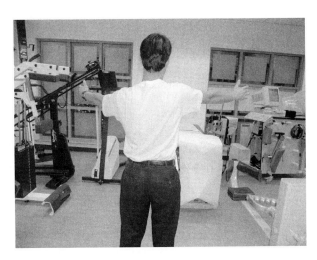

FIGURE **41-7** Compensatory motions to watch for during forward flexion in the scapular plane (shoulder hiking).

and infraspinatus has been found during this exercise.[37] This position also allows the greater tubercle to clear the acromion and minimizes the chance of impingement. Compensatory motions to watch for include shoulder hiking and anterior/superior translation of the humeral head[38] (Figure 41-7). Weights are added during this exercise to challenge the patient as strength improves. Progressive resistance exercises for more aggressive strengthening, using equipment, will begin toward the end of this phase (i.e., rows, chest press, latissimus pull-down).

Troubleshooting

One complication in this phase can be an increase in shoulder pain and stiffness. Frequently, when patients begin to feel a small improvement, they begin to overuse the arm before establishing adequate scapular stability

Postoperative Rehabilitation Phase II (Weeks 2 to 6)

GOALS

- Full ROM
- Strength 4/5 throughout the involved upper extremity
- Independent with light ADL (appropriate for preoperative functional level)
- Independent home exercise program
- Normal scapulohumeral rhythm <90 degrees elevation

PRECAUTIONS

- Avoid overhead reaching until appropriate ROM and strength have been achieved
- Avoid painful ROM

TREATMENT STRATEGIES

- ROM (active and passive)
- Pulleys
- Capsular stretching and joint mobilization
- Hydrotherapy
- Progress deltoid strengthening
- Progress rotator cuff strengthening
- Advance scapular strengthening below the horizontal
- Progressive resistance equipment (i.e., row, chest press, latissimus pull-down)
- Upper body ergometry
- Modalities as needed
- Progress to home exercise program

CRITERIA FOR ADVANCEMENT

- Minimal level of pain and swelling
- Full ROM
- Strength 4/5 throughout involved upper extremity
- Normal scapulohumeral rhythm <90 degrees elevation

and rotator cuff strength. This results in faulty mechanics, which can exacerbate symptoms. Patients are reminded that although they may use their arm for light activities, it will be several months before complete recovery. Patients must avoid any overhead motion or any heavy lifting that results in pain. The rehabilitation specialist should encourage pain-free use of the arm and avoidance of pain-provoking activities. The rehabilitation specialist should also encourage cryotherapy during this phase.

POSTOPERATIVE REHABILITATION PHASE III (WEEKS 6 TO 10)

In this phase, the goals are to return the patient to full overhead motion, strength, and flexibility. The patient continues to prepare for return to all previous ADL as well as work-related activities. For the athletic patient, activities continue to focus on preparing for eventual sports participation. As strength improves, more advanced activities can be incorporated. Rhythmic stabilization is used to improve upper extremity strength at multiple angles above 90 degrees. Diagonal patterns are introduced, using proprioceptive neuromuscular facilitation patterns. Initially, this is done with manual

resistance. Diagonal patterns progress to elastic bands or dumbbells once good scapulohumeral rhythm and rotator cuff strength have been established. For the overhead athlete, rotator cuff strengthening will advance to the elevated position. Internal and external rotation is performed using elastic resistance bands at 90 degrees of shoulder abduction. The patient is carefully monitored for any signs of pain with rotator cuff strengthening in the 90/90 position. Aggressive joint mobilization and posterior capsular stretching are performed to address any remaining joint stiffness or capsular tightness.

Troubleshooting

Before advancing to overhead activities and diagonal patterns, it is very important to make sure that the patient meets the criteria of full pain-free ROM, normal scapulohumeral rhythm throughout ROM, and 5/5 strength throughout the upper extremity. Failure to meet these criteria will lead to compensatory motion, poor mechanics, and increase the potential for reinjury.

One common movement fault that may contribute to pain with overhead movement is the failure of the scapula to upwardly rotate sufficiently. This can be the

Postoperative Rehabilitation Phase III (Weeks 6 to 10)

GOALS

- Full ROM
- Normal strength (5/5)
- Improved flexibility (surgical side equal to contralateral side)
- Normal scapulohumeral rhythm throughout ROM

PRECAUTIONS

- Avoidance of pain with therapeutic exercises and functional ADL
- Avoidance of sport activities until adequate flexibility and strength have been established

TREATMENT STRATEGIES

- Continue aggressive ROM activities
- Flexibility exercises
- Aggressive joint mobilization, capsular stretching
- Aggressive scapular strengthening
- Advanced rotator cuff strengthening
- Proprioceptive neuromuscular facilitation diagonal patterns (especially D2 flexion and extension, if appropriate)
- Advanced rotator cuff strengthening (elevated position, if appropriate)
- Rhythmic stabilization exercises
- Modalities as needed
- Modify and advance home exercise program as appropriate

CRITERIA FOR ADVANCEMENT

- Full PROM
- Strength 5/5 throughout upper extremity
- Good flexibility
- Normal scapulohumeral throughout ROM
- Pain-free AROM

result of many factors, such as poor posture (protracted shoulders and increased thoracic kyphosis), dominance of the upper trapezius during elevation, shortening of the latissimus dorsi, and insufficient synergistic recruitment of the serratus anterior and lower trapezius.[39,40] Limited upward rotation of the scapula is addressed by emphasizing strengthening exercises for the serratus anterior with exercises, such as scapular protraction supine or with a wall push-up emphasizing scapular protraction at end range. An exercise to emphasize the lower trapezius is performed by having the patient stand with his or her back against a wall, arms abducted to 70 degrees, elbows flexed to 90 degrees with the back of the hands against the wall. The patient abducts the arms from 70 to 100 degrees while actively pressing the back of the arms against the wall (Figure 41-8, *A* and *B*). Patient education emphasizing good posture is incorporated. Posture is addressed by emphasizing scapular retraction exercises with resistance bands, quadruped or prone arm lifts, abdominal, and gluteal strengthening. Latissimus dorsi tightness is addressed with supine wand exercises for shoulder flexion stretching. Patient education, emphasizing the importance of good posture, is reinforced.

POSTOPERATIVE REHABILITATION PHASE IV (WEEKS 10 TO 14)

The goal of this final phase is to return the patient to all of his or her previous functional activities and unrestricted sports participation. The criteria to return to sport activities are full strength, flexibility, and endurance appropriate to the patient's specific sport. Treatment strategies in this final phase will include dynamic strengthening, plyometrics, and sport-specific activities.

Dynamic strengthening exercises focus on the rotator cuff and scapula in varying planes of elevation. Scapular stabilization exercises are emphasized to improve dynamic stability of the shoulder. Advanced neuromuscular training includes both open and closed kinetic chain exercises as well as advanced proprioceptive exercises. Proprioceptive exercises that increase kinesthetic awareness are important for a patient who wishes to return to sports participation.[41,42] Exercises, including push-ups on unstable surfaces (ball/foam roller) or a quadruped exercise with manual perturbations for rhythmic stabilization, can be performed (Figure 41-9). Proprioceptive neuromuscular facilitation (PNF)

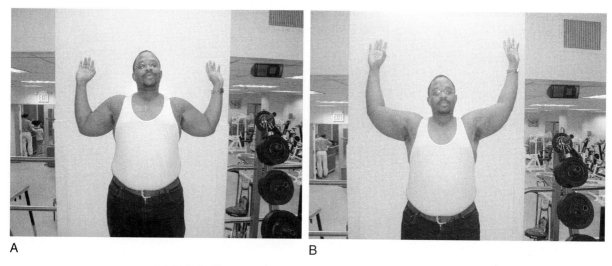

A   B

FIGURE **41-8** *A, B.* Abduction with active scapular retraction.

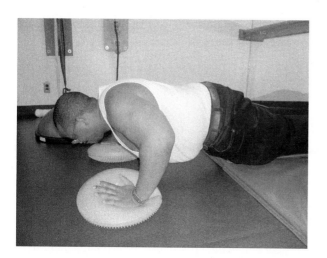

FIGURE **41-9** Push-ups on an unstable surface.

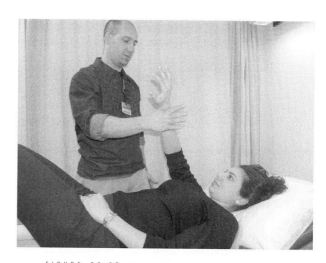

FIGURE **41-10** Manually resisted PNF patterns.

patterns and rhythmic stabilization exercises with isometric holds have shown to be an effective means of advancing rotator cuff musculature and developing kinesthetic awareness.[43,44] PNF patterns for the scapula and glenohumeral joint are initially performed on a treatment table with manual resistance by the therapist, with the patient supine or side-lying (Figure 41-10). In this final phase, PNF patterns advance to the standing position and are performed with resistance elastic bands to challenge the athlete. For an overhead athlete, isokinetic training for internal and external rotation is performed at speeds of 180 and 300 degrees per second to encourage strength and endurance. Initially, the athlete begins internal and external rotation training at 45 degrees of shoulder abduction, approximating the scapular plane. Overhead athletes are progressed to

training at 90 degrees of abduction for internal and external rotation.

Plyometric exercise is initiated during this final phase of rehabilitation. This advanced form of resistance training involves the quick stretching of muscle from an eccentric muscle action to a concentric muscle action.[45] Stretch-shortening muscle contractions use a prestretching of the muscle spindles and golgi tendon organs to produce a recoil action of the elastic tissues. This results in improved muscle performance by the combined effects of stored elastic energy and the myotactic reflex activation of the muscle.[46] Most overhead athletes use some form of plyometric movement in the performance of their sport.[47,48] Angular velocities of throwing average anywhere from 5000 to 9000 degrees per second.[49] Considering the angular velocities and forces applied to the shoulder during throwing motions (or other overhead motions, such as a tennis serve or volleyball serve), plyometrics is an essential component of an athlete's rehabilitation program. Plyometric exercise is initiated, first using a two-handed ball toss from chest level, advancing to a two-handed overhead soccer toss, and alternating two-handed, side-to-side throws using a 3- to 5-pound medicine ball. One-handed plyometrics begins with eccentric decelerations (Figure 41-11), progressing to PNF patterns, a one-handed side throw, and then, finally, to an overhead throw.

Near the end of the final phase, sport-specific drills are implemented. Before beginning any sport-specific drills, the athlete must have full pain-free ROM, at least 75% to 80% strength on an isokinetic test (both peak torque and total work) in the involved extremity during bilateral comparison, and at least 2 to 4 weeks of plyometric training. Isokinetic testing is performed for internal and external rotation. Normal internal to external rotation ratios have been reported to be 66% to 70% throughout the velocity spectrum.[50] Ratios that favor external rotation to internal rotation are desirable because a strong posterior shoulder reduces the chance of injury in throwing or racquet sports.[51,52]

For a throwing athlete, an interval throwing program is implemented. An athlete begins with a light-tossing program to gradually increase the distance and number of throws. Athletes begin at 45 feet and progress to longer throws of 60, 90, and 120 feet. A pitcher will progress to throw off of a mound, with a gradual

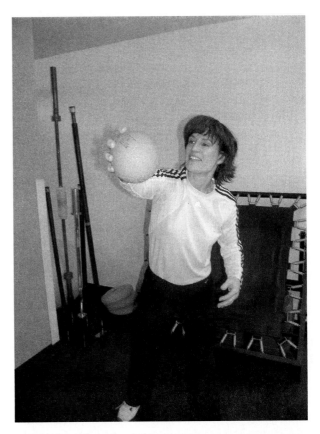

FIGURE **41-11** One-handed plyometrics with eccentric deceleration of a ball tossed against a wall.

Postoperative Rehabilitation Phase IV (Weeks 10 to 14)

GOALS
- Isokinetic testing to be >85% of the contralateral side (internal/external rotation)
- Pain-free during all sport-specific drills
- Functional strength, flexibility, and endurance to meet the demands of the individual's sport

PRECAUTIONS
- Avoidance of pain with therapeutic exercises and functional ADL
- Avoidance of sport activities until adequate flexibility and strength have been established

TREATMENT STRATEGIES
- Full upper extremity strengthening program
- Sport-specific plyometrics
- Isokinetic training and testing
- Advanced neuromuscular training
- Begin sport-specific drills/interval throwing program (surgeon directed)

CRITERIA FOR DISCHARGE/RETURN TO SPORT
- Patient has met strength, flexibility, and endurance goals specific to his or her sport
- Isokinetic testing to be >85% of the contralateral side (internal/external rotation), pain-free during all sport-specific drills

increase in the number of pitches and velocity. Position players progress to greater distances and positional drills. Tennis players initially practice ground strokes, such as forehands and backhands, progressing to volleys after two to three sessions. Last, the tennis player will advance to overhead serving. Sport-specific activities should be performed a maximum of only two to three times per week, depending on the sport, to allow for full recovery between sessions.

Criteria for returning to sport will vary, depending on the level of the athlete. A general rule is that isokinetic strength should be evaluated. An athlete should have >85% strength (both peak torque and total work) in the involved extremity during a bilateral comparison. In addition, the athlete will have to complete all of the sport-specific drills without pain and be able to meet the specific demands of the particular sport.

The rehabilitation specialist must carefully assess strength and ROM at the start of this phase to determine whether a patient is able to meet the demands of this part of the program.

Troubleshooting

Overaggressive advancement to plyometrics before full ROM and strength are achieved will lead to compensatory motion, poor mechanics, and increase the potential for reinjury. The rehabilitation specialist must carefully limit the volume of exercise to prevent an overuse injury. Although flexibility exercises can be performed daily, strengthening exercises for a specific muscle group should be performed only 3 to 4 days weekly. Sport-specific activities, such as an interval throwing program or overhead tennis serve, may require even longer rest periods (as long as 2 to 3 days rest, depending on patient response).

REFERENCES

1. Neer, C.S. *Anterior Acromioplasty for Chronic Impingement Syndrome in the Shoulder.* J Bone Joint Surg 1972;54A:41–50.
2. Neer, C.S. *Impingement Lesions.* Clin Orthop Relat Res 1983;173:70–77.
3. Wahl, C.J., Warren, R.F., Altchek, D.W. Shoulder Arthroscopy. In Rockwood, C.A., Matsen, F.A., Wirth, M.A., Lippitt, S.B. (Eds). *The Shoulder.* WB Saunders, Philadelphia, 2004, pp. 283–354.
4. Neer, C.S. II. *Anterior Acromioplasty for the Chronic Impingement Syndrome in the Shoulder: A Preliminary Report.* J Bone Joint Surg Am 1972;54:41–50.
5. Ellman, H. *Arthroscopic Subacromial Decompression.* Orthop Trans 1985;9:48.
6. Bunker, T.D. Impingement: Needle, Scope or Scalpel? In Bunker, T.D., Schranz, P.J. (Eds). *Clinical Challenges in Orthopedics: The Shoulder.* Mosby, St. Louis, 1998, p. 62.
7. Gartsman, G.M. Arthroscopy for Shoulder Stiffness. In Miller, M.D., Cole, B.D. (Eds). *Textbook of Arthroscopy.* WB Saunders, Philadelphia, 2004, p. 173.
8. Bigliani, L.U., Morrison, D.S. Subacromial Impingement Syndrome. In Dee, R., Mango, E., Hurst, L.C. (Eds). *Principles of Orthopedic Practice.* McGraw-Hill, New York, 1989, p. 627.
9. Burkhart, S. *Arthroscopic Debridement and Decompression for Selected Rotator Cuff Tears.* Orthop Clin North Am 1993;24:111–124.
10. Brox, J., Gjengedal, E., Uppheim, G., Bohmer, A.S., Brevik, J.I., Ljunggren, A.E., Staff, P.H. *Arthroscopic Surgery Versus Supervised Exercises in Patients with Rotator Cuff Disease (Stage II Impingement Syndrome): A Prospective, Randomized, Controlled Study in 125 Patients with a 2½ Year Follow-up.* J Shoulder Elbow Surg 1999;8:102–111.
11. Ellman, H. *Arthroscopic Subacromial Decompression: Analysis of One- to Three-year Results.* Arthroscopy 1987;3:173–181.
12. Esch, J. *Arthroscopic Subacromial Decompression and Postoperative Management.* Orthop Clin North Am 1993;24:161–171.
13. Beach, W., Caspari, R. *Arthroscopic Management of Rotator Cuff Disease.* Arthroscopy 1993;16:1007–1016.
14. Gleyze, P., Thomas, T., Gazielly, D.F., Bruyere, G., Kelberine, F., Kempf, J.F., Levigne, C., Marcillou, P., Nerot, G. Compared Results of the Different Treatments in Partial-thickness Bursal Side Tears of the Rotator Cuff. A Multi-center Study of 48 Shoulders. In Gazielly, D.F., Gleyze, P., Thomas, T. (Eds). *The Cuff.* Elsevier, Paris, France, 1997, pp. 257–259.
15. Hawkins, R.J., Abrams, J.S., Brock, R.M., Hobeika, P. *Acromioplasty for Impingement with an Intact Rotator Cuff.* J Bone Joint Surg Br 1988;70:795–797.
16. McShane, R.B., Leinberry, C.F., Fenlin, J.M. *Conservative Open Anterior Acromioplasty.* Clin Orthop 1987;223:137–144.
17. Olsewski, J., Depew, A. *Arthroscopic Subacromial Decompression and Rotator Cuff Debridement for Stage II and Stage III Impingement.* Arthroscopy 1994;10:61–68.
18. Paulos, L., Franklin, J. *Arthroscopic Shoulder Decompression Development and Application.* Am J Sports Med 1990;18:235–244.
19. Ryu, R.K. *Arthroscopic Subacromial Decompression: A Clinical Review.* Arthroscopy 1992;8:141–147.
20. Snyder, S.J., Pachelli, A.F., Del Pizzo, W., Friedman, M.J., Ferkel, R.D., Pattee, G. *Partial Thickness Rotator Cuff Tears: Results of Arthroscopic Treatment.* Arthroscopy 1991;7:1–7.
21. Speer, K.P., Lohnes, J., Garrett, W.E. Jr. *Arthroscopic Subacromial Decompression: Results in Advanced Impingement Syndrome.* Arthroscopy 1991;7:291–296.
22. Yamaguchi, K., Flatlow, E. *Arthroscopic Evaluation and Treatment of the Rotator Cuff.* Orthop Clin North Am 1995;26:643–659.
23. Lucas, D. *Biomechanics of the Shoulder Joint.* Arch Surg 1973;107:425.
24. Kapanji, I.A. *The Physiology of the Joints—Upper Limb,* vol 1. Churchill Livingstone, New York, 1970.
25. Weiner, D.S. *Superior Migration of the Humeral Head: A Radiological Aid in the Diagnosis of Tears of the Rotator Cuff.* J Bone Joint Surg 1970;52B:524.
26. Matsen, F.A., Arntz, C. Subacromial Decompression. In Rockwood, C.A., Matsen, F.A. (Eds). *The Shoulder.* WB Saunders, Philadelphia, 1998, pp. 795–833.
27. Kibler, W.B. *Role of the Scapula in the Overhead Throwing Motion.* Contemp Orthop 1991;22:525–533.
28. Kibler, W.B. *The Role of the Scapula in Athletic Shoulder Function.* Am J Sports Med 1998;26:325–336.

29. Ludewig, P.M. *Alterations in Shoulder Kinematics and Associated Muscle Activity in People with Symptoms of Shoulder Impingement.* Phys Ther 2000;80:276–291.

30. Sharkey, N.A. *The Rotator Cuff Opposes Superior Translation of the Humeral Head.* Am J Sports Med 1995;23:270–275.

31. Neer, C.S. *Anterior Acromioplasty for the Chronic Impingement Syndrome in the Shoulder. A Preliminary Report.* J Bone Joint Surg 1972;54A:41.

32. Nielson, K.E., Wester, J.U., Lorentsen, A. *The Shoulder Impingement Syndrome: The Results of Subacromial Decompression.* J Shoulder Elbow Surg 1994;3:12.

33. Speer, K.P., Cavanaugh, J.T., Warren, R.F., Day, L., Wickiewicz, T.L. *A Role for Hydrotherapy in Shoulder Rehabilitation.* Am J Sportsmed 1993;21(6):850–853.

34. Glousman, R., Jobe, F., Tibone, J., Moyner, P., Antonelli, D., Perry, J. *Dynamic Electromyographic Analysis of the Throwing Shoulder with Glenohumeral Instability.* J Bone Joint Surg 1998; 70:220–226.

35. Johnson, T.B. *The Movements of the Shoulder Joint. A Plea for the Use of the "Plane of the Scapula" as the Plane of Reference for Movements Occurring at the Humeri-Scapular Joint.* Br J Surg 1937;25:252–260.

36. Itoi, E., Kuechle, D.K., Newman, S.R. *Stabilizing Function of the Biceps in Stable and Unstable Shoulders.* J Bone Joint Surg 1993;75B:546.

37. Townsend, H., Jobe, F.W., Pink, M., Perry, J. *Electromyographic Analysis of the Glenohumeral Muscles During a Baseball Rehabilitation Program.* Am J Sportsmed 1991;19(3):264–272.

38. Burke, W.S., Vangsness, C.T., Powers, C.M. *Strengthening the Supraspinatus. A Clinical and Biomechanical Review.* Clin Orthop 2002;402:292–298.

39. Sahrmann, S. *Diagnosis and Treatment of Movement Impairment Syndromes.* Mosby, St. Louis, 2002.

40. Janda, V. Muscles, Central Nervous System Regulation and Back Problems. In Korr, I. (Ed). *The Neurobiologic Mechanisms in Spinal Manipulative Therapy.* Plenum Press, New York, 1978, pp. 27–41.

41. Davies, G.J., Dickhoff-Hoffman, S. *Neuromuscular Testing and Rehabilitation of the Shoulder Complex.* J Orthop Sports Phys Ther 1993;23:348.

42. Ellenbecker, T.S., Mattalino, A.J. *Comparison of Open and Closed Kinetic Chain Upper Extremity Tests in Patients with Rotator Cuff Pathology and Glenohumeral Joint Instability.* J Orthop Sports Phys Ther 1997;25(1):84.

43. Knott, M., Voss, D.E. *Proprioceptive Neuromuscular Facilitation.* Harper and Row, New York, 1956, pp. 27–76.

44. Wilk, K.E., Andrews, J. *Rehabilitation Following Arthroscopic Subacromial Decompression.* Orthopedics 1993;16(3):349–358.

45. Duda, M. *Plyometrics: A Legitimate Form of Power Training?* Phys Sportsmed 1988;16:213–218.

46. Wilk, K.E., Reinold, M.M. Specific Exercises for the Throwing Shoulder. In Sumant, K.G., Hawkins, R.J., Warren, R.F. (Eds). *The Shoulder and the Overhead Athlete.* Lippincott Williams & Wilkins, Philadelphia, 2004, pp. 95–121.

47. Pappas, A.M., Zawacki, R., Sullivan, T.J. *Biomechanics of Baseball Pitching: A Preliminary Report.* Am J Sports Med 1985;13: 216–221.

48. Flesig, G.S., Andrews, J.R., Dillman, C.J. *Kinetics of Baseball Pitching with Implications About Injury Mechanisms.* Am J Sports Med 1995;23:233–239.

49. Gainor, B.J., Piotrowski, G., Puhl, J., Allen, W.C., Hagen, R. *The Throw: Biomechanics and Acute Injury.* Am J Sports Med 1980;8:114–118.

50. Ivey, F.K., Calhoun, J.H., Rusche, K., Bierschenk, J. *Normal Values for Isokinetic Testing of Shoulder Strength.* Med Sci Sports Exerc 1984;16:127.

51. Ellenbecker, T.S. *Rehabilitation of Shoulder and Elbow Injuries in Tennis Players.* Clin Sports Med 1995;14(1):87.

52. Cain, P.R., Mutschler, T.A., Fu, F.H., Lee, S.K. *Anterior Stability of the Glenohumeral Joint: A Dynamic Model.* Am J Sports Med 1987;15(2):144.

42

Anterior Stabilization Surgery

MICKEY LEVINSON, PT

The etiology of anterior shoulder instability can be either the result of a traumatic, acute episode resulting in a dislocation that may have to be reduced by a physician or a chronic condition. The recurrence rate for anterior dislocations is extremely high, especially in the younger, active population.[1-4] The mechanism of injury for a traumatic anterior instability is usually some combination of shoulder external rotation, abduction, and extension. Common mechanisms include falling on an outstretched hand or planting a ski pole and falling forward. Instability can also be chronic, resulting from repetitive activities that can cause excessive laxity of the shoulder capsule and/or tearing of the labrum or individual general systemic laxity. Often the result of anterior shoulder instability is a "Bankart lesion," which is defined as an avulsion of the anteroinferior glenoid labrum.[5] Labral pathology and shoulder instability can be treated conservatively but often requires surgical intervention. This chapter will discuss the Hospital for Special Surgery (HSS) guidelines to rehabilitation following an anterior shoulder stabilization.

SURGICAL OVERVIEW

The labrum is a fibrocartilaginous structure that is attached to the glenoid rim (Figure 42-1). There is a great deal of anatomical variation.[6] The glenohumeral ligaments attach to the labrum. The labrum contributes to glenohumeral stability by increasing the surface contact area for the humeral head and provides resistance to humeral head translation.[6] An anterior stabilization may be performed open or arthroscopically. Patients with extreme laxity or who have multidirectional instability may need an open procedure. The most common open procedure performed is done by transecting a portion of the subscapularis muscle. The torn labrum is then repaired, and the capsule is tightened by making a cut through it and overlapping the margins of the cut (Figure 42-2).

In contrast to more traditional open procedures, which have greater morbidity, anterior stabilizations can now be performed arthroscopically. The arthroscopic procedure reduces the morbidity and risk of loss to range of motion (ROM). A Bankart lesion is commonly repaired with transglenoid suture anchors. In addition, any excess laxity in the capsule can be reduced by a similar procedure (Figure 42-3). The degree to which the capsule is shifted is based upon the patient's examination under anesthesia. Following the procedure, the patient's shoulder is placed in an immobilizer in adduction and internal rotation.

REHABILITATION OVERVIEW

The rehabilitation program following an anterior stabilization generally begins 1 to 3 weeks post-surgery. The patient constantly wears the immobilizer, except when performing exercises or bathing. The program

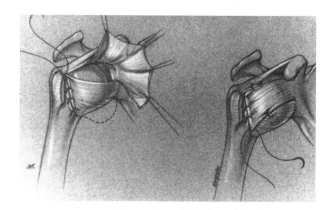

FIGURE **42-2** Open anterior stabilization.

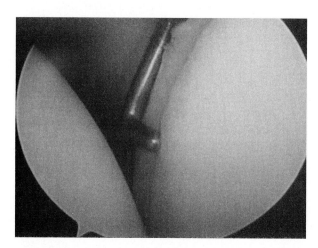

FIGURE **42-1** The labrum is a fibrocartilaginous structure that attaches to the glenoid rim.

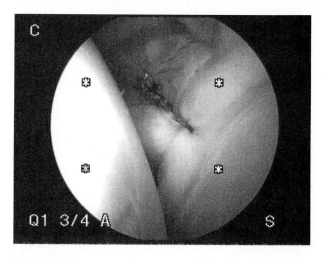

FIGURE **42-3** Arthroscopic anterior stabilization, using suture anchors.

emphasizes early, controlled motion to prevent contractures and avoid excessive passive stretching later in the program. External rotation and extension of the shoulder are progressed slowly to protect the repair of the labrum and avoid excessive stretching of the anterior capsule. Historically, there have been significant failure rates among arthroscopic procedures.[7-10] ROM progression following the arthroscopic procedure is slower than the open procedure secondary to the lesser fixation. Throughout the program a full upper extremity strengthening program will be progressed functionally to prepare the patient for return to activity. The goals are to restore normal strength, ROM, flexibility, and proprioception because loss of proprioception has been demonstrated with shoulder instability.[11-13] The program is based on the patient returning to sport-specific activities no earlier than 3 months post-surgery. Overhead activities are progressed last. Patient education is critical to avoid reinjury. Patients should understand the precautions associated with this surgery.

POSTOPERATIVE PHASE I (WEEKS 1 TO 3)

The primary goal of the first phase of rehabilitation is to gradually restore ROM while protecting the healing structures. The patient is advised to wear the immobilizer at all times, except when performing exercises or bathing. A goal is to minimize the adverse effects of immobilization and lessen the risk of contracture. Motion can stimulate mechanoreceptors that reduce pain and have a positive effect on collagen alignment and articular cartilage.[14-16] The patient is instructed to limit external rotation and extension to neutral to avoid overstressing the repair.

At postoperative weeks 1 to 3 the surgeon will allow passive forward flexion and external rotation ROM of the shoulder. For an arthroscopic procedure, external rotation is limited to neutral. For the open procedure, 30 degrees of external rotation is allowed.

Gripping exercises are initiated to promote circulation, and supported wrist and elbow ROM exercises are used to avoid any contractures caused by the immobilizer.

Based on the principle of proximal stability for functional stability, scapular isometrics are initiated[17] (Figure 42-4). In addition, submaximal, pain-free deltoid isometrics are initiated. It is important that the patient is aware that the amount of tension generated should not increase shoulder pain or inflammation. The patient is instructed in the use of cryotherapy to reduce any postoperative swelling, pain, or inflammation.

Postoperative Phase I (Weeks 1 to 3)

GOALS
- Promote healing: reduce pain, inflammation, and swelling
- Forward flexion to 90 degrees
- Arthroscopic: external rotation to neutral; open: 30 degrees
- Independent home exercise program

PRECAUTIONS
- Immobilizer at all times when not exercising
- External rotation and extension limited to neutral (30 degrees for open)

TREATMENT STRATEGIES
- Immobilizer
- Elbow/wrist active range of motion (AROM)
- Gripping exercises
- Scapular isometrics
- Pain-free, submaximal deltoid isometrics
- Active-assisted range of motion (AAROM): forward flexion (scapular plane)
- AAROM: external rotation to neutral
- Home exercise program
- Modalities as needed

CRITERIA FOR ADVANCEMENT
- External rotation to neutral (30 degrees for open)
- Forward flexion to 90 degrees
- Minimal pain or inflammation

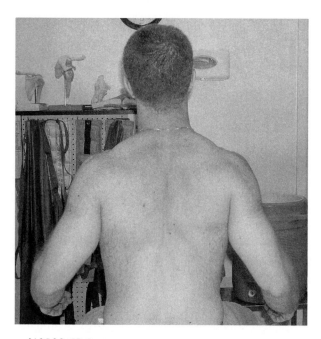

FIGURE **42-4** Isometrics for the scapular musculature.

Troubleshooting

During this phase, the clinician should carefully monitor the patient's ROM to assess whether the patient's motion is progressing too quickly and thus overstressing the repair. Second, especially with open procedures, monitoring the end feel is important to assess whether a possible contracture is developing. Either of these scenarios should be communicated to the surgeon.

The patient should be aware that isometrics for the deltoid should be pain-free and that any inflammation that occurs may slow the progression.

POSTOPERATIVE PHASE II (WEEKS 3 TO 6)

During this phase, the immobilizer will be discharged, and the patient will continue to progress with ROM. Generally, this phase lasts 3 to 4 weeks for the open procedure and 4 to 6 weeks for the arthroscopic. Wand exercises are used for AAROM. When the patient has achieved approximately 110 degrees of flexion in supine, a progression to pulleys is allowed. Patients who have difficulty restoring ROM may benefit from hydrotherapy. The buoyancy of the water is helpful in assisting elevation of the upper extremity.[18] Wand exercises are also used for external rotation. The arthroscopic patients will be allowed 45 degrees of external rotation and the open may progress to 60 degrees. Forward flexion is also progressed, as tolerated.

Scapular strengthening is progressed by performing manual side-lying stabilization exercises, and physio ball stabilization exercises are initiated when tolerated (Figure 42-5). Closed chain exercises, performed with

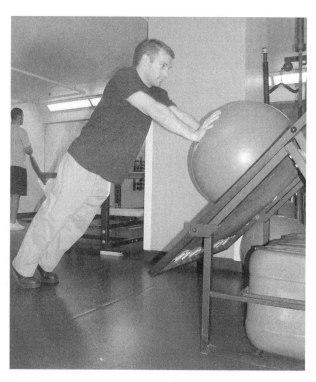

FIGURE **42-5** Physio ball stabilization exercises for closed chain strengthening.

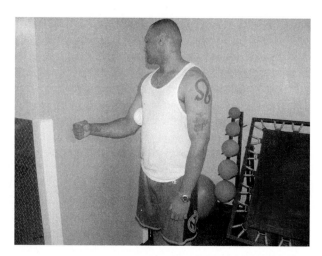

FIGURE **42-6** Submaximal internal and external rotation exercises performed in a modified neutral position.

distal end of the limb fixed, have been shown to promote stability and stimulate proprioception of the joint.[19,20] If the patient demonstrates adequate ROM and is relatively asymptomatic, submaximal internal/external rotation isometrics may be initiated in a modified neutral position (Figure 42-6). By beginning to activate the rotator cuff, the patient begins to restore dynamic stability to prepare the upper extremity for AROM. The patient should be aware that inflammation may result in a reflex inhibition of the rotator cuff.[21]

Postoperative Phase II (Weeks 3 to 6)

GOALS

- Continue to promote healing
- Arthroscopic: external rotation to 45 degrees; forward flexion to 120 degrees
- Open: external rotation to 60 degrees; forward flexion to 145 degrees
- Begin to restore scapula and rotator cuff strength

PRECAUTIONS

- Limit external rotation to 45 degrees (arthroscopic)
- Avoid excessive stretch to anterior capsule
- Avoid rotator cuff inflammation

TREATMENT STRATEGIES

- Discontinue immobilizer (surgeon directed)
- Continue AAROM, forward flexion: wand exercises, pulleys
- Continue AAROM, external rotation: wand exercises
- Hydrotherapy (if required)
- Manual scapula side-lying stabilization exercises
- Physio ball scapular stabilization exercises
- Internal/external rotation isometrics in modified neutral (submaximal, pain-free)
- Modalities as needed
- Modify home exercise program

CRITERIA FOR ADVANCEMENT

- Minimal pain and inflammation
- Arthroscopic: external rotation to 45 degrees; forward flexion to 120 degrees
- Open: external rotation to 60 degrees; forward flexion to 145 degrees
- Internal rotation/external rotation strength 4/5

Troubleshooting

During this phase, the patient's ROM should continue to be monitored carefully. For the open procedures, the clinician should be concerned with a slow progression of motion and continue to monitor the patient's end feel. With the arthroscopic procedures, too rapid a progression is monitored carefully. The patient must continue to be educated regarding the adverse effects of inflammation of the rotator cuff. Isometrics must continue to be pain-free.

POSTOPERATIVE PHASE III (WEEKS 6 TO 12)

During this phase, normal ROM is restored. Forward flexion and external rotation ROM may be progressed to tolerance. Wand exercises and pulleys are continued to be used. The patient begins to restore internal rotation. In addition, general flexibility exercises for the entire upper extremity are initiated. Excessive passive stretching should continue to be avoided.

During this phase, a normal strength base is established. This is a prerequisite for the sport or activity phase. Scapular strengthening is progressed in ranges that continue to protect the anterior capsule and labrum. By restoring normal scapulothoracic function, a stable

base for glenohumeral rotation is established. In addition, the scapular muscles tilt the glenoid in the proper position for maximal congruency with the humeral head. Finally, the proper length–tension relationship of the glenohumeral muscles is maintained.[22,23] Isotonic exercises are initiated to include the trapezius, rhomboids, serratus, and levator scapula. Exercises include rowing, shrugs, and serratus punch. In addition, closed chain exercises, such as wall push-ups with a plus, are incorporated (Figure 42-7).

If strength and ROM are adequate, internal/external rotation strengthening may be progressed to elastic resistance in a neutral position. A towel roll under the arm moves the patient into a position of comfortable abduction, which improves the blood supply to the shoulder.[24] In addition, it positions the arm closer to the plane of the scapula, where there is the optimal length–tension relationship of the glenohumeral muscles.[25]

Latissimus strengthening is initiated, using elastic resistance. The latissimus has been demonstrated to provide a compressive force to the glenohumeral joint, thus promoting stability and reducing the load of the glenohumeral muscles.[26] Initially, strengthening is limited to 90 degrees of flexion and not extended

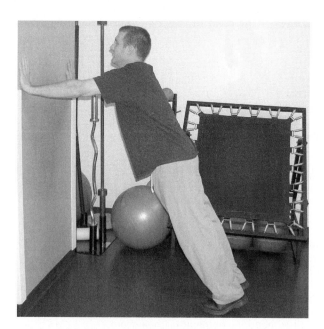

FIGURE 42-7 Wall push-ups with a plus. Exaggerated protraction emphasizes the serratus anterior.

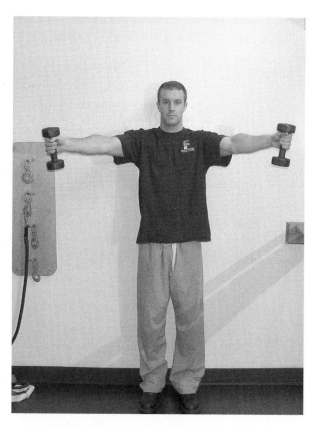

FIGURE 42-8 Scapular plane elevation performed in external rotation to avoid shoulder impingement.

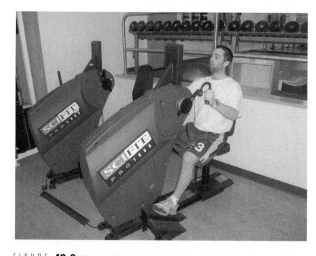

FIGURE 42-9 Upper body ergometry for endurance training.

beyond neutral to avoid stretching of the anterior capsule and labrum. As strength improves, the patient is progressed to the overhead position.

If the strength of the rotator cuff and scapula are adequate, active forward flexion is initiated in the scapular plane. Emphasis is placed on restoring normal glenohumeral rhythm. The scapular plane is used because it provides the greatest joint conformity and thus the least amount of capsular stress.[27] These exercises are performed with the thumb up to minimize the chance of rotator cuff impingement (Figure 42-8).

As this phase progresses, functional demands must be met. Eccentric strengthening should be emphasized because electromyographic (EMG) studies have demonstrated a great deal of eccentric muscle activity in certain sports.[28–30]

When strength and ROM are adequate, proprioceptive training is advanced. Neuromuscular exercises, such as rhythmic stabilization, are initiated. These are initiated in the scapular plane where stress to the capsule is minimized.[27] With adequate strength and ROM, proprioceptive neuromuscular patterns are initiated. In particular, the D2 flexion pattern emphasizes the musculature that is used in many overhead activities.[17]

It has been demonstrated that proprioception is compromised with fatigue.[31] Endurance training is incorporated into the program during this phase. As the patient progresses, neuromuscular drills are performed to fatigue. Upper body ergometry is used to restore endurance (Figure 42-9).

Isokinetic training is incorporated into the program to enable training at higher speeds and further build endurance. Following a training regime, isokinetic testing will provide an objective assessment, especially for rotator cuff strength, which plays an integral role in the stability of the glenohumeral joint. In addition, it provides specificity with regard to testing at faster and more functional speeds.[32]

Postoperative Phase III (Weeks 6 to 12)

GOALS

- Restore full shoulder ROM
- Restore normal scapulohumeral rhythm
- Upper extremity strength 5/5
- Restore normal flexibility
- Begin to restore upper extremity endurance
- Isokinetic internal/external rotation strength 85% of unaffected side

PRECAUTIONS

- Avoid rotator cuff inflammation
- Continue to protect anterior capsule
- Avoid excessive passive stretching

TREATMENT STRATEGIES

- Continue AAROM for forward flexion and external rotation to tolerance
- Begin AAROM for internal rotation
- Progress scapular strengthening (include closed chain exercises)
- Begin isotonic internal rotation/external rotation strengthening in modified neutral (pain-free)
- Begin latissimus strengthening (progress as tolerated)
- Begin scapular plane elevation (emphasis on correct scapulohumeral rhythm)
- Begin upper body ergometry to restore endurance
- Begin humeral head stabilization exercises (if adequate strength and ROM)
- Begin PNF patterns if internal/external rotation strength is 5/5
- Begin general upper extremity flexibility exercises
- Isokinetic training and testing
- Modalities as needed
- Modify home exercise program

CRITERIA FOR ADVANCEMENT

- Normal scapulohumeral rhythm
- Minimal pain and inflammation
- internal/external rotation strength 5/5
- Full upper extremity ROM
- Isokinetic internal rotation strength 85% of unaffected side

Troubleshooting

During this phase, the clinician continues to carefully monitor that the patient is not developing excessive inflammation that may result in a capsular contraction and reflex inhibition of the rotator cuff.[21] In such cases, the surgeon should be notified. Certain mobilization techniques may be indicated. Scapulohumeral rhythm is also monitored to avoid any development of abnormal movement patterns. The patient continues to be educated to avoid activities that evoke excessive pain and inflammation. Aggressive strengthening does not mean painful strengthening. In addition, flexibility exercises should not be performed in painful ranges. Patients often have the tendency to "overstretch." The clinician must also monitor that the patient has adequate strength and ROM to perform an exercise, such as a PNF pattern. This will avoid developing any muscular substitution or abnormal movement pattern.

POSTOPERATIVE PHASE IV (WEEKS 12 TO 18)

This is the transitional phase that prepares the patient for return to sport or other functional activities. During this phase, the demands of the functional activity are met and normal neuromuscular function is restored. For example, if the patient is returning to any overhead activities, internal/external rotation strengthening is advanced to the abducted "90/90" position. When the patient enters this phase, he or she must exhibit normal strength, adequate ROM, flexibility, and endurance. An isokinetic test will provide some objective data regarding strength. The patient's internal and external rotation strength should be at least 85% of the unaffected side. The patient must be pain-free. If these criteria are met, if required, an activity-specific plyometric program is initiated. The plyometric program should be functionally specific to the demands of the patient. Voight and Draovitch[33] advocate stressing the quality of the exercise and using a program that is progressive in overload. Exercises are progressed by increasing the challenge to the shoulder. In addition, the demands of the trunk and lower extremities should be met (Figures 46-10 and 46-11).

After being cleared by the surgeon, the patient may begin a sport or activity-specific program, if the patient has completed a plyometrics program without symptoms. These programs range from sport-specific activities, such as interval throwing and tennis programs, to work-hardening activities. Regardless, the program is designed to be progressed individually so as to minimize the risk of reinjury. Proper mechanics of the activity are emphasized. As the patient completes an individual program, return to the desired sport or activity is allowed.

During this phase, patients are also encouraged to maintain a strengthening and flexibility program and incorporate it into their normal exercise routine. The functional activity may result in a loss of strength and flexibility, thus resulting in reinjury. Upon discharge, internal/external rotation isokinetic strength should be at least equal to the unaffected side. In addition, an external rotation to internal rotation strength ratio of 66% has been demonstrated in the normal population.[34,35] This criteria should also be met.

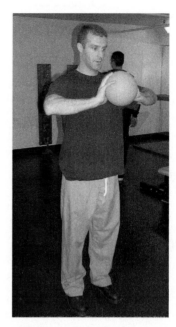

FIGURE **42-10** Plyometric chest pass exercise.

Postoperative Phase IV (Weeks 12 to 18)

GOALS
- Restore normal neuromuscular function
- Maintain strength and flexibility
- Isokinetic internal/external rotation strength at least equal to the unaffected side
- >66% Isokinetic external rotation/internal rotation strength ratio
- Prevent reinjury

PRECAUTIONS
- Pain-free plyometrics
- Significant pain with a specific activity
- Feeling of instability

TREATMENT STRATEGIES
- Continue full upper extremity strengthening program
- Advance internal rotation/external rotation strengthening to 90/90 position if required
- Continue upper extremity flexibility exercises
- Isokinetic strengthening and testing
- Activity-specific plyometrics program
- Address trunk and lower extremity demands
- Continue endurance training
- Begin sport or activity-related program
- Modify home exercise program

CRITERIA FOR DISCHARGE
- Pain-free sport or activity-specific program
- Isokinetic internal/external rotation strength to at least equal to unaffected side
- >66% Isokinetic external rotation/internal rotation strength ratio
- Independent home exercise program
- Independent sport or activity-specific program

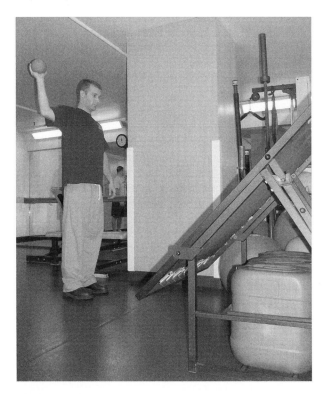

FIGURE **42-11** Plyometric exercise. More challenging overhead position.

Troubleshooting

Plyometric exercises must be monitored carefully, and the volume of work must be controlled. Any symptoms during or after these exercises may indicate that the patient is not prepared for them. Any symptoms should be reported to the surgeon. If the patient is unable to correctly perform a certain exercise and without symptoms, progression to the next level should not occur.

Any significant symptoms (sharp pain, instability) during the specific activity should be reported to the surgeon. However, the patient should be aware that muscle soreness is not uncommon as the activity level increases, and, at times, the program may have to be interrupted until symptoms have subsided. The patient is advised to continue the use of cryotherapy on a consistent basis. Occasionally, the patient may need to return to the previous phase of the program.

Although the volume of strengthening may be reduced during this phase, the patient should be educated as to the importance of maintaining strength and flexibility. Many sport or functional activities can result in selective strength and flexibility deficits that can result in injury. A common finding is that overhead athletes tend to lose flexibility of their posterior capsule and posterior rotator cuff. Harryman et al.[36] demonstrated that posterior tightness increases anterior and superior humeral head migration, thus leading to pathology,

such as a rotator cuff impingement. Patient education upon discharge is critical to avoiding reinjury or additional pathology.

REFERENCES

1. Hovelius, L. *Shoulder Dislocation in Swedish Hockey Players.* Am J Sports Med 1978;6:373–377.
2. Hovelius, L. *Recurrences after Initial Dislocation of the Shoulder.* J Bone Joint Surg 1983;65:343–349.
3. Hovelius, L. *Anterior Dislocation of the Shoulder in Teenagers and Young Adults.* J Bone Joint Surg 1987;69:393.
4. Rowe, C.R. *Acute and Recurrent Anterior Dislocation of the Shoulder.* Orthop Clin North Am 1980;11:252–269.
5. Bankart, A. *The Pathology and Treatment of Recurrent Dislocation of the Shoulder Joint.* Br J Surg 1938;26:23.
6. Levine, W.M. *The Pathophysiology of Shoulder Instability.* Am J Sports Med 2000;28:910–917.
7. Arciero, R.A., Taylor, D., Snyder, R.J., Uhorchak, J.M. *Arthroscopic Bioabsorbable Tack Stabilization of Initial Anterior Dislocations: A Preliminary Report.* Arthroscopy 1995;11:410–417.
8. Bacilla, P., Field, L.D., Savoie, F.H. *Arthroscopic Bankart Repair in a High Demand Population.* Arthroscopy 1997;13:51–60.
9. Burger, R.S., Shengel, D., Bonatus, T., Lewis, J. *Arthroscopic Staple Capsulorrhaphy for Recurrent Shoulder Instability.* Orthop Trans 1990;14:596–597.
10. Coughlin, L., Rubinovich, M., Johansson, A. *Arthroscopic Staple Capsulorrhaphy for Anterior Shoulder Instability.* Am J Sports Med 1992;20:253–256.
11. Lephart, S., Warner, J.P., Borsa, P.A., Fu, F.H. *Proprioception of the Shoulder Joint in Healthy, Unstable and Surgically Repaired Shoulders.* J Shoulder Elbow Surg 1994;3:371–380.
12. Smith, R.H., Brunolti, J. *Shoulder Kinesthesia after Anterior Glenohumeral Joint Dislocation.* Phys Ther 1989;69:106–112.
13. Zuckerman, J.D., Gallagher, M.D., Cuomo, F., Rokito, A. *The Effect of Instability and Subsequent Anterior Shoulder Repair on Proprioceptive Ability.* J Shoulder Elbow Surg 1997;6:180–186.
14. Wyke, B. *The Neurology of Joints.* Ann R Coll Surg Engl 1966;41:25.
15. Frank, C., Akeson, W.H., Woo, S.L., Amiel, D., Coutts, R.D. *Physiology and Therapeutic Value of Passive Joint Motion.* Clin Orthop 1983;185:113.
16. Salter, R., Simmonds, D., Malcom, B. *The Biologic Effects on Continuous Passive Motion on the Healing of Full Thickness Articular Cartilage Defects.* J Bone Joint Surg 1980;61A:1231–1251.
17. Knott, M., Voss, D. *Proprioceptive Neuromuscular Facilitation.* Harper and Row, New York, 1968.
18. Speer, K.P., Cavanaugh, J.T., Warren, R.F., Day, L., Wickiewicz, T.L. *A Role for Hydrotherapy in Shoulder Rehabilitation.* Am J Sports Med 1993;21:850–853.
19. Wilk, K.E., Arrigo, C., Andrews, J.R. *Closed and Open Chain Kinetic Exercise for the Upper Extremity.* J Sports Rehabil 1996;5:88–102.
20. Tippett, S. *Closed Chain Exercise.* Orthop Phys Ther Clin North Am 1992;1:253–268.
21. Timm, K. *The Isokinetic Torque Curve of Shoulder Instability in High School Baseball Pitchers.* J Orthop Sports Phys 1998;26:150–154.
22. Kibler, W.B. *Role of the Scapula in the Overhead Throwing Motion.* Contemp Orthop 1991;22:525–533.
23. Kibler, W.B. *The Role of the Scapula in Athletic Shoulder Function.* Am J Sports Med 1998;26:325–336.

24. Rathburn, J., MacNab, I. *The Microvasculature Pattern of the Rotator Cuff.* J Bone Joint Surg 1970;52B:540–553.

25. Saha, K. *Mechanism of Shoulder Movements and Plea for Recognition of the "Zero Position" of the Glenohumeral Joint.* Clin Orthop 1983;173:3–10.

26. Bassett, R., Browne, A., Morrey, B., An K.H. *Glenohumeral Muscle Force and Movement Mechanics in a Position of Shoulder Instability.* J Biomech 1988;23:401–415.

27. Johnson, T.B. *The Movements of the Shoulder Joint. A Plea for the Use of the "Plane of the Scapula" as the Plane of Reference for Movements Occurring at the Humeri-scapular Joint.* Br J Surg 1937;25:252–260.

28. Ryu, R.K., McCormick, J., Jobe, F.W. *An EMG Analysis of Shoulder Function in Tennis Players.* Am J Sports Med 1988;16:481–488.

29. Glousman, R., Jobe, F.W. *Dynamic Electromyographic Analysis of the Throwing Shoulder with Glenohumeral Instability.* J Bone Joint Surg 1988;70:220–226.

30. DiGiovine, N.M., Jobe, F.W., Pink, M. *An Electromyographic Analysis of the Upper Extremity in Pitching.* J Shoulder Elbow Surg 1992;1:15–25.

31. Carpenter, J.E., Blaiser, R.B., Pellizzon, G.G. *The Effects of Muscle Fatigue on Shoulder Joint Position Sense.* Am J Sports Med 1998;26:262–265.

32. Davies, G.J., Wilk, K.E., Ellenbecker, T.S. *Orthopedic and Sports Physical Therapy: Strength Assessment,* 3rd ed. Mosby, St. Louis, 1997.

33. Voight, M., Draovitch, P. *Eccentric Muscle Training in Sports and Orthopedics: Plyometric Training.* Churchill Livingstone, New York, 1991.

34. Ivey, F.M., Calhoun, J.H., Rusche, K., Bierschenk, J. *Normal Values for Isokinetic Testing of Shoulder Strength.* Med Sci Sports Exerc 1984;16:127.

35. Davies, G.J. *A Compendium of Isokinetics in Clinical Usage and Rehabilitation Techniques,* 4th ed. Simon & Schuster, LaCrosse, WI, 1992.

36. Harryman, D.T. II, Sidles, J.A., Clark, J.M., McQuade, K.J., Gibb, T.D., Matsen, F.A. III. *Translation of the Humeral Head on the Glenoid with Passive Glenohumeral Motion.* J Bone Joint Surg Am 1990;72(9):1334–1343.

43

Posterior Stabilization
Surgery

MICKEY LEVINSON, PT

Posterior shoulder instability is much less common than anterior instability. Incidence has been reported at 2% to 4% of all shoulder instability patients.[1,2] It has also been suggested that posterior instability may be related to multidirectional instability.[3] Pathological posterior translation of the humeral head may result in pain, instability, or detachment of the posterior and inferior capsulolabral complex.[4] The mechanism of injury varies; however, traumatic, acute dislocations are rare and usually result from a high energy posterior force to an outstretched arm or from a seizure.[3] More commonly, injury results from recurrent subluxations that occur with the shoulder in a forward flexed, adducted, and internally rotated position. Contact athletes, such as football linemen, who are subjected to posteriorly directed forces in this position, are often injured in this manner. In addition, activities such as bench pressing may exacerbate these symptoms.[5] Injury may also occur nontraumatically in overhead athletes, such as baseball pitchers or tennis players during the "follow through" phase of throwing, when the shoulder is horizontally adducted and internally rotated.[6] Labral pathology and shoulder instability can be treated conservatively but often requires surgical intervention. In this chapter, the Hospital for Special Surgery (HSS) rehabilitation guideline following posterior shoulder stabilization is presented.

ANATOMICAL OVERVIEW

The labrum is a fibrocartilaginous structure that, along with the glenohumeral ligaments, attaches to the glenoid.[7] It contributes to glenohumeral stability by increasing the contact area for the humeral head and provides resistance to humeral head translation.[7] The posterior capsulolabral complex is often detached with posterior instability.[3,4] At HSS, the posterior stabilization is done exclusively arthroscopically. An examination under anesthesia is performed to accurately determine the amount of capsular laxity. The posterior capsulolabral complex is then reattached to the glenoid labrum through an arthroscope, using either suture anchors or biodegradable tacks. At this time, any capsular redundancy is eliminated by placation and applying tension to the sutures[3,4] (Figure 43-1). Following surgery, the patient is immobilized for approximately 4 weeks and positioned in the scapular plane in neutral rotation.

REHABILITATION OVERVIEW

The rehabilitation program following a posterior stabilization generally begins 2 to 4 weeks post-surgery. The patient is protected with an immobilizer during the early phase of the program. The program emphasizes early, controlled motion so as to avoid contracture and need for excessive passive stretching later in the program. Internal rotation and horizontal adduction are

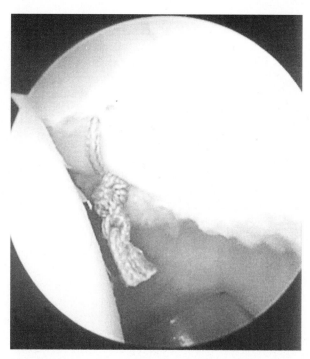

FIGURE **43-1** Posterior stabilization, using suture anchors to repair the labrum and eliminate capsular redundancy.

avoided during the early phases of the program and then progressed cautiously so as to avoid excessive stress to the posterior capsule. The reduced morbidity of the arthroscopic procedure should reduce the risk of range of motion (ROM) loss. Throughout the program a full upper extremity strengthening program will be progressed appropriately to prepare the patient for return to functional activity. However, particular emphasis will be placed on the posterior glenohumeral and scapular musculature to further assist in protecting the posterior capsulolabral complex. The goals are to restore normal strength, ROM, flexibility, and proprioception. The program is based on the patient returning to sport-specific activities no earlier than 16 weeks post-surgery, with contact sports and overhead activities progressed last. Patient education is critical to avoiding reinjury and adversely affecting the surgical procedure.

POSTOPERATIVE REHABILITATION

POSTOPERATIVE PHASE I (WEEKS 2 TO 4)

The emphasis of the first phase of the program is on beginning to gradually restore ROM while protecting the healing structures. The patient wears the immobilizer at all times, except when performing exercises or bathing. The goal is to minimize the adverse effects of immobilization and use the positive effects of early, controlled ROM, such as reducing pain, improving collagen alignment, and nourishing articular cartilage.[8-12]

Active-assisted range of motion (AAROM) is initiated for external rotation and forward flexion during this phase. Forward flexion is performed in the scapular plane (Figure 43-2). The scapular plane is used because it provides the most joint conformity and least capsular stress.[13,14] Motion should be relatively pain-free. Horizontal adduction and internal rotation are limited to neutral to avoid putting undue stress on the posterior capsule.

Gripping exercises and supported wrist and elbow ROM are initiated to promote circulation and avoid any contractures that may be caused by the immobilization.

Scapular isometrics and side-lying scapular stabilization exercises may be initiated to begin to establish a proximal strength base and improve patient posture. At 3 to 4 weeks postoperatively, submaximal deltoid and internal/external rotation isometrics may be initiated, if symptoms allow. It is important that the patient is aware that the amount of tension generated should not increase pain. The patient is instructed in the use of cryotherapy to reduce any postoperative pain or inflammation.

Troubleshooting

During this phase, the clinician should monitor the patient's pain and inflammation when performing iso-

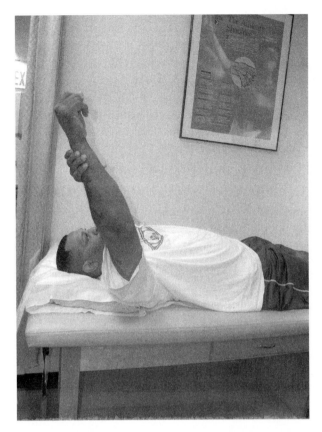

FIGURE 43-2 AAROM is initiated in the scapular plane.

Postoperative Phase I (Weeks 2 to 4)

GOALS
- Promote healing: reduce pain, inflammation, and swelling
- Restore ROM: forward flexion to 90 degrees, external rotation to 30 degrees
- Begin to regain humeral head and scapular control
- Independent home exercise program

PRECAUTIONS
- Immobilizer at all times when not exercising
- Internal rotation and horizontal adduction limited to neutral

TREATMENT STRATEGIES
- Immobilizer
- Elbow/wrist active range of motion (AROM)
- Gripping exercises
- Scapular isometrics
- AAROM for forward flexion
- AAROM for external rotation
- Manual side-lying, scapular stabilization exercises
- Pain-free, submaximal deltoid isometrics (3 to 4 weeks)
- Pain-free, submaximal internal/external rotation isometrics (3 to 4 weeks)
- Modalities as needed
- Home exercise program

CRITERIA FOR ADVANCEMENT
- External rotation to 30 degrees
- Minimal pain or inflammation

metric exercises and educate the patient, as to avoid performing them too vigorously. The patient should be educated that too strenuous exercise may prevent progression to the next phase.

The clinician should also be monitoring the patient's "end feel" to assess whether a possible contracture is developing. Any concern of this should be communicated to the surgeon. Patient compliance regarding the immobilizer and the home program should be monitored carefully.

POSTOPERATIVE PHASE II (WEEKS 4 TO 6)

During this phase, the immobilizer will be discharged, and the patient may continue to progress external rotation and forward flexion, as tolerated, within relatively pain-free guidelines. When performing ROM, internal rotation is limited to 45 degrees. Hydrotherapy may be used for patients who are having difficulty restoring ROM. The buoyancy of the water is helpful with upper extremity elevation.[15]

Scapular strengthening may be progressed to establish proximal stability for later phases of program. Exercises should continue to be performed in ranges that avoid stress to the posterior capsule. Horizontal adduc-

tion is limited to neutral. Isometrics for the rotator cuff and deltoid should be continued to restore dynamic stability and prepare the upper extremity for AROM. In contrast to anterior stabilization principles, closed chain exercises, performed with the distal end of the limb fixed, may stress the posterior capsule and should be modified.[16] During the early phases, any closed chain exercises should be performed in the plane of the scapula to maximize the congruency of the glenohumeral joint. Positioning the shoulder in abduction and external rotation will also reduce the load to the posterior capsule (Figure 43-3).

Troubleshooting

During this phase, the clinician should continue to monitor carefully the patient's ROM and "end feel" to make sure a contracture is not developing. On the other hand, one should be concerned that the patient's motion is not progressing too rapidly. Either scenario should be communicated to the surgeon. Excessive inflammation should also be monitored. In this case, a reflex inhibition of the rotator cuff may occur, and exercises may have to be reduced.[17]

Postoperative Phase II (Weeks 4 to 6)

GOALS
- Continue to promote healing
- Forward flexion to 90 degrees
- Internal rotation to 45 degrees
- Begin to restore strength internal/external rotation to 4/5

PRECAUTIONS
- Internal rotation limited to 45 degrees
- Horizontal adduction limited to neutral
- Protect posterior capsule
- Avoid rotator cuff inflammation

TREATMENT STRATEGIES
- Discontinue immobilizer
- Continue AAROM for external rotation
- Continue AAROM for forward flexion
- Hydrotherapy
- Continue deltoid and internal/external rotation isometrics
- Progress scapular strengthening protecting posterior capsule (modify closed chain exercises)
- Modalities as needed
- Modify home exercise program

CRITERIA FOR ADVANCEMENT
- Minimal pain and inflammation
- Forward flexion to 90 degrees
- internal/external rotation strength, 4/5

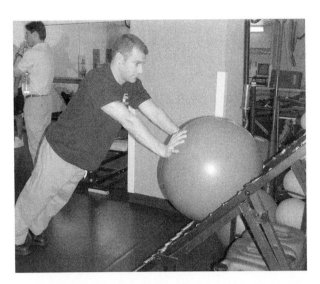

FIGURE **43-3** Closed chain exercises are performed in the scapular plane to maximize the congruency of the glenohumeral joint. Positioning the shoulder in abduction and external rotation also reduces the load to the posterior capsule.

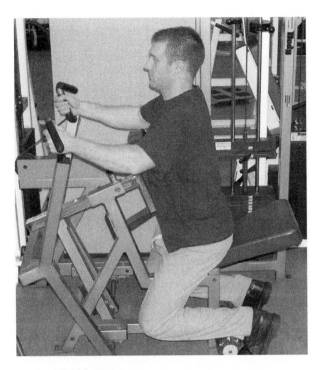

FIGURE **43-4** Rowing for scapular retraction.

POSTOPERATIVE PHASE III (WEEKS 6 TO 12)

The patient continues to progress external rotation and forward flexion ROM to tolerance in this phase. Wand exercises and pulleys are used. Internal rotation may be progressed, as tolerated. General upper extremity flexibility exercises are begun. Full ROM should be restored by the end of this phase. Excessive passive stretching should continue to be avoided. This phase should also be used to establish a normal strength base to prepare for the next phase—functional activity phase.

Scapular strengthening is progressed. Restoring normal scapulothoracic function provides a stable base for glenohumeral motion, tilts the glenoid in the proper position for humeral head congruency, and allows the proper length–tension relationship of the glenohumeral muscles.[18,19]

Isotonic exercises are initiated to include the rhomboids, serratus, trapezius, and levator scapula. Exercises include rowing (scapular retraction), shrugs (scapular elevation), and serratus punch (scapular protraction) (Figures 43-4 through 43-6).

Internal/external rotation strengthening is progressed to elastic resistance in a modified neutral position with a towel roll under the arm for a position of comfortable abduction, which improves the blood supply to the shoulder[20] (Figure 43-7).

If the strength of the rotator cuff and scapula is adequate, active forward flexion is initiated in the plane of the scapula (Figure 43-8). This exercise is performed in external rotation so as to minimize the chance of subacromial impingement. Emphasis is placed on restoring

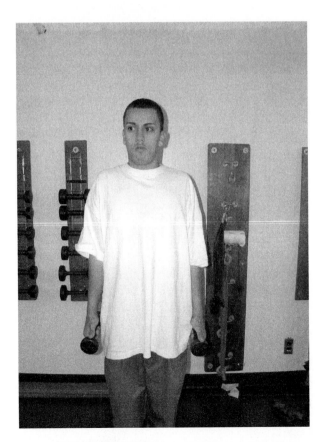

FIGURE **43-5** Shrugs for scapular elevation.

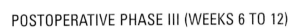

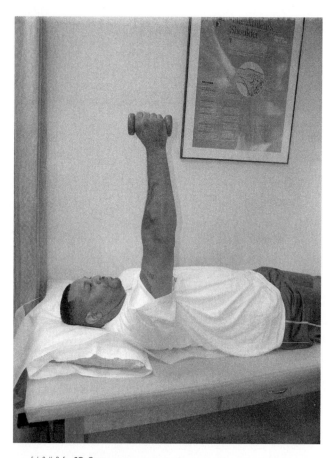

FIGURE 43-6 Serratus punch for scapular protraction.

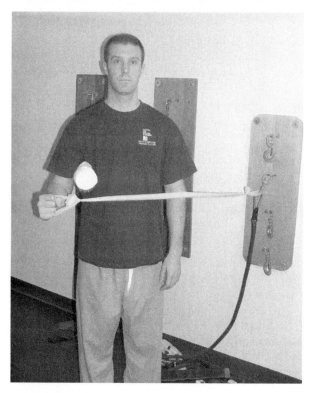

FIGURE 43-7 A towel roll is used for internal/external rotation strengthening to place the shoulder in comfortable abduction.

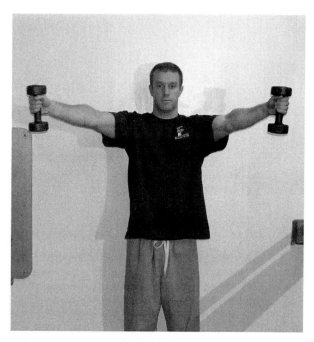

FIGURE 43-8 Forward flexion is performed in the scapular plane, where there is the optimal length tension relationship for the glenohumeral muscles.

normal glenohumeral rhythm. The plane of the scapula is used because it provides the optimal length–tension relationship for the glenohumeral muscles.[13]

Latissimus strengthening is initiated during this phase. Aside from being a core muscle group and an accelerator of the shoulder, the latissimus has also been demonstrated to provide a compressive force to the glenohumeral joint, thus reducing the load on the rotator cuff during many high level activities.[21,22] This should be initiated in a protective arc (0 to 90 degrees) to avoid overstressing the rotator cuff (Figure 43-9).

As the patient's strength improves, proprioceptive training is incorporated. Loss of proprioception with shoulder instability and surgery has been well documented.[23–25] If the rotator cuff strength is adequate, humeral head control drills, such as rhythmic stabilization, are initiated (Figure 43-10). These drills are functionally progressed to more challenging positions. With a good strength base, proprioceptive neuromuscular facilitation patterns are initiated. In particular, the D2 flexion pattern emphasizes a good deal of the posterior musculature that is critical after this surgery[26] (Figure 43-11). Fatigue has also been demonstrated to play a role in loss of proprioception.[27] Endurance training, such as upper body ergometry, is also incorporated into the program. Isokinetic training may be incorporated into this phase to train the shoulder, especially the rotator cuff, for speed and endurance. In addition, isokinetic testing will provide an objective assessment for progression to more functional activities.

Postoperative Phase III (Weeks 6 to 12)

GOALS

- Restore full ROM
- Upper extremity strength 5/5
- Restore normal scapulohumeral rhythm throughout ROM
- Restore normal upper extremity flexibility
- Isokinetic internal/external rotation, strength 85% of unaffected side

PRECAUTIONS

- Avoid rotator cuff inflammation
- Continue to protect posterior capsule
- Avoid excessive passive stretching

TREATMENT STRATEGIES

- Continue AAROM for external rotation and forward flexion
- Begin AAROM for internal rotation
- Continue progressive scapular strengthening program, protecting posterior capsule (avoid or modify closed chain exercises)
- Begin internal/external rotation isotonics in modified neutral
- Begin latissimus strengthening
- Begin scapular plane elevation, if scapula and cuff strength is adequate
- Begin humeral head stabilization exercises, if strength is adequate
- Begin PNF patterns, if internal/external rotation is 5/5
- Begin upper extremity flexibility exercises
- Begin upper body ergometry
- Isokinetic training and testing
- Modalities as needed
- Modify home exercise program

CRITERIA FOR ADVANCEMENT

- Pain-free
- Full shoulder ROM
- Normal glenohumeral rhythm
- Normal upper extremity flexibility
- Upper extremity strength 5/5
- Isokinetic internal/external rotation, strength 85% of unaffected side

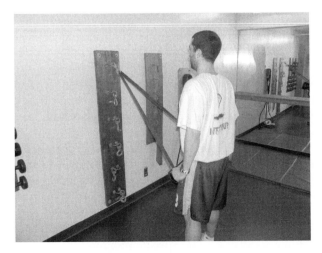

FIGURE **43-9** Latissimus strengthening is initiated in a protective arc (0 to 90 degrees).

Troubleshooting

In phase III, the clinician should continue to monitor the ROM progress to reduce the risk of a contracture. In the event that this is suspected, the surgeon should be notified and a decision will be made as to incorporate any more aggressive treatment, such as passive stretching, soft tissue techniques, and mobilization techniques. This will be based on the clinician's evaluation. For example, if the patient is having difficulty restoring forward flexion, it may be an indication that the inferior capsule has become contracted.[28] In this scenario, inferior glides of the humeral head may be introduced.

As the patient begins to perform scapular plane elevation, the clinician should monitor the patient's scapulothoracic function and scapulohumeral rhythm. If the patient does not have adequate scapular or rotator cuff strength, he or she can develop abnormal movement patterns and increased pain. In this case, the patient should not be progressed functionally. Active elevation

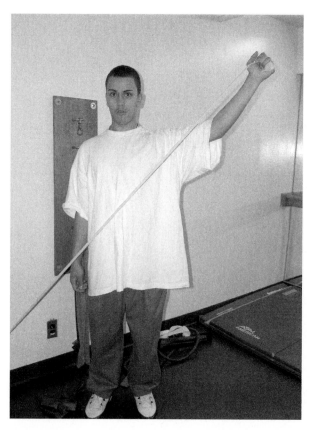

FIGURE **43-10** PNF D2 flexion pattern emphasizes a great deal of the posterior muscles.

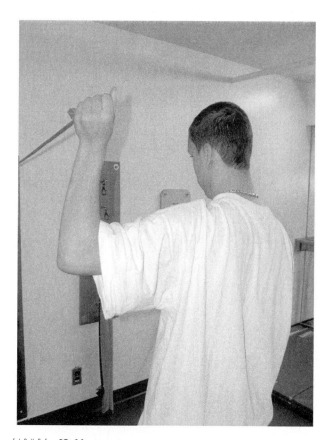

FIGURE **43-11** The 90/90 position is used for rotator cuff strengthening for overhead athletes.

should be avoided until adequate strength has been achieved. Excessive scapular "winging" or scapular substitution for scapulohumeral motion are prime examples.

When restoring flexibility, some patients have a tendency to stretch too aggressively. This should be monitored carefully. Patients must be educated on the risks of stretching into painful ranges, which can cause inflammation and muscle guarding that will prevent rehabilitative progression. Patients who experience inflammation will need to have their exercise program modified or held until their symptoms subside.

POSTOPERATIVE PHASE IV (WEEKS 12 TO 18)

Phase IV is the transitional phase that prepares the patient for return to sport or other functional activities. This phase is guided by the patient's functional demands. These demands should be reproduced, and normal neuromuscular function should be restored. For the athletic population, eccentric strengthening should be emphasized because it has been demonstrated to play a significant role in athletic activities, such as throwing and tennis.[29,30]

For the patient who will be performing overhead activities, rotator cuff strengthening is progressed to the 90/90 position (Figure 43-12). The patient should have 5/5 upper extremity strength and normal ROM. In addition, the patient should attain isokinetic internal and external rotation strength of at least 85% of the unaffected side.

If these criteria are met and the patient is pain-free, a functionally specific plyometric program may be initiated. A plyometric exercise program should be used only if it meets the functionally specific demands of the patient; quality of the plyometric exercise is stressed, and the program should be progressive in overload. For example, a patient is progressed from a two-hand chest pass to a two-hand overhead pass (Figure 43-13).

Endurance training is also progressed during this phase as neuromuscular drills are performed to fatigue. In addition, if the activity requires, the clinician must also be sure that trunk and lower extremity strengthening exercises are addressed.

After examination by the surgeon, the patient may begin a sport or activity-specific program. If indicated, the patient should have completed a plyometric program without symptoms. The functional program should be designed to be progressed individually so as to minimize the risk of reinjury. Proper mechanics of an

Postoperative Phase IV (Weeks 12 to 18)

GOALS

- Restore normal neuromuscular function
- Prevent reinjury
- Maintain strength and flexibility
- Isokinetic internal/external rotation strength at least equal to unaffected side
- >66% Isokinetic internal/external rotation ratio

PRECAUTIONS

- Plyometrics should be pain-free
- Significant pain with specific activity
- Feeling of instability
- Avoid loss of strength and instability
- Avoid overtraining

TREATMENT STRATEGIES

- Continue full upper extremity strengthening (emphasize eccentrics)
- Continue upper extremity flexibility exercises
- Advance internal/external rotation strengthening to the 90/90 position (if required)
- Isokinetic training and testing
- Continue endurance training
- Begin activity-specific plyometric program
- Address trunk and lower extremities as required
- Begin sport or activity-specific program
- Modify home exercise program
- Modalities as needed

CRITERIA FOR DISCHARGE

- Isokinetic internal/external rotation strength at least equal to unaffected side
- Pain-free
- Independent home exercise program
- Independent sport or activity-specific program

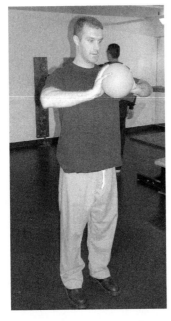

FIGURE **43-12** Plyometrics are initiated with a two-hand chest pass.

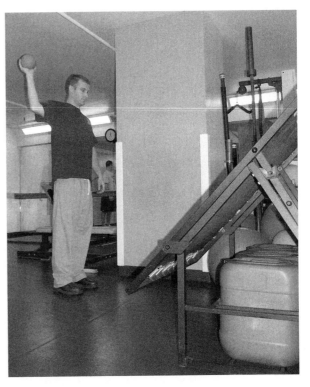

FIGURE **43-13** Plyometrics are progressed functionally to the overhead position.

activity should be emphasized. As the patient completes the functional program, he or she may return to the desired activity. During this phase, patients are encouraged to maintain a strengthening and flexibility program. This program can be incorporated into their normal exercise routine. Before discharge, an isokinetic test is again performed. At this point, internal and external rotation strength should at least equal the unaffected side. Finally, an external rotation to internal rotation ratio of 66% has been established.[31,32]

Troubleshooting

Obviously, any significant symptoms, such as pain or a feeling of instability, should be noted and the referring surgeon notified. However, the patient should be aware that muscle soreness is not uncommon as more functional activities are progressed. At times, a patient may have to decrease or interrupt a specific program until pain and inflammation have subsided. Patients are encouraged to continue the use of cryotherapy throughout their return to functional activity.

Patients must be made aware that sport or functional specific programs may result in selective strength and flexibility deficits. Although the volume of exercise may be reduced toward the end of this phase, the patient must maintain a program for strength and flexibility.

REFERENCES

1. Boyd, H.B., Sisk, T.D. *Recurrent Posterior Dislocation of the Shoulder.* J Bone Joint Surg 1972;54A:779–785.
2. Schwartz, E., Warren, R.F., O'Brien, S.J. *Posterior Shoulder Instability.* Clin Orthop 1987;18:409–419.
3. Arciero, R.A., Mazzocca, A.D. *Traumatic Posterior Shoulder Subluxation with Labral Injury: Suture Anchor Technique.* Tech Shoulder Elbow Surg 2004;5:13–24.
4. Williams, R.J., Strickland, S., Cohen, M., Altchek, D.W., Warren, R.F. *Arthroscopic Repair for Traumatic Posterior Shoulder Instability.* Am J Sports Med 2003;31:203–209.
5. Mair, S.D., Zarzour, R., Speer, K.P. *Posterior Labral Injury in Contact Athletes.* Am J Sports Med 1998;26:753–758.
6. Perry, J. *Anatomy and Biomechanics of the Shoulder in Throwing, Swimming, Gymnastics and Tennis.* Clin Sports Med 1983;2:247–254.
7. Levine, W.N., Flatow, E.L. *The Pathophysiology of Shoulder Instability.* Am J Sports Med 2000;28:910–917.
8. Wyke, B. *The Neurology of Joints.* Ann R Coll Surg Engl 1966;41:25.
9. Frank, C., Akeson, W., Woo, S., Amiel, D., Coutts, R.D. *Physiology and Therapeutic Value of Passive Joint Motion.* Clin Orthop 1983;185:113.
10. Akeson, W., Woo, S., Amiel, D. *The Connective Tissue Response to Immobility: Biomechanical Changes in Periarticular Connective Tissue of the Immobilized Rabbit Knee.* Clin Orthop 1973;93:356–362.
11. Salter, R., Simmonds, D., Malcom, B. *The Biologic Effects on Continuous Passive Motion on the Healing of Full Thickness Articular Cartilage Defects.* J Bone Joint Surg 1980;61A:1231–1251.
12. Salter, R., Bell, R., Keely, F. *The Protective Effect of Continuous Passive Motion on Living Articular Cartilage in Acute Septic Neuritis.* Clin Orthop 1981;159:223–247.
13. Johnston, T.B. *The Movements of the Shoulder Joint. A Plea for the Use of the "Plane of the Scapula" as the Plane of Reference for Movements Occurring at the Humeri-scapular Joint.* Br J Surg 1937;25:252–260.
14. Saha, A.K. *Mechanism of Shoulder Movements. A Plea for Recognition of the "Zero Position" of the Glenohumeral Joint.* Clin Orthop 1983;173:3–10.
15. Speer, K.P., Cavanaugh, J.T., Warren, R.F., Day, L., Wickiewicz, T.L. *A Role for Hydrotherapy in Shoulder Rehabilitation.* Am J Sports Med 1993;21:850–853.
16. Timm, K. *The Isokinetic Torque Curve of Shoulder Instability in High School Baseball Pitchers.* J Orthop Sports Phys Ther 1998;26:150–154.
17. Sutter, J.S. *Conservative Treatment of Shoulder Instability.* In Andrews, J.R., Wilk, K.E. (Eds). *The Athlete's Shoulder.* Churchill Livingstone, New York, 1994, pp. 589–604.
18. Kibler, W.B. *Role of the Scapula in the Overhead Throwing Motion.* Contemp Orthop 1991;22:525–533.
19. Kibler, W.B. *The Role of the Scapula in Athletic Shoulder Function.* Am J Sports Med 1998;26:325–336.
20. Rathburn, J., MacNab, I. *The Microvascular Pattern of the Rotator Cuff.* J Bone Joint Surg 1970;52B:540–553.
21. Bassett, R., Browne, A., Morrey, B., An, K. *Glenohumeral Muscle Force and Movement Mechanics in a Position of Shoulder Instability.* J Biomech 1988;23:401–415.
22. Dillman, C., Fleisig, G., Werner, S., Andrews, J.R. *Biomechanics of the Shoulder in Sports: Throwing Activities. Post Graduate Advances in Sports Medicine.* Forum Medicum, Inc., Berryville, VA, 1991.
23. Smith, R.H., Brunolti, J. *Shoulder Kinesthesia after Anterior Glenohumeral Joint Dislocation.* Phys Ther 1989;69:106–112.
24. Lephart, S., Warner, J.P., Borsa, P.A., Fu, H. *Proprioception of the Shoulder Joint in Healthy, Unstable, and Surgically Repaired Shoulders.* J Shoulder Elbow Surg 1994;3:371–380.
25. Zuckerman, J.D., Gallagher, M.A., Cuomo, F., Rokito, A. *The Effect of Instability and Subsequent Anterior Shoulder Repair on Proprioceptive Ability.* J Shoulder Elbow Surg 2003;12(2):105–109.
26. Knott, M., Voss, D. *Proprioceptive Neuromuscular Facilitation.* Harper and Row, New York, 1968.
27. Carpenter, J.E., Blaiser, R.B., Pellizzon, G.G. *The Effects of Muscle Fatigue on Shoulder Joint Position Sense.* Am J Sports Med 1998;26:262–265.
28. Paris, S.V. *Extremity Dysfunction and Mobilization.* Institute Press, Atlanta, GA, 1980.
29. Fleisig, G.S., Dillman, C.J., Andrews, J.R. Biomechanics of the Shoulder During Throwing. In Andrews, J.R., Wilk, K.E. (Eds). *The Athlete's Shoulder.* Churchill Livingstone, New York, 1994, pp. 355–368.
30. Ryu, R.K., McCormick, J., Jobe, F.W. *An EMG Analysis of Shoulder Function in Tennis Players.* Am J Sports Med 1988;16:481–488.
31. Ivey, F.M., Calhoun, J.H., Rusche, K., Bierschenk, J. *Isokinetic Testing of Shoulder Strength: Normal Values.* Arch Phys Med Rehabil 1985;66(6):384–386.
32. Davies, G.J. *A Compendium of Isokinetics in Clinical Usage and Rehabilitation Techniques,* 4th ed. Simon & Schuster, New York, NY, 1992.

C H A P T E R

44

Superior Labrum Anterior to Posterior (SLAP) Repair

MICKEY LEVINSON, PT

Superior labral lesions were first described by Snyder et al.[1] and termed *superior labrum anterior to posterior* (SLAP) lesions. They defined a SLAP lesion as a labral detachment, which originated posteriorly to the long head of the biceps tendon insertion and extended anteriorly[1] (Figure 44-1). The lesions were classified into four types, according to their arthroscopic appearance.[1] The mechanism of injury of a SLAP lesion is unclear. It has been described by Andrews et al.[2] as a chronic traction injury of the biceps on the superior labrum in overhead athletes because stimulation of the biceps has been demonstrated to pull the labrum off the superior glenoid. Conversely, Snyder et al.[1] describes an axial compression force from a fall on an outstretched arm. Pain is the most common complaint; however, some patients may complain of "catching" or "locking."[3] SLAP lesions can be treated conservatively; however, in cases in which the labrum is detached, especially in the athletic population, surgical intervention is required. Complete SLAP lesions have been shown to result in significant increases in anterior and inferior humeral head translation.[4]

SURGICAL OVERVIEW

The labrum is a fibrocartilaginous structure that surrounds the glenoid. It contributes to glenohumeral stability by increasing the contact area for the humeral head and provides resistance to humeral head translation.[5] The superior labrum is loosely attached to the glenoid rim and may overlap the glenoid surface.[6] The superior labrum also inserts into the long head of the biceps.[7] The biceps has also been shown to contribute to the stability of the glenohumeral joint.[8-10] Pathology resulting from the previously described mechanism of injury can include labral fraying, detachment of the labrum, the labrum being displaced into the joint, and partial rupture of the biceps.[11] Surgical intervention for SLAP lesions is dictated by the extent of the injury. In cases in which the biceps attachment is intact, the frayed labrum may simply be debrided. For cases in which the labrum is detached from the glenoid and the long head of the biceps is unstable, a repair is often necessary.[12] Currently, this procedure can be done arthroscopically. The labrum and the long head of the biceps are reattached, using either suture anchors or bioabsorbable tissue tacks (Figure 44-2). The patient is then immobilized in a sling until rehabilitation begins.

REHABILITATION OVERVIEW

The rehabilitation program following a SLAP repair generally begins 1 to 3 weeks post-surgery. The patient constantly wears the immobilizer, except when performing exercises or bathing. Early, controlled range of motion (ROM) is allowed to optimize healing and avoid excessive passive stretching later in the program. Throughout the program, the patient is progressed slowly into abduction and external rotation so as to avoid excessive stretch to the labrum and traction to the long head of the biceps. The reduced morbidity associated with new, improved surgical techniques will reduce the incidence of motion loss. However, the rate of progression is determined by the functional demands of the patient. Patients who require a great deal of external rotation, such as overhead athletes, will be progressed more aggressively.

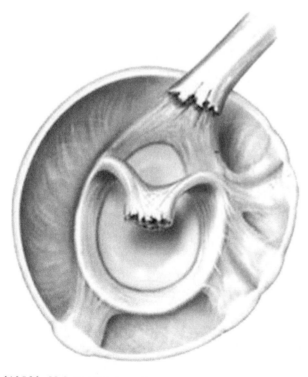

FIGURE **44-1** SLAP lesion. Superior labral repair anterior to posterior.

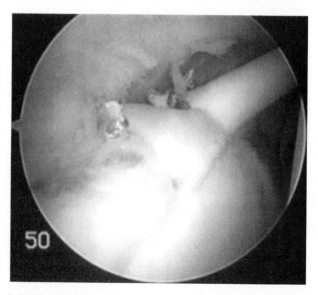

FIGURE **44-2** Repair of a SLAP lesion, using suture anchors.

Throughout rehabilitation, a full upper extremity strengthening program will be progressed functionally and independently to prepare the patient for return to activity. Biceps strengthening is progressed very slowly because biceps activity can cause traction to the labrum and thus jeopardize the repair.[2] The goals of rehabilitation are to restore normal strength, ROM, flexibility, and normal neuromuscular function. The program is based on the patient returning to sport-specific activities no earlier than 3 to 4 months post-surgery.

POSTOPERATIVE PHASE I (WEEKS 1 TO 4)

During phase I of rehabilitation, the emphasis is on restoration of ROM and avoidance of any possible capsular restrictions later in the program. Although allowing motion, the clinician must protect the healing tissues. Benefits of early motion include improving pain perception, nourishing articular cartilage, and enhancing collagen alignment.[13-15] External rotation and extension are limited to neutral to avoid overstressing the healing repair.

During this phase, the patient will be allowed to perform active-assisted forward flexion and external rotation. Forward flexion is performed in the plane of the scapula (Figure 44-3). In this plane, approximately 30 to 45 degrees anterior to the frontal plane, the capsule is

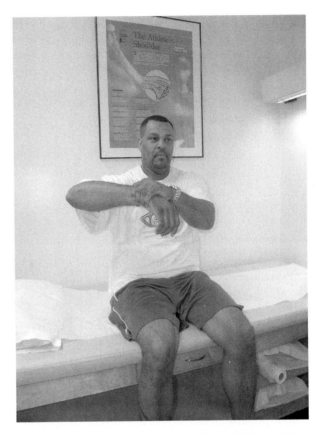

FIGURE **44-3** Elevation in the plane of the scapula, minimizing capsular stress.

Postoperative Phase I (Weeks 1 to 4)

GOALS

- Promote healing: reduce pain and inflammation
- Forward flexion to 90 degrees
- External rotation to neutral
- Independent home exercise program

PRECAUTIONS

- Immobilizer at all times, except when exercising or bathing
- External rotation and extension limited to neutral

TREATMENT STRATEGIES

- Immobilizer
- Gripping exercises
- Active range of motion (AROM): wrist/elbow (supported to avoid biceps stress)
- Scapular "pinches"
- Pain-free, submaximal deltoid isometrics
- Active-assisted range of motion (AAROM): forward flexion (scapular plane)
- AAROM: external rotation to neutral
- Modalities as needed
- Home exercise program

CRITERIA FOR ADVANCEMENT

- External rotation to neutral
- Forward flexion to 90 degrees
- Minimal pain or inflammation

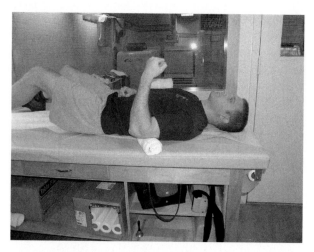

FIGURE **44-4** Elbow AROM. Arm is supported to minimize stress to the biceps.

stressed the least, and there is the greatest degree of conformity between the glenoid and the humeral head.[16]

Gripping exercises are initiated to promote circulation. Wrist and elbow ROM are initiated to avoid any contractures resulting from immobilization. Elbow ROM is performed in a supported position to avoid any stress to the biceps tendon (Figure 44-4).

Patients often develop postural problems while in the immobilizer. Scapular "pinches" are initiated to improve posture and tone. In addition, as symptoms allow, submaximal, pain-free deltoid isometrics are initiated (Figure 44-5). The patient is instructed in the use of cryotherapy to minimize the effects of pain and inflammation.

Troubleshooting

Generally, arthroscopic procedures for SLAP lesions do not result in ROM loss; however, the clinician should cautiously monitor the end feel of the patient, who is having difficulty attaining the ROM goals. If assessment determines that a possible contracture is developing, the surgeon should be notified.

Excessive pain and inflammation may be an indication that the patient is being too aggressive with the exercise program. In this scenario, the patient needs to modify or reduce the program until symptoms have subsided.

POSTOPERATIVE PHASE II (WEEKS 4 TO 8)

During this phase, the immobilizer will be discharged by the surgeon. The patient will continue to progress ROM with forward flexion progressed, as tolerated, and external rotation limited to 30 degrees until approximately 6 weeks (for overhead athletes, this may be progressed more rapidly, if the shoulder seems to be

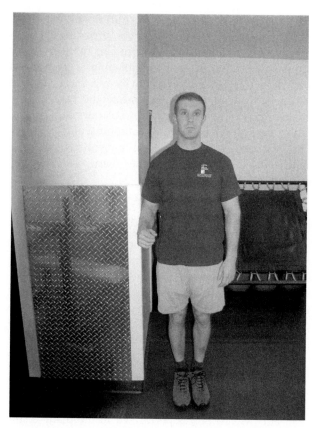

FIGURE **44-5** Deltoid isometric. Performed submaximally with the elbow flexed.

becoming too tight). Wand exercises are used in supine (Figure 44-6). As the patient reaches approximately 110 degrees of forward flexion, pulleys are incorporated for ROM (Figure 44-7). At 6 weeks, ROM is progressed, as tolerated; however, the abducted and externally rotated position should continue to be avoided. Patients who are progressing slowly may benefit from the addition of hydrotherapy (Figure 44-8), in which the buoyancy of the water assists in elevation of the upper extremity.[17]

The patient should begin establishing good proximal stability. Scapular strengthening is initiated with side-lying stabilization exercises (Figure 44-9). Manual resistance is applied to provide tactile feedback to the patient. In addition, low-level closed chain activities are used. Closed chain activities, performed with the distal end of the limb fixed, provide a compressive, axial load that enhances stability and proprioception.[18,19] Proprioception has been demonstrated to be compromised with shoulder instability.[20,21]

During phase I, dynamic stabilization activities should begin with submaximal, pain-free internal/external rotation isometrics. These can be performed with a small towel roll under the arm to place the patient

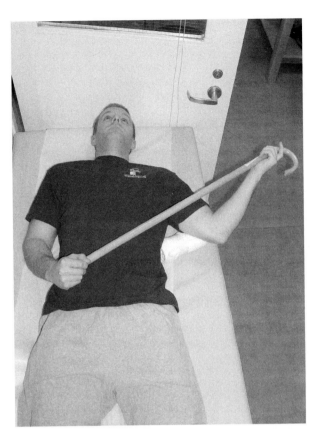

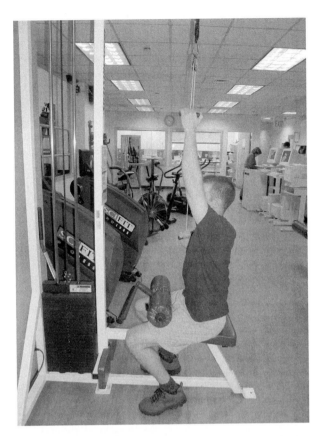

FIGURE **44-6** Wand exercises performed in supine for active assistive external rotation.

FIGURE **44-7** Pulleys used for active assistive forward flexion.

in comfortable abduction, which may improve the circulation to the rotator cuff.[22] The patient should be reminded that excessive force with isometrics will result in inflammation and subsequent reflex inhibition of musculature.[23] As the patient progresses with ROM and symptoms subside, internal/external rotation isotonics can be initiated, using elastic resistance.

Scapular strengthening is progressed to isotonics at approximately 6 weeks. Normal scapulothoracic function is critical to successful rehabilitation because it provides a stable base for humeral rotation, maintains the proper inclination angle of the glenoid, and maintains the proper length–tension relationship for the glenohumeral muscles.[24,25] Exercises include rowing, shrugs, and serratus punch. As ROM allows, wall push-ups with a plus are initiated.

Latissimus strengthening is initiated in ranges that continue to protect the repair. Initially, the range is limited to 90 degrees of elevation and neutral extension. Aside from being a strong extensor of the shoulder, the latissimus has also been shown to provide a compressive load to the glenohumeral joint, thus reducing stress to the rotator cuff.[26]

If rotator cuff strength is adequate, scapular plane elevation is initiated. Emphasis is placed on restoring

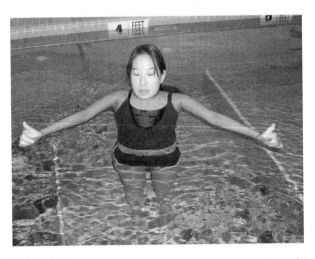

FIGURE **44-8** Patient uses the buoyancy of the water to assist with forward flexion.

normal scapulothoracic and scapulohumeral rhythm. The plane of the scapula is used because it provides the optimal length–tension relationship of the glenohumeral muscles.[27] Elevation in this plane also recruits the scapular musculature, including the upper and lower trapezius, rhomboids, and serratus anterior.[28] The exercise is performed with the thumb up in

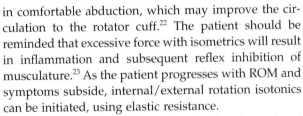

Postoperative Phase II (Weeks 4 to 8)

GOALS

- Continue to promote healing
- Forward flexion to 145 degrees
- External rotation to 60 degrees
- Begin to restore scapular and upper extremity strength
- Restore normal scapulohumeral rhythm

PRECAUTIONS

- Limit external rotation to 30 degrees until 6 weeks
- Avoid excessive stretch to the labrum and biceps
- Avoid rotator cuff inflammation

TREATMENT STRATEGIES

- Discontinue immobilizer (surgeon directed)
- Continue AAROM forward flexion: wand exercises, pulleys
- Continue AAROM external rotation: limited to 30 degrees until 6 weeks
- Hydrotherapy as required
- Manual scapular side-lying stabilization exercises
- Physio ball stabilization exercises
- Internal/external rotation isometrics (submaximal, pain-free)
- Progress scapular strengthening in protective arcs
- Isotonic internal/external rotation strengthening at 6 weeks
- Scapular plane elevation (emphasis on scapulohumeral elevation)
- Begin latissimus strengthening, limited to 90 degrees forward flexion
- Begin humeral head stabilization exercises
- Modalities as needed
- Modify home exercise program

CRITERIA FOR ADVANCEMENT

- Forward flexion to 145 degrees
- External rotation to 60 degrees
- Normal scapulohumeral rhythm
- Minimal pain and inflammation
- Internal/external rotation strength 5/5

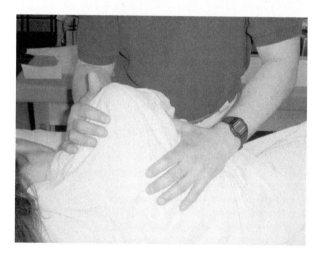

FIGURE 44-9 Patient performs side-lying scapula stabilization exercises with manual resistance.

external rotation to minimize the risk of subacromial impingement. Humeral head control exercises, such as rhythmic stabilization, are initiated to improve dynamic stability.

Troubleshooting

SLAP lesions are often associated with rotator cuff pathology.[3] A thorough history is critical to identifying a patient who may be predisposed to inflammation. During this phase, the clinician should carefully monitor the patient of any developing excessive inflammation that may result in a capsular contraction and reflex inhibition. In such cases, the surgeon should be notified and certain mobilizations or soft tissue techniques may be indicated. Scapulohumeral rhythm should also be assessed carefully to avoid development of abnormal movement patterns.

POSTOPERATIVE PHASE III (WEEKS 8 TO 14)

The goals of this phase are to restore normal strength, ROM, and flexibility. AAROM for internal rotation is initiated (Figure 44-10). Forward flexion, internal rotation ROM, and external rotation ROM are continued until normal. General upper extremity flexibility exercises are initiated.

Aggressive strengthening continues for the scapular musculature and the entire upper extremity. The scapular plane should continue to be emphasized for reasons mentioned previously.[16,27] Eccentric strengthening should be included, because this type of muscle action clearly plays a large role in many sport-specific activities.[29,30] During this phase, it is now safe to initiate biceps strengthening, but it must be progressed cautiously to avoid excessive stress to the repair (Figure 44-11). Biceps strengthening is included in the program because of the stabilizing function it plays at the glenohumeral joint in the abducted and externally rotated position.[8-10] In this phase, a normal strength base of 5/5 of the entire upper extremity should be established to prepare for more functional activities later.

Proprioceptive and functional training is advanced. Humeral head stabilization exercises are advanced to more challenging positions. At approximately 12 weeks, if the patient's demands require overhead activities, internal/external rotation strengthening is progressed to the abducted 90/90 degree position.

Finally, in phase III, endurance and speed training are incorporated. Endurance training is important, as Wickiewicz[31] has demonstrated increased humeral head migration with fatigue. In addition, loss of proprioception has been associated with fatigue.[32] Upper body ergometry is used, and neuromuscular drills are performed while the patient is fatigued. In addition, isokinetic training is used to provide a speed or activity-specific component to the program (Figure 44-12). Isokinetic testing will also provide an objective assessment for progression to more functional activities.

Troubleshooting

In phase III, the patient who has not achieved full ROM must be monitored very carefully. Any possible capsular restriction should be communicated to the surgeon. As always, excessive passive stretching should be avoided. However, other techniques, such as joint mobilization, soft tissue techniques, or continuous passive motion, may be indicated. The clinician should also monitor the patient's scapulohumeral rhythm to avoid any abnormal movement patterns. In addition, the patient is educated to perform flexibility exercises in nonpainful ranges because many patients have a tendency to overstretch.

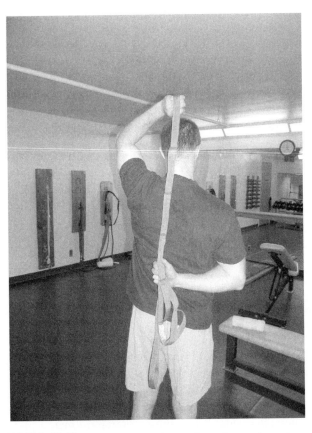

FIGURE **44-10** Active assistive internal rotation, using strap.

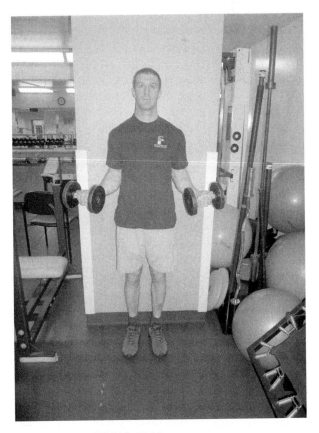

FIGURE **44-11** Biceps curls.

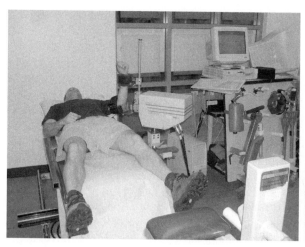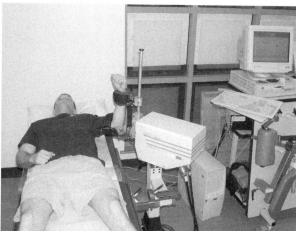

FIGURE **44-12** Isokinetic training for the internal and external rotators.

Postoperative Phase III (Weeks 8 to 14)

GOALS

- Restore full shoulder ROM
- Restore normal scapulohumeral rhythm
- Isokinetic internal/external rotation: strength 85% of uninvolved side
- Restore normal flexibility

PRECAUTIONS

- Avoid rotator cuff inflammation
- Avoid excessive passive stretching

TREATMENT STRATEGIES

- Continue AAROM for forward flexion and external rotation
- AAROM for internal rotation
- Aggressive scapular and latissimus strengthening
- Begin biceps strengthening
- Begin PNF patterns if internal/external rotation strength is 5/5
- Progress humeral head stabilization exercises
- Progress internal/external rotation to 90/90 position if required
- General upper extremity flexibility exercises
- Upper body ergometry
- Isokinetic training and testing
- Modalities as needed
- Modify home exercise program

CRITERIA FOR ADVANCEMENT

- Normal scapulohumeral rhythm
- Minimal pain and inflammation
- Full upper extremity ROM
- Isokinetic internal/external rotation strength 85% of uninvolved side

POSTOPERATIVE PHASE IV (WEEKS 14 TO 18)

The emphasis of this phase is to restore normal neuro-muscular function and prepare the patient for return to the desired sport or functional activity. During this phase, the functional demands of the desired activity must be reproduced. The patient should have normal strength, ROM, and flexibility, and the patient should be asymptomatic. An isokinetic test should demonstrate internal/external rotation strength, at least 85% of the uninvolved side. When these criteria are met, a plyometric program may be implemented. Plyometrics uses the stretch reflex of the muscle to produce powerful contractions.[35] Several authors have outlined certain guidelines for plyometric exercises[36,37]: (1) They should be functionally specific, (2) the quality of exercise should be stressed, and (3) they should be progressive in overload (Figure 44-13). In addition to the upper extremity, any sport or activity-related demands of the trunk and lower extremities should be addressed.

Upon successful completion of a plyometric program, the patient is given approval by the surgeon to initiate a sport or activity-specific interval program. Regardless of the activity, the patient should be progressed individually and monitored carefully for symptoms and proper mechanics, to minimize the risks of reinjury. Sport or activity-specific programs may often result in a loss of strength, ROM, and flexibility. Before discharge, an isokinetic test is again performed to monitor progress. The goals at this point of rehabilitation are to have equal internal/external rotation strength to the uninvolved side and a 66% external to internal rotation ratio, which has been demonstrated in the normal population.[33,34] Upon discharge, the patient must be instructed in a home exercise or training program that will maintain strength and flexibility as he or she returns to normal activity. The patient must also be educated on modifications that can be made to a previous exercise routine to protect the shoulder from future injury.

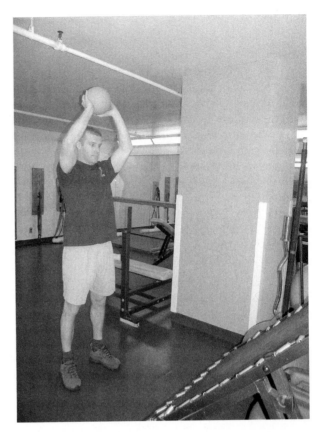

FIGURE 44-13 Overhead plyometric exercise.

Postoperative Phase IV (Weeks 14 to 18)

GOALS
- Restore normal neuromuscular function
- Isokinetic internal/external rotation strength equal to unaffected side
- Maintain strength and flexibility
- Prevent reinjury

PRECAUTIONS
- Pain-free plyometrics
- Significant pain with specific activity
- Feeling of instability

TREATMENT STRATEGIES
- Continue full upper extremity strengthening program
- Continue upper extremity flexibility exercises
- Activity-specific plyometrics program
- Address trunk and lower extremity demands
- Continue endurance training
- Begin sport or activity-related program
- Modify home exercise program

CRITERIA FOR DISCHARGE
- Isokinetic internal/external rotation strength equal to uninvolved side
- Independent home exercise program
- Independent, pain-free sport or activity-specific program

Troubleshooting

Once a plyometrics program is initiated, symptoms must be monitored carefully. Any significant symptoms may indicate that the patient is not prepared for a particular activity or the volume of work is too great. Also, sports or activity programs may result in soreness that does not indicate serious injury. The patient may need to take only a step back in the program or rest for a period of time. However, if any significant symptoms persist or recur, the program must be stopped and the patient referred back to the surgeon. Finally, when beginning a sport or activity-specific program, some patients may choose to stop their home exercise program. They must be educated that doing so can result in a selective loss of strength and flexibility, leading to potential reinjury. Thus, patients must be aware that a home exercise program should be maintained to avoid this scenario.

REFERENCES

1. Snyder, S.J., Karzel, R.P., Del Pizzo, W., Ferkel, R., Friedman, M. *SLAP Lesions of the Shoulder.* Arthroscopy 1990;6:274–279.
2. Andrews, J.R., Carson, W.G., Mcleod, W.D. *Glenoid Labrum Tears Related to the Long Head of the Biceps.* Am J Sports Med 1985;13:337–341.
3. Snyder, S.J., Banas, M.P., Karzel, R.P. *An Analysis of 140 Injuries to the Superior Glenoid Labrum.* J Shoulder Elbow Surg 1995;4:243–248.
4. Pagnani, M.J., Deng, X.H., Warren, R.F. *Effect of Lesions of the Superior Portion of the Glenoid Labrum on Glenohumeral Translation.* J Bone Joint Surg 1995;77:1003–1010.
5. Levine, W.N., Flatow, E.L. *The Pathophysiology of Shoulder Instability.* Am J Sports Med 2000;28:910–917.
6. Cooper, D.E., Arnoczky, S.P., O'Brien, S.J., Warren, R.F., DiCarlo, E., Allen, A.A. *Anatomy, Histology and Vascularity of the Glenoid Labrum. An Anatomical Study.* J Bone Joint Surg 1992;74:46–52.
7. Mileski, R.A., Snyder, S.J. *Superior Labral Lesions in the Shoulder: Pathoanatomy and Surgical Management.* J Am Acad Orthop Surg 1998;6:121–131.
8. Itoi, E., Kuechle, D.K., Newman, S.R., Morrey, B.F. An, K.N. *The Stabilizing Function of the Biceps in Stable and Unstable Shoulders.* J Bone Joint Surg 1993;75:546–550.
9. Itoi, E., Motzkin, N.E., Morrey, B.F., An, K.N. *Stabilizing Function of the Long Head of the Biceps in Stable and Unstable Shoulders.* J Shoulder Elbow Surg 1994;3:135–142.
10. Rodosky, M.W., Harner, C.D., Fu, F.H. *The Role of the Long Head of the Biceps Muscle and Superior Glenoid Labrum in Anterior Instability of the Shoulder.* Am J Sports Med 1994;22: 121–130.
11. McGlynn, F.J., Caspari, R.B. *Arthroscopic Findings in the Subluxating Shoulder.* Clin Orthop 1984;183:173–178.
12. DiRaimondo, C.A., Alexander, J.W., Noble, P.C. *A Biomechanical Comparison of Repair Techniques for Type II SLAP Lesions.* Am J Sports Med 2004;32:727–733.
13. Wyke, B. *The Neurology of Joints.* Ann R Coll Surg Engl 1966; 41:25.
14. Frank, C., Akeson, W., Woo, S., Amiel, D., Coutts, R.D. *Physiology and Therapeutic Value of Passive Joint Motion.* Clin Orthop 1983;185:113.
15. Salter, R., Simmonds, D., Malcom, B. *The Biologic Effects on Continuous Passive Motion on the Healing of Full Thickness Articular Cartilage Defects.* J Bone Joint Surg 1980;61A:1231–1251.
16. Johnston, T.B. *The Movements of the Shoulder Joint. A Plea for the Use of the "Plane of the Scapula" as the Plane of Reference for Movements Occurring at the Humeri-scapular Joint.* Br J Surg 1937;25:252–260.
17. Speer, K.P., Cavanaugh, J.T., Warren, R.F., Day, L., Wickiewicz, T.L. *A Role for Hydrotherapy in Shoulder Rehabilitation.* Am J Sports Med 1993;21:850–853.
18. Wilk, K.E., Arrigo, C., Andrews, J.R. *Closed and Open Chain Kinetic Exercise for the Upper Extremity.* J Sports Rehabil 1996;5: 88–102.
19. Tippett, S. *Closed Chain Exercise.* Orthop Phys Ther Clin North Am 1992;1:253–268.
20. Lephart, S., Warner, J.P., Borsa, P.A., Fu, F.H. *Proprioception of the Shoulder Joint in Healthy, Unstable and Surgically Repaired Shoulders.* J Shoulder Elbow Surg 1994;3:371–380.
21. Smith, R.H., Brunolti, J. *Shoulder Kinesthesia after Anterior Glenohumeral Joint Dislocation.* Phys Ther 1989;69:106–112.
22. Rathburn, J., MacNab, I. *The Microvasculature Pattern of the Rotator Cuff.* J Bone Joint Surg 1970;52B:540–553.
23. Timm, K. *The Isokinetic Torque Curve of Shoulder Instability in High School Baseball Pitchers.* J Orthop Sports Phys Ther 1998; 26:150–154.
24. Kibler, W.B. *Role of the Scapula in the Overhead Throwing Motion.* Contemp Orthop 1991;22:525–533.
25. Kibler, W.B. *The Role of the Scapula in Athletic Shoulder Function.* Am J Sports Med 1998;26:325–336.
26. Bassett, R., Browne, A., Morrey, B., An, K. *Glenohumeral Muscle Force and Moment Mechanics in a Position of Shoulder Instability.* J Biomech 1988;23:401–415.
27. Saha, K. *Mechanism of Shoulder Movements and Plea for Recognition of the "Zero Position" of the Glenohumeral Joint.* Clin Orthop 1983;173:3–10.
28. Moseley, J., Jobe, F., Pink, M., Perry, J., Tibone, J. *EMG Analysis of Scapular Muscles During a Shoulder Rehabilitation Program.* Am J Sports Med 1992;20:128–134.
29. Ryu, R.K., McCormick, J., Jobe, F.W. *An EMG Analysis of Shoulder Function in Tennis Players.* Am J Sports Med 1988;16: 481–488.
30. DiGiovine, R., Jobe, F.W., Pink, M. *An Electromyographic Analysis of the Upper Extremity in Pitching.* J Shoulder Elbow Surg 1992;1:15–25.
31. Wickiewicz, T. *Radiographic Evaluation of the Glenohumeral Kinematics: A Muscle Fatigue Model.* American Academy of Orthopedic Surgeons, Sports Medicine Specialty Meeting, Washington, DC, 1994.
32. Carpenter, J.E., Blaiser, R.B., Pellizzon, G.G. *The Effects of Muscle Fatigue on Shoulder Joint Position Sense.* Am J Sports Med 1998;26:262–265.
33. Ivey, F.M., Calhoun, J.H., Rusche, K., Bierschenk, J. *Isokinetic Testing of Shoulder Strength: Normal Values.* Arch Phys Med Rehabil 1985;66(6):384–386.
34. Davies, G.J. *A Compendium of Isokinetics in Clinical Usage and Rehabilitation Techniques,* 4th ed. Simon & Schuster, LaCrosse, WI, 1992.

35. Chu, D. *Jumping into Plyometrics.* Leisure Press, Champaign, IL, 1992.
36. Voight, M., Draovitch, P. *Eccentric Muscle Training in Sports and Orthopedics: Plyometric Training.* Churchill Livingstone, New York, 1991.
37. Wilk, K.E., Voight, M.L., Keirns, M.A., Gambetta, V., Andrews, J.R., Dillman, C.J. *Stretch-shortening Drills for the Upper Extremities: Theory and Clinical Application.* J Orthop Sports Phys Ther 1993;17:225–239.

45

Ulnar Collateral Ligament Reconstruction

MICKEY LEVINSON, PT

Injury of the ulnar collateral ligament (UCL) is almost exclusively limited to the competitive throwing population. More specifically, it is most common in baseball players. The UCL of the elbow has been shown to contribute 54% of the resistance to valgus stress while throwing.[1] Injury is a result of the extreme valgus forces placed on the elbow, especially during pitching. Tearing of the UCL can result in pain and instability. Conservative treatment has not been seen to be successful for this injury, especially with pitchers.[2] Continued pitching with this injury can lead to arthritic changes.[3] To restore stability, a reconstruction is often indicated. The most common graft choice for the reconstruction is the palmaris longus tendon. In the absence of this muscle, the graft is generally taken from the patient's gracilis. Graft choice does not affect the Hospital for Special Surgery (HSS) guideline. The HSS UCL reconstruction guideline is based on the "docking technique" described by Altchek et al.[4]

ANATOMICAL OVERVIEW

A UCL reconstruction, using a palmaris longus tendon graft, is performed using a combination of open and arthroscopic surgery. Most commonly, the graft is harvested from the ipsilateral palmaris longus tendon. Exposure is created by splitting the flexor carpi ulnaris muscle (Figure 45-1). Bone tunnels are created in the humerus and ulna. The graft is "docked" securely into the tunnels, using sutures (Figure 45-2). The elbow is then taken through a full range of motion (ROM) to determine final graft tension and placed in a splint at 60-degree flexion.[4]

REHABILITATION OVERVIEW

The rehabilitation program following UCL reconstruction begins immediately after surgery, with the patient instructed in a home exercise program. Formal physical therapy usually does not begin until approximately 4 to 6 weeks post-surgery. Care must be taken to protect the graft throughout the progression of the rehabilitation program. The program emphasizes early, controlled motion so as to avoid any excessive passive stretching later in the program. This will allow the graft to remain as tight as possible until the patient is allowed to return to activity. The program also limits excessive stress to the wrist and elbow during the early phases to allow optimal soft tissue healing. Shoulder and scapular strengthening are a key component of the program. Following kinetic chain principles, improved proximal strength and efficiency should reduce stress on the elbow. The program is based on the patient beginning an interval throwing program at 4 months post-surgery and a hitting program at 5 months.

POSTOPERATIVE PHASE I (WEEKS 1 TO 4)

Emphasis of the first phase of the program is on beginning to gradually restore ROM without placing excessive forces on the healing graft. Early ROM will help minimize the adverse effects of immobilization, such as articular cartilage degeneration and contracture of the elbow joint.[5-7] In addition, it should have a positive effect on pain and collagen formation.[8-10] The nature of the surgical technique and its fixation allows for immediate motion. On postoperative day (POD) 1, the patient is placed in a hinged brace set at 30 degrees of extension and 90 degrees of flexion (Figure 45-3). Active range of motion (AROM) is initiated in the brace, and this range should be achieved during this phase. The patient is advised to wear the brace at all times to avoid any valgus stress to the elbow.

Gripping and wrist ROM exercises are initiated to promote circulation and avoid stiffness, as the ipsilateral palmaris longus tendon is most commonly used for the graft.

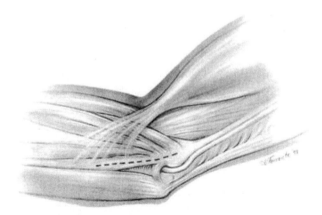

FIGURE 45-1 Exposure is created by splitting the flexor carpi ulnaris muscle.

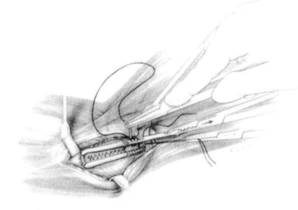

FIGURE 45-2 Docking technique: The graft is "docked" securely into the bone tunnels, using sutures.

Postoperative Phase I (Weeks 1 to 4)

GOALS

- Promote healing: reduce pain, inflammation, and swelling
- Begin to restore ROM to 30 to 90 degrees
- Independent home exercise program

PRECAUTIONS

- Brace should be worn at all times
- No PROM of the elbow

TREATMENT STRATEGIES

- Brace set at 30 to 90 degrees of flexion
- Elbow AROM in brace
- Wrist AROM
- Scapular isometrics
- Gripping exercises
- Cryotherapy
- Home exercise program

CRITERIA FOR ADVANCEMENT

- Elbow ROM: 30 to 90 degrees
- Minimal pain or swelling

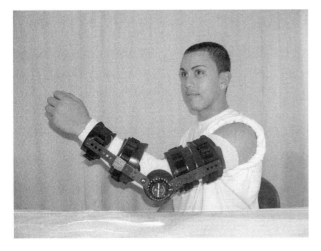

FIGURE 45-3 Hinged brace set at 30 to 90 degrees on POD 1.

Scapular isometrics are initiated to maintain some proximal tone, and the patient is encouraged to maintain ROM of the shoulder without placing any valgus stress on the elbow.

The patient is instructed in cryotherapy to reduce any postoperative swelling, inflammation, and pain, which may inhibit ROM restoration. In the author's experience swelling has not been a significant factor with this technique. However, additional procedures, such as spur removal or scar tissue removal, may increase postoperative swelling.

Troubleshooting

The patient's ROM should be monitored during this phase. If the patient's motion does not appear to be progressing well, the surgeon should be notified. At this point, the surgeon may elect to further open the brace to avoid the need for aggressive passive motion later in the program. On the other hand, if the patient's motion appears to be progressing too quickly, or excessive swelling or inflammation persists, the patient must be advised to limit activity, at this point, and must have the brace worn at all times. Modalities, such as cryotherapy, may be used to control pain and swelling.

POSTOPERATIVE PHASE II (WEEKS 4 TO 6)

During this phase, the brace is continued to be used to protect the healing graft. ROM must be continually monitored to assure that a flexion contracture is not developing. In the case of a flexion contracture, the surgeon should be notified and the brace may be opened to 15 to 115 degrees. This reduces the risk of a joint contracture.

Upper extremity strengthening may be initiated to begin to establish a strength base for later, more functional phases. The patient continues to wear the brace while exercising, to protect the healing graft. Pain-free deltoid isometrics are initiated. If pain and swelling have been minimized, pain-free isometrics for wrist flexion/extension and elbow flexion/extension are initiated. Manual scapular stabilization exercises are initiated in side-lying with manual, proximal resistance to

Postoperative Phase II (Weeks 4 to 6)

GOALS
- ROM: 15 to 115 degrees
- Minimal pain and swelling

PRECAUTIONS
- Continue to wear brace at all times
- Avoid PROM
- Avoid valgus stress

TREATMENT STRATEGIES
- Continue AROM in brace
- Begin pain-free isometrics in brace (deltoid, wrist flexion/extension, elbow flexion/extension)
- Manual scapular stabilization exercises with proximal resistance
- Modalities as needed
- Modify home exercise program

CRITERIA FOR ADVANCEMENT
- ROM: 15 to 115 degrees
- Minimal pain and swelling

avoid any stress to the elbow. Initiating this program gives the patient a "head start" on normalizing upper extremity strength and preparing for later functional phases.

Pain and swelling should be continued to be monitored to assure that the patient is not exercising too much and is able to advance to the next phase. Modalities should be continued to minimize any adverse effects of exercise.

Troubleshooting

As mentioned previously, the patient should be monitored to be certain that a flexion contracture is not developing or that the range is not progressing too quickly, which may stretch the graft. The surgeon must be made aware of either of these scenarios so as to determine how aggressive the patient should be. Isometric exercises should be initiated individually, because some patients may become symptomatic. Patients must be educated as to working within pain guidelines to prevent any risks that may interfere with their progress.

POSTOPERATIVE PHASE III (WEEKS 6 TO 12)

Upon meeting the established criteria for advancement, the patient enters a phase designed to restore full ROM, normalize upper extremity strength, and begin to restore endurance. Motion should continue to be restored actively. The brace is discharged at 6 weeks; however, aggressive passive stretching should continue to be avoided. For extension, a low intensity, long duration stretch has been shown to be effective and has positive effects (Figure 45-4).[11-15] Mobilization techniques may be used when motion progresses at a slower pace.

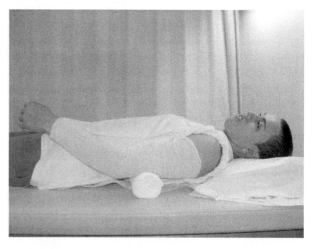

FIGURE 45-4 Low load, long duration stretch is used to achieve passive extension.

Full ROM should be restored during this phase. As ROM allows, upper body ergometry is initiated.

Isotonic exercise can be initiated for the scapula, shoulder, elbow, and wrist muscles at 6 weeks and progressed individually. Internal and external rotation exercises are avoided until approximately 8 weeks, to avoid any excessive valgus stress on the elbow. These may begin isometrically and advance to elastic resistance, as tolerated. Resistance should be progressed slowly and individually to avoid any exacerbation of symptoms.

As a good strength base is established, eccentric strengthening should be incorporated into the program. A good portion of the muscular activity at the scapula,

Postoperative Phase III (Weeks 6 to 12)

GOALS

- Restore full ROM
- All upper extremity strength 5/5
- Begin to restore upper extremity endurance

PRECAUTIONS

- Minimize valgus stress
- Avoid PROM by the clinician
- Avoid pain with therapeutic exercise

TREATMENT STRATEGIES

- Continue AROM
- Low intensity, long duration stretch for extension
- Isotonics for scapula, shoulder, elbow, forearm, wrist
- Begin internal/external rotation strengthening at 8 weeks
- Begin forearm pronation/supination strengthening at 8 weeks
- Upper body ergometer (if adequate ROM)
- Neuromuscular drills
- PNF patterns when strength is adequate
- Incorporate eccentric training when strength is adequate
- Modalities as needed
- Modify home exercise program

CRITERIA FOR ADVANCEMENT

- Pain-free
- Full elbow ROM
- All upper extremity strength 5/5

shoulder, elbow, forearm, and wrist has been shown to be eccentric during the different phases of throwing.[16–18] For example, the elbow flexors must work eccentrically to control the rapid rate of elbow extension during a throw.[16–18]

Proprioceptive neuromuscular facilitation patterns are initiated when adequate scapular and rotator cuff strength have been established. These patterns should be initiated manually to avoid excess valgus stress and then progressed to elastic resistance. In particular, the D2 flexion pattern incorporates a great deal of the musculature used in throwing (Figure 45-5).[19] In addition, neuromuscular drills, such as rhythmic stabilization, are incorporated (Figure 45-6).

Troubleshooting

As a full upper extremity strengthening program is developed, the patient must be educated as to allowing the healing process to continue. Pain at either the elbow or the shoulder may indicate that the patient is trying to progress too rapidly. Patients should be advised to avoid excessive volumes of work and progress their program only when they are ready. They should understand that pain will delay their progression to a throwing program.

POSTOPERATIVE PHASE IV (WEEKS 12 TO 16)

This is the preparation phase for return to activity. During this phase, the goal is to restore full upper extremity strength and flexibility. Rotator cuff strengthening is progressed to the overhead (90/90) position, because this is a more functional position for a throwing athlete (Figure 45-7). Aggressive strengthening is continued for strength, power, and endurance.

Flexibility exercises should be performed for the entire upper extremity to avoid any secondary pathology as the patient's activity level increases.

Upon manual muscle testing, upper extremity strength should be at least equal to the unaffected side. In addition, flexibility should also be equal. If these criteria are met, then plyometric exercises are initiated and progressed functionally to prepare the upper extremity for the forces placed on it while throwing or hitting. Plyometric exercises use the stretch reflex of the muscle. An eccentric contraction is performed to prestretch the muscle before a concentric contraction. This stimulates the muscle spindle to create a greater reaction.[20,21] These exercises should be monitored carefully and limited in frequency (two to three times per week, maximum). They should also follow a functional progression, beginning with positions of low difficulty,

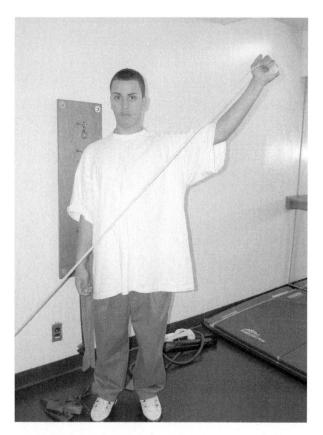

FIGURE 45-5 PNF D2 flexion patterns incorporate a great deal of the musculature used in throwing.

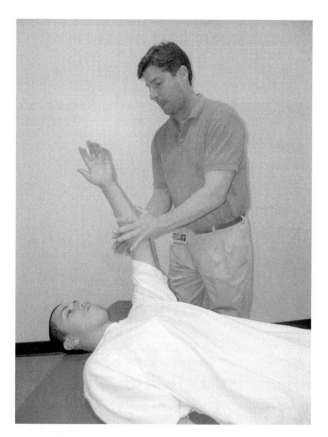

FIGURE 45-6 Rhythmic stabilization drills.

Postoperative Phase IV (Weeks 12 to 16)

GOALS

- Restore full strength and flexibility
- Restore normal neuromuscular function
- Prepare for return to activity

PRECAUTIONS

- Pain-free plyometrics

TREATMENT STRATEGIES

- Advance internal/external rotation to 90/90 position
- Full upper extremity flexibility program
- Neuromuscular drills
- Plyometrics program
- Continue endurance training
- Address trunk and lower extremities
- Modify home exercise program

CRITERIA FOR ADVANCEMENT

- Complete plyometrics program without symptoms
- Normal upper extremity flexibility

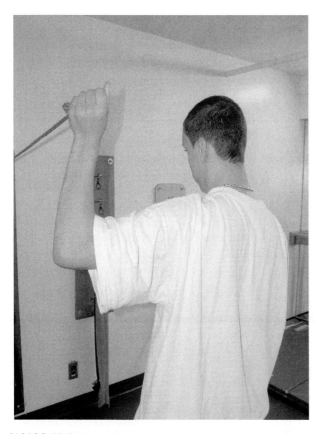

FIGURE **45-7** The rotator cuff is strengthened in a more functional 90/90 position.

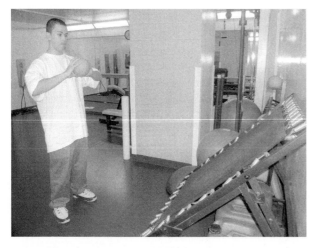

FIGURE **45-8** Plyometric training is initiated in a less challenging position, such as a two-hand chest pass.

such as a two-hand chest pass and progressing to overhead positions. In addition, these exercises should incorporate the legs, hips, and trunk because they are vital components of the kinetic chain (Figures 45-8 and 45-9).

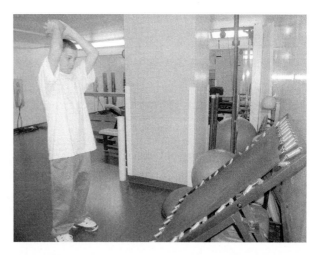

FIGURE **45-9** Plyometric training is progressed to an overhead position.

Troubleshooting

Plyometric exercises must be monitored carefully, and the volume of work must be controlled. Any symptoms that occur during or after these exercises may indicate that the patient is not prepared for them or to progress functionally. Any symptoms should be reported to the surgeon. If the patient is unable to adequately perform a certain exercise and without symptoms, progression to the next level may not occur.

POSTOPERATIVE PHASE V (MONTHS 4 TO 9)

At the beginning of this phase, the patient will be examined by the surgeon. If the examination is satisfactory and the patient is asymptomatic, an interval throwing program may be initiated. Upper extremity strength, flexibility, and endurance must be normal. The patient must have completed a plyometrics exercise program without symptoms. Interval throwing programs are generally progressed individually by volume and distance. For example, the patient will begin by throwing a set number of throws at a set distance. The volume of throws will be progressed, as tolerated. As this is achieved successfully without symptoms, the patient then progresses to the next distance. The patient must complete each phase of the program successfully before advancing to the following phase. Proper warm-up and mechanics are emphasized while building up arm strength. During this phase, the volume of strengthening exercises is generally reduced. However, the patient is encouraged to continue a strengthening and flexibility program as the throwing program progresses. Only when the throwing program has reached its target distance may the pitcher begin to throw off a pitching mound. This usually does not occur before 7 months post-surgery.[4] When applicable, a hitting program may be initiated at 5 months.

Postoperative Phase V (Months 4 to 9)

GOALS
- Return to activity
- Prevent reinjury

PRECAUTIONS
- Significant pain with throwing or hitting
- Avoid loss of strength or flexibility

TREATMENT STRATEGIES
- Begin interval throwing program at 4 months
- Begin hitting program at 5 months
- Continue flexibility exercises
- Continue strengthening program (incorporate training principles)

CRITERIA FOR DISCHARGE
- Pain-free
- Independent home exercise program
- Independent throwing/hitting program

Troubleshooting

Any sharp pain or swelling in the elbow must be addressed and communicated to the surgeon. However, the patient should be aware that elbow or shoulder soreness is not uncommon, and, often, the throwing program may have to be interrupted until symptoms have subsided. The patient is advised to continue the use of cryotherapy on a consistent basis. Occasionally, the patient may have to return to the previous phase of the throwing program.

Although the volume of strengthening is often decreased during this phase, the patient should be aware of the importance of maintaining upper extremity strength and flexibility. Throwers tend to lose strength as they increase their volume of work. In addition, throwers tend to develop tight posterior capsules and rotator cuff contractures, which can lead to functional shoulder impingement or chronic subluxation.[22] Finally, as throwing increases, the wrist flexors and pronator teres have a tendency to tighten and cause pain.

REFERENCES

1. Kal-Nan, A., Morrey B.F. Biomechanics of the Elbow. In Morrey B.F. (Ed). *The Elbow and its Disorders.* WB Saunders, Philadelphia, 1993, pp. 53–72.
2. Jobe, F.W., Elattrache, N.S. Diagnosis and Treatment of Ulnar Collateral Ligament Injuries in Athletes. In Morrey B.F. (Ed). *The Elbow and its Disorders.* WB Saunders, Philidelphia, 1993, pp. 566–572.
3. Timmer, L.A., Andrews, J.R. *Histology and Arthroscopic Anatomy of the Ulna Collateral Ligament of the Elbow.* J Sports Med 1994;22:667–673.
4. Altchek, D.W., Hyman, J., Williams, R., Levinson, M., Paletta, G.A., Dines, D.M., Botts, J.D. *Management of MCL Injuries of the Elbow in Throwers.* Tech Shoulder Elbow Surg 2000;1:73–81.
5. Hettinga, D. *Normal Joint Structures and Their Reaction to Injury.* J Orthop Sports Phys Ther 1979;1:16–21.
6. Hettinga, D. *Normal Joint Structures and Their Reaction to Injury. II* J Orthop Sports Phys Ther 1979;1:83–87.
7. Booth, F. *Physiological and Biomechanical Effects of Immobilization on Muscle.* Clin Orthop 1987; 219:15–20.
8. Wyke, B.D. *The Neurology of the Joints.* Ann Coll Surg Eng 1966;41:25.
9. Akeson, W.H., Woo, S.L.Y., Amiel, D. *The Connective Tissue Response to Immobility.* Clin Ortop 1973;93;356–362.
10. Franks, C., Akeson, C.J., Woo, S. *Physiology and Therapeutic Value of Passive Joint Motion.* Clin Orthp 1984;185:113.
11. Wilk, K.E., Arrigo, C.A., Andrews, J.R. *Rehabilitation of the Elbow in the Throwing Athlete.* J Ortho Sports Phys Ther 1993;17:305–317.
12. Hepburn, G., Carvelli, R. *Use of Elbow Dynasplint for Reduction of Elbow Flexion Contracture: A Case Study.* J Orthop Sports Phys Ther 1984;5:269–274.
13. Ihara, H., Nakiayama, A. Dynamic Joint Control Training for Knee Ligament Injuries. Am J Sports Med 1986;14:309–315.
14. Bonutti, P.M., Windav, J.E., Ables, B.A., Miller, B.G. *Static Progressive Stretch to Reestablish Elbow Range of Motion.* Clin Orthop 1994;303:128–134.
15. Nuismer, B.A., Ekes, A.M., Holm, M.B. *The Use of Low Load, Long Stretch Devices in Rehabilitation Programs in the Pacific Northwest.* Am J Occup Ther 1997;51:538–543.
16. DiGiovine, M.N., Jobe, F.W., Pink, M. *An Electromyographic Analysis of the Upper Extremity in Pitching.* J Shoulder Elbow Surg 1992;1:15–25.
17. Pappas, A.M., Zawacki, R.M., Sullivan, T.J. Biomechanics of Baseball Pitching; A Preliminary Report. AM J Sports Med 1985;13:216–222.
18. Glousman, R.E., Baron, J., Jobe, F. *An Electromyographic Analysis of the Elbow in Normal and Injured Pitchers with Medial*

Collateral Ligament Insufficiency. Am J Sports Med 1992;20: 311–317.

19. Knott, M., Voss, D.E. *Proprioceptive Neuromuscular Facilitation.* Harper and Row, New York, 1968.

20. Chu, D.A. *Jumping into Plyometrics.* Leisure Press, Champaign, IL, 1992.

21. Chu, D.A. *Plyometric exercise.* Natl Strength Cond Assoc J 1984;6:56.

22. Harryman, D.T., Sidles, J.A., Clark, J.M., McQuade, K.J., Gibb, T.D., Matsen, F.A. *Translation of the Humeral Head on the Glenoid with Passive Glenohumeral Motion.* J Bone Joint Surg 1990;72:1334–1343.

Index